Health Informatics

Vimla L. Patel • David R. Kaufman • Trevor Cohen
Editors

Cognitive Informatics in Health and Biomedicine

Case Studies on Critical Care, Complexity and Errors

Springer

Editors
Vimla L. Patel
New York Academy of Medicine
New York, NY
USA

Trevor Cohen
University of Texas
Health Science Center
Houston, TX
USA

David R. Kaufman
Arizona State University
Scottsdale, AZ
USA

ISBN 978-1-4471-5489-1 ISBN 978-1-4471-5490-7 (eBook)
DOI 10.1007/978-1-4471-5490-7
Springer London Heidelberg New York Dordrecht

Library of Congress Control Number: 2013956008

Printed on acid-free paper

Springer is part of Springer Science+Business Media (www.springer.com)

To Walter Kinstch and Robert Glaser
Who inspired me to push the boundaries
of my thought,
but to do so with style and grace

–Vimla L. Patel

Foreword

In 2000 the James S. McDonnell Foundation initiated a program to support research on complex systems. The purpose of the program is to develop new methods and mathematical tools for advancing complexity science. The particular problem area in which the tools and methods are developed, while not irrelevant, is of secondary interest. However, when a project emerges that combines methodological advances with the promise of addressing a pressing social problem, Foundation support is even more appropriate. This was the case for the proposal submitted to the Foundation by Dr. Vimla Patel and her collaborators – Cognitive Complexity and Error in Critical Care, ER, and Trauma. The research presented in this volume was principally supported by a five-year grant awarded by the McDonnell Foundation beginning in 2007.

The project was funded as a collaborative activity which requires that the funds be used to support the work of a multidisciplinary, multi-institutional team. The grants are intended to encourage collaboration on new or persisting problems that might benefit from being viewed from a new, multidisciplinary perspective. Often the initial years of the grant support the cross-disciplinary discussions and deliberations that are required to develop a new research agenda. Those deliberations developed rapidly among the project collaborators, allowing, as the following chapters attest, a significant body of research to be completed during the first five years of the grant.

As mentioned in the chapters, the stimulus to develop a new research program on the problem of medical errors was the 1999 Institute of Medicine report.

To Err is Human

This report documented the tens of thousands of deaths annually in the United States attributable to preventable medical errors. Medical errors cause more deaths each year than motor vehicle accidents, breast cancer, or HIV. The Institute's report resulted in an unprecedented focus of attention on the problem of errors in medical practice. Even so, follow-up studies by other organizations have found only modest improvements in patient safety since the report's publication.

Cognitive Complexity and Error in Critical Care, ER, and Trauma brings the perspectives of cognitive informatics, complexity science, and clinical practice to bear on the problem of medical errors. Cognitive informatics, a field with its roots in cognitive psychology, provides a framework and methods for understanding and modeling human cognition and behaviors, particularly in technology-mediated environments. In such environments, information flow and human limitations on information processing are fundamental to successful functioning. Research in cognitive informatics is applied in the design of better information and communication systems that enhance rather than impede human cognition.

A most elegant introduction to complexity science is the brief, reader-friendly volume *Thinking in Systems: A Primer* (1993) by Donella Meadows. She writes: "A system is an interconnected set of elements that is coherently organized in a way that achieves something." A system consists of elements, interconnections among the elements, and a function or purpose. As one often hears, a system is more than the sum of its parts and as Meadows states, "it may exhibit adaptive, dynamic, goal-seeking, self-preserving, and sometimes evolutionary behavior." Many interconnections between system elements are flows of information or signals connecting decision or action points in the system. The importance of information flow in a system renders systems science and cognitive informatics, the study of human information processing, highly complementary in understanding a complex system, such as an emergency room or intensive care unit.

These complementary disciplines are well suited to provide answers to the fundamental research question: Why does medical error seem resistant to correction? The reason is that these errors arise within highly complex medical care systems. The traditional culture of medicine holds that individuals are responsible when mistakes occur and it is sensible to look for and blame error on a single individual. In fact, medical error is rarely the result of the actions of a single person. If error reduction methods are focused on identifying, blaming, and correcting the individuals responsible for errors, it is not surprising that conventional approaches to error reduction have resulted in at best minimal gains. Thinking in systems points to a different strategy to error. The traditional approach fails because the settings in which errors occur are complex systems. As Meadows points out, some of the most serious and intractable problems arise not from external causes, but are rooted in the internal structure of the complex system. The solutions to these problems will not yield to identifying and blaming the individuals responsible, they will only yield to solutions when we can see the system as the source of its own problems. Its structure can generate errors. Solving the problem requires understanding the system and restructuring it; it requires understanding and restructuring information flow within the system. Cognitive science, and its cousin cognitive informatics, can tell us about the processing capabilities of the system elements, and complexity science can tell us about the effects of sub-optimal versus optimal information-bearing interconnections within the system. The work presented here thus combines two ideas, the importance of understanding how errors occur in a complex system and the need to understand the cognitive demands of medical decision making. Human error will always be a factor, but errors arising out of recurring systemic weaknesses are amenable to intervention, mitigation, and correction.

The work reported in this volume begins to develop methods and approaches that will allow us to apply both systems thinking and cognitive science to address the problem of medical errors. The research is presented as organized around three themes. The first theme emphasizes the cognitive processes that underlie decision-making in critical care, how errors are generated, and how a system can recover from errors. One might say this research looks at the elements of the complex system. The second research theme addresses team interactions and clinical workflow, and the ways in which the unpredictable nature of these interactions may affect patient safety. One might say this research examines the interconnections within the system. The third theme is concerned with issues pertaining to the generation of interventions to improve patient safety, based on the improved understanding of the system's elements and inter-connections. One might say this work addresses the purpose or goal of the complex system that provides medical care.

As for the clinical medicine perspective, one of the strengths of this collaborative project was the inclusion of expert medical practitioners, such as Dr. Timothy Buchman and his colleagues, who kept the work grounded in the realities of practice and facilitated interactions between cognitive scientists and clinicians in the medical workplace. Hospitals and clinicians in Phoenix, Houston, St. Louis, Atlanta and New York made profound contributions to the work reported here. Thanks to this involvement, research-based changes in clinical practice and changes in medical training for work in high-risk settings have been developed, evaluated, and refined.

The initial findings and results of this new research program are encouraging. We can expect further advances and as research is translated into practice, a reduction in medical error and improved patient outcomes.

John T. Bruer, PhD, President
Department of Philosophy
Washington University in St. Louis
St. Louis, MO
USA

Reference

Meadows DH. Thinking in systems: a primer. White River Junction, Vermont: Chelsea Green Publishing; 1993.

Preface

Early in my career, I became fascinated with the area of Cognition and Education, influenced heavily by my interactions with my mentors and colleagues, such as Guy Groen, Carl Frederikson, Walter Kintsch and Robert Glaser. I became especially intrigued by the notion of exploring how research on cognition and education could be applied to and advanced in the medical domain. I wholeheartedly embraced this combination of cognitive science, education, and medicine starting in 1985, when our work at McGill University, titled "Cognitive Foundations of Medication Education," was funded by the Josiah Macy Jr. Foundation. I owe a debt of gratitude to John T. Bruer, then at Macy, who recognized that education and training decisions for medical education were too often made on an ad hoc basis rather than on the basis of science. The recognition that accompanied this grant, and the funds themselves, gave me an opportunity to explore a process-oriented approach to understanding medical cognition and expertise. It also allowed me to conduct empirical investigations that influenced curricular decisions at our medical school. In addition to the support I received from John Bruer and the Macy Foundation, I was fortunate to have enthusiastic support from Richard Cruess, McGill's Dean of Medicine at the time. He was an extremely powerful force behind my continuing interest in the topic and my belief that, through studies of medical cognition, we can gain a great deal of insight into understanding how doctors reason, and how they make decisions with incomplete information and under conditions of uncertainty. These studies also brought insight into the role that the basic biomedical sciences play in supporting clinical practice.

Over time I realized the myriad of ways in which my chosen field of cognitive science interacted and overlapped with the fields of linguistics and computer science, as well as with anthropology and philosophy. These insights were largely due to my interactions with Herbert Simon, Earl (Buzz) Hunt, David Evans, Alan Lesgold, Anders Ericsson, Henk Schmidt, Paul Feltovich, James Greeno, and Bill Clancey. Also during this period, my laboratory-based studies extended to include semi-naturalistic and naturalistic studies of clinical environments. I found that each of these study types contributed something different to the building of cognitive models of medical decision-making. I still hold this view today and I still conduct studies across this spectrum. It became apparent that, to understand medicine and the role of medical training, we first have to understand how people who practice medicine think about the problems that they solve as they go about their tasks.

My involvement with Biomedical Informatics was serendipitous, commencing in 1991 when I was asked to speak at the European Artificial Intelligence (AI) in Medicine conference in Maastricht, The Netherlands. My invited talk was intended to discuss cognitive models of medical decision-making and their implications for AI systems. I was excited about building bridges to this new field of biomedical informatics, having become convinced that my understanding of the medical field necessitates a multi-disciplinary approach. Scholars and colleagues such as Ted Shortliffe, Mario Stefanelli, Jean Raoul Sherrer, Jan Van Bemmel, and Jim Cimino greatly influenced the direction of my work towards the application of cognitive informatics in medicine. This was particularly timely, given that use of health information technology (HIT) was becoming more widely adopted in healthcare. In addition, patient care by individual practitioners was also moving in the direction of team-based care. Both of these shifts led me to reconsider my research program and set out in new directions.

Our early studies involving computing technology began to show how HIT mediates human performance. Technology does not merely augment, enhance or expedite performance, but rather it transforms the ways individuals and groups think and behave. The difference is not one of quantitative change, but is qualitative in nature. My cognitive studies also began moving towards investigations of such "real-world" phenomena. The constraints of controlled laboratory-based work tended to prevent our team from capturing the dynamics of real-world problems. This problem is particularly salient in high-velocity critical-care environments. Over the years, my studies used a multi-method approach (bench to the bedside and vice versa), which has shown synergy between laboratory-based research and cognitive studies in the "wild." An important question about how studies of individual cognition scale to teams and the real world environment where clinicians function forced me to think about the relationship between individual and team cognition.

By early 2007, coinciding with my move from Columbia University to Arizona State University, there was growing recognition that medical errors were frequent and often life-threatening. The complex nature of healthcare work was also seen as a primary barrier to the implementation of effective safety measures. Having spent long periods of time working in the clinical environment, I also came to believe that common approaches to error, which were generally based on individual accountability, could not possibly address this complexity. Strategies to eradicate error proposed by the medical community failed to appreciate that error detection and recovery are integral to the function of complex cognitive workflow. Here, I was also influenced by the work of Rene Amalberti and David Woods. Through investigations of the emergence of and recovery from error, I believed we could identify new approaches, which could capture errors and recovery processes in real time and would help identify conditions that push clinicians to the boundaries that compromise safe practices. This led me and my colleagues to submit a collaborative proposal on *Cognitive Complexity and Error in Critical Care* to the James S. McDonnell

Foundation (JSMF). The funding support that followed was once again a major breakthrough in my career and has provided me with an opportunity to explore the underlying cognitive mechanisms of error, ways to mitigate these errors in a complex healthcare setting, and ways to help bridge the underlying science to the real-world practice.

JSMF funding has been made available through their *Collaborative Complex System* program. With their support we have created a multi-site collaboratory consisting of an interdisciplinary team of cognitive scientists, clinicians, biomedical informaticians, computer scientists and psychologists. The team is geographically distributed across several research institutions – Arizona State University, the University of Texas Health Science Center at Houston, Columbia University, Emory University, Washington University in St. Louis, and the New York Academy of Medicine (NYAM). The multi-year collaboratory has evolved over the course of the research project, adapting not only to external influences such as national initiatives (e.g., the Affordable Care Act of 2009; the IOM Patient Safety Report of 2011), but also re-aligning the research agenda based on the early results obtained from each of the multiple sites.

This collaboratory brought together an eclectic group of researchers, fellows and students. In addition, the collaboratory employed an approach, which gave investigators ample freedom to pursue their research while sharing a common set of high-level goals, which converged on similar research themes. While the specific research topics varied across the different collaborating sites, the central themes remained consistent: identifying, characterizing, explaining and mitigating errors that occur in a complex critical-care environment. This was achieved by conducting research on conceptual topics that significantly overlapped across multiple sites. For example, communication, a key aspect of critical-care work activities and workflow, was addressed at three of the collaborating sites: Columbia, Emory, and NYAM. Though the projects varied in their focus, design and implementation, the outcomes were aligned to address the key challenges arising out of communication complexity. Similar innovative thinking was manifested in the research projects related to our analyses of errors and error recovery, resulting in integrated outcomes through investigations at multiple sites.

The key researchers who led the projects at the various sites include Timothy Buchman, Trevor Cohen, David R. Kaufman, Kanav Kahol, Amy Franklin, Jiajie Zhang, Thomas Kannampallil, Joanna Abraham and Lena Mamykina. Besides the critical roles of the clinicians at each site, many postdoctoral fellows, students and research associates worked closely as members of our team. Over the five-year period, my ideas were shaped by my interaction with the team, who constantly challenged me through the different perspectives that they brought to the table. The energy and insights generated through this collaborative endeavor were both gratifying and exciting.

Our research activities over this period were monitored and guided by an Advisory Board, whose members were chosen for their multidisciplinary expertise: Michael Shabot, MD, PhD (chairman), Rene Amalberti, MD PhD, Edward H. Shortliffe, MD, PhD; Alan Lesgold, PhD, William J Clancey, PhD. Each year, informed by our annual report, the Board evaluated the performance of the collaboratory during our annual Symposium. A very special thanks goes to Susan Fitzpatrick, Vice President James S. McDonnell Foundation, for her patience and her guidance over the past five years, as we maneuvered through multisite complex budget issues and researchers transferred from one institution to another.

Most of the chapters in this volume are derived from the James S. McDonnell Foundation-funded research. In the foreword to this book, the foundation's president, John T. Bruer, discusses the JSMF program background, explaining their motivation for the supported work we present in these pages. Many individuals have aided in preparing the manuscripts and copy formatting, but none more than my team from the *Center for Cognitive Studies in Medicine and Public Health* at NYAM: Lora Liharska, Corinne Brenner and Sana Khalid, all working under the careful guidance of Joanna Abraham (who also assisted with reviewing and finalizing the manuscripts). I am indebted to my co-editors and colleagues, David Kaufman and Trevor Cohen, as well as to Thomas Kannampallil, for their intellectual contributions, and for their support in dealing with the occasional inevitable challenges that occurred in the collaboratory. Finally, I wish to thank all the chapter authors. They worked diligently to generate documents from various stages of their completed or ongoing research, and then managed to meet most of my constant demands in a timely manner.

This volume does not generically represent the domain of error or complexity in medicine, but rather focuses specifically on the unifying themes of cognition, complexity, and the generation and correction of error in critical care practice. The implications of cognitive processes captured at one level of complexity in critical care provide us with an opportunity to investigate the extent to which these implications also apply to primary care practice, where the complexity level is different. The results reflect the interdisciplinary strengths of cognitive science, and offer a fresh insight into ways to investigate and mitigate errors in complex, dynamic environments such as the emergency room and the intensive care unit.

On behalf of my team, I wish to thank John T. Bruer and the James S. McDonnell Foundation for having the vision to recognize the need to invest in research that addresses the role of cognition in managing clinical errors in complex healthcare environments. We believe that this kind of work will become even more important as we introduce a new generation of technologies to support clinical practice in dynamic patient-care settings.

New York, NY, USA Vimla L. Patel

Contents

1 **Complexity and Errors in Critical Care** 1
Vimla L. Patel, David R. Kaufman, and Trevor Cohen

Part I Cognition and Errors

2 **A Framework for Understanding Error and Complexity in Critical Care** 17
Trevor Cohen and Vimla L. Patel

3 **Failed Detection of Egregious Errors in Clinical Case Scenarios** 35
Vimla L. Patel, Trevor Cohen, and Vafa Ghaemmaghami

4 **Teamwork and Error Management in Critical Care** 59
Vimla L. Patel, Trevor Cohen, Suchita Batwara, and Khalid F. Almoosa

5 **Error Recovery in the Wilderness of ICU** 91
Vimla L. Patel, Alisabeth L. Shine, and Khalid F. Almoosa

6 **Training for Error Detection in Simulated Clinical Rounds** 113
Elie Razzouk, Trevor Cohen, Khalid F. Almoosa, and Bela Patel

7 **Characterizing the Nature of Work and Forces for Decision Making in Emergency Care** 127
Amy Franklin, David J. Robinson, and Jiajie Zhang

8 **Adaptive Behaviors in Complex Clinical Environments** 147
Mithra Vankipuram, Vafa Ghaemmaghami, and Vimla L. Patel

9 **Standard Solutions for Complex Settings: The Idiosyncrasies of a Weaning Protocol Use in Practice** 183
Sahiti Myneni, Trevor Cohen, Khalid F. Almoosa, and Vimla L. Patel

10 **Enhancing Medical Decision Making When Caring for the Critically Ill: The Role of Cognitive Heuristics and Biases** 203
Velma L. Payne and Vimla L. Patel

Part II Communication

11 **Communication and Complexity: Negotiating Transitions in Critical Care** 235
David R. Kaufman, Joanna Abraham, and Lena Mamykina

12 **Falling Through the Cracks: Investigation of Care Continuity in Critical Care Handoffs** 243
Joanna Abraham and Khalid F. Almoosa

13 **Bridging Gaps in Handoff Communication: A Comparative Evaluation of Information Organization Tools** 271
Joanna Abraham, Thomas G. Kannampallil, and Bela Patel

14 **Investigating Shared Mental Models in Critical Care** 291
Lena Mamykina, R.Stanley Hum, and David R. Kaufman

15 **Clinical Artifacts as a Treasure Map to Navigate Handoff Complexity** 317
Sarah A. Collins, Lena Mamykina, Desmond A. Jordan, and David R. Kaufman

Part III Clinical Workflow

16 **Re-thinking Complexity in the Critical Care Environment** 343
Thomas G. Kannampallil, Trevor Cohen, David R. Kaufman, and Vimla L. Patel

17 **Automated Workflow Analysis and Tracking Using Radio Frequency Identification Technology** 357
Mithra Vankipuram, Thomas G. Kannampallil, Zhe (Eric) Li, and Kanav Kahol

18 **Sub-optimal Patterns of Information Use: A Rational Analysis of Information Seeking Behavior in Critical Care** 389
Thomas G. Kannampallil, Amy Franklin, Trevor Cohen, and Timothy G. Buchman

19 The Effects of Structuring Clinical Rounds on Communication and Efficiency 409
Laura K. Jones, Amy Franklin, Thomas G. Kannampallil, and Timothy G. Buchman

Part IV Looking into the Future

20 Clinical Implications of Cognitive Complexity in Critical Care 423
Khalid F. Almoosa, R. Stanley Hum, Timothy G. Buchman, Bela Patel, Vafa Ghaemmaghami, and Trevor Cohen

21 Large Scale Cognitive Error in Critical Care: The Adoption of "Best Practices" That Are Either Ineffective or Harm Patients 441
Timothy G. Buchman

22 Newly-Acquired Complex Performance Competence and Medical Errors 455
Alan Lesgold

23 Reflections on the Role of Cognitive Science in Biomedical Informatics 467
Edward H. Shortliffe

Epilogue 477

Glossary 481

Index 491

Contributors

Joanna Abraham, PhD Department of Biomedical and Health Information Sciences, College of Applied Health Sciences, University of Illinois, Chicago, IL, USA

Khalid F. Almoosa, MD, MS, FCCP University of Texas Health Science Center, Houston, TX, USA

Transplant Surgery ICU, Memorial Hermann Hospital, Texas Medical Center, Houston, TX, USA

Suchita Batwara, MBBS, MPH University of Iowa Hospitals and Clinics, Iowa City, IA, USA

Timothy G. Buchman, PhD, MD, FACS, FCCP, MCCM Emory University School of Medicine, Atlanta, GA, USA

Emory Center for Critical Care, Woodruff Health Sciences Center, Emory University, Atlanta, GA, USA

Trevor Cohen, MB ChB, PhD School of Biomedical Informatics, University of Texas Health Science Center, Houston, TX, USA

Sarah A. Collins, RN, PhD Harvard Medical School and Brigham and Women's Hospital, Boston, MA, USA

Partners Healthcare Systems, Boston, MA, USA

Amy Franklin, PhD School of Biomedical Informatics, University of Texas Health Science Center, Houston, TX, USA

National Center for Cognitive Informatics and Decision Making in Healthcare (NCCD), Houston, TX, USA

Vafa Ghaemmaghami, MD, FACS Trauma Division, Department of Surgery, Banner Good Samaritan Hospital, Phoenix, AZ, USA

University of Arizona College of Medicine, Phoenix, AZ, USA

R. Stanley Hum, MD, FRCPC Department of Pediatrics, College of Physicians and Surgeons, Columbia University, New York, NY, USA

Laura K. Jones, PhD Department of Surgery, Emory University School of Medicine, Atlanta, GA, USA

Desmond A. Jordan, MD Columbia University College of Physicians and Surgeons, New York, NY, USA

Kanav Kahol, PhD Affordable Health Technologies Division, Public Health Foundation of India, New Delhi, India

Thomas G. Kannampallil Center for Cognitive Studies in Medicine and Public Health, New York Academy of Medicine, New York, NY, USA

David R. Kaufman, PhD Department of Biomedical Informatics, Arizona State University, Scottsdale, AZ, USA

Alan Lesgold, PhD School of Education, University of Pittsburgh, Pittsburgh PA, USA

Zhe (Eric) Li, MS Drchrono Inc., Mountain View, CA, USA

Lena Mamykina, PhD Department of Biomedical Informatics, Columbia University, New York, NY, USA

Sahiti Myneni, MSE School of Biomedical Informatics, University of Texas Health Science Center, Houston, TX, USA

Bela Patel, MD, DABSM, FCCP University of Texas Health Science Center, Houston, TX, USA

Division of Critical Care Medicine, Memorial Hermann Hospital, Texas Medical Center, Houston, TX, USA

Vimla L. Patel, PhD, DSc, FRSC Center for Cognitive Studies in Medicine and Public Health, New York Academy of Medicine, New York, NY, USA

Department of Biomedical Informatics, Columbia University, New York, NY, USA

Department of Biomedical Informatics, Arizona State University, Scottsdale, AZ, USA

Velma L. Payne, PhD, MS (BMI), MBA, MS (CIS) Houston Veterans Affairs, Health Services Research and Development Center of Excellence, Houston, TX, USA

School of Biomedical Informatics, University of Texas Health Science Center, Houston, TX, USA

Elie Razzouk, MD, MS Internal Medicine, Miller School of Medicine, University of Miami, West Palm Beach, FL, USA

David J. Robinson, MD, MS, FACEP Department of Emergency Medicine, University of Texas Medical Center, Houston, TX, USA

Alisabeth L. Shine, MA Center for Cognitive Studies in Medicine and Public Health, New York Academy of Medicine, New York, NY, USA

Edward H. Shortliffe, MD, PhD, MACP College of Health Solutions, Arizona State University, Phoenix, AZ, USA

Department of Biomedical Informatics, Columbia University, New York, NY, USA

Department of Public Health, Weill Cornell Medical College, New York, NY, USA

Mithra Vankipuram, MS, PhD Analytics Lab, Hewlett-Packard (HP) Labs, Palo Alto, CA, USA

Jiajie Zhang, PhD, MS School of Biomedical Informatics, University of Texas Health Science Center, Houston, TX, USA

National Center for Cognitive Informatics and Decision Making in Healthcare (NCCD), Houston, TX, USA

Chapter 1
Complexity and Errors in Critical Care

Vimla L. Patel, David R. Kaufman, and Trevor Cohen

Introduction

This volume is unique in its focus on cognitive informatics (CI), a flourishing discipline that cuts across several academic and professional sectors. The chapters in this volume focus on motivating examples drawn from the application of methods and theories from CI to challenges pertaining to the practice of critical-care medicine. Informatics is a discipline concerned with the basic and applied science of information, the practices involved in information processing, and the engineering of information systems. Cognitive Informatics is the multidisciplinary study of cognition, information and computational sciences that investigates all facets of human computing, including design and computer-mediated intelligent action [1]. The basic scientific discipline of CI is strongly grounded in the methods and theories of cognitive science. As an applied discipline, it also draws on the methods and theories from human factors and human-computer interaction. The healthcare domain has provided significant challenges and a fertile test bed for theories from these

V.L. Patel, PhD, DSc, FRSC (✉)
Center for Cognitive Studies in Medicine and Public Health,
New York Academy of Medicine, New York, NY 10029, USA

Department of Biomedical Informatics, Columbia University,
New York, NY 10032, USA

Department of Biomedical Informatics, Arizona State University,
Scottsdale, AZ 85259, USA
e-mail: vpatel@nyam.org

D.R. Kaufman, PhD
Department of Biomedical Informatics, Arizona State University,
Scottsdale, AZ 85259, USA

T. Cohen, MB ChB, PhD
School of Biomedical Informatics, University of Texas Health Science Center,
Houston, TX 77054, USA

V.L. Patel et al. (eds.), *Cognitive Informatics in Health and Biomedicine*,
Health Informatics, DOI 10.1007/978-1-4471-5490-7_1, © Springer-Verlag London 2014

disciplines. CI provides a framework for the analysis and modeling of complex human performance in technology-mediated settings and contributes to the design and development of better information systems.

Overview

The research presented in this volume is motivated by the harmful consequences of medical error, a problem that persists despite substantial efforts toward safety in the 12 years since the publication of the influential Institute of Medicine Report entitled "To Err is Human" [2]. To its credit, the IOM report was prescient in that it strongly emphasized that the majority of factors contributing to preventable adverse events are systemic and not due to the negligence of poorly performing clinicians [3]. However, observers have noted that while the report raised awareness of medical errors, little evidence exists to indicate that there have been substantial systematic improvements in healthcare safety in the time since its publication [4]. In assessment of the progress towards safety since the release of this report, Leape and his colleagues note that while the report raised awareness of medical error, "little evidence exists that systematic improvements in safety are widely available." Leape points out barriers to improved healthcare safety, amongst which "the first (such) challenge is complexity."

The work we have drawn together in this volume aims to identify new paths toward patient safety, as directed by awareness of the complexity of clinical care practice. We focus our investigations in the domain of critical care, which includes both the emergency department and the Intensive Care Unit. These environments are characterized by the need for rapid response by multidisciplinary teams with shifting priorities driven by the needs of patients that are inherently unpredictable, on account of the complex physiology underlying their disease states and the ever-present possibility of the transfer of unstable patients into the unit concerned. Thus, the interpretation of error in such environments requires an understanding of the interrelationships between the entities and artifacts that mediate patient care, and between these entities and the outside world.

In the sections that follow, we describe some characteristics of complex systems that relate to critical care environments, and their implications for the study of these environments.

Interdependencies and Open-Endedness

As is the case with complex biological and ecological systems, a healthcare environment cannot be understood by focusing exclusively on its individual components, as these components are interrelated [5]. Consequently, the framework of individual accountability that is typical of institutional, medico-legal and media responses to medical error [6], is not adequate for explaining or addressing the issue of error as it occurs in complex healthcare systems. How then, are we to approach the study and mitigation of error in such environments? Proponents of a systems-centered approach argue that significant improvements in quality and safety are most likely to be realized by attending to and correcting the misalignments among interdependent levels of care, and focusing not only on members of the clinical team and the tasks performed, but also on the broader environmental factors that constitute the workplace [3]. Negotiating the system interdependencies of care, as evidenced by continued breakdowns such as inadequate transitions of patient care, is a significant challenge faced by providers and researchers alike [3]. It should be noted that not all of the chapters in this volume are focally concerned with error; rather, they cover a range of topics such as workflow, decision-making, information seeking and communication. A systems-centered approach informs all of the research described in the volume.

The study of performance in critical settings is conducive to a systems-centered or complexity approach given the high velocity of work, the interdependence on multiple agents in the care process and the potential gravity of medical care in the setting. Systems thinking involves studying phenomena in a holistic way and understanding the causal dependencies and emergent processes among the elements that comprise the whole system [7]. Complex systems are said to have the property of emergence, in which some behaviors and patterns result from interactions among elements. The systems are also characterized by feedback loops, both positive ones which serve to amplify an effect and negative ones which serve to dampen it. The boundaries of a system can be construed as open-ended and observer-defined. For example, an intensive care unit can be studied in terms of teamwork activity that focuses on the care of a single patient, workflow in the entire unit at a given point in time, and communication that stretches beyond the boundary of the unit. One may also choose to situate the unit within the sociocultural or economic boundaries of the hospital, the local community or even within the greater healthcare system. Of course, different research questions necessitate different units of analysis.

Methodological Imperatives for Taming Complexity

Given the degree of interrelatedness of a complex entity, how can we render it a proper subject of inquiry? How can we make the study of a given a phenomenon, such as handoff communication, tractable? One such strategy is functional decomposition in which complex systems can be decomposed into smaller functional components and the relations between them [8]. The objective is to cut a system at its seams, thus rendering the problem tractable without doing violence to the system as a whole. Another strategy is based on the figure-ground metaphor. One may choose to shine a bright light on the foreground, illuminating a phenomenon of interest, and a dimmer light on the background. In this regard, one never loses sight of the context and one may choose to bring different facets of context to the foreground in sharp view, as their relevance becomes apparent. It is also possible to invert the image where the foreground recedes and the background surfaces as the focal point for scrutiny. A case in point is the study of handoff as a verbal exchange between a clinician finishing a shift and one just beginning a shift. One may also situate the handoff event within the stream of clinical communication including other handoffs and patient rounds. It can also be connected to the ongoing activity/workflow involved in taking care of the patient who is the subject of the handoff communication. Both the functional decomposition (FD) and the figure-ground (FG) research strategy are employed in the research described in this volume. The FD strategy is particularly useful for in-vitro or laboratory-based studies, whereas the FG study supports naturalistic or ethnographic field studies.

The authors of the chapters in this volume provide a range of methodological alternatives, each of which provides new insight into important but sparsely investigated issues such as the nature of error recovery and communication in critical care, the ways in which interactions between individuals direct the course of clinical work, and the applicability of interventions based on normative models of clinical decisions such as guidelines, which are often constructed without consideration for the environment in which they are to be implemented.

One line of research focuses on the study of error recovery, motivated by work in other error-critical domains, which suggests that development of error tolerance is a more practical safety goal than the outright of error [9]. The framework of individual accountability, predominant within the medical community, is further reinforced by the litigious nature of healthcare practice in the United States. Implicit in this framework is the assumption that human error in medicine *should not* occur. This assumption is flawed, as complex work environments are not conducive to the definition of normative models of optimal task performance. Furthermore, it is incompatible with current thinking on the role of error as a component of "learning the ropes" in such environments [10]. This suggests the need to shift focus from the elimination of error toward the mechanisms through which the potentially harmful consequences of error are eliminated. Error is viewed as something that cannot be eliminated, but is usually negotiated in complex environment [11]. However, the mechanisms of error detection and recovery in complex clinical settings are currently poorly understood. This provides further motivation for this line of research, which evaluates the ability of clinicians to recover from errors using a range of complementary methodologies, from laboratory-based studies involving case scenarios with embedded errors to naturalistic studies of spontaneous error recovery as it occurs during clinical rounds. Our studies in this area suggest that focused individual attention [12], the availability of expertise [11] and team interaction [13–16] all play important roles. However, the distribution of attention, expertise and team members in a complex healthcare system is inherently unpredictable, as this distribution is an emergent property of a workflow that is directed by circumstance and patient needs [8, 17].

Therefore, a deeper understanding of workflow in such environments is desirable. However, this presents its own methodological challenges. Methodologies evaluated as a means to characterize this workflow include human-intensive observation supplemented by technological tools to mediate rapid and consistent annotation of workflow activities [17]. However, human observers are largely constrained to a single stream of attention, as well as to a specific spatiotemporal location, and as such are limited in their ability to capture the interactions between multiple team members that underlie the complexity of clinical workflow. Automated approaches in which the movements of multiple team members are monitored using Radio Frequency Identification (RFID) tags are evaluated, and shown to contribute new insights into clinical workflow [8, 18], including the characterization of team aggregation and dissemination as emergent properties of the system as a whole.

The non-linear nature of the flow of activity demonstrated in these studies raises issues for the design of interventions intended to enhance patient safety in clinical settings. Interventions based on a static, normative model of clinical decision making such as practice guidelines and checklists have been successful in addressing medical error in certain circumstances [19]. However, outcome measures aside, little is known about the ways in which such interventions are implemented in the context of an existing sociotechnical ecosystem. The results discussed in this volume show considerable variability in the ways in which these interventions are implemented in practice [20, 21], suggesting opportunities for customization and training to further improve outcomes.

Research in workflow has increasingly focused on particular communication events, which are instrumental in coordinating clinical practice. In recent years, handoff has been the subject of many investigations [22]. However, researchers have often focused on understanding handoff as a discrete communication event, independent of other activities in the clinical workflow. Abraham and colleagues argue that handoff must be examined within the overall context of the clinician workflow, considering activities prior to, during, and after information transfer [23]. The developed methodological framework situates handoff within a broader temporal stream of clinical workflow activity. The clinician-centered approach is predicated on capturing the contextual factors that impact the continuity of care across multiple clinicians providing care for a patient. The focus is on continuity of care as realized in a "day in the life" approach.

The clinician-centered approach employs a series of methods with a particular focus on shadowing clinicians. The objective is to develop a "more accurate and nuanced representation of the overall handoff process with respect to a temporal sequence of the clinician's information management and transfer activities as they relate to patient care events" ([23] p.242). This approach, which characterizes the interdependencies between the various workflow components, can yield insights into a range of contextual factors that mediate quality of care. It also serves to surface and identify the source of breakdowns in communications and clinical errors.

In the sections that follow, we provide an overview of the research described in this volume, grouped in accordance with four themes that emerged during the course of this research. The first of these relates to the cognitive processes that underlie decision-making in critical care. Motivated by the inadequacy of normative models to account for the relationship between variability of clinical practice and patient safety, these studies focus on the recovery from error in critical care, and the cognitive and environmental factors that drive decision making in this context. The second and third themes relate to communication and clinical workflow, and the ways in which the unpredictable nature of these interactions may impact patient safety. The final theme provides overall lessons learned from clinical, education and informatics perspectives.

Error Recovery, Standardization and Decision-Making

It has been argued that the tendency to strive toward perfection is inherent to the culture of medical practice, and that this tendency has made it difficult for practitioners to acknowledge, and hence learn from, errors [6]. Arguably, this tendency has also impacted the efforts taken toward improving patient safety, many of which have proposed error reduction, or even error elimination, as goals. While these are laudable goals, the implied "quest for zero defect" has been largely abandoned by researchers in other safety critical domains [24]. This shift in perspective, and its implications for the study of error, are discussed in Chap. 2 of this volume. This chapter addresses the theoretical rationale for the set of error chapters to follow, and concerns contemporary approaches to error that are able to address the complex nature of critical care work. The complex nature of healthcare work has been proposed as a primary barrier to the implementation of effective safety measures. Approaches to error based on individual accountability cannot address this complexity. Patel and Cohen introduced the phrase 'error in evolution' that denotes the progression of a series of small mistakes towards a cumulative adverse event. This progression is not inevitable: erroneous decisions undergo a selection process based on their anticipated consequences [15]. The authors of this chapter argue that focusing on this process of recovery, rather than producing situation-specific 'quick fixes,' is more likely to reveal generalizable mechanisms of error recovery that can support widely applicable solutions.

The authors of Chaps. 3, 4, 5, and 6 develop new experimental paradigms for investigating the nature of error recovery in the critical care context. While two of the three experimental approaches concern the presentation of cases with embedded errors to clinicians, they all differ from one another in important ways.

Chapter 3 documents studies of error-recovery by individuals in a laboratory setting, using written case scenarios, as described earlier. A striking finding from this research is that error detection by both domain experts and trainees under these conditions, was on the whole, alarmingly poor. While experts did show some advantage in dealing with more complex errors, it was possible that the use of paper-based cases in a laboratory environment may be sufficiently removed from the real world practice environment that cognitive cues and other factors promoting error recovery in practice may be lost.

The research described in Chap. 4 investigates another aspect of this problem, the role of team interaction in error recovery. Clinical rounds have previously been identified as high-yield activities for error detection and recovery [13, 14], as they provide a focal point of information exchange and the opportunity to address errors made by other clinicians. In order to investigate the effects of these aspects of the clinical environment on error recovery, case scenarios with embedded errors were presented in the context of real-world clinical rounds, while recording the interactions between team members that occurred in response to these scenarios. The overall trend indicates that teams of physicians are better able to detect errors than individuals. More interaction between team members was associated with more effective error recovery, and detailed qualitative analysis of these interactions revealed instances in which the detection of and recovery from an embedded error was accomplished collaboratively. This indicates that interaction promotes recovery; an unexpected finding of this research was that new errors were introduced during the process of interaction. Recovery from these errors did not always occur, suggesting that in a complex environments when trainees are present, it is essential that adequate supervision occur, such that the potential for learning is realized, and the potential for adverse events averted.

Extensions of this study were performed in naturalistic settings (Chap. 5) where the data from three morning rounds were audio-recorded in real time in a medical ICU environment covering 35 patient beds. Using methods of conversational analysis, this study showed that teams working at the bedside optimized performance with little room for generating and explicating any mistakes. There appears to be an inherent check within the team (with time pressure) in a naturalistic environment to correct any mistakes quickly. This ability to correct errors also supports the results from our previous naturalistic study [13]. These results and their relationship to competent performance and learning are discussed in this chapter.

Chapter 6 documents an alternative approach to addressing the gap between the laboratory setting and real-world clinical rounds. To better approximate clinical case presentation in remove a controlled experiment, Razzouk and colleagues generated simulated clinical rounds in the context of a computer-based three-dimensional immersive virtual world created with the OpenSimulator development platform. In addition, knowledge-based questions related to each embedded error were added, to distinguish between failure to detect errors on account of ignorance and failure on account of some other cause. Finally, the notion of priming was introduced, which in this context refers to alerting participants to the presence of errors in the case. This suggests the possibility of the development of training modules with this task in mind, an idea that has been proposed in the context of aviation [25]. To this end, the chapter also discusses the development and evaluation of an online tool that adapts the cases used in our experiments for the purpose of training physicians to detect and recover from error.

In summary, the results of our studies on error recovery suggest that both directed attention and team interaction contribute to recovering from errors. However, in a complex work environment the distribution of attention and team members is unpredictable. In Chap. 7, Franklin and colleagues aim to quantify this unpredictability by characterizing the forces that drive clinicians in an Emergency Department (ED) toward a particular course of action. An important finding of this research is that choices made in the ED are more often driven by situations in the environment, rather than by conscious selection. That is to say, rather than being guided by protocol, situational factors such as spatial proximity to a particular patient or colleague direct the course of action in the ED in many cases. This degree of non-deterministic behavior strengthens the analogy between critical care units and complex systems. In general, it also raises issues relevant to intervention in such settings, as the non-linear nature of this workflow may be poorly suited to standardized treatment protocols.

The extent to which standardized protocols, such as treatment guidelines, are effective in a complex workspace is a recurring theme in this volume. In Chap. 8, Vankipuram and colleagues investigate this issue by observing and characterizing deviations from standard protocol in the context of a trauma unit. While some of these deviations represented errors, it was observed that in many cases they represent dynamic adjustments to the operating conditions within the unit, made in order to enhance efficiency by being responsive to the surroundings. Such adjustments, termed "innovations," were found to account for a substantial proportion of deviations by experts; deviations made by trainees, on the other hand, generally represented errors. Guidelines may serve to provide assistance for trainees, but the improvisations observed during this study suggest that excessive standardization may impede the efficiency of expert practice [20].

Myneni and colleagues (Chap. 9) similarly address the utility and limitations of standardization with respect to weaning patients off of ventilators in an ICU setting. Standardizing a care process through the use of health information technologies is seen as a viable way to reduce medical errors by diminishing unnecessary variation in the care delivery. However, the dynamic nature of critical care environments demands context-specific and complexity-inclusive assessment of these standardization strategies for optimal results. The authors describe three studies that focus on the safety assessment of a Computerized Weaning Protocol (CWP), which has been used to standardize the weaning process of mechanically ventilated critically ill patients. The studies employed a range of methods and identified several risk factors that were either inherent to the particular protocol or externalized in the environment. This chapter provides an overview of techniques that can be used for fine-tuning and optimizing HIT-based standardization interventions such as the weaning protocol, thus improving patient safety.

The majority of studies described in this volume employ a naturalistic decision making (NDM) approach. However, Payne and Patel (Chap. 10) develop a hybrid approach that embraces the study of heuristics and biases, more typical of the classical decision-making approach with ethnographic methods more exemplary of NDM. Critical care settings are complex environments that are stressful, time-sensitive and interruption-laden, where clinicians, influenced by factors such as extended work hours and sleep-deprivation, make life-critical decisions. In such settings, decision-making requires the use of cognitive heuristics in order to sustain the required pace. The authors demonstrate a method for eliciting heuristics and biases in critical care settings and use the illustrative study to develop a framework. The authors then demonstrate that the framework can be used to facilitate identification of specific actions associated with heuristics and biases that result in better decisions, as well as actions with the potential for causing patient harm. They conclude that development of an automated detection and correction system is essential for advancing health information technology within healthcare and for enhancing patient safety.

Communication in Critical Care

Chapter 11 in this section presents three interrelated in-situ studies of handoff communication [12–14]. They all engage methods which frame the communication problem in the context of workflow and related factors that constitute work in these settings. Handoffs, as used in this volume, refer to the transfer of care from one clinician to the next during shift change. They involve a transfer of information, responsibility and authority for patient care [26]. Successful handoff in a given setting is predicated upon substantial common ground. Communication failures during handoff may lead to uncertainty in decisions on patient care. These may result in suboptimal care leading to an adverse event. The quality and safety of the handoff process has come under increasing scrutiny because of efforts to reduce duty hours for residents, resulting in increased number of shift changes and potential gaps in communication.

The findings described in Chap. 12 suggested the need for a new approach for supporting handoff and team communication as discussed above. In Chap. 13, the authors compared the effectiveness of two paper-based tools for supporting handoffs: the SOAP note and HAND-IT (Handoff Intervention Tool). The SOAP note is based on a widely used mnemonic, which stands for *subjective*, *objective*, *assessment*, and *plan* of care. It follows a problem-based format commonly used in a range of clinical settings. HAND-IT employs a body system-oriented format and summarization using a problem-case narrative format. The objective is to introduce a format grounded in clinical experience with the belief that it will serve to reduce communication complexity and reduce transition errors. The study indicated that use of the HAND-IT tool resulted in fewer transition breakdowns. It was hypothesized that the tool also led to better learning outcomes for less-experienced clinicians as compared to the current (SOAP) tool. The chapter considers the implications for improving patient safety through a continuity of care-based approach.

Chapters 11 and 14 situate handoff within a particular temporal context that includes the activities and communication events preceding and following the handoff event in question. A property of complex systems is that they can be situated within a particular historical trajectory [7]. For example, past interaction between different parts has modified the parts themselves as well as what constitutes their system environment. The history is realized at multiple time scales. For example, two residents communicating at the time of shift change have a particular history; they know each other variably well and may or may not have cared for the patient in past shifts. Their common experience constitutes part of the process of establishing common ground. For example, two senior residents who have ample familiarity with each other and with the patient who is the subject of the handoff communication can assume a great deal of tacit knowledge and adjust their conversation accordingly.

Patient care in intensive care settings is characterized by a rich and complex interplay between clinicians, mediated by both verbal discussions and a range of tools that support coordinated clinical activity. As previously discussed, clinical care in this setting is a highly collaborative enterprise [27]. In Chap. 14, Mamykina and colleagues employ a shared mental models approach to characterize handoff communication events in a cardio-thoracic ICU. Mental models are used to characterize, explain, and predict events in the environment. In the literature, handoff is typically studied as an interaction between clinicians within the same discipline and position (e.g., resident to resident handoff). However, poor communication within clinical teams is a common cause of sentinel events, clinical errors and "near misses" [28]. Mamykina and colleagues observed and recorded verbal handoffs by different members of patient care teams (e.g., residents, nurses, attendings and fellows) during transitions of care. Records of verbal handoffs were coded for clinical content and language form using a handoff communication taxonomy [29]. Structural analysis focused on frequencies of categories for different clinicians on patient care teams. The analysis showed considerable divergence between clinicians in both the structure and content of their handoffs. The study illustrated the potentially disruptive impact of transitions of care on clinicians' ability to maintain shared mental models of their patients.

Collins and colleagues aimed to understand the structure, functionality, and content of nurses' and physicians' handoff artifacts (Chap. 15). They analyzed nurses' and physicians' handoff artifacts from a Cardiothoracic Intensive Care Unit (CTICU) at a large urban medical center. The authors combined artifact analysis with semantic coding based on Collins and colleagues' [30] Interdisciplinary Handoff Information Coding (IHIC) framework. The study found a high degree of structure and overlap in the content of nurse and physician artifacts. The findings demonstrated a non-technical yet sophisticated system with a high degree of structure in the organization and communication of patient data, which functions to coordinate the work of multiple disciplines in a highly specialized unit of patient care. The findings indicate that the development of semi-structured patient-centered interdisciplinary handoff tools with discipline-specific views customized for specialty settings may effectively support handoff communication and patient safety.

Work and Information Flow

Kannampallil and colleagues (Chap. 16) provide a methodological approach to understanding, describing, predicting and managing complexity in critical care settings. Using multiple examples based on research reported in this book, they describe the various methodological and analytic approaches, and technical innovations that have helped in studying complexity in critical care settings.

The following section is concerned with the dynamics of team interaction in complex critical care settings. Threats to patient safety have been linked to unexpected disturbances in clinical workflow. The effectiveness of workflow analysis is critical to understanding the impact of these perturbations on patient outcomes. Although ethnographic observations and interviews are useful tools for capturing workflow, they are limited in their ability to capture simultaneous activities.

Vankipuram and colleagues (Chap. 17) characterize a quantitative method for capturing and analyzing workflow. In order to model activities in critical care environments using a supervised machine-learning component, the approach employs recordings of motion and location of clinical teams that are gathered using radio identification tags and observations. The detected activities can then be replayed in 3D virtual reality environments for further analysis and training. The proposed system augments existing methods of workflow analysis, allowing for the capture of workflow in complex and dynamic environments. The machine-learning component of the system was tested using data gathered during a laboratory simulation of the clinician movements corresponding to a set of 15 clinical activities, with a mean recognition rate of 87.5 %.

As in most clinical settings, information in critical care environments is distributed across multiple sources such as paper charts, electronic records, and support personnel. Physicians must seek, gather, filter and organize information from various sources in a timely manner to make decisions. Kannampallil and colleagues (Chap. 18) characterize the nature of physicians' information seeking process. They conducted a study in which clinicians were asked to think aloud while performing a clinical diagnosis task. The study focused on the verbal descriptions of physicians' activities, sources of information they used, time spent on each information source, and interactions with other clinicians, which were all captured for analysis. The authors found that the information-seeking process was exploratory and iterative and driven by the contextual organization of information. While there were no significant differences between the overall time spent on paper or electronic records, there was marginally greater relative information gain (i.e., more unique information retrieved per unit time) from electronic records. Additionally, information retrieved from electronic records was at a higher level (i.e., observations and findings) in the knowledge structure than paper records, reflecting differences in the nature of knowledge utilization across resources. Physicians tended to use information that maximized their information gain even though it required significantly more cognitive effort. The authors discuss implications for the design of health information technology solutions that seamlessly integrate information-seeking activities within the workflow; enriching the clinical information space and supporting efficient clinical reasoning and decision-making are discussed. Jones and colleagues (Chap. 19) discuss the effects of different rounding mechanisms on the structure and effectiveness of rounding communication. The intricate differences in remove communication patterns between a structured "team theater" and a "bedside" rounding practice are provided in terms of the content of clinical communication and their effectiveness is provided.

Implications

The final four chapters constitute the work of invited discussants asked to explore the implications for clinical practice, education and HIT design. Timothy Buchman explores the prospects for redesigning and re-conceptualizing clinical workflow in critical care settings. Alan Lesgold examines the significance of this work for education and training, with a particular focus on developing cognitive competencies in the complex critical care workplace. Khalid Almoosa and remove clinical colleagues consider how to bridge research and practice and thereby mitigate errors in the ED and ICU. Edward Shortliffe explores the potential impact of cognition, error and complexity within the context of biomedical informatics and considers the challenges for the next decade. The final chapter is an epilogue by remove Patel, Kaufman, Cohen and Kannampallil, which describes some future projections of this research.

Emergent Themes and Common Threads

The purpose of this volume is to draw together a set of studies and experiments that utilize a range of methodological approaches to address the inherent complexity of critical care practice. While these approaches vary in their methodological emphasis and scale of analysis, they are unified by a rejection of the notion that a top-down, normative, deterministic model of critical care practice can account for the forces that drive decision-making, and consequently error, in such contexts. Rather, these approaches acknowledge the intrinsic variability of critical care practice, and attempt to understand the positive and negative consequences of this variability for patient safety, and the ways in which it might be leveraged or controlled to enhance the quality of critical care practice. Consequently the volume includes work that focuses on the ability of a critical care team to tolerate and recover from error; studies of the unpredictable forces that drive decision making in this context; studies of critical interactions between clinicians; and the characterization of the "environmental" effects of interventions that seek to control the variability of clinical practice.

References

1. Patel VL, Kaufman DR. Cognitive science and biomedical informatics. In: Shortliffe EH, Cimino JJ, editors. Biomedical informatics: computer applications in health care and biomedicine. 3rd ed. New York: Springer; 2006. p. 133–85.
2. Kohn LT, Corrigan JM, Donaldson MS. To err is human: building a safer health system. Washington, DC: National Academy Press; 2000.
3. Henriksen K, Albolino S. Towards a safer healthcare system. Qual Saf Health Care. 2010;19 Suppl 3:i1–2.
4. Leape L, Berwick D. Five years after to err is human: what have we learned? J Am Med Inform Assoc. 2005;293:2385–90.
5. Berg M. Patient care information systems and health care work: a sociotechnical approach. Int J Med Inform. 1999;55:87–101.
6. Leape LL. Error in medicine. JAMA. 1994;272(23):1851–7.

7. Clancey WJ. Scientific antecedents of situated cognition. In: Robbins P, Aydede M, editors. Cambridge handbook of situated cognition. New York: Cambridge University Press; 2008. p. 11–34.
8. Kannampallil T, Schauer GF, Cohen T, Patel VL. Considering complexity in healthcare systems. J Biomed Inform. 2011;44(6):943–7.
9. Amalberti R. The paradoxes of almost totally safe transportation systems. Saf Sci. 2001; 37(2–3):109–26.
10. Rasmussen J. The role of error in organizing behaviour. Ergonomics. 1990;33:377–85.
11. Patel VL, Cohen T, Murarka T, Olsen J, Kagita S, Myneni S, et al. Recovery at the edge of error: debunking the myth of the infallible expert. J Biomed Inform. 2011;44(3):413–24.
12. Razzouk E, Cohen T, Almoosa K, Patel VL. Approaching the limits of knowledge: the influence of priming on error detection in simulated clinical rounds. AMIA Annu Symp Proc. 2011;2011:1155–64.
13. Kubose TT, Patel VL, Jordan D. Dynamic adaptation to critical care medical environment: error recovery as cognitive activity. In: Proceedings of the 24th annual meeting of the cognitive science society. Fairfax, Virginia; 2002. p. 43–4.
14. Cohen T, Blatter B, Almeida C, Patel VL. Reevaluating recovery: perceived violations and preemptive interventions on emergency psychiatry rounds. J Am Med Inform Assoc. 2007; 14(3):312–9.
15. Patel VL, Zhang J, Yoskowitz NA, Green RA, Sayan OR. Translational cognition for decision support in critical care environments: a review. J Biomed Inform. 2008;41(3):413–31.
16. Patel VL, Batwara S, Myneni S, Cohen T, Gilmer A, Patel B, et al. Teamwork and error in critical care: safety in numbers? Technical Report, Center for Cognitive Studies in Medicine and Public Health, New York Academy of Medicine. April 2013.
17. Franklin A, Liua Y, Li Z, Nguyen V, Johnson RR, Robinson D, et al. Opportunistic decision making and complexity in emergency care. J Biomed Inform. 2011;44(3):469–76.
18. Vankipuram M, Kahol K, Cohen T, Patel VL. Visualization and analysis of activities in critical care environments. AMIA Annu Symp Proc. 2009;2009:662–6.
19. Hales BM, Pronovost PJ. The checklist-a tool for error management and performance improvement. J Crit Care. 2006;21(3):231–5.
20. Kahol K, Vankipuram M, Patel VL, Smith ML. Deviations from protocol in a complex trauma environment: errors or innovations? J Biomed Inform. 2011;44(3):425–31.
21. Myneni S, McGinnis D, Almoosa K, Cohen T, Patel B, Patel VL. Effective use of clinical decision support in critical care: using risk assessment framework for evaluation of a computerized weaning protocol. Annals of Information Systems (in press) [Forthcoming Special Issue on Healthcare Informatics].
22. Cohen MD, Hilligoss PB. The published literature on handoffs in hospitals: deficiencies identified in an extensive review. Qual Saf Health Care. 2010;19(6):493–7.
23. Abraham J, Kannampallil T, Patel VL. Bridging gaps in handoffs: a continuity of care approach. J Biomed Inform. 2012;45(2):240–54.
24. Morel G, Amalberti R, Chauvin C. Articulating the differences between safety and resilience: the decision-making process of professional sea-fishing skippers. Hum Factors. 2008;50(1):1–16.
25. Naikar N, Pearce B, Drumm D, Sanderson PM. Designing teams for first-of-a-kind, complex systems using the initial phases of cognitive work analysis: case study. Hum Factors. 2003; 45(2):202–17.
26. Arora V, Johnson J, Meltzer DO, Humphrey HJ. A theoretical framework and competency-based approach to improving handoffs. Qual Saf Health Care. 2008;17(1):11–4.
27. Vazirani S, Hays RD, Shapiro MF, Cowan M. Effect of a multidisciplinary intervention on communication and collaboration among physicians and nurses. Am J Crit Care. 2005;14(1):71–7.
28. Coiera EW, Jayasuriya RA, Hardy J, Banna A, Thorpe ME. Communication loads on clinical staff in the emergency department. Med J Austr. 2002;176(9):415–8.
29. Apker J, Mallak LA, Gibson SC. Communicating in the "gray zone": perceptions about emergency physician-hospitalist handoffs and patient safety. Acad Emerg Med. 2007;14(10):884–94.
30. Collins SA, Bakken S, Vawdrey DK, Coiera E, Currie LM. Agreement between common goals discussed and documented in the ICU. J Am Med Inform Assoc. 2011;18(1):45–50.

Part I
Cognition and Errors

Chapter 2
A Framework for Understanding Error and Complexity in Critical Care

Trevor Cohen and Vimla L. Patel

The Enduring Problem of Medical Error

In 1999, the Institute of Medicine published a widely cited report [1] that suggested between 44,000 and 98,000 people die each year because of preventable medical error. Even the more conservative estimate suggests that medical error causes more death annually than motor vehicle accidents, breast cancer, or AIDS. This report resulted in unprecedented focus of attention on the issue of error in medicine. However, there is little evidence of widely available improvements in patient safety. According to leading patient safety researcher Lucian Leape, of the primary barriers to progress 'the first such challenge is (the) complexity' of medical practice [2].

Limitations of Traditional Approaches

Conventional approaches to medical error are poorly suited to address this complexity. Within the culture of medicine, the traditional approach to error involves assigning blame to a single individual. This attitude towards error is exemplified by

T. Cohen, MB ChB, PhD (✉)
School of Biomedical Informatics,
University of Texas Health Science Center, Houston, TX 77030, USA
e-mail: trevor.cohen@uth.tmc.edu

V.L. Patel, PhD, DSc, FRSC
Center for Cognitive Studies in Medicine and Public Health,
New York Academy of Medicine, New York, NY 10029, USA

Department of Biomedical Informatics,
Columbia University, New York, NY 10032, USA

Department of Biomedical Informatics,
Arizona State University, Scottsdale, AZ 85259, USA
e-mail: vpatel@nyam.org

V.L. Patel et al. (eds.), *Cognitive Informatics in Health and Biomedicine*,
Health Informatics, DOI 10.1007/978-1-4471-5490-7_2, © Springer-Verlag London 2014

the litigious climate and medical malpractice claims in the United States. However, the framework of individual accountability is poorly suited to address the problem of medical error, as it fails to address the complexity of the system within which medical error occurs. The role of latent systemic flaws as mediators of error is well established [3]. In addition, and in keeping with research on human error in other domains [4], we propose that approaches seeking to eradicate error fail to recognize that error recovery is integral to any cognitive work. The critical role of error recovery mechanisms in the maintenance of system safety is neglected by approaches that focus exclusively on completed errors. Furthermore, the retrospective analysis of completed error is vulnerable to bias, as actions that have led to error tend to be viewed as incorrect even though they may have been the best alternative with the information available at the point of decision. In the sections that follow, we will consider the ways in which these traditional approaches have limited progress toward safer healthcare practice.

The Framework of Individual Accountability

Media attention to high-profile medical malpractice cases has raised public awareness of the occasionally disastrous consequences of medical error. Not only are clinicians expected to perform flawlessly, the litigious nature of society in the United States raises the possibility of severe, often career-altering consequences in the event of an error. Even in the absence of such consequences, clinicians are faced with the personal expectation that they perform flawlessly: failing to meet this expectation is associated with burnout and significant emotional distress that manifests with symptoms of clinical depression [5]. The societal pressure to perform without error was highlighted by Dr. Albert Wu in a *British Medical Journal* editorial:

> Strangely, there is no place for mistakes in modern medicine. Society has entrusted physicians with the burden of understanding and dealing with illness. Although it is often said, "doctors are only human," technological wonders, the apparent precision of laboratory tests, and innovations that present tangible images of illness have in fact created an expectation of perfection. Patients, who have an understandable need to consider their doctors infallible, have colluded with doctors to deny the existence of error. Hospitals react to every error as an anomaly, for which the solution is to ferret out and blame an individual, with a promise that "it will never happen again" [6].

Perhaps on account of this expectation, physicians are reluctant to acknowledge their errors, or to discuss them with supervisors. House-staff have been shown to resort to a range of socio-psychological mechanisms such as denial, discounting and externalization of blame, suggesting a reluctance to acknowledge or take responsibility for error [7]. Only 54 % of house-staff report discussing errors with their supervising attending physician, and 28 % acknowledge a fear of repercussions on account of a committed error [8]. The reluctance to discuss error with colleagues has also been shown in studies that include attending physicians as well as residents [9]. While residents have been shown to attribute their errors to lack of training, supervision by attending physicians is considered an important check for error [10]. There have also been recent efforts to acknowledge errors and disclose them to patients and their families in the hope to reduce liability claims and costs, given that physicians are reluctant to acknowledge errors [11].

While there is evidence that attitudes amongst recently qualified physicians are changing [12], these obstacles to open discussion of medical errors present obstacles that impede progress toward safer healthcare practice. While there are without a doubt significant differences between the aviation and healthcare domains, it has been argued that the non-punitive error reporting systems implemented in this latter domain provide important and actionable information about safety risks that are not available in healthcare [13]. From a teaching perspective, evidence exists that committed errors provide valuable opportunities for instruction, and evidence exists that methods of instruction that draw attention to common errors lead to better outcomes than those that provide instruction concerning ideal performance only [14].

The Quest for Zero Defects

Perhaps of greater concern than either of these missed opportunities for improvement is the implicit assumption that human error *should not* occur, that underlies this reluctance to acknowledge its existence. This notion relates to the "zero defects" philosophy originated by Crosby [15], which has at times been embraced by leaders in the automotive and computer hardware industries as a performance goal. However, the analogy between an industrial assembly line and a complex workspace, such as those that exist in the critical care domain, is flawed as the dynamic nature of these complex work environments makes for a poor fit with normative models of optimal task performance. Furthermore, as argued by Rasmussen [16], within these work environments, errors serve a *functional purpose*, as new recruits define the boundaries of acceptable practice by considering and sometimes committing erroneous actions. This last issue is clearly a concern in academic medical settings, where trainees are responsible for hands-on clinical care, so much so that the evidence of a July spike in fatal medical errors has been sought and found [17] to substantiate anecdotal reports of the so-called "July Effect:" an increase in medical errors upon arrival of new medical residents.

However, as illustrated by our empirical work ([18] and Chap. 3 of this volume), even experts cannot be expected to perform perfectly at all times. While considerable evidence exists that experts exhibit vastly improved knowledge organization, solution strategies, performance efficiency, a highly refined ability to recognize and integrate the pertinent features of problems and an improved ability to predict the consequences of decisions taken (for a review, see [19]), there also exists compelling evidence that experts are by no means immune from committing errors. For example, studies of expertise in medicine reveal experts are prone to making particular sorts of error in diagnosis and management: experts are shown to be vulnerable to premature closure, rapidly reaching a conclusion and ignoring evidence in support of competing hypotheses [20]. Recent research in air traffic control simulations has shown that no demonstrable reduction in the rate of committed errors occurs after the preliminary stages of training [21]. However, as we will subsequently discuss, the nature of these errors and the propensity to recover from them differ with expertise.

The Role of Recovery: Insights from Aviation

Given that neither experts nor trainees can realistically be expected to perform without error, this raises the issue of error recovery and its role in patient safety. The perspective that the elimination of error is an impractical goal is well established in the European aviation and transport industries, as noted by safety researchers in these areas:

> The total eradication of human error was quickly abandoned as an objective (being unrealistic from a simple theoretical viewpoint) and safety naturally evolved toward a more systemic perspective [22].

This shift in perspective allowed for the characterization of systemic causes of error [3], as well as the recognition that the exploration of the boundaries of error has a functional role in the acquisition of expertise [3]. This acknowledgment of the inevitability of human error suggested avenues for safety research also, including research into the ability of institutions to tolerate perturbation (for a review of this line of research, see [23]), and investigations of the nature of error recovery by individuals and teams [21]. The first of these avenues, relates to the concept of resilience that has emerged in contemporary studies of human error. Hollnagel [23] draws the analogy between the ability of materials to accommodate stress and the ability of a system to maintain performance under high production pressure. This approach represents a promising line of inquiry into both the qualities of a system that confer resilience, and the nature of the production pressures that push a system to its limits. The second avenue is directly related to the research direction we have pursued. It concerns the cognitive underpinnings of error recovery by individuals and teams, and the role of error recovery in safety critical environments.

The critical role of error recovery in aviation safety was demonstrated by Amalberti and Wioland [21] in a study of error commission and recovery by crews over 44 flight hours. Rates of error production and detection were studied as a function of task demand. Three levels of demand are considered; very demanding (e.g. flight incidents, landing), busy (e.g. planning), low workload (e.g. cruising). While it might seem intuitive that more errors would occur at high workload, the results of this study showed the greatest number of errors at low workload, with the least errors at high workload. However, at high workload, error detection was reduced, leading to a much higher rate of actual incidents (or completed errors). These results suggest a different perspective, in which safety is a function of the balance between error commission and error detection.

Studying the performance of trainees using simulations of air traffic control scenarios provided further evidence for the role of error recovery. With training, raw error rate eventually stabilized at around 12 errors per hour. However, the rate of error detection continued to improve with practice. Similar findings were subsequently seen in a preliminary study in the critical care environment [24], where both expert and non-expert physicians were found to generate errors, but the experts were better able to detect and recover from their errors. Kubose et al. conducted a study of error detection and recovery in the ICU, using methods of observation, shadowing of ICU team members, audio recording, and analysis of infusion pump keystroke logs [24]. Four handovers (in which information is exchanged between clinicians at shift change) and rounds (in which the team gathers and reassess the management plan for a particular patient) for six patients were captured. Recorded protocols were analyzed and coded for error detection and recovery. Both handovers and rounds exhibited error detection, with a mean of 10.5 errors per handover and 5.6 per round. Most errors detected were recovered (mean of 5.25 per round and 7.25 per handover, respectively). Further studies were conducted to determine the relationship between expertise and error correction, by selectively shadowing clinicians of different levels of experience. The results suggest that clinicians of all levels of expertise make mistakes; however, experts are better able to detect and recover from error. While these findings challenge the common perception that experts are somehow infallible, they are consistent with error research in other domains, which shows a constant rate of error regardless of expertise (with the exception of absolute beginners), but that experts tend to make types of errors that are more readily recovered [21]. Nyssen and Blavier' investigate the role of error detection in anesthesiology using retrospective analysis data obtained from an accident reporting system employed in two university hospitals in Belgium [25]. Their results emphasize the importance of standard checks in error detection, and show significant relationships between type of error and error detection mode, as well as type of error and the level of expertise of the anesthetist concerned. As noted by Klein, expert ability to recognize patterns that underlie multiple cues provides an advantage in the detection of subtle errors [26], an observation that is consistent with the differences across expertise noted in our laboratory based studies ([18] and Chap. 3 of this volume).

Motivated by these studies, and prior to the studies discussed in this volume, we proceeded to study error recovery prospectively. We chose as our domain a Psychiatric Emergency Department (PED), for a number of reasons aside from our interest in psychiatry as a clinical domain. We had established collaborators in this area in a previous research project, in which we characterized the PED [27] in accordance with the framework of distributed cognition [28]. So we had already committed many hours of ethnographic observation toward the goal of understanding this environment. In addition, the PED seemed a particularly interesting as a study site in and of itself. The PED is a unique critical care environment. It is mandated to provide acute-phase psychiatric care, with license to hold patients for observation and acute management for up to 72 h. It differs from other psychiatric contexts: patients present in crisis, and limited information is available at the outset to guide management. It also differs substantially from other critical care contexts: patients are cared for by multidisciplinary teams that address a broad range of psychosocial issues in addition to the patient's immediate clinical problem. These teams would frequently meet with one another in a central location, to discuss patient care, which allowed for convenient audio recording of these interactions for subsequent transcription and analysis once approval from the local institutional review board and the clinicians concerned was obtained. We studied evidence of the evolution of error in audio-recorded data capturing discussions between colleagues on clinical rounds [29]. Excerpts from recordings suggesting perceived violations of the accepted bounds of safe practice or incidents of miscommunication were extracted and analyzed using qualitative coding methods. This analysis reveals a variety of perceived violations, many of which have potentially serious consequences for patient safety. Of these incidents, only one had been formally reported. However, ten incidents were considered by physicians with domain experience to have potentially dangerous consequences. Frequently, perceived violations were followed by corrective actions, such as the prescription of a previously neglected medication, revealing both the apparent boundaries of acceptable practice and the mechanisms in place to correct a violation of these boundaries. Such analysis of the detection and prevention of potential error during patient rounds expands the data available for error analysis beyond the occasional reported adverse event. These findings are consistent with contemporary error research, which suggests that the detection and correction of potential error are an integral part of cognitive work in the complex, modern-day workplace.

Our literature review during this period revealed that the issue of error recovery had been largely neglected in the medical domain, where an older paradigm focusing on error reduction or elimination still predominated. The prominent role of recovery in the promotion of safety suggested by Amalberti's work, and the vast yield of otherwise unreported corrected errors we had observed during our ethnographic work indicated the need for a new framework for the study of medical error better suited to the demands of the complex workspace. In the sections that follow, we will attempt to further define the characteristics of our approach to this problem.

The Temporal Evolution of Medical Error

Motivated by Rasmussen's characterization of error as a violation of the bounds of acceptable practice norms [16], we defined an area of interest for our research based on a model of the temporal evolution of error, as depicted in Fig. 2.1. As we had observed in our ethnographic work, error is initiated by a violation of the bounds of safe practice, which make up the first boundary in the figure. It is not necessarily the case that an individual is at fault, as it is possible that circumstantial factors led to the error. For example critical clinical information may not have been available at the point of care. Subsequently, and of particular interest for our purposes, there

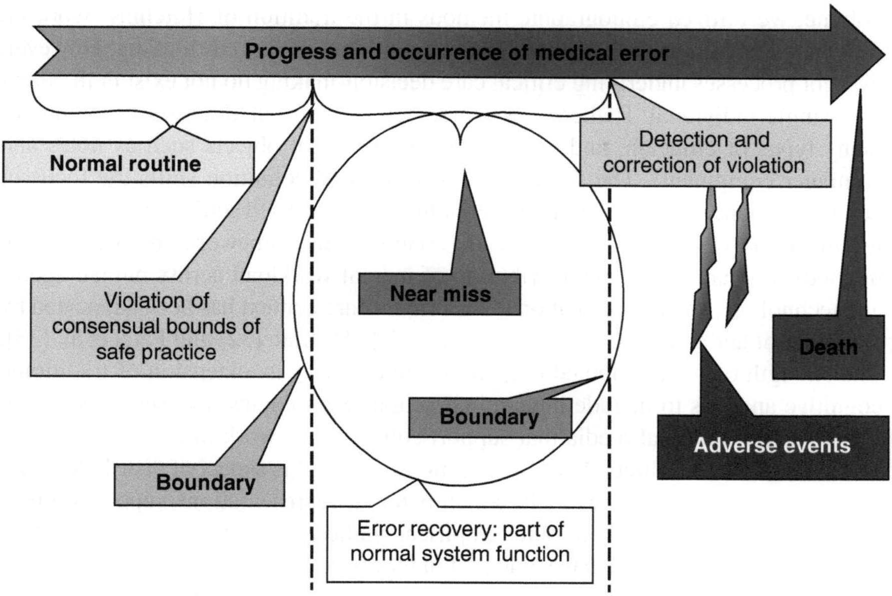

Fig. 2.1 The evolution of medical error (Adapted from Patel and Cohen [30])

exists a period of time in which there is an opportunity to detect and recover from this error before an adverse event has occurred. For example, an excessive dose of a particular medication may have been prescribed, but not yet administered to a patient. If recovery does not occur, the error proceeds to the stage where it has affected the patient concerned, violating the second boundary in the figure. At this stage, there is often still opportunity for recovery before an adverse event occurs. For example, it may be possible to monitor for, or reverse the effect of the excessive dose that was administered. In fact, recoveries at this point in the process are more common than one might imagine: the observation of unintended effects on the physiology of a patient has been identified a prominent mechanism of error detection in anesthesiology, where the effects of the administration of a particular drug may be immediately apparent [25]. However, it is clearly desirable to avert adverse events entirely, and so we elected to focus our attention on the important yet neglected issue of error detection in medicine.

Capturing Error Correction

Distributed Cognition and Vulnerability to Error

With this point of focus in mind, the question arises of how one might go about studying error recovery. In the work prior to that discussed in the contents of this volume, we utilized ethnographic methods in the tradition of Hutchins' work on distributed cognition [28]. Faulty action is a product of flawed thinking. However, thought processes underlying critical care decision-making do not exist in the mind of a single individual. Rather, they are spread or distributed across the minds of many types of clinician, and across artifacts (physical objects such as notes and computer equipment). The framework of distributed cognition shifts the focus of cognitive science from the study of individuals in controlled settings to the study of groups of individuals in their real-world context. This framework provides a set of methods to characterize the distribution of mental workload across human agents and technology, and its application to the critical care context has been advocated by a number of authors including Hazlehurst et al. [31], Xiao [32] and Patel et al. [33]. The strength of the distributed cognition framework is its extension of traditional cognitive analysis to include human interaction technologies (external representations) such as physical media that support collaborative work in complex contexts and tasks. Xiao [32] direct their investigations toward this aspect of distributed cognition, characterizing the ways in which external representations support clinical care in practice. A number of other empirical studies employing this framework in the context of critical care have emerged in recent years.

While research on distributed cognition tends to focus on the advantages conferred by the distribution of cognitive tasks, the methods and theoretical framework have also been employed in the study of error. A series of cognitive ethnographic studies were conducted in parallel in three critical care environments at Columbia University Medical Center: the ICU [34] and the medical [35] and psychiatric emergency departments (PEDs) [27]. The primary objective was to characterize the cognitive system underlying decision-making, and consequently error, in critical care medicine. Ethnographic and interview data were analyzed to characterize the distribution of cognitive work and information flow in each context, revealing latent systemic flaws that are vulnerable to error. This characterization was enriched by cognitive analysis of recorded verbal protocols, including collaborative decision-making during rounds. The analysis of these data required the development of novel methodologies, and resulted in the characterization of the cognitive mechanisms underlying error in each domain. Malhotra et al. [34] present a methodology for the modeling of workflow within the complex cognitive systems that underlie critical care work. This methodology involves the detailed characterization of individual work-flows, with the identification of events of critical clinical importance. A collective workflow is then reconstructed from events of critical importance that are temporally or spatially correlated, and performed collaboratively. The methodology is implemented in order to construct a detailed workflow model of an intensive care unit. Cohen et al. [27, 29] interpret psychiatric emergency data using the distributed cognition framework. While the distribution of cognitive processes across groups and individuals generally enhances the capacity of a cognitive system, it may introduce additional vulnerabilities to error. This analysis focuses on the identification of the vulnerabilities conferred by the distribution of cognitive work in the emergency department (ED), revealing several latent flaws in the system related to the underlying distribution of cognition across teams, time, space and artifacts. Laxmisan et al. [35] focus their analysis of data from the medical emergency room on the cognitive demands imposed by multitasking, interruptions and handovers during shift change. Within the captured data, on average, interruptions occur every 9 min for attending clinicians, and every 14 min for residents. In addition, gaps in information flow are found to occur during handoffs at shift change. The studies described above illustrate methods for the characterization and modeling of the distributed cognitive systems that underlie critical care work, enabling the prediction of their vulnerability to error. A recent paper reviews the cognitive dimensions of complex critical care environments [36].

Types of Knowledge Involved

One needs to have sufficient domain knowledge to make judgments of various things, including detecting and correcting mistakes. However, we know that knowledge alone is not sufficient, since despite knowledge of a problem, we cannot always correct errors. This dissociation between action (correction) and judgment (detection), which can be viewed in terms of declarative and practical knowledge, is a well-established aspect of human cognition [37]. Practical or working knowledge works towards generating actions to reach a goal (for example, patient care during clinical rounds), while declarative knowledge is considered more prescriptive, and the cognitive functions supported by this knowledge are more judgment-oriented (for example, error evaluation during teaching clinical rounds). Because these two knowledge types have different bases, an individual may have the ability to use generic declarative knowledge but not have the practical knowledge to specify its application in a specific case, as seen in the ICU.

The idea that shifts from concrete and specific knowledge structures toward abstract ones occur as expertise is acquired has been expressed repeatedly in a variety of ways in different cognitive theories. For example, contemporary theories of skill acquisition envision a process of generalization that can be applied to production rules to generate more abstract rules (e.g., [38, 39]) and to descriptions to generate more abstract mental representations, which are often called schemas [40]. The fundamental principle behind these and many other cognitive theories is that knowledge moves from concrete and specific to abstract and general in the course of learning. In team interaction, it is possible for different members of the team to have complementary types of knowledge and to support each other during interaction so that the error detection and correction process is more efficient and effective. Thus we hypothesize that teams will detect both their own errors and the errors of others more effectively than what we observed in individual problem-solving situations. The role of senior attending physicians as tutors in these situations will also be explored.

Relationship to Learning

Learning from errors is well known. It has been argued that error commission is an essential component of the learning process in complex work environments, one through which the consensually defined boundaries of acceptable practice are learned [41]. In an academic setting, critical care units are intended to support patient care and provide a learning environment for trainees, such as residents and interns, who arrive in these clinics with generic expertise in medicine and face the challenge of developing specific expertise related to the performance of tasks particular to this clinical environment. The difference between the nature of generic and specific expertise in medicine has been documented with respect to diagnostic decision making [42], and the implication is that trainees in such settings generate and correct errors as they develop competency. There are accepted norms and guidelines for safe practice and any deviation from these norms in a complex work setting provides the opportunity to re-evaluate the assumptions upon which the deviation is based. So the commission of error, if appropriately corrected, is likely to play an important role in the learning of safe practices. This is where expert mentors are known to play significant part.

The acquisition and adaptation of knowledge and skills begins with general problem-solving methods (such as those one learns in medical school). An example would be learning the general pathophysiology of cancer and then applying this knowledge to the specific care of colon cancer [43]. The rules that govern such methods may generate errors since they are too general and are applied with minimal constraints in a specialized situation. Error detection is recognized as constraint violation; error correction is a specialization of that rule by adding conditions that restrict its application in a situation where constraints are violated [44].

Error correction (EC) is an opportunity to learn. Little or no learning will occur unless errors are corrected. If the recovery action is incorrect, even though the error is correctly detected, then the practical knowledge on which the decision is based is probably erroneous. Brown, Burton and Van Lehn liken this type of errors to *bugs* in a computer program [45, 46]; this is similar to what is called a *misconception* in science, health and education [47]. To learn from an action that generates an undesirable outcome (such as giving the incorrect dosage of medication to a patient that results in an adverse event) would be to eradicate or correct the fault in practical knowledge that prompted the action. This, in turn, would lower the probability of the learner committing further errors of same type. Therefore, the key question that emerges is: what is the best learning mechanism for correcting errors? During team interactions in ICU patient rounds, an attending physician with practical knowledge of the domain usually acts as a tutor and guides discussions in resolving conflicts, and promoting new knowledge acquisition. This is a classical example of learning on the job, where a fine line exists between providing competent patient care (without errors) and learning from errors through team interaction at the bedside. Patel and her colleagues address some of these issues in Chaps. 4 and 5 of this volume.

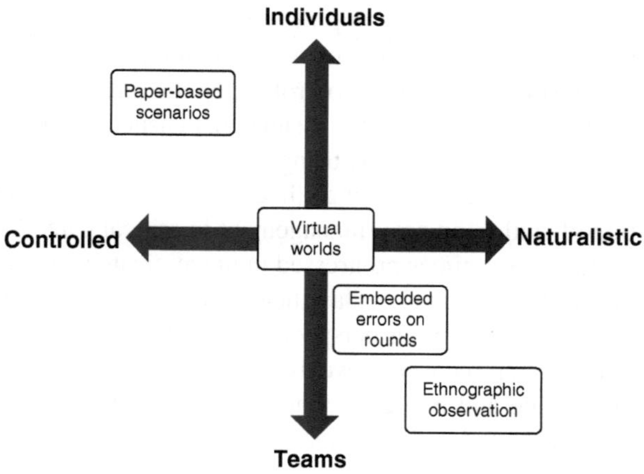

Fig. 2.2 Summary of error recovery work

Embedding Errors to Capture Recovery

The approaches taken to the study of error recovery we have described so far in this chapter can be broadly categorized as prospective. Prospective studies depend on the observation of the process of error recovery, often in a naturalistic setting (e.g., [29]). Retrospective studies (e.g. [48, 49]) utilize error reports and interviews in an effort to analyze reported adverse events. These approaches are complementary, and each has its respective advantage. Retrospective studies allow for a focused analysis of large numbers of events that have been identified as violations of the accepted standards of practice by clinicians during the course of their work. In contrast, prospective studies in naturalistic settings require the investment of many hours of ethnographic observation by a trained observer in order to capture incidents of error recovery in process. In order to capture error recovery more efficiently, and complement our existing naturalistic studies, we developed a new paradigm for the study of error recovery in medicine that involved embedding errors in clinical case scenarios, and presenting these to clinicians in various ways.

As shown in Fig. 2.2, this work can be characterized along two axes. The first of these involves the environment, starting on the left with controlled studies using paper-based cases in a laboratory setting with individual subjects as discussed in Chap. 3 of this volume. In an attempt to better approximate the verbal presentation of cases on clinical rounds, we subsequently used a similar experimental paradigm, but rather than presenting cases on paper these were presented in the context of an immersive three-dimensional virtual world, in which the roles of various team members were played by digital scripted avatars, and clinicians immersed themselves in the world to participate in the round. These studies are discussed in Chap. 6 of this volume. As is the case with the paper-based studies, it is ensured that each participant will experience an identical case presentation. Next, we conducted experiments of this nature in a semi-naturalistic setting, in which an attending physician presented scenarios during the course of normal rounds and the reactions of team members to these scenarios were recorded and analyzed, as discussed in Chap. 4. These studies were less controlled, as the information any individual was exposed to, depended upon the discussions that ensued amongst the members of the clinical team concerned. Finally, using a completely naturalistic paradigm, data were collected at the bedside during clinical rounds, adding another dimension to our collection of studies on error management in critical care. As discussed in Chap. 5. these discussions at times progressed in unanticipated and occasionally worrisome directions. The other axis of classification concerns the study of individuals as compared with teams. From our perspective these foci are complementary. The study of individual error recovery reveals aspects of individual cognition such as attention, knowledge and inference that are prerequisite to detection of, and recovery from error. The study of error recovery by teams is complementary, as it reveals other components such as communication, negotiation, hierarchy and the generation of new errors that are pertinent to the process of recovery as it occurs in multidisciplinary teams. All of these aspects could potentially inform the design interventions to enhance error recovery in order to improve patient safety.

A Cycle of Error Generation and Recovery

Averting the progression of error requires both the detection of possible error and some corrective action, the effects of which must then be evaluated. Consequently, the process of error recovery contains stages of both execution and evaluation, and this cyclical process can be modeled using Norman's well established and generic seven-stage model of interaction [50]. Norman's model was originally applied to the problem of system usability, but on account of its generic nature, has also been used to model a broad range of cognitive interactions in which interpretation and action are tightly connected. Figure 2.3 presents an adaptation of Norman's generic model to the process of error recovery, first described by Patel and Cohen [30]. This process incorporates the stages of *triggering*, *diagnosis* and *correction* described by Allwood in an earlier work [51]. However, we have presented these in the context of a decision and action cycle so as to include additional aspects of clinical decision making such as risk mitigation and cultural barriers to acting on a detected error, and the possibility of generating new errors while recovering from others. This perspective is discussed within the experimental context in Chap. 4 of this Volume.

Error perception is a critical step in the cycle, since without it the error will not be noticed. Error detection can be viewed as a type of problem detection (the problem in this case originates in human action). Klein and his colleagues enumerate several factors affecting problem detection [26]. These include expert ability to recognize the pattern underlying multiple subtle cues, expectancies based on the ability to recognize chains of events using a causal framework, expert mental models (including models of the instruments used to collect observed data) and a sense of *typicality*, which provides a baseline for the detection of anomalies. Allwood notes

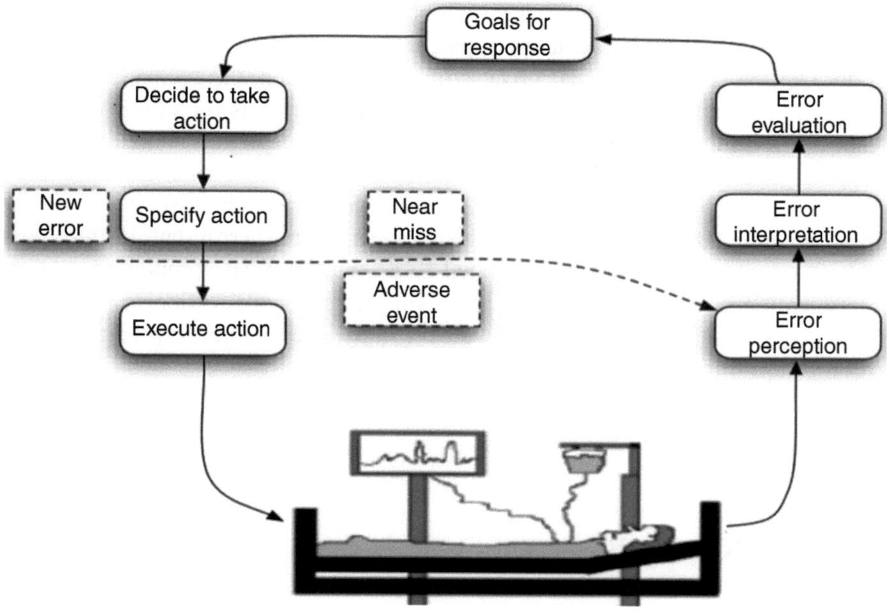

Fig. 2.3 Seven-stage model of error generation and recovery

that this process of error detection, or *triggering* [51] can be either spontaneous (in response to some perceived discrepancy) or systematic (for example, the use of a checklist to prevent procedural errors [52]).

The next step in the cycle is the **interpretation** of the perceived potential error in context (sometimes referred to as error *diagnosis*). For example, what appears on the surface to be an inadequate dose of a drug may in fact be an appropriate dose in the presence of renal failure. Once the error has been interpreted, and detected in fact to be an error, **evaluation** of the potential consequences of the error occurs. This is a critical stage, as research from other domains suggests that often times, even though an error has been recognized, no action may be taken because other concerns take higher priority in the overall case management [22]. In the critical care environment, these concerns may include (a) the priority of other errors; (b) the need to address emergent consequences of a given error at hand; and (c) other urgent care priorities in the unit within narrow time constraints. Nonetheless, a **new goal** is likely to be set in response to the error, even if this is as simple as closer observation for potential consequences. In some cases, this goal may require taking action. Once this intention has been set, a plan of action is **specified and then executed**, and its effects are observed. In studies of statistical problem solving Allwood notes that error detection occurs when "the problem solver perceives a discrepancy between the results produced and his expectations" [51]. So it appears that one is applying knowledge of the domain in order to anticipate the outcome of executed actions. As mentioned previously, the perception of a discrepancy between the actual and intended outcomes of a decision has been found to be an important mechanism of error detection in anesthesiology [25] where the effects of the administration of a particular drug may be immediately apparent.

In addition to this idealized process of error detection and recovery, we have included in the cycle the potential to generate new errors, based on the observation from our recent work (detailed in Chap. 4) that both teams and individuals were prone to generate new errors while attempting to manage the errors we had embedded during our clinical cases. In Fig. 2.3, we have illustrated the case of a new error being generated during the process of managing a detected error, but it is also possible that such errors might be generated on account of misperception, inaccurate interpretation or poor evaluation of an existing error, or the setting of misguided goals in response to this error. If, as we have illustrated, the new error leads to the specification of an action, this constitutes a violation of the first safety boundary depicted in Fig. 2.1, and the opportunity to recover exists until the action is executed, violating the second boundary.

Review of Key Findings

Much of our research to date has focused on the issue of error perception and interpretation. The issues attached to evaluating the importance of correcting a particular error in the context of larger operational priorities, such as the needs of other patients, are not addressed by our studies aside from those that are entirely naturalistic. However we were able at times to capture the specification of actions to be taken in response to an error, as well as the generation of new errors in our laboratory-based, semi-naturalistic and naturalistic studies.

In our initial experiments, we utilized paper-based case scenarios relating to traumatic injury ([18], Chap. 3), and captured verbal protocols as participants read and interpreted the scenarios without forewarning that errors were present. We found that participants at all levels of expertise detected fewer errors than anticipated, and in many instances the undetected errors were egregious with harmful or fatal consequences. This experimental paradigm was also employed in the context of a dialysis unit, with participant population of 31 Registered Nurses (RNs) of different levels of expertise [53], with similar findings. In both cases further characterization of the nature of the errors detected by each group revealed advantages for domain experts with respect to the time frame of error detection, and the detection certain error types.

In recognition of fact that case reports are seldom read as written text in isolation in the context of real-world critical care, we extended these studies using a virtual world environment to more accurately capture the verbal presentation of information by multiple team members that occurs on critical care rounds ([54], Chap. 4). In addition, we included a set of knowledge-based questions that evaluated the clinical knowledge required to detect each error, in order to enable us to distinguish between failure to detect errors that occurred on account of inadequate clinical knowledge, and those that occurred for some other reason. In addition, we introduced an additional experimental parameter in which participants were primed (i.e. alerted beforehand to the presence of errors) to detect error ahead of their second case. Similarly to our other controlled experiments, overall error detection was poorer than anticipated. However improvements in performance occurred with priming. These results are discussed in detail in Chap. 4 of this volume. An optimistic interpretation of this finding suggests opportunities for intervention, as while training programs are deliberately designed to impart knowledge; it is not generally the case that training directed specifically at error recovery is incorporated.

To complement our paper-based and virtual-world studies, we developed an approach to capturing error recovery in its natural environment (Chap. 4), the clinical unit in the context of a collaborative round. To do so, we again created cases with embedded errors. However, in contrast to our work in controlled settings, these cases are presented for discussion at the conclusion of a clinical round with several members of the clinical team present. Consequently, we are able to characterize team interactions, and their role in error recovery. We created two clinical cases, each with several embedded errors. These cases were presented by a clinical collaborator to clinical teams, consisting of interns in their first year of residency training (post-graduate training), residents in second and third years, and fellows-the specialists training after completion of their residency. As compared to individuals in both laboratory-based and virtual world studies, teams of physicians appear to detect and correct more errors. Though the results are not strictly comparable on account of the different cases used in each experiment, this result is intuitive on account of the greater resources of attention and expertise that are available to an entire team, as well as the possibility that the real-world setting and presence of a peer group serve to promote engagement with the scenario. It is also encouraging, as the rates of recovery observed in our laboratory- based and virtual world experiments would have disturbing implications for patient safety. However, it was also the case that new errors were generated during the ensuing discussions, some of which remained undetected. These findings raise issues related to the balance between team interaction and patient discussion that are discussed in further detail in Chap. 5.

Conclusion

Despite unprecedented attention to the issue of medical error over the last 12 years, there is little evidence of its impact on patient safety. It has been argued that the framework of individual accountability, reinforced by both professional attitudes toward error and the litigious nature of healthcare practice, is an obstacle to progress in this regard as, errors cannot be understood in isolation from the context in which they have occurred. This chapter concerns alternative approaches to the study of human error that shift the focus from error to error recovery. The complex nature of healthcare work has been proposed as a primary barrier to the implementation of effective safety measures. Approaches to error, based on individual accountability, cannot address this complexity. Strategies to eradicate error fail to appreciate that error detection and recovery are integral to the function of complex cognitive systems. Through investigation of the emergence of and recovery from error, one can identify new approaches for error management. In the chapters that follow, we discuss key findings and new avenues for future research that have emerged from this shift in perspective in our own research.

References

1. Kohn LT, Corrigan JM, Donaldson MS. To err is human: building a safer health system. Washington, DC: National Academy Press; 2000.
2. Leape L, Berwick D. Five years after to err is human: what have we learned? J Am Med Inform Assoc. 2005;293:2385–90.
3. Reason J. Human error. Cambridge: Cambridge University Press; 1990.
4. Amalberti R. The paradoxes of almost totally safe transportation systems. Saf Sci. 2001; 37(2–3):109–26.
5. West CP, Huschka MM, Novotny PJ, Sloan JA, Kolars JC, Habermann TM, et al. Association of perceived medical errors with resident distress and empathy: a prospective longitudinal study. J Am Med Inform Assoc. 2006;296(9):1071.
6. Wu AW. Medical error: the second victim. West J Med. 2000;172(6):358–9.
7. Mizrahi T. Managing medical mistakes: ideology, insularity and accountability among internists-in-training. Soc Sci Med. 1984;19(2):135–46.
8. Wu AW, Folkman S, McPhee SJ, Lo B. Do house officers learn from their mistakes? J Am Med Inform Assoc. 1991;265(16):2089–94.
9. Kaldjian LC, Forman-Hoffman VL, Jones EW, Wu BJ, Levi BH, Rosenthal GE. Do faculty and resident physicians discuss their medical errors? J Med Ethics. 2008;34(10):717–22.
10. Schenkel SM. Resident perceptions of medical errors in the emergency department. Acad Emerg Med. 2003;10(12):1318–24.
11. Kachalia A, Kaufman SR, Boothman R, Anderson S, Welch K, Saint S, et al. Liability claims and costs before and after implementation of a medical error disclosure program. Ann Intern Med. 2010;153(4):213–21.
12. Varjavand N, Bachegowda LS, Gracely E, Novack DH. Changes in intern attitudes toward medical error and disclosure. Med Educ. 2012;46(7):668–77.
13. Helmreich RL. On error management: lessons from aviation. Br Med J. 2000;320(7237): 781–5.
14. Rogers DA, Regehr G, MacDonald J. A role for error training in surgical technical skill instruction and evaluation. Am J Surg. 2002;183(3):242–5.
15. Crosby PB. Quality is free: the art of making quality certain. New York: McGraw-Hill; 1979.
16. Rasmussen J. The role of error in organizing behaviour. Ergonomics. 1990;33:377–85.
17. Phillips DP, Barker GEC. A July spike in fatal medication errors: a possible effect of new medical residents. J Gen Intern Med. 2010;25(8):774–9.
18. Patel VL, Cohen T, Murarka T, Olsen J, Kagita S, Myneni S, et al. Recovery at the edge of error: debunking the myth of the infallible expert. J Biomed Inform. 2011;44(3):413–24.
19. Chi MTH, Glaser R, Farr MJ. The nature of expertise. Hillsdale: Lawrence Erlbaum Associates; 1988.
20. Patel VL, Arocha JF, Kaufman DR. Diagnostic reasoning and medical expertise. Psychology of Learning and Motivation. 1994;31:187–252.
21. Amalberti R, Wioland LL. Human error in aviation. In: Soekkha H, editor. Aviation safety: human factors, system engineering, flight operations, economics, strategies, management. Utrecht: VSP; 1997. p. 91–108.

22. Morel G, Amalberti R, Chauvin C. Articulating the differences between safety and resilience: the decision-making process of professional sea-fishing skippers. Hum Factors. 2008;50(1):1–16. Epub 2008/03/22.
23. Hollnagel E. Resilience engineering concepts and precepts. Burlington: Ashgate Publishing Limited; 2006.
24. Kubose TT, Patel VL, Jordan D. Dynamic adaptation to critical care medical environment: error recovery as cognitive activity. In: Proceedings of the 24th Annual Conference of the Cognitive Science Society. Virginia: Fairfax; 2002. p. 43–4.
25. Nyssen AS, Blavier A. Error detection: a study in anaesthesia. Ergonomics. 2006;49:517–25.
26. Klein G, Pliske R, Crandall B, Woods DD. Problem detection. Cogn Technol Work. 2005;7(1):14–28.
27. Cohen T, Blatter B, Almeida C, Shortliffe E, Patel VL. Distributed cognition in the psychiatric emergency department: a cognitive blueprint of a collaboration in context. Artif Intell Med. 2006;37:73–83.
28. Hutchins E. Cognition in the wild. Cambridge: MIT Press; 1995, xviii, 381 p.
29. Cohen T, Blatter B, Almeida C, Patel VL. Reevaluating recovery: perceived violations and preemptive interventions on emergency psychiatry rounds. J Am Med Inform Assoc. 2007; 14(3):312–9.
30. Patel VL, Cohen T. New perspectives on error in critical care. Curr Opin Crit Care. 2008; 14(4):456–9.
31. Hazlehurst B, Gorman PN, McMullen CK. Distributed cognition: an alternative model of cognition for medical informatics. Int J Med Inform. 2008;77:226–34.
32. Xiao Y. Artifacts and collaborative work in healthcare: methodological, theoretical, and technological implications of the tangible. J Biomed Inform. 2005;38:26–33.
33. Patel VL, Kaufman DR, Arocha JF. Emerging paradigms of cognition in medical decision making. J Biomed Inform. 2002;35:52–75.
34. Malhotra S, Jordan D, Shortliffe E, Patel VL. Workflow modeling in critical care: piecing together your own puzzle. J Biomed Inform. 2007;40(2):81–92.
35. Laxmisan A, Hakimzada AF, Sayan OR, Green RA, Zhang J, Patel VL. The multitasking clinician: decision-making and cognitive demand during and after team handoffs in emergency care. Int J Med Inform. 2007;76:801–11.
36. Patel VL, Zhang J, Yoskowitz NA, Green R, Sayan OR. Methodological review: translational cognition for decision support in critical care environments: a review. J Biomed Inform. 2008;41(3):413–31.
37. Perkins DN. The mind's best work. Cambridge: Harvard University Press; 1981.
38. Ohlsson S. Restructuring revisited. Scand J Psychol. 1984;25(2):117–29.
39. Sun R, Merrill E, Peterson T. From implicit skills to explicit knowledge: a bottom-up model of skill learning. Cognit Sci. 2001;25(2):203–44.
40. Gick ML, Holyoak KJ. Schema induction and analogical transfer. Cogn Psychol. 1983; 15(1):1–38.
41. Rasmussen J. The role of error in organizing behaviour. Qual Saf Health Care. 2003;12(5): 377–85. PubMed PMID: 14532371. Pubmed Central PMCID: 1743771. Epub 2003/10/09.
42. Patel VL, Groen GJ. The general and specific nature of medical expertise: a critical look. In: Ericsson A, Smith J, editors. Towards a general theory of expertise: prospects and limits. Cambridge: Cambridge University Press; 1991. p. 93–125.
43. Patel VL, Evans DA, Groen GJ. Biomedical knowledge and clinical reasoning. In: Evans DA, Patel VL, editors. Cognitive science in medicine: biomedical modeling. Cambridge: MIT Press; 1989. p. 53–112.
44. Holyoak KJ, Thagard P. Analogical mapping by constraint satisfaction. Cognit Sci. 1989;13(3):295–355.
45. Brown JS, Burton RR. Diagnostic models for procedural bugs in basic mathematical skills. Cognit Sci. 1978;2(2):155–92.
46. Brown JS, VanLehn K. Repair theory: a generative theory of bugs in procedural skills. Cognit Sci. 1980;4(4):379–426.

47. Keselman A, Kaufman DR, Kramer S, Patel VL. Fostering conceptual change and critical reasoning about HIV and AIDS. J Res Sci Teach. 2007;44(6):844–63.
48. Kanse L, van der Schaaf TW, Vrijland ND, van Mierlo H. Error recovery in a hospital pharmacy. Ergonomics. 2006;49(5–6):503–16. PubMed PMID: 16717007.
49. Kessels-Habraken M, Van der Schaaf T, De Jonge J, Rutte C. Defining near misses: towards a sharpened definition based on empirical data about error handling processes. Soc Sci Med. 2010;70(9):1301–8.
50. Norman DA. The psychology of everyday things. New York: Basic Books; 1988.
51. Allwood CM. Error detection process in statistical problem solving. Cognit Sci. 1984;8(4): 413–37.
52. Hales BM, Pronovost PJ. The checklist-A tool for error management and performance improvement. J Crit Care. 2006;21(3):231–5. PubMed PMID: 16990087.
53. Wilkinson WE, Cauble LA, Patel VL. Error detection and recovery in dialysis nursing. J Patient Saf. 2011;7(4):213–23. PubMed PMID: 22064625. Epub 2011/11/09.
54. Razzouk E, Cohen T, Almoosa K, Patel VL. Approaching the limits of knowledge: the influence of priming on error detection in simulated clinical rounds. In: AMIA annual symposium proceedings. 2011. p. 1155–64.

Chapter 3
Failed Detection of Egregious Errors in Clinical Case Scenarios

Vimla L. Patel, Trevor Cohen, and Vafa Ghaemmaghami

Reevaluating Recovery

The notion that human error should not be tolerated is prevalent in both the public and personal perception of the performance of clinicians. However, researchers in other safety-critical domains have long since abandoned the quest for zero defects as an impractical goal, choosing to focus instead on the development of strategies to enhance the ability to recover from error. This holistic perspective motivated the studies of error detection and recovery described in this chapter. As we have argued in Chap. 2, the expectation of flawless performance is misguided, as it fails to take into account the systemic factors that promote error [1], the role of error in the

---

This section has been adapted from Patel et al. Recovery at the Edge of Error: Debunking the Myth of the Infallible Expert. *Journal of Biomedical Informatics. 44*(3), 413–424.

V.L. Patel, PhD, DSc, FRSC (✉)
Center for Cognitive Studies in Medicine and Public Health,
New York Academy of Medicine, New York, NY 10029, USA

Department of Biomedical Informatics, Columbia University,
New York, NY 10032, USA

Department of Biomedical Informatics, Arizona State University,
Scottsdale, AZ 85259, USA
e-mail: vpatel@nyam.org

T. Cohen, MB ChB, PhD
School of Biomedical Informatics, University of Texas Health Science Center,
Houston, TX 77054, USA
e-mail: trevor.cohen@uth.tmc.edu

V. Ghaemmaghami, MD, FACS
Trauma Division, Department of Surgery, Banner Good Samaritan Hospital,
Phoenix, AZ 85006, USA

University of Arizona College of Medicine, Phoenix, AZ USA

V.L. Patel et al. (eds.), *Cognitive Informatics in Health and Biomedicine*,
Health Informatics, DOI 10.1007/978-1-4471-5490-7_3, © Springer-Verlag London 2014

acquisition of expertise [2], and the characterization of cognitive mechanisms of error at all levels of expertise (for example [3]). So while the elimination of error is a laudable goal, we elected to focus instead on the goal of promoting error recovery, following both the lead of researchers in other domains and the evidence of error recovery observed in our prior ethnographic studies [4].

The Myth of the Infallible Expert

Media attention to high-profile medical malpractice cases has raised public awareness of the occasionally disastrous consequences of medical error. Not only are clinicians expected to perform without error; but also the litigious nature of society in the United States raises the possibility of severe, often career-altering consequences in the event of an error. Even in the absence of such consequences, clinicians are faced with the personal expectation that they perform flawlessly: failing to meet this expectation is associated with burnout and significant emotional distress, which manifests with symptoms of clinical depression [5]. However, while considerable evidence exists that experts exhibit vastly improved knowledge organization, solution strategies, performance efficiency, a highly refined ability to recognize and integrate the pertinent features of problems and an improved ability to predict the consequences of decisions taken (for a review, see [5]), there also exists compelling evidence that experts are by no means immune to error. For example, studies of expertise in medicine reveal experts are prone to making particular sorts of error in diagnosis and management: experts are shown to be vulnerable to premature closure, rapidly reaching a conclusion and ignoring evidence in support of competing hypotheses [3]. Furthermore, and as discussed in Chap. 2, research in the domain of air traffic control has shown that no demonstrable reduction in the rate of committed errors occurs after the preliminary stages of training [6].

Human beings use innovative and economical strategies to aid in problem solving and decision-making, known as heuristics. These strategies are even more critical when the large number of patients and high degree of uncertainty exhibited in certain medical contexts further tax the processing capacities of physicians. The utility of heuristics lies in limiting the extent of purposeful search through the problem space of possible solutions, and instead basing reasoning largely on past experience. By increasing efficiency in this way, they have substantial practical value. Heuristics are rules of thumb, which develop with familiarity in the domain of application. While decisions based on heuristics have high levels of confidence associated with them, there is often no way of checking the validity of a heuristic decision against the evidence, as the cognitive mechanisms underlying the use of heuristics are often not available for conscious processing. These rules of thumb can result in errors in several ways, including the use of the *availability heuristic*, judgment on the basis of how easily previous examples spring to mind; the *anchoring heuristic*, in which clinicians stick to their initial impression of a case and ignore evidence to the contrary; and *framing effects*, in which decisions are biased by the manner in which information is presented [7]. Combinations of these types of heuristics have been shown to produce serious misdiagnoses.

Experts use heuristic reasoning, which is valuable from a practical point of view, but the use of these heuristics also introduces considerable bias in medical reasoning, resulting in a number of conceptual and procedural errors. These include misconceptions about laws governing probability, inaccurate instantiation of general rules to a specific patient's problem, failure to consider prior probabilities, perceptual illusions, and delusions of validity. These factors are described in studies reported by Croskerry and colleagues [8, 9]. Patel and her colleagues have conducted a number of studies examining the use of heuristics by expert physicians and medical students [10]. Most of these studies are summarized in Patel, Arocha and Kaufman [3]. A frequently used heuristic is the reliance on disease schemata during clinical diagnosis. Disease schemata are knowledge structures that have been formed from previous experience with diagnosing diseases, and contain information about relevant signs and symptoms. When physicians and medical students diagnose patients, they tend to rely on their schemata and base their reasoning on the apparent similarity of patient information with these schemata, instead of a more objective analysis of patient data. The schemata that are used in diagnosis often guide future reasoning about the patient, affecting what diagnostic tests are requested and how data are interpreted [10]. This strategy is consistent with the fast and frugal heuristic approach in which decision makers look for recognizable patterns and cues in order to narrow the space for making decisions [11]. This is an effective strategy for an expert, who has the domain knowledge. However, this strategy does not work when the nature of the problem is complex [12]. This is also similar to the "Satisficing" principle put forth by Herbert Simon [13], which describes the tendency of human problem solvers to seek a solution that is satisfactory, but not optimal. It also appears that there is a downside to expert diagnostic reasoning [14]. Specialists tend to diagnose cases outside their domain as though they fall within their areas of expertise, often assigning higher probabilities to diagnoses that are familiar to them than do clinicians who are expert in other areas [15]. Studies of medical trainees show that they maintain their initial hypotheses, even if the subsequent data are counter-indicative. If the initial hypothesis is inaccurate, errors are likely to occur in final diagnosis and treatment regimen [10].

Error Recovery in Other Domains

While an exhaustive review of the literature on error detection and recovery in other domains is beyond the scope of this chapter, we provide here a brief summary of key findings that motivate our research. As described previously, the research presented in this paper is motivated by some surprising findings from the aviation and transport domain, as presented by Amalberti and his colleagues [6]. In the studies on aviation and training of pilots, it was clear that the flight crews made fewer errors when confronted with demanding conditions (such as weather changes) then when their workload is low. However, the rate of error detection and recovery under demanding conditions was also reduced, with the end result being a higher frequency of incidents despite fewer raw errors. Amalberti and his colleagues' interpretation of these data is that under high workload cognitive resources are focused on the task at hand, resulting in fewer raw errors. Diversion of these resources means that they are no longer available for error recovery, and thus results in fewer error recoveries (and error detections). In these studies, reduction in recovery rate had a greater influence on safety than the number of raw errors committed. Other domains in which error recovery was also investigated include the maritime domain, in which the research emphasizes the need for crewmembers to use knowledge-based strategies for efficient error recovery and decision-making in novel and unfamiliar situations [16]. Similarly, a study in the chemical process industry has shown that error recovery and contingent decision-making responses at skill-based and knowledge-based levels play important roles in mitigating the adverse effects of any error [17]. At the time during which our studies were being conducted, we knew little about the nature of error recovery in medicine. This motivated our initial investigations of this issue in the clinical environment using ethnographic methods.

A Cognitive Model of Error Recovery

In our previous work, we have defined the following categories of evolving error in relation to violation of constraints [18]. We summarize the definitions of these categories here, since they are necessary for the interpretation of our results:

- **Near-Miss**: A violation of normal routine, from which it is still possible to recover without consequences (for example, a patient is prescribed a drug he/she is allergic to, but this erroneous treatment is not yet delivered).
- **Miss**: The action cycle is complete, and some adverse consequences are possible due to the missed error (for example, the treatment is given).
- **Adverse Event**: An untoward consequence of the error occurs (for example, an allergic reaction ensues).

These categories relate to the temporal evolution of medical error, described in further detail in Chap. 2. The process of error recovery may occur at different stages of this model of error evolution. Although the error ideally would be detected at the 'near miss' stage, some intervention may be possible even after the 'miss' has actually occurred. We note that in order to avert this progression, not only is the detection of possible error required, there is also a need to take some corrective action.

The process of error recovery contains stages of both execution and evaluation, and consequently this cyclical process can be modeled using Donald Norman's well-established and generic seven-stage model of interaction [19]. Norman's model was originally applied to the problem of system usability, but has also, on account of its generic nature, been used to model a broad range of cognitive interactions in which interpretation and action are tightly connected. When adapted to the

Table 3.1 Mean number of errors detected and corrected during patient handovers and clinical rounds in a cardio-thoracic ICU

	Handovers (n=4)	Rounds (n=6)
Errors	10.5	5.6
Recoveries	7.25	5.25
Recovery through interactions	1.75	5.25
Clarification questions	16.5	13.75

modeling of error recovery, the seven stages in the cycle are: (1) Error Perception; (2) Error Interpretation; (3) Error Evaluation; (4) Setting Goals for Response; (5) Decision to Take Action; (6) Action Specification; and (7) Execution of this Action. The first three two stages have to do with the detection of error, the third relates to the issue of risk mitigation (in particular the decision whether to respond to the detected error or not), and the last four stages concern the issue of correction of a detected error. The mapping between these stages of evolution, Norman's model and other cognitive research on error recovery (for example [20]) is discussed in detail in Chap. 2.

Early Indicators of Error Recovery

Kubose, Patel and colleagues conducted 3 months of ethnographic observations and audio recordings of interactions between core members of the clinical team in a cardiothoracic intensive care unit (ICU) [21]. Analysis of these data showed that the highest degree of team interaction occurred during clinician-to-clinician handover, during clinical rounds and in the admission of new patients to the ICU. These studies were conducted to better understand the mechanism by which errors are detected and corrected in this dynamic, high velocity, time-pressured environment, and to investigate the strategies for error management and risk assessment as a function of expertise. These foci of increased interactivity were also identified as most likely to produce a high yield of incidents of error detection and recovery. Consequently, four patient handovers and six team discussions from clinical rounds were audio-recorded and analyzed using qualitative coding methods to identify incidents of an error being detected and corrected. Error recoveries were further categorized into those affected by an individual, and those requiring teamwork. Table 3.1 below shows the number of errors detected and corrected during these sessions.

A mean of 10.5 and 5.6 errors were detected in handovers and clinical rounds respectively. Of note, a higher proportion of recovered errors occurred during the rounds, which provides some support for the intuitive notion that the chances of error detection are greater during interactions between multiple team members. However, other factors, in particular the presence of experts on rounds and the differences between rounds and handovers with respect to their purpose and duration are also likely to contribute toward differences in error detection. The relationship between expertise and error was also examined in this study. An ICU expert, a resident and a student were identified and shadowed by an observer for a total of 10 h.

Table 3.2 Number of errors during ICU practice in a 10-h period

Subject	Error detection	Recovery
Expert	18	15
Resident	13	8
Student	8	2

The entire session was audio recorded and transcribed for analysis. Incidents of error detection and recovery by each subject are shown in Table 3.2.

Experts were shown to detect as well as recover from 75 % of the errors made during the 10-h period. On further analysis, it was found that 70 % of the errors identified required expert knowledge for recovery and were likely to have serious consequences if uncorrected. The resident detected fewer errors than the expert subject, and corrected a smaller proportion of these (61 %) errors. The student detected the least number and those that were corrected were mostly routine errors that did not require detailed medical knowledge.

Further Prospective Studies of Error Recovery in Medicine

These studies were prospective in nature, which is to say that incidents of error recovery were captured as they occurred, rather than attempting retrospective analysis of historical incidents of error or error recovery. Prospective error recovery studies have also been conducted in the context of the psychiatric emergency department (PED). Clinical rounds were audio-recorded and transcribed in order to document the evolution of error during discussions among colleagues on clinical rounds [4]. Excerpts from these recordings, suggesting perceived violations of the accepted bounds of safe practice or incidents of mis-communication, were extracted and analyzed using qualitative coding methods. The results were interpreted in relation to prior research on vulnerabilities to error in the PED. In addition to confirming the predictions of this prior research, the data revealed a variety of perceived violations, many of which have potentially serious consequences for patient safety. Ten of these incidents were considered by physicians with specific domain experience to have potentially dangerous consequences, but only one incident was formally reported. Frequently, perceived violations were followed by corrective actions, such as the prescription of a previously neglected medication, revealing both the apparent boundaries of acceptable practice and the mechanisms in place to correct a violation of these boundaries. Such analysis of the detection and prevention of potential error during patient rounds expands the data available for error analysis beyond the occasional reported adverse event. These findings are consistent with contemporary error research, which suggests that the detection and correction of potential errors are integral parts of cognitive work in the complex, modern-day workplace [2].

Retrospective Studies of Error Recovery in Medicine

In contrast to these prospective approaches, Nyssen and Blavier investigated the role of error detection in anesthesiology using retrospective data obtained from an accident reporting system employed in two university hospitals in Belgium [22]. Their results emphasized the importance of standard checks in error detection, and showed significant relationships between type of error and error detection mode, as well as type of error and the level of expertise of the anesthetist concerned. The following modes of error detection were identified: standard checks, detection on the basis of outcome (the effect on the patient), suspicion based on knowledge, detection by another operator, detection on the basis of an alarm and detection by chance. Of these modes, standard checks contributed most to detection of error (27.7 % of 216 analyzed error reports), followed by detection based on outcome (24.8 %). They also observed that more experienced anesthetists used a broader range of error detection modes than their younger colleagues [22].

Retrospective data analysis is vulnerable to bias towards final outcomes since one uses the outcome (positive or negative) to interpret the event, showing post-hoc bias. In a study of error recovery in the pharmacy setting, Kanse and his colleagues supplement near-miss reports with confidential interviews, to provide further insight into the recovery process [23]. This study identifies several factors associated with successful and unsuccessful recovery efforts. Many of the successful recovery efforts in this environment were associated with planned checks, and similarly failure to complete systematic checks was associated with failure to recover in many instances. Checklist-based implementation of systematic checks in procedural tasks has been shown to be similarly effective for error reduction [24]. However, the question remains as to what sorts of interventions might improve the chances of error detection in the kind of dynamic decision-making processes that occur in critical care and that cannot be characterized as a set of normative "correct" steps. Adherence to checklists and some evidence-based standards is very important, but given the nature of the work in critical care, decision making on the fly requires one to know exactly when to deviate from a protocol.

Retrospective studies offer certain advantages, as they allow for the analysis of a pre-existing pool of data related to incidents relevant to error recovery. However, as discussed previously the interpretation of these data is vulnerable to bias, and they are limited in their ability to capture the *process* of error recovery. From the perspective of cognitive science, the essence of task performance, effective or otherwise, lies in the thought processes that underlie it. In order to capture this essence, prospective studies that occur during task performance are necessary. Consequently, while it is in many respects fortunate that incidents of commission, detection and recovery occur relatively infrequently when compared with incidents of routine care, this raises logistical issues that make it difficult to approach this problem using a traditional ethnographic approach. Furthermore, as every incident of error recovery occurs in a unique clinical context, ethnographic fieldwork precludes meaningful comparison between physicians with respect to their ability to detect the same error.

Experimental Approach: Embedding of Errors, Sometimes Egregious

Development of Clinical Cases

Consequently, in order to provide a degree of experimental control, and focus our attention on error recovery, we developed an experimental paradigm that involved creating case scenarios containing embedded errors, and asking physicians to read through and interpret these without alerting them beforehand to the presence of error. In-vitro or laboratory-based studies offer scientists the opportunity to investigate aspects of a phenomenon of interest under controlled conditions. Insights into thought processes of Individuals under study are often gathered using a "think-aloud" method, which documents verbalizations of thoughts as subjects perform cognitive tasks [25]. We conducted laboratory-based studies of experts (attending physicians) and non-experts (residents at various levels of training) and assessed their ability to detect, correct and justify their interpretation of errors embedded in a set of realistic written clinical case scenarios. Two problem cases, with a range of management errors embedded in them were developed with the assistance of our clinical collaborators. The cases resembled clinical situations encountered in practice and were expressed in a format similar to those used during the clinical rounds. Each case provided a brief clinical history followed by several management decisions. In order to set the stage for the description of our experiments, we will describe these cases with an emphasis on the errors embedded in each of them.

Case 1: Mismanaged Diverticulitis

The first of these cases concerns a patient with suspected diverticulitis. Diverticulitis involves the inflammation of an extrusion of a pouch of colon through a weakening in the abdominal wall. On account of this inflammation, perforation may occur, resulting in the dissemination of infective organisms from the colon into the abdominal cavity. So management of a patient with suspected diverticulitis requires the administration of broad-spectrum antibiotics that includes coverage for the anaerobic organisms that occupy the colon. The first error in this hypothetical scenario involved the administration of an inappropriate antibiotic without this coverage, which would be dangerously ineffective in the event that bowel perforation occurs.

The second error involved the use of colonoscopy in an attempt to make a diagnosis. Colonoscopy is contraindicated in this scenario on account of the risk of perforation presented by the weakened wall of the colon that occurs in diverticulitis. Arguably, these first two errors are egregious in nature: the need to cover anaerobic organisms in the event of bowel perforation is emphasized repeatedly during medical training, and the erroneous application of colonoscopy may cause perforation of the bowel with potentially fatal consequences.

In addition to these two egregious errors, a further two procedural errors of a less serious nature were included. The first involved failure to obtain a plain X-ray before ordering a CT scan of the abdomen. In situations in which perforation may be an issue, it is important to recognize this expediently, and a plain X-ray is inevitably faster obtained than a CT scan. Sometimes when perforation of the bowel has occurred, a bubble of air is seen under the diaphragm on chest X-ray. When visible, this as a pathognomonic radiological finding, enabling rapid and accurate diagnosis of the urgent problem of bowel perforation. As the situation deteriorates (arguably on account of the erroneously applied colonoscopy) the patient is taken to the Operating Room. Upon exploration of the abdomen, a mass of inflammatory tissue known as a *phlegmon* is encountered in the Left Lower Quadrant of the abdomen. Unfortunately for our hypothetical patient, this area of the abdomen is also the location of the left ureter, a muscular tube that carries urine from the left kidney to the bladder. In the presence of such dense inflammatory tissue, it is advisable to obtain assistance from urology for the pre-operative placement of a ureteral stent, to make it easier to dissect the area around the ureter inflammatory tissue without the danger of injuring it.

While not stated explicitly, injury to the ureter during surgery is extremely likely in this case scenario, particularly as the patient proceeds to develop pain and a fever after surgery, and upon investigation with a CT scan, a fluid collection is revealed at the site of the operation. Draining this collection of fluid revealed clear straw-colored fluid. The patient is discharged with a drain in place, which at the time of discharge was still draining around 200 cc/day of fluid. This strongly suggests the surgeon had injured the ureter, resulting in urine leaking into the abdominal cavity. Injuries to the ureter are associated with significant morbidity, including the loss of kidney function, and the most important controllable factor resulting in adverse outcomes is delayed diagnosis of the injury [26].

Case 2: The Anatomy of an Attempted Murder

The second case concerns a traumatic injury, in which a 23-year-old man is brought to the trauma unit after being stabbed twice on the left side. One wounds occurs at the anterior axillary line at the level of the nipple, and the other occurs 3 cm below it. The anterior axillary line runs vertically in front of the armpit, just medial to the shoulder joint, and extends down the side of the abdomen. So even without specialized training, the fact that these penetrating injuries might have affected the left lung and heart are readily apparent. The first of the two errors included in this case has to do with the heart. One possibility in a penetrating injury at this location is that the *pericardium*, the membranous sac surrounding the heart has been injured. The pericardium usually contains a small amount of fluid, but the danger with a stab wound at this location is that bleeding into the pericardium can occur. When this is severe, it can mechanically restrict the heart's ability to pump blood, a condition known as *cardiac tamponade*, which is frequently fatal. The error in this case was that the trauma team did not rule out the possibility of pericardial injury using sonography. As treatment is a matter of urgency in this condition, this error could have had fatal consequences.

Fortunately for the patient and the management team, this was not the case in this scenario. After insertion of a chest tube to drain blood from the membrane that surrounds the left lung, the patient was taken to the Operating Room, where a laparoscopic examination of the abdomen showed that one of the stab wounds (presumably the lower of the two) had penetrated the abdomen. Consequently, surgical exploration of the abdomen was conducted, which revealed a number of injuries including a 2-cm defect in the left diaphragm, and a laceration of the left lobe of the liver. In addition, and of particular importance for our purposes, a *hematoma*, a localized collection of blood, was found in a region of the abdomen known as *zone one*. This region is found at the back of the abdomen, in the midline, and contains the two largest blood vessels in the abdomen, the abdominal aorta and the inferior vena cava. As these are the major conduits of blood between the heart and the lower half of the body, injury to either of these structures has dire consequences. The hematoma in this case was neither expanding rapidly nor pulsing, as one might anticipate if the abdominal aorta had been injured. However, the inferior vena cava may have been injured, and injury of this vessel is associated with a severe mortality rate. The surgical team in this case elected to repair the diaphragm, suture the liver, and close the patient. This was an error, as operative exploration of the hematoma is indicated to rule out the possibility of injury to the abdominal aorta and inferior vena cava.

Prerequisites to Detection

Identification of several of the embedded errors requires not only factual knowledge, but also the generation of a specific inference from the problem information provided. For example, without the recognition that the first case suggests acute diverticulitis, the contra-indication to colonoscopy is not evident. A breakdown of the nature of the errors included in the problem cases is shown in Table 3.3.

Study Procedure

The study was conducted in makeshift laboratory settings in two hospitals (Banner Good Samaritan Medical Center in Phoenix, AZ and Washington University School of Medicine in St. Louis, MO). The developed clinical scenarios, parts of which

Table 3.3 Prerequisites for detection of embedded errors

Error	Required inference	Prerequisite knowledge
C1E1 Inappropriate antibiotics	Anaerobic organisms likely to be involved Perforation possible	Anaerobic organisms exist in the colon Prescribed antibiotics do not cover anaerobic organisms
C1E2 Colonoscopy performed	Presentation suggests acute diverticulitis	Diagnostic features of diverticulitis Colonoscopy contraindicated in acute diverticulitis
C1E3 No chest x-ray before CT scan	Perforation possible	Procedural: management guidelines
C1E4 No stent placed	A ureter is at risk because of proximity to the inflammation.	Anatomical: proximity of ureter Procedural: place stent prior to dissection
C1E5 Undiagnosed injury to ureter	Draining clear fluid + surgery in vicinity of ureter suggests ureteral injury	Ureteral injury demands active management
C2E1 No pericardial ultrasound	Risk of pericardial injury	Anatomical: location of stab wound Fast U/S scan should be performed when at risk for cardiac injury
C2E2 Hematoma not explored	Possible large vessel injury	Anatomical: zone 1 of abdomen contains Abdominal Aorta & Inferior Vena Cava Hematomata in this area should be explored

CxEy = Case x, Error y

were based on real situations, were presented to participants in paper form, and the following instructions were provided:

- Read the case and "think aloud" (verbalize your thoughts without interpreting or editing them) as you are reading through the case. You may take notes on the writing paper provided.
- Answer the questions that follow the case.
- All of the responses will be audio recorded.

These instructions were followed by a second set of instructions for summarizing and making the final evaluation:

- Summarize the case from memory and your notes.
- Discuss the resident's evaluation, including any additional information you may wish to request.
- Summarize your own final evaluation of the case management.

The participants were not allowed to refer back to the case, except for their written notes. The participants were not warned of the errors present in the cases. This facet of the experimental design encouraged participants to interpret the case as they might interpret a similar situation presented by a colleague on clinical rounds. All the responses were audio recorded and transcribed anonymously. After completing

Table 3.4 An example of recall and inference analysis from the transcripts

Original text	Recall	Inference	Errors detected
The patient is discharged home with the drain in place	"Discharged home with the drain in place"	"Shouldn't have done so. Should have worked up ureteral injury"	Did not diagnose ureteral injury

the first case, participants were asked to complete the second case using the same set of instructions. The sequence of case presentation was counterbalanced to make sure that there was no order effect.

Method of Analysis

We employed our usual method of natural language protocol analysis, using propositional and concept representations. The details of these analyses are reported elsewhere [27]. In summary, the Subjects' responses were analyzed for spontaneity (time), error detection, error correction, and the provision of justification for clinical decisions. Transcribed subject responses were used to identify specific concepts used by the participants in their responses. The stimulus text (problem case given to each subject) was also divided into a set of propositional concepts. A detailed manual mapping of the propositions (basic units of representation of text) between the subject's response transcript and the stimulus text was performed, where the presence or absence of a particular concept in the transcribed protocol was matched against the corresponding concept in the original text in terms of recall and inference as described by Patel and Groen [27]. The errors detected and corrected at each stage of analysis were noted. Table 3.4 shows an example of a part of the analysis of the transcript for recall and inference.

The responses of all the participants were characterized as error detection, partial error correction, complete error correction, doubtful detection and justification. These are shown on Table 3.5, along with the definition of each category.

Expertise and Expectations

The study was conducted at two sites- in Phoenix, Arizona (Site #1) and in St. Louis, Missouri (Site #2). The sample for the study consisted of 25 participants (13 surgical attendings, 11 surgical residents and one anesthesiology resident). The attendings practiced both general surgery and trauma, and varied in their level of experience from one to over 20 years since specialization. Residents included were from all 5 years of training. On account of our observations of more efficient error detection by experts in a critical care context [21], and the relatively efficient and

Table 3.5 Definition and characterization of error categories based on participants' responses

Category	Example	Comments
Detection: Error detected and fully specified.	"That drug would not have been my first choice"	The participant questions the use of the drug, an inappropriate antibiotic (C1E1).
Partial detection: A reference to some discrepancy related to the error, without fully specifying the error.	"With the clear straw-colored fluid without knowing whether they sent amylase or lipase, it is likely to be a pancreatic leakage".	The participant was not sure that it was ureteral injury but points out that there is something amiss (C1E5).
Doubtful detection: Some doubt exists as to the presence of error.	"Probably explore the hematoma, but to be honest I actually do not know if it is the correct thing to do or not".	The participant detected the error, but was not certain about this. (C2E2)
Correction: An alternative is proposed after detecting the error.	"I wouldn't have sent her home anticipating a ureteral injury. I probably would have studied her with IvP or urogram, with urology involved."	Participant not only points out the C2E5, but also defines a course of corrective action.
Justification: Error detection accompanied by an explanation of the nature of the error.	"Wouldn't have scoped her so early, because two days into her treatment that is already giving her quite a bit of trouble and maybe has a little perforation, I don't think that it adds to the management."	Not only was C1E1 detected, an explanation of the rationale behind this critique is also provided.

accurate processing of information that is characteristic of expertise in medicine [3] and in general [28], we anticipated that experts would have little difficulty detecting the more egregious errors we had embedded. However, our results were somewhat surprising.

Results: Error Detection

Figure 3.1 shows the percentage of expert ($n=13$) and non-expert participants ($n=12$) that detected each of the embedded errors. A striking finding is that none of the errors were detected by more than half of the participants, regardless of expertise. Contrary to expectations, the number of errors detected by each subject was poorly correlated with their years of clinical experience (Pearson's $r=0.117$, $p=0.58$), and while the mean number of errors detected was higher for expert subjects (mean = 1.77) than non-expert subjects (mean = 1.5) this difference was not statistically significant as there was considerable variability in performance within each group. However, despite these global trends, large differences between expert and novice performance were observed for specific errors.

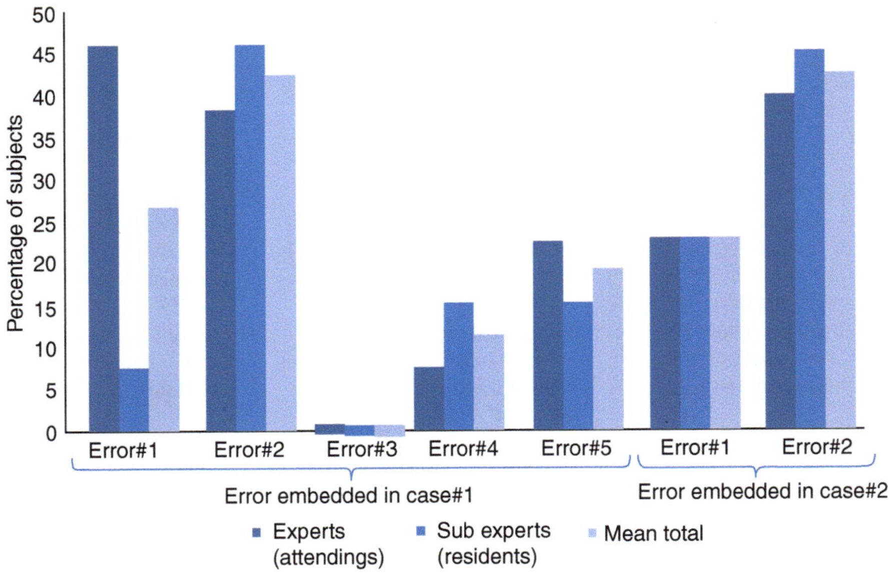

Fig. 3.1 Percentage of expert and non-expert participants detecting each of the errors (Reprinted with permission from Patel et al. [36])

Of the five errors in case #1, two of the errors (#2 and #5) are major errors and if undetected, they can be fatal. Errors #1, 3 and 4 are not as critical in terms of patient outcome. A detailed interpretation of errors described in Fig. 3.1. The description of each of these errors is given below.

C1E1: Inappropriate Antibiotics

This error was detected by only 7 of the 25 participants and all seven of them mentioned broadening antibiotic coverage with high confidence. Six of these seven participants were experts, and the error revealed the greatest disparity between experts and novices of any of the errors in our experiment. As this is a knowledge-based error, this disparity is to be expected, as it has been shown in other domains that knowledge-based errors decrease with expertise [16]. Intuitively, one would not expect error recovery without the knowledge required to recognize a particular error, an issue we will revisit in Chap. 6 of this volume. This finding is also consistent with our studies with nurses, where nurses detected more knowledge-based errors than technicians working in a renal dialysis unit [29].

Further analysis of the responses showed that the experts could promptly detect the error with certainty while reading the case and did not need to go back to the case or their notes, while the single non-expert subject that detected this error was doubtful initially but re-affirmed the conviction this was indeed an error upon review of the case after reading through it. Information processing by an expert functioning at a heuristic level is fairly obvious in this situation (we envision a heuristic along the lines of "provide good coverage for the anaerobic organisms that occupy the bowel when bowel perforation is suspected").

C1E2: Contraindicated Colonoscopy

This was the one of the serious errors introduced in the first case, as colonoscopy in this situation can (and quite possibly did) lead to perforation with dire consequences for the patient. Twelve out of 25 participants detected the problem and suggested the colonoscopy was not appropriate. Many also referred to the risk of perforation as a result of colonoscopy. More than half of our expert subjects did not identify this error despite the severe clinical consequences involved. Nonetheless, this was the most frequently identified of all of the embedded errors across cases, which may be explained by the fact that the clinical consequences were already apparent during presentation occurred, given that detection of errors based on patient outcomes has been identified as a prominent mechanism of recovery in previous work [22].

C1E3: No X-Ray Before CT Scan

This error was not detected by any of the participants. Given that any findings visible on x-ray are also likely to be noted on CT scan (in particular, the lack of a clear indication for surgery), this error is less dangerous than other embedded errors. In the event that free air under the diagram was visible on a plain x-ray, the result would have been more rapid treatment of the same nature. This may be explained by the well-established tendency of problem-solvers to satisfice rather than to seek optimal solution. Another possible explanation is that the nature of this error is primarily procedural: the abdominal x-ray is one of a series of sequential steps that are expected in the investigation of penetrating abdominal trauma. These types of errors may be more difficult to detect when a case is presented on paper (for example, our clinical scenarios discussed in the previous sections are paper-based) as a snapshot in time after of the temporal context in which the error occurred.

C1E4: Did Not Consider Preoperative Stent

Three of the 25 participants detected the presence of this error. Two were residents, and one was an attending with a maximum of 6 years of experience, suggesting that this may be a recently popularized treatment protocol, and thus this precaution was not taken by more experienced surgeons. It is also possible that more experienced surgeons do not feel this precaution is necessary. In any event, the importance of this procedure is debatable and its significance as an error to the patient is minimal. However, the perception that the ureter is in danger at this point is of relevance to the detection of error C1E5, below. While an individual error may not be harmful in and of itself, when combined with other errors it may lead to an adverse event.

C1E5: Undiagnosed Ureteral Injury

Only 5 of the 25 participants "completely" detected this error by explicitly and with confidence mentioning ureteral injury, which has significant consequences if left untreated as was the case in this scenario. In addition, one non-expert subject "doubtfully" detected this error, and interestingly five of the expert subjects exhibited partial detection in which they did not explicitly mention ureteral injury but suspected something had been missed. This would be characterized as "spontaneous triggering" in Allwood's cognitive model of error detection. There were several clues to the presence of this error, and it is interesting to note that in some cases subjects recognized the ureter was at risk during dissection without connecting this to the fact that the clear fluid present was likely to be urine. However, the majority of the subjects that were concerned about the absence of a ureteral stent did detect this error.

C2E1: No Pericardial Sonogram

Only 5 of 25 participants "completely" detected this error, which has potentially fatal consequences if left undetected. One explanation for this may be that, similarly to error three in case one, this can be considered to be a procedural error in which focused sonography to rule out pericardial injury is part of a sequence of management steps that would have occurred earlier in time than the point in which the case was presented, and it may be difficult to detect this sort of error out of its temporal context.

C2E2: Hematoma Not Explored

Ten participants detected the error of which nine were confident about their judgments. Qualitative analysis of our think-aloud protocols showed that five of the participants (who did not detect the error) lacked knowledge about the location of "zone 1", which was discussed in the case. Lack of the appropriate knowledge was clearly a problem with detection of error in this scenario.

Experts and Complex Errors

Experts were better able to detect errors one and five in case one (C1E1 and C1E5), and error two in case two (C2E2). From a problem solving perspective, these are arguably the most complex errors, as in all cases integration of multiple elements of the case narrative with background clinical knowledge is required. In the first error in case one (C1E1), participants must infer both the likely diagnosis (diverticulitis with perforation) from the patient's symptoms, and the organisms likely to be involved in this case, in order to recognize that these organisms are not covered by the antibiotic prescribed. In the case of the fifth error (C1E5), participants must infer that the ureter lies amongst the anatomical structures in the region of the inflammatory mass (left lower quadrant), and is therefore likely to be injured during surgery. This inference supports the diagnosis that the clear fluid draining post-operatively is likely to be urine. In the second error in case 2 (C2E2), participants must infer that the patient's stab wound is likely to have penetrated the diaphragm, and that the hematoma in zone one may involve the large vessels in this region in order to detect the life-threatening consequences of the failure to explore it. This ability to integrate multiple cues is characteristic of problem detection by experts [30], and suggests the presence of a well-organized and highly interconnected knowledge base. Successful error detection by residents was focused on those errors with the greatest potential impact on patient outcome. This finding is consistent with a recent study of error detection in the context of general medicine [31], in which residents and nurses were more likely to detect error-related adverse events than attending physicians. Residents may be sensitized to these issues on account of the intensity of their involvement in hands-on patient care.

Error Correction and Justification

Table 3.6 summarizes the proportion of detected errors that were corrected and justified across all subjects that detected errors. Attending physicians more frequently provide justifications for their detected errors than residents, which may be a reflection of their involvement in teaching activities. Experts on average corrected 36.4 % of their detected errors, while residents corrected on average 66.7 %. This differs from our previous data that showed experts corrected a higher proportion of their errors, though this case the scenario involved detecting errors committed by others. However, this finding may be an artifact of our experimental design, as in many cases the error was only encountered at a point in time at which correction was no longer possible. Error detection is a prerequisite to error correction, although not all subjects articulated clearly that an error was detected, even if it was corrected. These findings, as well as emerging research on risk mitigation [32] suggest a need for further research into the features of a detected error that determine whether or not corrective action is taken.

Detection and Recovery in Dialysis Nursing

In a subsequent study, we used the same experimental paradigm to evaluate the ability of dialysis nurses to detect and recover from errors embedded in paper-based case scenarios [29]. Dialysis nursing is a complex specialty area that necessitates focused training and experience and it requires enhanced skills because during

Table 3.6 Correction and justification of detected errors (participants detecting no errors are excluded)

Attendings	Years of experience	Errors detected	% Errors corrected	% Errors justified
3	34	1	0	100
5	30	1	0	0
2	21	4	25	0
4	21	4	75	75
1	19	3	33.3	66.7
7	12	1	100	100
8	7	1	0	100
9	6	2	50	100
11	6	3	66.7	66.7
12	6	1	0	100
13	6	2	50	100
Mean		2.1	36.4	73.5
Residents	**Years in training**	**Errors detected**	**% Errors corrected**	**% Errors justified**
1	4	3	33.3	33.3
12	4	1	100	100
4	3	1	100	0
5	3	2	0	0
7	3	2	50	100
8	3	2	50	100
11	3	1	100	100
9	3	3	100	66.7
10	3	1	100	100
3	1	1	0	0
6	1	1	100	0
Mean		1.6	66.7	54.6

treatment patients can suffer severe fluid and electrolyte imbalances, or can develop cardiac, pulmonary and other fatal complications. The most important professional role for dialysis nurses is to foster an environment of continuous kidney patient safety at the point of care. As was the case in our trauma studies, we embedded management errors within two clinical case scenarios based on real events that Registered Nurses (RNs) were asked to detect and recover during subjects' oral readings of the cases. RNs from five clinical dialysis settings that were part of a single national dialysis chain in Southern Arizona were invited to participate as subjects in this research. Four of the clinical locations were outpatient dialysis clinics and one site was an in-patient hospital hemodialysis setting. A total of 31 participants were recruited from these sites.

The two constructed clinical cases reflected a constructed, realistic composite of chronic-care dialysis patients and treatment events that have happened or could happen with any patient who received dialysis treatments. There were eight errors in the first case, and four errors embedded within the second case. A domain expert

Table 3.7 Summary of results from dialysis nursing study

Case/error number	Total errors detected (n=31)	Expert RN (n=16)		Non-expert RN (n=15)		Total errors recovered (n=31)
Case # 1	# (%)	D	R	D	R	# (%)
K 1	3 (10 %)	3	3	0	0	3 (10 %)
K 2	8 (26 %)	7	7	1	1	8 (26 %)
K 3	8 (26 %)	6	6	2	2	8 (26 %)
P 4	8 (24 %)	7	7	1	1	8 (26 %)
P 5	11 (27 %)	9	7	2	1	8 (26 %)
P 6	5 (15 %)	4	3	1	0	3 (10 %)
P 7	8 (20 %)	5	4	3	3	7 (23 %)
P 8	17 (47 %)	9	9	8	8	17 (55 %)
Case # 2						
K 1	16 (52 %)	9	8	7	6	24 (44 %)
K 2	29 (94 %)	15	15	14	14	50 (91 %)
P 3	17 (55 %)	12	12	5	5	31 (56 %)
P 4	8 (26 %)	4	4	4	4	12 (22 %)

categorized these embedded errors as either procedural or knowledge-based errors. Detection of errors in both categories requires general and specific nursing domain knowledge. The distinction between the categories is that the procedural category requires the class of nursing information involving technical and procedural information while the knowledge-based category requires the underlying knowledge that drives the procedures. Procedural errors are defined as errors made while performing nurse care giving derived from *routine schema-driven and protocol-driven activities*. These activities are typically performed by RNs. Procedural errors incorporate both of the categories described in the human error literature as rule-based errors (managed by rules and procedures that may be wrong or recalled inaccurately) and skill-based errors (using mental models of tasks automatically). Knowledge-based errors require care-specific, specialized knowledge linked to dialysis nursing domain tasks.

The experimental procedure was identical to those used in our previous experiments in trauma, including the details of the instructions given to each participant. Transcripts of the audio-recorded data were evaluated for evidence of detection or correction of any of the 12 errors.

Results

The results for this study are summarized in Table 3.7. As is evident in the table, in many cases the errors were detected by a minority of participants only. As all of the participants were qualified nurses rather than trainees, expertise was defined on the basis of ten or more years of experience in practice. The number of errors detected were computed against the subjects' years of experience in dialysis specialty care, where nurses with experience of 10 years or more (n = 16) were considered experts, and experience of less than 10 years non-experts (n = 15).

The overall rate of error detection by expert nurses (P = .448) and non-expert nurses (P = .289) were significantly different, χ^2 (1) = 9.94, p < .01. Similarly, The rate of errors recovered by expert nurses was (P = .433) and the rate of errors recovered by non-expert nurses (P = .267) were significantly different, χ^2 (1) = 9.75, p < .01. However, upon further investigation it was found that the difference in detection rate with respect to detection of, or recovery from, knowledge-based errors was not statistically significant (although the rate was marginally higher for experts). In contrast, the difference in rates of both detection of, and recovery from procedural errors was statistically significant.

The results clearly show there is significant growth in the ability of dialysis nurses to detect procedural errors after 10-years of experience in practice. However, assuming though that the laboratory-based findings generalize to the field, the fact that no significant difference between expert and non-expert dialysis nurses in the detection and recovery of errors which are conceptual, knowledge-based errors raises concern for patient safety. If conceptual errors are missed and if the development of expertise does not improve the ability of dialysis nurses to detect and recover these types of errors then the management of this class of error will never be affected with many years of practice. Since nursing harbors a knowledge domain filled with procedures it is not surprising that procedural expertise develops with years of practice as expertise is attained. In dialysis nursing procedures are emphasized because the nature of dialysis nursing practice includes very detailed procedural knowledge and skill to care for patients in this setting. At the sites studied, a focus on continued training for procedural knowledge and skills development is provided and encouraged because it is necessary for professional growth in this area to improve nurses' ability to practice dialysis nursing. However, the same focus is not present for continued growth in the conceptual, knowledge-based area of dialysis nursing beyond what is learned in the basic training program at the beginning of practice in this specialty area. The initial training is deemed sufficient to practice at a minimum safe level. Based on our research findings, we believe the encouragement of enhanced continuing nursing education programs focused on the conceptual, knowledge-based areas of dialysis nursing practice is needed to rectify this now identified deficit.

Summary and Implications

In this chapter, we have discussed research concerning the issue of error recovery from complementary perspectives. Research in naturalistic critical care environment, and in other domains, suggests that experts are better able to detect and recover from errors. However, in our laboratory based experiments both expert and non-expert subjects were limited overall in their ability to detect errors. When analyzing these data, we were surprised by the low rate of error detection across all levels of expertise. Our surprise was mirrored by the groups we presented this research to, and audience members at times pointed out the alarming implications of this research if this rate of error detection were consistent with the rate of error detection in real-world clinical practice. Our conclusion at this point was that further research was required, as our laboratory-based studies with paper-based scenarios differed from the way in which information is presented on clinical rounds in a number of ways. For example, on rounds information is presented verbally by multiple presenters, requiring online processing and information integration. While laboratory-based studies allow us to focus on more general aspects of the error detection and recovery process, they have certain inherent limitations as they isolate this process from its larger context. Consequently, the impact of team interaction on error recovery cannot be captured (as subjects are evaluated independently), and one would anticipate presenting patients to a team of clinicians with complementary expertise increasing the odds of successful detection. This presents some limitations, given that previous research suggests that situations in which many team members interact are most productive for error recovery [21]. Subsequently we extended our paradigm for the study of error to accommodate both verbal presentation by multiple presenters (using a virtual world environment); as well as the detection of error by teams of clinicians in the context of their work domain. These studies are discussed in the chapters that follow.

Informatics Implications

Taken at face value, these studies suggest the need for informatics interventions that automatically detect human error, as human detection of medical error appears haphazard at best. A number of such interventions already exist, in the form of automated alerts and reminders integrated with the Electronic Health Record [33]. However, the rigid computational rules that underlie such systems cannot account for the variability of clinical practice, and as such their application may be limited to basic decision support to do with detecting potential drug interactions, and preempting overdoses and allergic reactions. The question therefore arises of how information technology might support the detection of more complex errors by clinicians during the course of patient care. It has been suggested that expert problem detectors are distinguished by their ability to recognize complex cues that involve multiple disparate data points [30]. Might it be possible, then, to design technology that aggregates these disparate data points in an expert-like manner so as to facilitate error detection? In previous research we have shown that computers can learn to organize elements of clinical cases in psychiatry in accordance with higher-level knowledge structures utilized by expert problem solvers [34], and that organizing knowledge in accordance with expert emphasis leads novice practitioners to interpret cases in an expert-like manner [35]. This suggests it may be possible to reorganize the data elements of a clinical case in a manner that would facilitate error detection, by supporting the recognition of meaningful connections between disparate data points. In summary, the flexible and dynamic nature of critical care limits the applicability of fully automated error detection systems. However, the deficiencies in detection displayed by clinicians in our studies suggest the need for other forms of informatics support. One possibility might be the development of interventions that reorganize information so as to highlight clinically meaningful implicit associations, thereby mediating, rather than replacing, the detection of error by clinicians.

Discussion Questions

1. What are the implications of the alarmingly low rates of error observed in these laboratory studies for patient safety?
2. What factors might contribute toward the failure to detect egregious errors in laboratory studies such as these?
3. What differences in knowledge organization and pattern recognition account for the improved ability of experts to detect certain sorts of errors?
4. How might clinical case elements be reorganized so as to facilitate error detection?
5. How might educational and other interventions be designed to improve the ability of clinicians to detect error?

References

1. Reason J. Human error: models and management. Br Med J. 2000;320:768–70.
2. Rasmussen J. The role of error in organizing behaviour. Ergonomics. 1990;33:377–85.
3. Patel VL, Arocha JF, Kaufman DR. Diagnostic reasoning and medical expertise. In: The psychology of learning and motivation: advances in research and theory, vol. 31. San Diego: Academic Press; 1994. p. 187–252.
4. Cohen T, Blatter B, Almeida C, Patel VL. Reevaluating recovery: perceived violations and preemptive interventions on emergency psychiatry rounds. J Am Med Inform Assoc. 2007;14(3):312–9.
5. Wu AW. Medical error: the second victim. West J Med. 2000;172(6):358–9.
6. Amalberti R, Wioland LL. Human error in aviation. In: Soekkha H, editor. Aviation safety: human factors, system engineering, flight operations, economics, strategies, management. Utrecht: VSP; 1997. p. 91–108.
7. Kahneman D, Slovic P, Tversky A. Judgment under uncertainty: heuristics and biases. New York: Cambridge University Press; 1982. p. 1124–31.
8. Croskerry P. The importance of cognitive errors in diagnosis and strategies to minimize them. Acad Med. 2003;78(8):775–80.
9. Croskerry P, Shapiro M, Campbell S, LeBlanc C, Sinclair D, Wren P, et al. Profiles in patient safety: medication errors in the emergency department. Acad Emerg Med. 2004;11(3): 289–99.
10. Patel VL, Groen GJ, Patel YC. Cognitive aspects of clinical performance during patient workup: the role of medical expertise. Adv Health Sci Educ. 1997;2:95–114.
11. Gigerenzer G, Todd PM. Fast and frugal heuristics: the adaptive toolbox. In: Gigerenzer G, Todd PM, editors. Simple heuristics that make us smart. New York: Oxford University Press; 1999. p. 3–34.

12. Arocha JF, Patel VL. Novice diagnostic reasoning in medicine: accounting for evidence. J Learn Sci. 1995;4(4):355–84.
13. Simon HA. Models of man: social and rational. New York: Wiley; 1957.
14. Hashem A, Chi MTH, Friedman CP. Medical errors as a result of specialization. J Biomed Inform. 2003;36(1–2):61–9.
15. Patel VL, Groen GJ, Arocha JF. Medical expertise as a function of task difficulty. Mem Cogn. 1990;18:394–406.
16. Mörel G, Amalberti R, Chauvin C. Articulating the differences between safety and resilience: the decision-making process of professional sea-fishing skippers. Hum Factors. 2008; 50(1):1–16.
17. Kanse L, van der Schaaf TW. Recovery from failures in the chemical process industry. Int J Cogn Ergon. 2001;5(3):199–211.
18. Patel VL, Cohen T. New perspectives on error in critical care. Curr Opin Crit Care. 2008; 14(4):456–9.
19. Norman DA. The psychology of everyday things. New York: Basic Books; 1988.
20. Allwood CM. Error detection process in statistical problem solving. Cognit Sci. 1984; 8(4):413–37.
21. Kubose TT, Patel VL, Jordan D. Dynamic adaptation to critical care medical environment: error recovery as cognitive activity. In: Proceedings of the 24th annual meeting of the Cognitive Science Society. Virginia: Fairfax; 2002. p. 43–4.
22. Nyssen AS, Blavier A. Error detection: a study in anaesthesia. Ergonomics. 2006;49(5–6): 517–25. PubMed PMID: 16717008. Epub 2006/05/24.
23. Kanse L, van der Schaaf TW, Vrijland ND, van Mierlo H. Error recovery in a hospital pharmacy. Ergonomics. 2006;49(5–6):503–16. PubMed PMID: 16717007.
24. Hales BM, Pronovost PJ. The checklist-a tool for error management and performance improvement. J Crit Care. 2006;21(3):231–5.
25. Ericsson KA, Simon HA. Protocol analysis: verbal reports as data. Cambridge: Harvard University Press; 1993.
26. Ghali AM, El Malik EM, Ibrahim AI, Ismail G, Rashid M. Ureteric injuries: diagnosis, management, and outcome. J Trauma. 1999;46(1):150–8.
27. Patel VL, Groen GJ. Knowledge-based solution strategies in medical reasoning. Cognit Sci. 1986;10(1):91–116.
28. Chi MTH, Glaser R, Farr MJ. The nature of expertise. Hillsdale: Lawrence Erlbaum Associates; 1988.
29. Wilkinson WE, Cauble LA, Patel VL. Error detection and recovery in dialysis nursing. J Patient Saf. 2011;7(4):213–23. PubMed PMID: 22064625. Epub 2011/11/09.
30. Klein G, Pliske R, Crandall B, Woods DD. Problem detection. Cogn Technol Work. 2005;7(1):14–28.
31. Chaudhry SI, Olofinboba KA, Krumholz HM. Detection of errors by attending physicians on a general medicine service. J Gen Intern Med. 2003;18(8):595–600.
32. Amalberti, R. Navigating Safety: Necessary Compromises and Trade-Offs-Theory and Practice. Dordrecht. Springer Netherlands. 2013.
33. Kuperman GJ, Bobb A, Payne TH, Avery AJ, Gandhi TK, Burns G, et al. Medication-related clinical decision support in computerized provider order entry systems: a review. J Am Med Inform Assoc. 2007;14:29–40.
34. Cohen T, Blatter B, Patel VL. Simulating expert clinical comprehension: adapting latent semantic analysis to accurately extract clinical concepts from psychiatric narrative. J Biomed Inform. 2008;41(6):1070–87.
35. Sharda P, Das AK, Cohen T, Patel VL. Customizing clinical narratives for the electronic medical record interface using cognitive methods. Int J Med Inform. 2006;75:346–68.
36. Patel VL, et al. Recovery at the edge of error: debunking the myth of the infallible expert. J Biomed Inform. 2011;44:413–24.

Chapter 4
Teamwork and Error Management in Critical Care

Vimla L. Patel, Trevor Cohen, Suchita Batwara, and Khalid F. Almoosa

Introduction

Our earlier studies show that physicians' ability to detect errors in clinical problems in the intensive medical care domain is limited when tested individually in laboratory-based conditions (Chaps. 3 and 6). We extended this study to explore the mechanism of error detection and recovery when working in teams, using (a) semi-naturalistic and (b) naturalistic empirical paradigms. The data were collected in an intensive care unit and were analyzed to reveal the process of patient management and the frequency and the nature of errors generated and corrected. The results show that teams perform better than individuals, due to advantages conferred by the distribution of cognitive tasks across multiple team members. Attending and trainee

V.L. Patel, PhD, DSc, FRSC (✉)
Center for Cognitive Studies in Medicine and Public Health,
New York Academy of Medicine, New York, NY 10029, USA

Department of Biomedical Informatics, Columbia University,
New York, NY 10032, USA

Department of Biomedical Informatics, Arizona State University,
Scottsdale, AZ 85259, USA
e-mail: vpatel@nyam.org

T. Cohen, MB ChB, PhD
School of Biomedical Informatics, University of Texas Health Science Center,
Houston, TX 77054, USA

S. Batwara, MBBS, MPH
University of Iowa Hospitals and Clinics, Iowa City, IA 52242, USA

K.F. Almoosa, MD, MS, FCCP
Transplant Surgery ICU, Memorial Hermann Hospital, Texas Medical Center,
Houston, TX 77030, USA

University of Texas Health Science Center, Houston, TX, USA

V.L. Patel et al. (eds.), *Cognitive Informatics in Health and Biomedicine*,
Health Informatics, DOI 10.1007/978-1-4471-5490-7_4, © Springer-Verlag London 2014

clinicians were found to generate the most errors as well as recover from most of them in the real world, as compared to other conditions. Error detection and correction in a situation closer to complex real world practice appears to induce certain urgency for quick action resulting in rapid detection and correction. Furthermore, teams working at the bedside in the real world optimize performance with little room for explicating any mistakes and thus little learning from errors. There is a close relationship between competency in delivery of patient care and the need to minimize errors. This is juxtaposed with the competing demand for learning from errors, an essential part of the apprentice training process. The challenge of managing the balance between these two modes, professional practice and learning, for delivery of efficient and safe care in complex critical care settings, are discussed.

In previous chapters, we discussed a series of studies of the ability of individual clinicians to detect errors embedded in case scenarios presented on paper and in a virtual world. These studies show that physicians' ability to detect errors in clinical problems in the intensive medical care domain is limited when tested individually in laboratory-based conditions. The purpose of the studies described in this chapter is to evaluate mechanisms of error detection and recovery by teams of physicians operating in their natural habitat, the Intensive Care Unit (ICU). For the first of these studies we adapted our previous paradigm, involving the presentation of cases with embedded errors, such that cases were presented verbally to clinical teams in the context of a clinical round. This allowed for the capture of interaction between team members as they considered the case scenario. We refer to this approach as "semi-naturalistic" in contrast to the "naturalistic" approach we applied in the second of these studies, in which the process of error detection and recovery was observed as it occurred during the process of clinical care, without our provocation.

Errors in any practice, including medicine are inevitable since most often errors are ingrained in the nature of a cognitive task. The 1999 Institute of Medicine (IOM) report, "*To Err is Human*" was the harbinger of an unprecedented focus on medical errors and their prevention [1, 2]. Extrapolating from studies preceding it by nearly a decade, the IOM report proclaimed that between 44,000 and 90,000 people died each year as a result of medical errors. This report included all levels and settings of medical practice. However, studies focusing on complex critical care environments, such as intensive care units (ICUs) and emergency rooms, provide a relatively acute view of errors committed in these domains [3]. Donchin et al. reported that, on average, an ICU patient had 178 *activities* performed on them daily with a 99 % success rate that resulted in 1.78 errors per patient, per day [4]. Adverse events and serious errors involving critical care patients are common, and can often be potentially life threatening.

Although human beings are erratic and err in unexpected ways, they are also resourceful and innovative and have the potential to recover from errors and crises [5, 6]. The clinical environment is also a place where trainees learn "on the job" and generating errors and correcting them is a part of the learning process. Thus there is a close relationship between competent performance for delivery of safe care and learning during this process. This chapter discusses the issue of fine balance between these two aspects of modern clinical care in complex environments, where teamwork is becoming a common practice.

Error Recovery: Prospective and Retrospective Studies

In recognition of the inevitable occurrence of human error in a complex work setting, recent work on medical errors in critical care medicine has focused on error recovery by physicians [7–10], nurses [7, 11], and hospital pharmacists [12]. This shift in focus sees precedent in the aviation and transport industries [13, 14], where it has long been recognized that the elimination of human error is not an attainable goal. Approaches taken to the study of error recovery can be broadly categorized as prospective and retrospective. Prospective studies depend on the observation of the process of error recovery in either naturalistic (e.g., [13, 14]) or laboratory (e.g., [9] settings. Retrospective studies (e.g., [15] and [12]) utilize error reports and interviews in an effort to analyze reported adverse events so as to learn from these mistakes. These approaches are complementary, and each has its respective advantages. Retrospective studies allow for a focused analysis of large numbers of events that have been identified as violations of the accepted standards of practice by clinicians during the course of their work. In contrast, prospective studies in naturalistic settings require the investment of many hours of ethnographic observation by a trained observer in order to capture incidents of error recovery in process. In prospective studies incidents are captured as they occur, so the captured data are not vulnerable to recall and reporting bias as is the case with interview data and data in event reporting systems respectively. The nature of factors that contribute to the generation of errors and recovery from errors are captured more directly.

Studying Recovery with Embedded Errors

In our recent research we have used a specific approach to studying the process of error recovery [9–11]. This approach involves presenting simulated case scenarios containing embedded errors to clinicians, and evaluating their ability to detect and remove recover from (correct) these errors. Consequently, this approach provides a means of studying the process of error recovery in a controlled setting, where problem cases and embedded errors are pre-determined. In our initial experiments, we used paper-based case scenarios related to traumatic injury [9], and captured verbal protocols as participants individually read and interpreted the scenarios without prior warning that errors were present. A striking finding from this research was that error detection and recovery in this setting was alarmingly poor across all levels of expertise. For example, none of the participants detected more than half of the embedded errors, regardless of their level of training [9]. In many instances the errors were egregious with harmful or fatal consequences. In recognition of the fact that case reports are seldom exclusively read as isolated written text in the context of real-world critical care, we extended these studies using a virtual world environment in order to more accurately capture the verbal presentation of information by multiple team members that occurs on critical care rounds [10]. In addition, we included a set of knowledge-based questions that evaluated the clinical knowledge required to detect each error, in order to enable us to distinguish between failure to detect errors that occurred on account of inadequate clinical knowledge and failure to detect errors that occurred for some other reason. We introduced an additional experimental parameter in which participants were primed (i.e. alerted beforehand to the presence of errors) to detect error ahead of their second case. This step was shown to dramatically improve error detection, with many participants achieving rates of error detection approaching the limits of their knowledge once primed. However, detection by unprimed participants was relatively poor, suggesting that physicians are likely to fail to detect errors unless they are interpreting clinical cases with this goal in mind [10]. In practice, this is often the role of a tutor, such as an attending physician. These results show the important role a tutor plays in clinical care practice, as in any learning environment.

Teamwork and Error Detection

While this work has provided insights into the process of individual error detection, it does not address the role of clinical teams in the error detection and recovery process. The critical care environment has been characterized as a high velocity, high urgency environment, which necessitates quick decision making, often with incomplete information, and demands effective coordination among stakeholders including patients and clinicians [16]. Clinical decisions are influenced by interactions between the clinicians, the patient, and the sociocultural milieu as well as by biomedical considerations. A growing body of research in other fields such as the military [14] and aviation [13] have lent considerably to our understanding of constraints faced by organizations, such as critical care units, operating in fast-paced environments. One common theme that emerges across these complex environments is the importance of teamwork. Clinical rounds in which multidisciplinary teams gather to discuss cases have been identified as a high-yield activity for error detection and recovery [7, 17]. However, little is known about the process of error management in this context, even though research from other domains suggests that the quality of communication during team interaction is important. For example, in an analysis of 67 events from the nuclear, aviation and shipping industries, Sasou and Reason identified inadequate team communication as a key factor related to failed error detection, and an important factor related to the failure to recover from detected errors [5]. Conversely, frequent communication leading to corrective action has been found to be a defining characteristic of outstanding pilots [18].

Summary of Theoretical Background

Cognitive research from a number of other domains such as aviation and engineering has contributed insights that relate to the processes underlying error detection in general. It has been proposed that errors that are near misses suggest that there must exist some monitoring mechanism that checks for errors before they manifest as adverse events [19]. In order to monitor or regulate, one would need to evaluate both intention and outcome, and the difference between the two can account for error correction or recovery processes.

In Chap. 2 of this volume, we introduced a mapping between the stages of error detection and recovery and Norman's well established and generic seven-stage model of interaction [20]. This process includes the steps of *error perception*; *error interpretation*; *error evaluation*; *setting response goals*; *a decision to take action*, *specification of the action to be taken* and *execution of this action*. The cyclical nature of this process is of particular importance to the research described in this chapter. In addition, we introduced a distinction between the goal-directed nature of practical (or working) knowledge and the generic nature of declarative (colloquially "book") knowledge, and the notion that experts' well-organized knowledge structures may confer an advantage with respect to the recognition of certain sorts of error. We also discussed the apparent contradiction between the need for patient safety and the educational role of error, which is thought to be an inherent part of the learning process as trainees define the bounds of safe practice in a complex workspace [21]. Consequently, expert mentors are required to ensure that safe practice occurs without suppressing the learning process.

In this study we focus on the collaborative nature of team interaction and its impact on error management in critical care. Error management can be defined as a process beginning initially with error detection and continuing on to error recovery. This process is activated after error production and involves two stages: error diagnosis and error recovery. Error diagnosis includes both error detection and error explanation, while error recovery involves planning and execution of recovery action [22].

The Nature of Teamwork in Critical Care

Teams in the ICU have fixed day-to-day activities and are composed of people at various levels of training and sensibilities. The diagnosis, monitoring and treatment of patients are interrelated, and iterate rapidly. This process often includes real-time implementation of care by an integrated team in addition to writing orders for later execution. In the ICU, care provision to patients involves continuous allocation of attention, use of redundant information, and repeated situational evaluation [23].

Research reported in this chapter builds on laboratory-based studies conducted by Patel et al. on error detection and recovery by physicians working individually on critical care problems [9] including studies conducted in virtual worlds [10]. These prior studies focused on characterization of systemic causes of error as well as exploration of error boundaries. The importance of teamwork in providing support to mitigate and check medical errors has motivated several naturalistic studies in critical care and is the motivation for our current study [17]. In this research we

Table 4.1 Subject demographics by team

	Team 1	Team 2	Team 3	Team 4	Team 5	Total
	N (%)	N (%)	N (%)	N (%)	N (%)	N (%)
Gender						
Male	2 (28.6)	2 (28.6)	6 (75.0)	3 (75.0)	3 (50.0)	16 (48.5)
Female	5 (71.4)	5 (71.4)	2 (25.0)	2 (25.0)	3 (50.0)	17 (51.5)
Training level						
Intern	3 (42.9)	3 (42.9)	3 (37.5)	2 (40.0)	2 (33.3)	13 (39.4)
Resident PGY2	1 (12.3)	0 (0)	2 (25.0)	1 (20.0)	1 (16.7)	5 (15.1)
Resident PGY3	2 (28.6)	3 (42.9)	2 (25.0)	1 (20.0)	2 (33.3)	10 (30.4)
Fellow	1 (14.3)	1 (14.3)	1 (12.5)	1 (20.0)	1 (16.7)	5 (15.1)

characterize the process of error management by clinical teams within an environment as close to a real-life ICU as possible, and investigate the nuances of team dynamics that underlie this error management process.

Method

Participants

The study was conducted at a tertiary-level teaching hospital with a 16-bed ICU. All trainees in Internal Medicine at our study site went through at least1 month of ICU training per year. We identified clinical teams that were posted each month in the ICU for the duration of our study. Teams consisted of interns in their first year of residency training (post-graduate training), residents in their second and third years of training, and fellows (specialists training after completion of their residency). We included 5 teams with a total of 32 subjects comprised of 15 residents at different post-graduate year (PGY) levels (5 PGY2 residents and 10 PGY3 residents), 13 medical interns and 4 clinical fellows. We excluded medical students, nurses, pharmacists, and other staff from the study in order to best procure subjects that were consistent from team to team and representative of the day-to-day medical decision-making teams in the medical ICU. Table 4.1 illustrates the subject demographics in each team. Team 1 and Team 2 have more female participants, while Team 3 and Team 4 have more male participants. With respect to the level of medical training, the teams were comprised of more interns and PGY3 residents than PGY2 residents and fellows. Furthermore, every team had at least 2 medical interns, 2 residents (PGY1 and PGY2 combined), and 1 clinical fellow, including the attending physician.

Clinical Case Development

Two clinical cases based on actual patients with diabetic ketoacidosis (DKA) and upper gastro-intestinal bleeding were developed in collaboration with our clinical

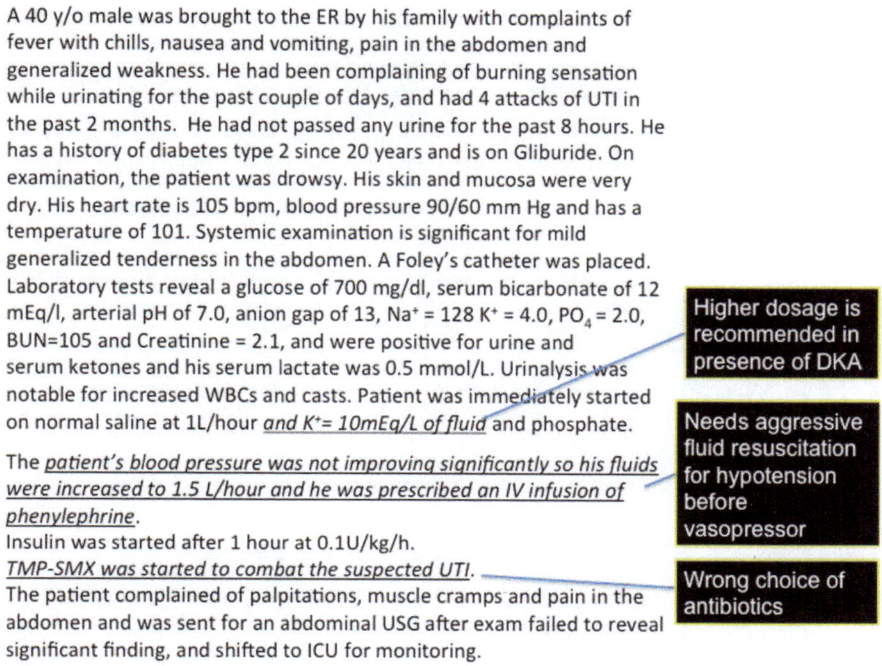
A 40 y/o male was brought to the ER by his family with complaints of fever with chills, nausea and vomiting, pain in the abdomen and generalized weakness. He had been complaining of burning sensation while urinating for the past couple of days, and had 4 attacks of UTI in the past 2 months. He had not passed any urine for the past 8 hours. He has a history of diabetes type 2 since 20 years and is on Gliburide. On examination, the patient was drowsy. His skin and mucosa were very dry. His heart rate is 105 bpm, blood pressure 90/60 mm Hg and has a temperature of 101. Systemic examination is significant for mild generalized tenderness in the abdomen. A Foley's catheter was placed. Laboratory tests reveal a glucose of 700 mg/dl, serum bicarbonate of 12 mEq/l, arterial pH of 7.0, anion gap of 13, Na^+ = 128 K^+ = 4.0, PO_4 = 2.0, BUN=105 and Creatinine = 2.1, and were positive for urine and serum ketones and his serum lactate was 0.5 mmol/L. Urinalysis was notable for increased WBCs and casts. Patient was immediately started on normal saline at 1L/hour *and* K^+*= 10mEq/L of fluid* and phosphate.

The *patient's blood pressure was not improving significantly so his fluids were increased to 1.5 L/hour and he was prescribed an IV infusion of phenylephrine*.

Insulin was started after 1 hour at 0.1U/kg/h.

TMP-SMX was started to combat the suspected UTI.

The patient complained of palpitations, muscle cramps and pain in the abdomen and was sent for an abdominal USG after exam failed to reveal significant finding, and shifted to ICU for monitoring.

Fig. 4.1 Clinical Case 1 with embedded errors

experts. Since DKA and upper GI bleeding are two conditions commonly seen in the ICU, all subjects were expected to have had some degree of experience in dealing with them. The cases were modified based on feedback from a pilot study conducted using randomly selected interns, residents and attending physicians. Each scenario provided a brief clinical history followed by several patient management decisions. Errors of a different nature were then embedded into both cases. Some errors were simple and required only a single-step inference for detection, while others were complex and required integration of multiple data elements from the case for detection. Figures 4.1 and 4.2 provide the brief clinical histories and explanations of the embedded errors for each case. Tables 4.2 and 4.3 provide detailed explanations of the errors and the corresponding inferences and knowledge required by the medical team to solve the errors. The tables also classify the errors based on the nomenclature provided below.

I. Simple errors: Errors that require single step inference along with factual knowledge during problem solving
II. Complex errors: Errors that require integration of multiple data elements (including factual knowledge) from the given case during problem solving
III. Knowledge-based errors: Errors caused by incorrect or incomplete medical knowledge
IV. Procedural errors: Errors caused by deviations from standard task-oriented clinical guidelines and procedures

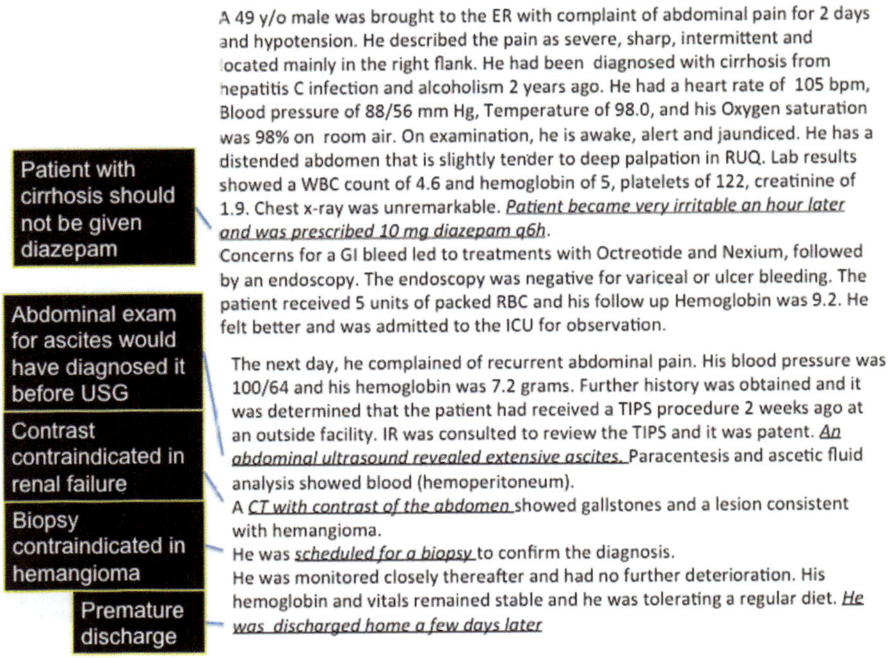

A 49 y/o male was brought to the ER with complaint of abdominal pain for 2 days and hypotension. He described the pain as severe, sharp, intermittent and located mainly in the right flank. He had been diagnosed with cirrhosis from hepatitis C infection and alcoholism 2 years ago. He had a heart rate of 105 bpm, Blood pressure of 88/56 mm Hg, Temperature of 98.0, and his Oxygen saturation was 98% on room air. On examination, he is awake, alert and jaundiced. He has a distended abdomen that is slightly tender to deep palpation in RUQ. Lab results showed a WBC count of 4.6 and hemoglobin of 5, platelets of 122, creatinine of 1.9. Chest x-ray was unremarkable. *Patient became very irritable an hour later and was prescribed 10 mg diazepam q6h*.
Concerns for a GI bleed led to treatments with Octreotide and Nexium, followed by an endoscopy. The endoscopy was negative for variceal or ulcer bleeding. The patient received 5 units of packed RBC and his follow up Hemoglobin was 9.2. He felt better and was admitted to the ICU for observation.

The next day, he complained of recurrent abdominal pain. His blood pressure was 100/64 and his hemoglobin was 7.2 grams. Further history was obtained and it was determined that the patient had received a TIPS procedure 2 weeks ago at an outside facility. IR was consulted to review the TIPS and it was patent. *An abdominal ultrasound revealed extensive ascites.* Paracentesis and ascetic fluid analysis showed blood (hemoperitoneum).
A *CT with contrast of the abdomen* showed gallstones and a lesion consistent with hemangioma.
He was *scheduled for a biopsy* to confirm the diagnosis.
He was monitored closely thereafter and had no further deterioration. His hemoglobin and vitals remained stable and he was tolerating a regular diet. *He was discharged home a few days later*

Fig. 4.2 Clinical Case 2 with embedded errors

Table 4.2 Required inferences and knowledge necessary for error recovery as well as error classification for Case 1

Problems from Case 1	Error	Classification	Required inference	Required knowledge
1	Dose of KCl = 10 mEq/L is very low.	Simple Knowledge based	Insulin treatment in DKA will cause an intracellular shift of K+ and cause severe hypokalemia.	Recommended dose of K+ is 20–40 mEq/L. K+=4.0 is very low to begin within presence of DKA
2	Inappropriate antibiotic.	Complex Knowledge based	History of frequent UTIs (four in past 2 months) suggests a resistant organism.	TMP-SMX will not be useful in cases of infection with resistant organism and renal insufficiency.
3	Patient is not given enough fluids but prescribed vasopressors instead.	Complex Knowledge based	Severe dehydration or hypovolemia (anuria, dry skin and drowsiness) and high creatinine of 2.0 mg/dl suggests impending renal failure.	In impending renal failure vasopressors will increase the risk of renal injury. The patient needs to be adequately hydrated first.

Table 4.3 Required inferences and knowledge necessary for error recovery as well as error classification for Case 2

Problems from Case 2	Error	Error classification	Required inference	Required knowledge
1	Abdominal examination for ascites, including fluid thrill and percussion, was not done	Simple Procedural		Given h/o Cirrhosis distended abdomen could be due to ascites and physical exam could have diagnosed that before the CT.
2	CT with contrast done	Complex Procedural	High creatinine of 1.9 mg/dl is indicative of renal insufficiency.	Contrasts are contraindicated in case of renal insufficiency as they may lead to contrast induced nephropathy.
3	Benzodiazepines (diazepam)	Complex Knowledge	Benzodiazepines (BZD) cause CNS depression.	In a patient with low BP and signs of liver decompensation BZD should not be given.
4	Biopsy scheduled for hemangioma	Simple Procedural	Hemangiomas may cause severe bleeding.	Biopsy is contraindicated for hepatic hemangiomas.
5	Premature discharge from ICU undiagnosed liver decompensation	Complex Knowledge	H/o cirrhosis, hepatitis C and TIPS, jaundice, bleeding, mental status change suggests liver decompensation and signs of early hepatic encephalopathy.	Liver decompensation needs to be managed before discharge from ICU.

Procedure

The study protocol was approved by the local Institutional Review Board and conducted between August 2010 and February 2011. Confidentiality of the data was maintained throughout the process and informed consent of the subjects was obtained. The two case scenarios described previously were presented by an attending physician to each of the five teams as part of their daily morning clinical rounds. To avoid priming of the subjects, the task instructions were kept neutral but specific: "*This case evaluation is based on a real patient in the ICU. Please discuss the case evaluation from another hospital as a team like you would in your usual rounds, and*

Table 4.4 An example of text analysis and coding

Original text	Recall	Inference	Justification	Errors detected
Cirrhosis from hep C and alcohol abuse. Patient became very irritable an hour later and was prescribed 10 mg diazepam q6h	*"Cirrhosis from hep C and alcohol abuse"*	*"Shouldn't have prescribed diazepam"*	*"Benzodiazepines cause CNS depression"*	Patient with Cirrhosis should not be given diazepam

come up with your own assessment and plan for this patient." The attending physician was instructed to read the case clearly and slowly. At the end of each case presentation, the attending was instructed to ask the subjects: "*How would you assess this case? Given the patient's presentation and management at another hospital please discuss your evaluation*." All discussions were audio recorded along with details of field note recordings from the observers, and these were all transcribed for analysis.

Data Analysis

The transcribed audio recordings were analyzed using a method of natural language representation, propositional analysis and thematic coding, which has been successful in previous research by Patel and Groen [24]. This particular method permits the integration of propositional analysis and observation data into key concepts, themes and patterns that can then be extrapolated, categorized and combined to form a cohesive and comprehensive qualitative data set. The two original problem cases were divided into a set of basic concepts, namely, propositional concepts. A detailed manual mapping of the propositions (basic units of representation of text) between the subject's response transcript and the stimulus text was performed, where the elaborations of any particular concept in the transcribed protocol was matched against the corresponding concept in the original text in terms of recall and inference as described by Patel and Groen [24]. The errors detected and corrected at each stage of analysis were noted. The coding taxonomy used was based on previous research [25]. Table 4.4 displays an excerpt from the coding scheme used for the analysis of the audio transcripts. The qualitative data were quantified and analyzed statistically to look for relationships between error management and multiple variables in the ICU. Error management included the steps of detection ("I don't think he should get this antibiotic again"), error justification ("He might be resistant to it with his history of multiple urinary tract infections treated with this") and error correction ("I think he needs to be started on a broad spectrum or culture specific antibiotic").

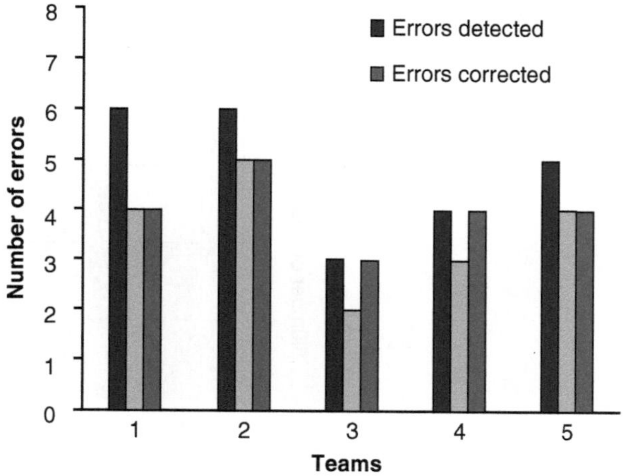

Fig. 4.3 Number of errors, detected, corrected and justified by each of five teams

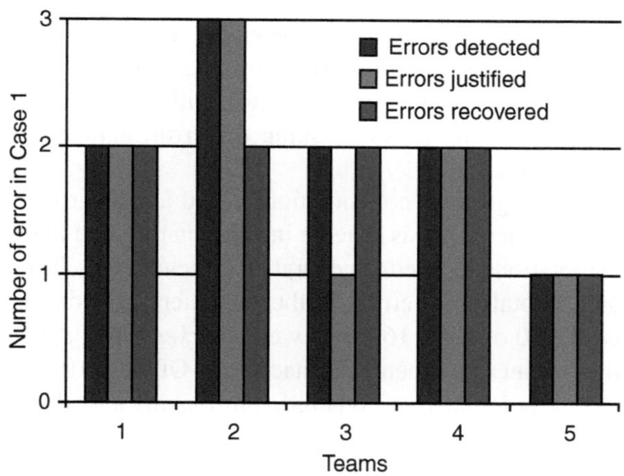

Fig. 4.4 Analysis of errors in Case 1

Results

Error Management

The results showed that the teams detected a mean of 4.8 (S.D. = 1.3) out of a total of 8 errors in both cases, accounting for 60 % of all errors. Figure 4.3 illustrates error management (detection, correction and justification) for each team.

Figures 4.4 and 4.5 give the number of errors detected, justified, and recovered from by each team for the errors embedded in Case 1 and Case 2, respectively.

In summary, the teams detected an average of 60 % of the errors. The teams performed better than individuals in detecting and correcting errors as a result of the reduced cognitive load and natural error checks realized through collaboration. Error detection increased as the level of team interaction increased throughout

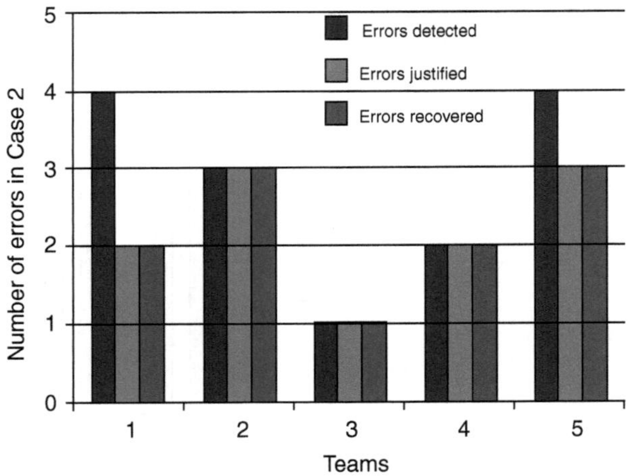

Fig. 4.5 Analysis of errors in Case 2

case discussion. However, new errors were generated as a result of increased discussion and elaboration. Many of these errors were corrected but some remained uncorrected. Several variables were identified as affecting the correction of an error, including person making the error, nature of the error, and level of team interaction.

Although team collaboration played a major role in error detection and correction, further analysis of team interaction revealed that longer team discussions with elaborations resulted in generation of new errors. Taken together, the 5 teams generated a total of 16 errors in the 10 patient case discussions (5 teams with 2 cases each); 10 of these 16 errors were *checked* when a team member explicitly pointed out that an assessment was inaccurate. Of these 10 checked errors, 9 were corrected (recovered) and 1 was ignored, thus making a total of 7 newly generated errors that crossed a *boundary* of safe practice and progressed from *near-misses* to actual *adverse events*, as defined by Patel and Cohen [8]. It is important to note that one of the uncorrected errors, which led to subsequent propagation into the delivery of patient care, was originally detected by an intern. However both the fellow and the resident on the team ignored the necessary correction, and thus overrode the intern's suggestion. This finding is consistent with previous research in which the hierarchical nature of clinical teams has been identified as an obstacle to error recovery and team performance [18, 26].

Figure 4.6 illustrates the progression and occurrence of medical error in the ICU in terms of error generation, detection, recovery and propagation. Breaching the first boundary can be considered a violation of the consensual bounds of safe practice. At this stage (the near miss), an opportunity exists to detect and correct the error before the second boundary is reached. The exclusive analysis of adverse event reports fails to attend to the incidents of near miss and recovery that are an integral part of cognitive work in critical care [8].

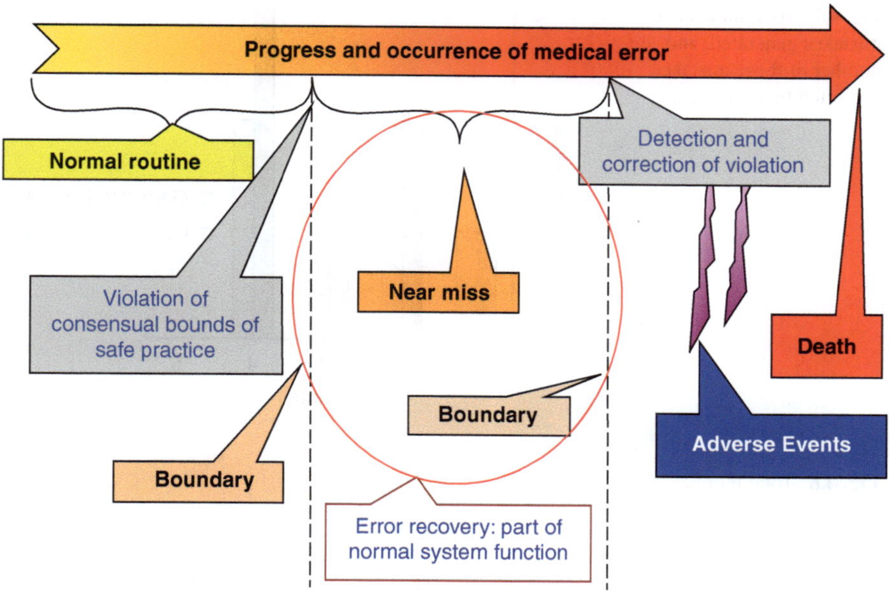

Fig. 4.6 Error generation and progress (Adapted from Patel and Cohen [8])

Classification of the Newly Generated Errors

As discussed earlier, new errors were generated irrespective of the nature of the embedded errors. We used the taxonomy described in the existing literature [27–29] to divide these new errors into *slips* and *mistakes*. The intention of this taxonomy is to classify errors according to their underlying mechanisms. *Slips* are related to the inaccurate execution of a correct process; for example, a slip occurred when a serum bicarbonate value was mistaken for an "anion gap" value. This is a kind of action specification slip where the underlying cognitive mechanisms include failure of retrieval of the action sequence concerned, mutation of this sequence and so forth. *Mistakes* occur on account of incorrect or incomplete knowledge or interpretation; for example, a mistake occurred when one of the subjects said that the patient with DKA did not need potassium supplementation because his serum potassium was normal at that point (indicating incorrect knowledge of the relevant reference range), and that with insulin therapy his serum potassium would rise (indicating incorrect knowledge of the effect of insulin administration on serum potassium).

Analysis of newly generated errors revealed that 56 % were slips and 44 % were mistakes. Corrections for slips and mistakes were marginally different. As seen with correction of the errors embedded in the case, correction of these new errors also correlated significantly with team interaction (r = 0.8). When these new errors were analyzed for their correction with respect to the expertise of the subjects, all subjects

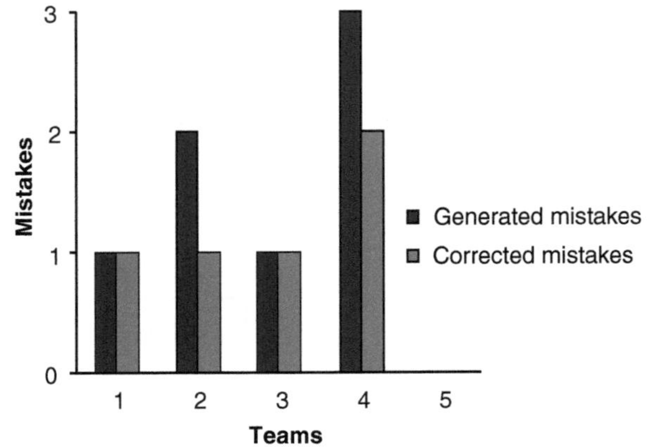

Fig. 4.7 Total number of mistakes generated, and number of these mistakes corrected by each team

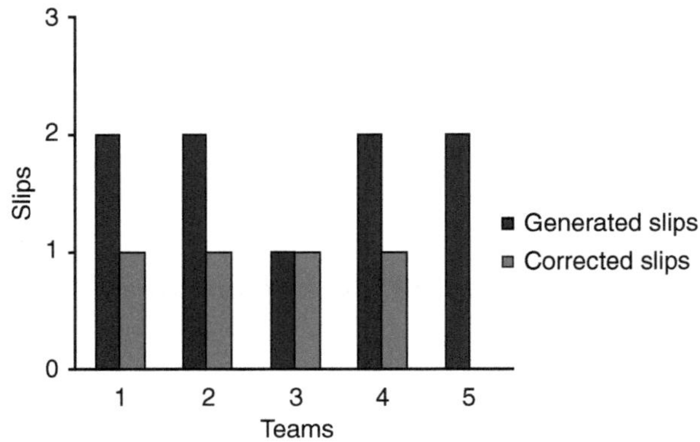

Fig. 4.8 Total number of slips generated, and number of these slips corrected by each team

corrected an equal number of slips. However, mistakes (wrong interpretation or wrong knowledge) made by interns were not corrected by anyone, while mistakes made by seniors (residents and fellows) were all corrected. Figures 4.7 and 4.8 illustrates error generation and management by each team for mistakes and slips, respectively.

Qualitative Nature of Team Interaction and Error Management

The transcripts of the protocols from clinical rounds were further analyzed to explicate the precise nature of interactions among the team members. The transcripts were segmented into events and episodes, and detection and resolution of errors were traced as a function of team interaction. For example, one team member identified an area of concern for further discussion. This issue was added to or built upon by other team members who continued the theme, using their content

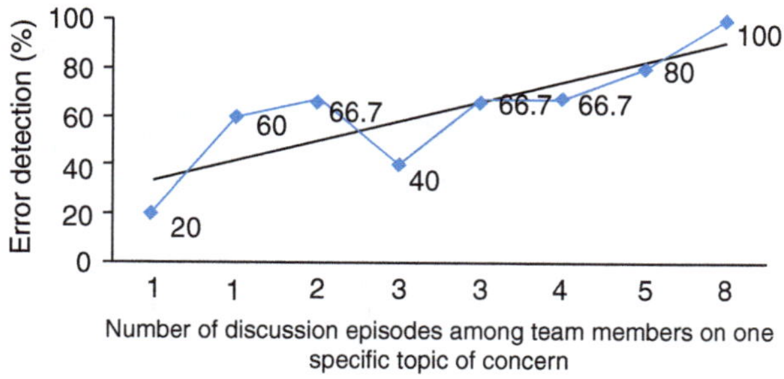

Fig. 4.9 Error detection and elaboration and discussion surrounding the error

knowledge and utilizing other members' understanding of the concern to create a rich dialogue. Members of the team identified different cues from various parts of the cases to trigger team interaction, which facilitated collective error detection and correction.

The working definition used for a unit of interaction was an *episode of direct communication between team members in response to dialogue relevant to the case*. Several such interactive episodes were identified among the various teams. When team interaction (number of episodes of discussion) was evaluated against the performance (error detection and error correction), it strongly correlated ($r=0.8$) with the number of errors detected by the team. While increased discussion and elaboration also led to the generation of new errors, the likelihood of recovering from an error (error correction) *increased as a function of the number of interactive dialogue episodes*. This means that percent error correction increased as a function of increased team dialogue during clinical rounds. Figure 4.9 illustrates this finding.

Schematic Representations of Error Detection, Correction, Generation and Recovery

In the following section we provide illustrative examples of embedded error detection, embedded error correction and new error generation (resulting from clinical team interaction). The abbreviations referenced by the examples are as follows: DKA: diabetic ketoacidosis; DM: diabetes mellitus; UTI: urinary tract infection; DDx: differential diagnosis; URTI: upper respiratory tract infection; BUN: blood urea nitrogen; PSA: prostate-specific antigens; BPH: benign prostatic hypertrophy. Green flags indicate errors detected from the case; orange flags indicate newly generated errors recovered by the individual or the team; red flags indicate newly generated errors that were never corrected, thus compromising patient care. The inscribed numerals on the left side denote the clinician number. Figure 4.10 provides a schematic network of Team 1 working through Case 2. The transcript from which the schema was generated is given in Fig. 4.11.

In the following illustrated example of Team 1 working on Case 2, *the Fellow* presented the clinical case and *Resident 2* initiated the discussion by recalling or summarizing the following important observations regarding the patient:

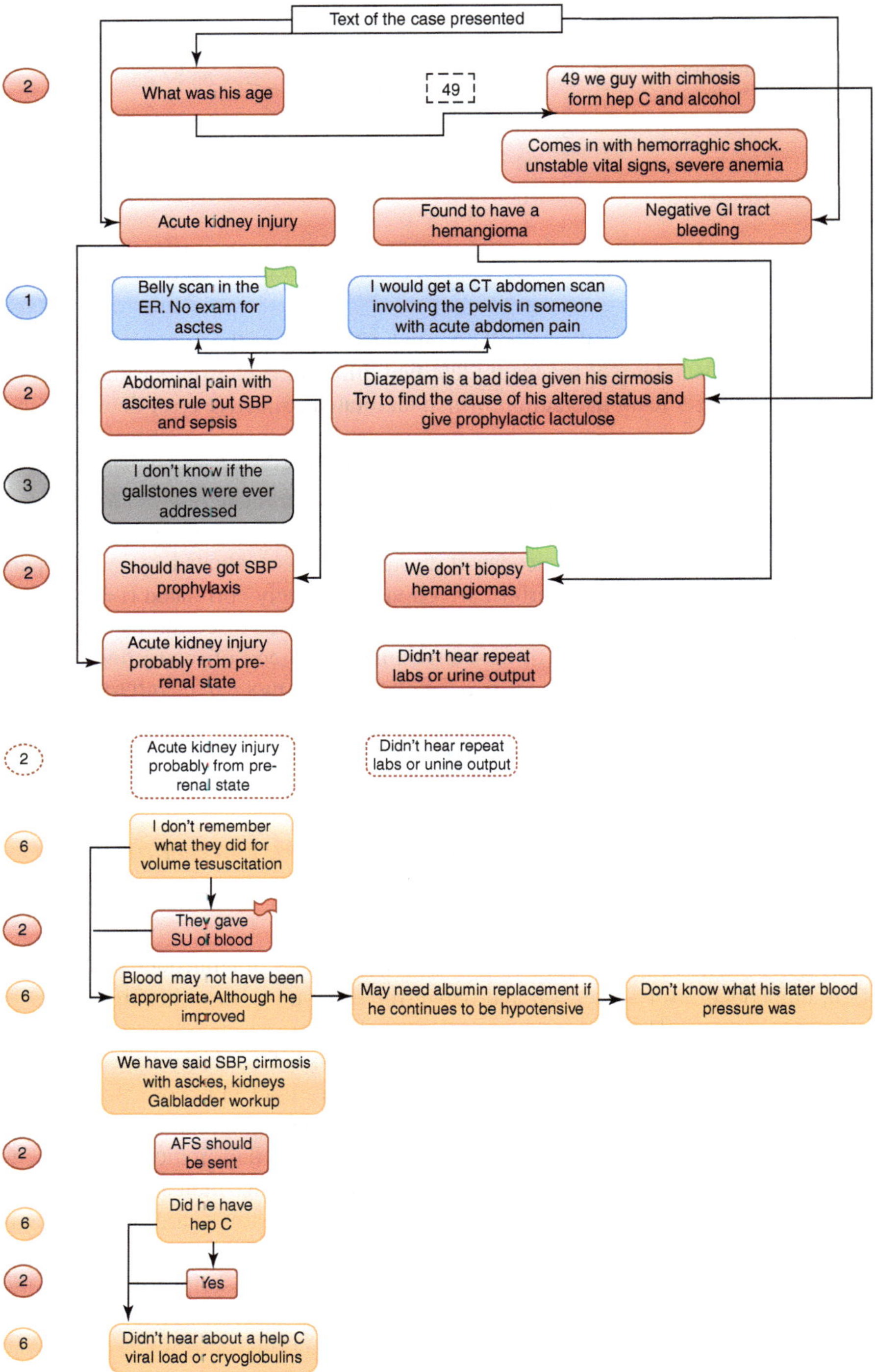

Fig. 4.10 Team 1, Case 2 schematic network of discussion

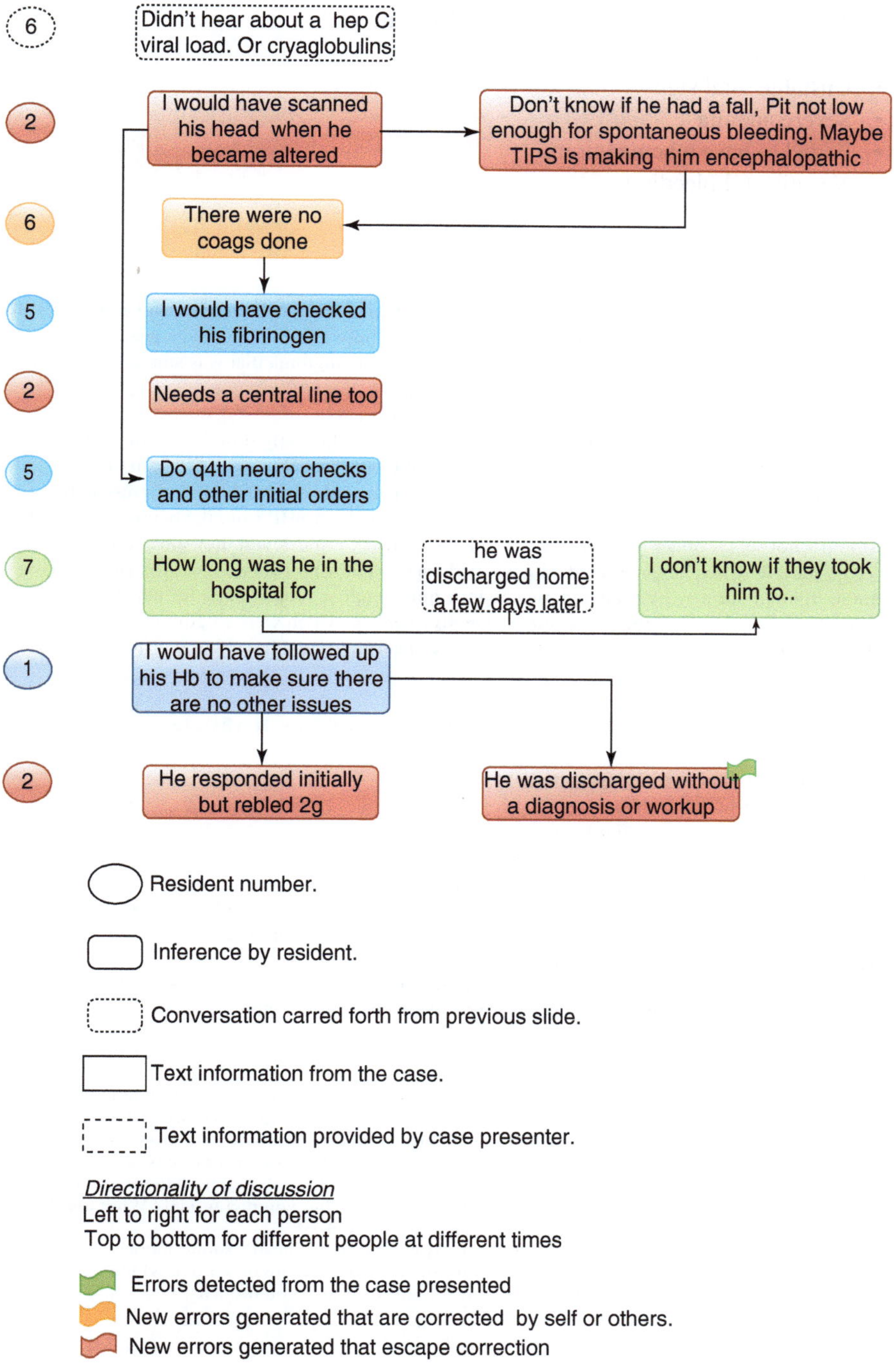

Fig. 4.10 (continued)

- 49 year-old with cirrhosis from hep C and alcohol
- Has hemorrhagic shock
- Unstable vital signs
- Severe anemia
- Found to have a hemangioma,
- Negative GI bleeding

2: What was his age?
A: 49
2: So we have a 49 year-old-guy with cirrhosis from hep C and alcohol abuse who comes in with what sounds like hemorrhagic shock hemoperitoneum and with unstable vital signs, severe anemia, acute kidney injury, jaundice, found to have a hemangioma that was supposedly what was bleeding with negative GI tract bleeding as far as we can tell.
B: OK. What are you thoughts on analysis and management?
1: I can't remember but I think the ER person they scanned his belly initially... with that kind of abdominal pain make sure it wasn't ascites... I would have probably got a CT scan of the abdomen involving the pelvis specially someone with an acute abdomen kind of presentation.
2: And abdominal pain with ascites they should have ruled out SBP from the beginning to make sure it's not sepsis rather than what looked like hemorrhagic shock and they gave him diazepam 10 q6 initially when he got altered with his cirrhosis... that is probably a bad idea. Should have rather figured out why he is altered, maybe give him lactulose prophylactic for hepatic encephalopathy and find the cause rather than give benzos, which weren't going to clear anyway.
3: I don't know if it was addressed but I remember hearing something about gallstones; I don't know if that was ever addressed...
B: No.
2: He should have gotten SBP prophylaxis extra initially with pro- or whatever.
B: OK, what else?
2: And I don't think we biopsy hemangiomas.
B: OK, what else?
1: They could do a biopsy to rule out cancer.
2: Yes I don't think they biopsy hemangiomas.
B: OK, what else? Other assessments of the case?
2: Acute kidney injury probably from a pre-renal state, can't say if it's a hepatorenal because that's a diagnosis of exclusion. Didn't hear repeat labs or a urine output.
B: OK, what else? Other assessments of the case?
2: Acute kidney injury probably from a pre-renal state, can't say if it's a hepatorenal because that's a diagnosis of exclusion. Didn't hear repeat labs or a urine output.
6: I don't remember what they did for volume resuscitation.
2: They gave 5 units of blood.
B: Correct.
6: I don't know if blood is appropriate in this case but he is hypotensive with probable ascites. It wasn't determined right away whether he had ascites... but he was given volume which sounds like it helped, but he could also have had low albumin and maybe needed albumin replacement if he continues to be hypotensive. I don't remember what his later blood pressure was.
A: His initial blood pressure was 88/56. That's all we have. Other thoughts? Management? Anything you would do differently or additionally besides what you mentioned? What are the possible differential diagnoses for this case that you can think of?
6: We have said a couple SBP, alcoholic cirrhosis with ascites, doesn't sound like he has hepatorenal syndrome, because his kidneys I think ...gall bladder involvement, which wasn't worked up... so he may have a cholecystitis resulting from his cholelithiasis.
2: AFB should be sent.
6: I think... did he have hep C?
A: Yes.
6: I didn't hear anything about the hep C or viral load, whether he is being treated for that or whether it was necessary. Nothing about cryoglobulins; he may have had cryoglobulinemia contributing to the abdominal distension.
B: OK

Fig. 4.11 Excerpt from transcript of Team 1 working through Case 2

6: I didn't hear anything about the hep C or viral load, whether he is being treated for that or whether it was necessary. Nothing about cryoglobulins; he may have had cryoglobulinemia contributing to the abdominal distension.
B: OK.
2: I probably would have scanned his head too initially when he became altered.
B: OK, the reason for that?
2: I don't know before presentation if he had trauma or a fall. He is not thrombocytopenic enough for me to think he bled spontaneously. Most likely the TIPS is making him encephalopathic.
6: There were no coags done.
5: I would have liked to check his fibrinogen.
2: Probably needs a central line too.
B: OK.
5: You could do the q4h neuro checks. Just order up the initial orders.
A: Did you all have any questions? Or any last thoughts?
7: How long was he in the hospital for?
B: All information that is given has been given to you.
7: So I don't know if they took him....
1: I mean I would have followed up his Hb to make sure he is not having any anemia issues. I think he kind of ...
B: So he was discharged home a few days later.
2: Because he responded to the 5U initially almost responded and then rebled 2 grams and then he was stable but if this is a hemangioma they said they were going to do a biopsy but didn't and they sent him home really with not a diagnosis of what it was that was bleeding. Presumably something from the liver, whether it's an HCC instead of hemangioma. Overall he did not really have a completely satisfying diagnosis.

Transcript Key	
Text Formatting	**Corresponding Depiction in the Semantic Network**
Underlined	Text with green flags in the semantic network figure; indicates errors detected from the case
Bold	Text with red flags in the semantic network figure; indicates newly generated errors that were never corrected
Italicized	Text with orange flags in the semantic network figure; indicates newly generated errors that were corrected by the individual or the team
Clinician Symbol	**Corresponding Clinician**
A	Attending Physician
B	Fellow
1-6	Residents 1 through 6

Fig. 4.11 (continued)

From this information, *Resident 1* continued and **identified the first error**, "Belly scan in the ER. No exam for ascites." *Resident 2* then followed by **detecting another embedded error**, "Diazepam is a bad idea given his cirrhosis," and corrected this error by stating, "Try to find the cause of his altered status and give prophylactic lactulose." Using the information that the patient has a hemangioma (as mentioned by *Resident 1*), *Resident 2* **discovered the third embedded error**, "We don't biopsy hemangiomas." He/she then moved on to discuss renal issues, "Acute kidney injury probably from pre-renal state," and "I didn't hear repeat labs or urine output." As the discussion progressed, *Resident 6* picked up this thread and commented, "I don't remember what they did for volume resuscitation." *Resident 2* responded, "They gave 5U of blood." **This was a new error generated by the resident**- 5U of blood was never presented in the case. Additionally, **this error was never corrected**. The team continued to discuss issues regarding the hepatitis C, neurological checks, and possible central line insertion. Towards the end of the discussion, *Resident 7* asked, "How long was he in the hospital for?" When the answer

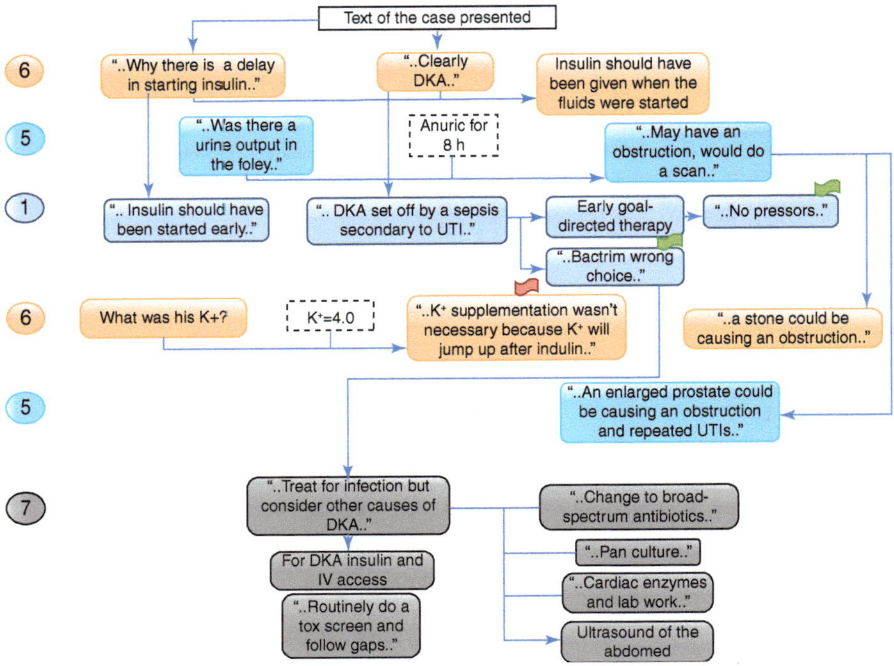

Fig. 4.12 Schematic network of Team 3 working through Case 1 and generating a new and uncorrected error

to the question was recalled, "He was discharged home a few days later," *Resident 2* identified the **fourth embedded error**, "He was discharged without a diagnosis or workup."

In summary, four of the five embedded errors were identified and corrected through team interaction. As reported earlier, the probability of an error being detected and corrected was higher during team interaction than during individual assessment. However, the probability of new errors being generated increased as the length of discussion and its associated elaboration increased. In the illustrated case, one new error was generated that was never corrected. Figure 4.12 shows another example of a new error generated and never corrected by Team 3.

Using the same case and a different team (Case 1 and Team 3), we illustrate how new errors are generated. This is given in Fig. 4.12. The transcript of team communication is given in Fig. 4.13. *Resident 6* started off the discussion by stating, "this is clearly DKA," and "Why is there a delay in starting insulin…insulin should have been given when the fluids were started." *Resident 1* responded, "insulin should have been started early," and "DKA set off by a sepsis secondary to UTI." He then **identified two embedded errors**, "Early goal directed therapy…no pressors," and "Bactrim was the wrong choice." *Resident 6* then asked, "What was his K+?" When the information was given as K+ = 4.0, the resident **generated the new error**, "K+

6: I don't see why there is the delay in the insulin? The sugar is 700 and what did they say, an hour...?
B: An hour and a half.
6: Yes, so why the delay in insulin? It seems to be a pretty straightforward presentation of DKA. Insulin should have been started earlier, they started with a liter of fluid, they could have bolused insulin then initially with the fluids.
B: Other comments?
5: Did the foley actually show urine? Did we hear a urine output?
B: Did not say.
5: If he has been anuric for 8 hours I would be concerned about a possible obstruction. Probably do some kind of a scan or...
B: OK, other thoughts?
1: There could be sepsis secondary to UTI, which probably set off his DKA. So I would start him on goal-directed therapy, start him on broad-spectrum antibiotics not Bactrim. Not for his UTI or sepsis. He doesn't require pressors at this point and I agree with XXX insulin drip should have been started a little early.
6: What was his potassium?
B: Initial potassium is 4.0?
6: So was potassium supplementation with the IV fluids necessary because the potassium as he would come out of DKA will jump up and they are above the 3.3 level so I don't think it is necessary to supplement.
6: We could also think of kidney stones causing obstruction.
5: He could also have an enlarged prostate causing obstruction and repeated UTIs.
7: So you start with a broad differential and narrow it down through results of tests so I think we have to treat for infection, but keep in mind other causes of DKA; in fact, stroke neglect other infections so pan cultures and treat accordingly with antibiotics and fluids. Until then, broad-spectrum antibiotics as you said. Insulin and IV access tests-wise, ultrasound of the abdomen to start with is indicated. The cardiac enzymes and all the lab work then based on his response. I would routinely ask for a toxicology screen in acidemia patient, urine tox and follow the gaps.

Fig. 4.13 Excerpt from transcript of Team 3 working through Case 1

supplementation wasn't necessary because K+ will jump up after insulin." This new error was not corrected. Instead *Resident 7* moved on to discuss treatments for infection, lab work, toxicology screens and ultrasound tests.

In summary, Team 3 identified and corrected two of the five embedded errors as a result of their further discussions and generated one additional error that was not embedded in the case. Figure 4.14 provides an example of problem solving in a clinical case, where team interaction generated an additional error, but was then able to correct it.

A schematic representation of generation and correction of error by Team 2 is given in Fig. 4.14, and the transcript from which schema was generated in given in Fig. 4.15. After the presentation of Case 1, *Resident 5* started the discussion by stating his ideas about the patient's diagnosis, "Patient has DKA," and "Very hypotensive and tachycardic. I would conclude sepsis." *Resident 4* added his opinion of possible diagnosis, "Pyelonephritis." *Resident 5* then stated, "He also has pre-renal

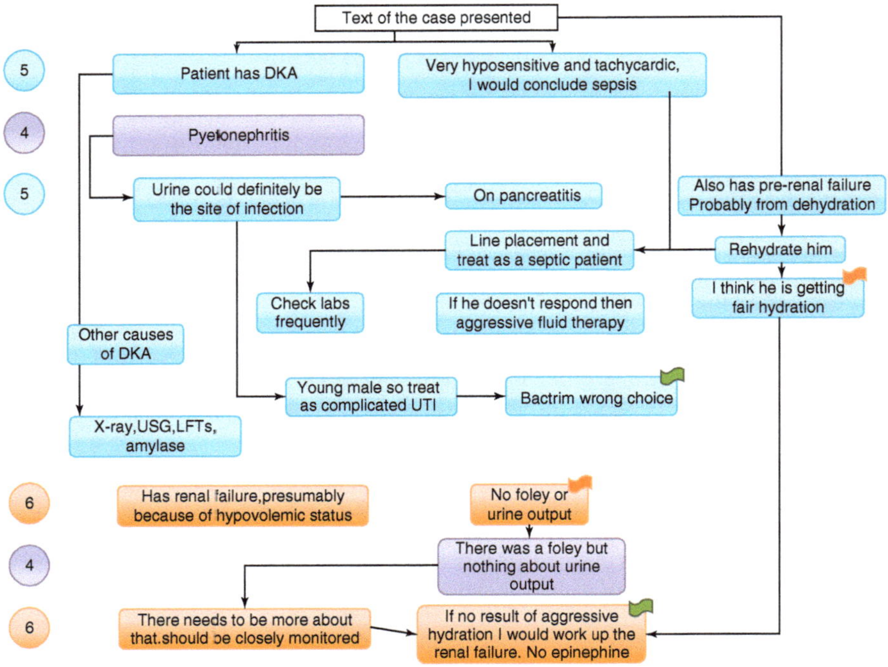

Fig. 4.14 Schematic network of Team 2 working through Case 1

failure. Probably from dehydration." With this statement, *Resident 5* **generated the following new error**, "Rehydrate him." However, he was quickly able to recover from his error, "I think he is getting fair hydration." Following this, *Resident 5* continued with the issues of infection, "Urine could definitely be the site of infection," and "young male so treat as complicated UTI." He then **caught an embedded error** by stating, "Bactrim was the wrong choice." *Resident 6* then stated, "his renal failure, presumably because of hypovolemic status." *Resident 6* then **generated a new error** by stating, "No foley put in place or urine output." **This error was quickly corrected** by *Resident 4* who stated, "There was a foley, but nothing about urine output." In summary, the residents of Team 2 generated new errors, but were able to identify and correct these errors through team interaction.

We summarize and illustrate patient safety evaluation and decision making in the context of collaborative teamwork by utilizing an adapted version of Norman's seven-stage model of interaction [20]. This is given in Fig. 4.16. The original model was applied to the problem of system usability, but its generic nature allowed us to apply it to the process of error recovery. Described in Allwood's earlier model (1984), the process incorporates the stages of triggering, diagnosis and correction, but presents them in the context of a decision-action cycle so as to include additional aspects of clinical decision making, such as distributed cognition during collaborative teamwork acting on error detection, correction, and recovery [30].

6: Evidently the patient has DKA. He also is very hypotesive and tachycardic overall, so I would conclude sepsis…
4: Pyelonephritis.
6: And definitely the possible site of infection could be the urine, on my differential would be pyelo, also pancreatitis. He also has pre-renal failure probably from the dehydration; I would *rehydrate him.*
In terms of the management I think he is getting fair hydration… definitely the insulin regimen is something important... One thing I don't agree with is choice of antibiotic, because to start with Bactrim, at least in Houston the most common causative organism is E. coli and most are resistant to Bactrim. Also I feel like he has a septic picture so I would have actually used a broader spectrum antibiotic and send lab cultures until they come back and then we escalate later on. I didn't hear anything about line placement, I think he should get both a subclavian and a central line and treated as a septic patient unless he responds quickly to fluids because his initial vital signs are very concerning… So I would have been very aggressive with fluid hydration and cardiovascular monitoring in case he doesn't respond to the fluids initially. I didn't hear anything about checking the labs frequently on him... and the other thing is the workup that we need to do to figure out what's causing his DKA because he sounds like he's had diabetes for a while now. Like I said, we thought that there might be a UTI but there are plenty of things that could be causing it. I didn't hear about a chest X-ray so we need to get that. He probably needs an abdominal USG and a CT scan; he needs LFTs and amylase lipase, most likely he is Bactrim resistant. The other thing is if he does have a UTI, he is 40, he is a very young guy so we will treat it as a complicated UTI and also a workup because that's not normal... that could be done once the situation is resolved. We can send a lipid profile to see… calcium; also I didn't hear to see… what could be causing for instance a pancreatitis and then… picture.
7: I agree the other thing is the renal failure although we presume this because of his hypovolemic status. He has been anuric for 8 hours, which is a long time *and I didn't hear anything about a foley being placed* or how much urine was…
4: There is a foley but it didn't say how much was the urine output…
7: Yes after the foley, how much was output. I think there needs to be more about that… after I didn't hear if there was any benefit with his aggressive hydration for his urine output. I think that should be monitored pretty closely. **And if there was no result with the aggressive IV hydration within a short period of time then I would not give epinephrine and go forward with the renal ultrasound urine electrolytes to try to work up the renal failure.**

Fig. 4.15 Excerpt from Transcript of Team 2 working through Case 1

Error Detection Factors

Person Attributed to the Error

Tacit boundaries imposed by hierarchy in a group can inhibit transfer of critical information and confound communication. We show that social/organizational hierarchy can interfere with team performance and can lead to error generation. In this study we also found that it was the residents who made most errors, a finding that fits with the Intermediate Effect Theory for mid-level trainees (residents) [24], which predicts a fall in performance as new knowledge is integrated during the learning process. The finding is also consistent with expectations that residents are prone to generating more errors, as they are usually the ones responsible for initiating and sustaining the discussion during clinical rounds, where errors increase with the number of elaborations. However, as opposed to interns, residents were more likely to correct errors as well.

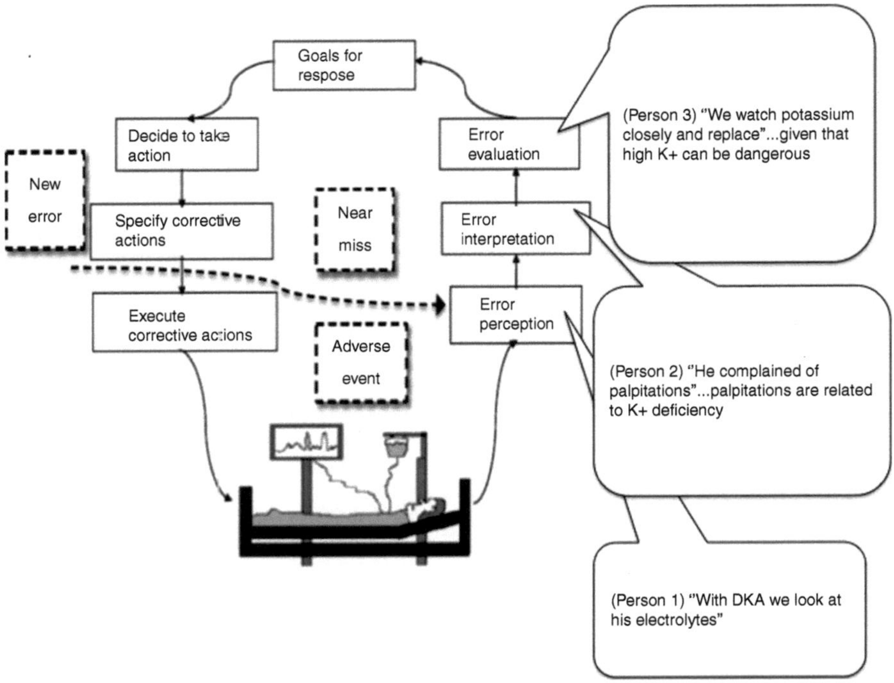

Fig. 4.16 Example of collaborative thinking where more than one person contributed to error detection

Nature of the Error

As previously stated, this study identified four types of error: knowledge-based, procedural, simple, and complex. Teams performed better at detecting *knowledge-based* and *complex* errors than at detecting *simple* or *procedural* errors. One reason for this could be that mental alerts in complex situations provide inherent checks, and simple and procedural errors may go undetected due to the presence of distracting knowledge-based and complex errors. Interns may become distracted by the knowledge-based and complex errors that they are not sufficiently experienced to solve, and residents may become distracted by their natural tendency to focus on higher priority errors that require their expertise.

Team Interaction

Teams collaborated at different stages of the error detection process. Some collaborated during the trigger phase, while others collaborated during error detection and error evaluation. Residents generated more *inferences* and recalled more *clinical information*, while fellows generated more *requests for clarifications*. In other words, residents had a greater share in error management focusing on patient care, while fellows mostly served an educational role within the discussion and contributed more towards further management instead of error detection.

This study found that increased team discussion and interaction created an iterative process that provided varying results. For instance, while team discussion and interaction increased the detection and correction of errors, they also resulted in new errors that required additional monitoring and resolution. The study also found that as teams continued to interact, their ability to recover from the errors improved. A recent work investigating error among team-based acute care scenarios produced similar results regarding error generation. Tallentire et al. found that some new errors were the result of preceding errors, which resulted from previous errors as well as from misunderstandings between team members, including junior doctors' misperceptions or misinterpretations of information [31].

Comparison of Semi-Naturalistic and Laboratory-Based Studies

Our previous studies in a laboratory setting focused on error recovery by individuals. The study assessed the ability of experts (attending physicians) and non-experts (residents at various levels of training) to detect, correct and justify their interpretations of errors embedded in a set of realistic written clinical case scenarios. It was found that error detection by both domain experts and trainees was on the whole alarmingly poor – no participant from either of these groups managed to detect more than half of the errors embedded in either of the two case scenarios, despite many of these errors being egregious with severe consequences for the hypothetical patients concerned. In these laboratory-based studies, subjects committed errors that included recalling incorrect information and incorrectly assessing embedded errors as appropriate steps. Of the 25 total individual participants, 52 errors were generated, 6 of which were corrected (11 %), while the remaining 46 errors (89 %) were propagated, potentially compromising patient safety.

In this semi-naturalistic study remove the 5 teams generated 16 new errors. The percentages of corrected errors show a difference of 41 %, with individuals correcting only 15 % of the errors, and teams correcting 56 %. Figures 4.17 and 4.18 illustrate these results.

Discussion

Reducing the consequences of errors does not only depend on detecting them, but also on recovering from them. To that end, it can be said that recovery from errors initially depends on their detection and associated mechanisms leading up to detection [22]. Edmonson maintains that the unintended perpetuation of error that leads to negative patient outcomes is frequently the result of addressing the superficial problems/errors that occur in a complex environment without addressing the underlying problems, which can then be exacerbated if the solutions feed into a vicious

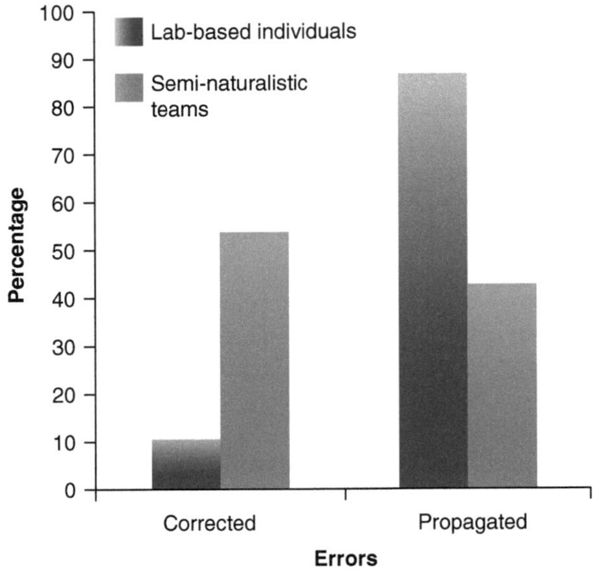

Fig. 4.17 Percentage of error correction and propagation in two experimental settings

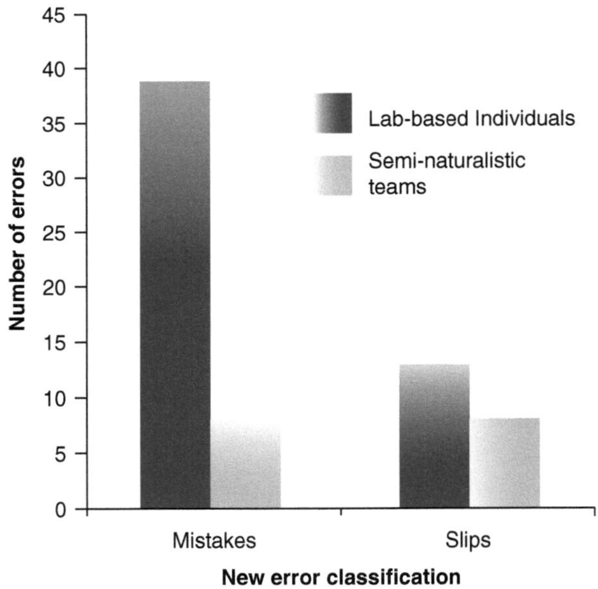

Fig. 4.18 Frequency and classification of newly generated errors in two experimental settings

cycle [32]. The use of semi-naturalistic data collection and qualitative techniques for error management analysis as well as group discussion have served to uncover those underlying issues relative to the cognitive processes that occur during team interaction. The ICU teams in this semi-naturalistic study performed well when compared to previous laboratory-based work on individuals, in which neither experts nor trainees detected more than half the embedded errors.

These results are not surprising when considered from the perspective of distributed cognition [33], which considers team members as part of a computational system with greater capacity than any of its individual components. As illustrated in Figs. 4.10, 4.11, 4.12, 4.13, 4.14, and 4.15, error detection was often achieved as a collaborative effort integrating the knowledge of multiple individuals. So our results support the proposal that clinical teams have greater capacity for error recovery than their individual members. The positive results of collaborative problem solving or learning may also be attributed to the fact that social interaction stimulates elaboration of conceptual knowledge [34]. From the perspective of complexity science, this capacity for error recovery can be viewed as an emergent property of the team that is contingent upon interactions between its component members. These interactions are innately unpredictable, as they are influenced by a myriad of personal and social factors that are difficult to characterize, such as the hierarchical nature of clinical roles. Consequently, error detection and recovery does not proceed in the orderly manner one might anticipate in the context of fault detection on the production line. Rather, the process of detection and recovery is non-linear, and includes the generation of new errors that may elude recovery.

In order to achieve a lasting cultural shift towards safe practice, medical education needs to be restructured with a focus on improved ability to manage increasing amounts of information, improved understanding of the concepts of human interaction and patient safety, and improved acquisition of communication and teamwork skills, in addition to the current focus on acquisition of expertise in clinical and scientific knowledge. Over the past decades many studies have compared aviation to critical care, positing that heightened alertness in environments such as these improves performance [35]. Furthermore, research in aviation has illustrated that fatigued flight crews produced significantly less errors when compared to rested flight crews who had not yet worked together [36]. These findings are congruent with our own research, since most errors in critical care are generated when units are busiest and slowest, thus implicating other factors, including teamwork, in error reduction and correction in complex environments.

Our results indicate a correlation between team interaction through verbal communication and error correction, as well as knowledge elaboration. This finding is consistent with previous research in the aviation domain, which found that the best performing pilots spent more time discussing problems and errors with their crew [35]. It has been suggested that while talking out loud, knowledge becomes more elaborate because communication implies the need to be understood by others, which therefore results in more coherent explanations [37]. Elaborative talk also stimulates reorganization and awareness of knowledge gaps and inconsistent reasoning. This in turn leads to more elaborated concepts, which result from creating new examples, reformulating theories or approaches, and reinforcing past experiences [38]. Therefore, the significance of group discussion should be emphasized and the role of team interaction through verbal communication should be highlighted. (Organizational and group interventions may be necessary to stimulate detection and discussion of error [32]).

Furthermore, new errors are generated as teams interact and continue to elaborate patient problems, resolve conflicts and generate new hypotheses. Similar to our finding, Brown and Palincsar found that with appropriate teamwork, the results of the conflict and controversy that arises can in fact generate clarifications, explanations, justifications and a search for new information or a new solution [39]. In our study, the individuals in the team engaged in elaborative activities by not only reflecting upon and elaborating upon their own understanding, but by also integrating/elaborating the input of their team members. This emphasizes an important aspect of learning through knowledge elaboration and conflict resolution. However, efforts are required to supervise learners in team-based care activities and to correct mistakes as they occur; otherwise, serious errors can go unresolved and cause severe consequences. This finding is also consistent with the research on clinical teamwork discussed previously [18], as well as with research from other studies on teamwork skills and performance in simulated trauma teams [40] where communication failure was attributed to a lack of shared understanding among team members in their respective roles. It is now accepted in the literature that mistakes are more difficult to correct than slips. Detection of mistakes is more difficult irrespective of error complexity and may require more time with less success, as well as more frequent external intervention [28, 41]. The nature of errors changes with expertise: routine-based errors increase with expertise whereas knowledge-based errors decrease with expertise [42].

Our study illustrates that longer discussions and greater elaboration in team interactions occur as discussions move away from the direct patient problem, which leads to the possibility of generating new errors (Cf [43]). The generative nature of continued elaboration [44] performed on an idea during discussion opens itself up to distortion of recent memory (of patient care) and to creeping in of erroneous decisions. This raises the issue of tension and trade-off between simultaneous learning and delivering of competent performance. It is therefore essential to look for ways to mitigate generation of new errors and induce learning. Although we must train health professionals to deliver competent care in a timely manner to their patients, opportunities must be created, either through simulations or group discussion with *near misses*, where learning (under little time pressure or no multitasking) is encouraged. The discussions around these near miss scenarios allow trainees to focus on real-world problems rather than artificially created problems. This is important because what is learned (using causal reasoning) will eventually be proceduralized and automated to be available for quick use in a time-critical environment. On account of the potential consequences of errors in practice, the clinical environment provides limited opportunity to learn and thus must be supplemented by other training situations.

Informatics Implications

In addition to education and training, health information technologies will provide some of these solutions. Creating a simulated virtual environment that genuinely mimics a real-life critical care setting will help in this endeavor; this is an avenue that we have already begun to explore [10]. While research suggests that computer-based physician order entry systems can reduce medication error rates [45], the safety features of such systems focus on the detection of potential errors generated by individual physicians, and the poor fit between the rigidity of the rules used to detect these errors and the flexibility of clinical practice has led to dissatisfaction with the large numbers of false alerts that occur [46]. Given our finding that team interaction promotes error detection, we suggest a role for technology that mediates team interaction in patient safety. It has been argued previously that methods and insights from the field of Computer-Supported Cooperative Work (CSCW) may be applicable to the problem domain of clinical informatics [47]. In particular, CSCW techniques that aim to raise awareness of the activities of other team members may help to promote error detection in practice. Ethnographic methodologies have been employed by CSCW researchers as a means of characterizing the ways in which existing artifacts support collaborative work in practice (for a clinically oriented review, see [48]). Our findings provide further motivation for the design of technology with an awareness of the ways in which existing artifacts mediate communication in context, since impeding this flow of information may be detrimental to error recovery.

Conclusion

Plutarch famously said, "To make no mistakes is not in the power of man; but from their errors and mistakes the wise and good learn wisdom for the future." Good teamwork is shown to be better than individuals working alone in detecting and correcting errors. This requires individual expertise in keeping up to date with the latest information as well as willingness to communicate with other members of the team. Clinical environments such as rounds are opportune places for learning from each other during the delivery of care.

One of the consequences of a long team dialogue on any particular patient-related issue is that new errors are generated. In this case the details of the problem discussion interfere with the utility of making quick patient care decisions. However, results show that even though new errors are generated, they are also detected and corrected quickly. Some errors are not corrected and propagate through the system, and it is this potential for generation of new errors during team discussion that underscores the importance of supervision by an expert mentor. This finding is consistent with studies in problem-based learning conditions, where expert tutors play an important role in learning. Simulation of team clinical practice under careful supervision can ensure that healthcare providers are adept at exchanging high-quality information among themselves with minimal errors.

The analysis and understanding developed through this study provide an opportunity to characterize team interaction in situations of error detection and recovery. However, the relationship between error detection and correction and learning needs to be further explored. Additionally, this analysis reinforces the importance of the various factors that contribute heavily to error etiology and recovery within a team. An individual's knowledge, attention and comprehension are all crucial to successful error detection and resolution as well as to subsequent acquisition of new knowledge.

Questions for Discussion

1. What do these findings suggest about the relationships between the rigid hierarchical structures that have been observed in some practice settings, patient safety and education?
2. How might one encourage trainees to engage in the sorts of collaborative error detection that were observed to occur on occasion in this study?
3. How might one re-structure clinical rounds in order to encourage collaborative error detection of this nature?
4. What manner and degree of mentoring would promote learning through error correction without compromising patient safety?

References

1. Kohn LT, Corrigan JM, Donaldson MS. To err is human: building a safer health system. Washington, DC: National Academy Press; 2000.
2. Stelfox HT, Palmisani S, Scurlock C, Orav EJ, Bates DW. The "to err is human" report and the patient safety literature. Qual Saf Health Care. 2006;15:174–8.
3. Brennan TA, Localio AR, Leape LL. Identification of adverse events occurring during hospitalization. Ann Intern Med. 1990;112:221–6.
4. Donchin Y, Gopher D, Olin M, Badihi Y, Biesky M, Sprung CL, et al. A look into the nature and causes of human errors in the intensive care unit. Crit Care Med. 1995;23(2):294–300.
5. Sasou K, Reason J. Team errors: definition and taxonomy. Reliability Eng Syst Saf. 1999;65(1): 1–9.
6. Bates WD, Cohen M, Leape LL, Overhage JM, Shabot MM, Sheridan T. Reducing the frequency of errors in medicine using information technology. J Am Med Inform Assoc. 2001; 8(4):299–308.
7. Cohen T, Blatter B, Almeida C, Patel VL. Reevaluating recovery: perceived violations and preemptive interventions on emergency psychiatry rounds. J Am Med Inform Assoc. 2007; 14(3):312–9.
8. Patel VL, Cohen T. New perspectives on error in critical care. Curr Opin Crit Care. 2008; 14(4):456–9.
9. Patel VL, Cohen T, Murarka T, Olsen J, Kagita S, Myneni S, et al. Recovery at the edge of error: debunking the myth of the infallible expert. J Biomed Inform. 2011;44(3):413–24. PubMed PMID: 20869466.
10. Razzouk E, Cohen T, Almoosa K, Patel V. Approaching the limits of knowledge: the influence of priming on error detection in simulated clinical rounds. AMIA Annu Symp Proc. 2011; 2011:1155–64.
11. Wilkinson WE, Cauble LA, Patel VL. Error detection and recovery in dialysis nursing. J Patient Saf. 2011;7(4):213–23. PubMed PMID: 22064625.

12. Kanse L, van der Schaaf TW, Vrijland ND, van Mierlo H. Error recovery in a hospital pharmacy. Ergonomics. 2006;49(5–6):503–16.
13. Orasanu J. Training for aviation decision making: the naturalistic decision making perspective. Proc Human Factors Ergon Soc Annu Meet. 1995;39(20):1258–62.
14. Oser RL, McCallum GA, Salas E, Morgan Jr BB. Toward a definition of teamwork: an analysis of critical team behaviors. Orlando: Naval Training Systems Center; 2005.
15. Kessels-Habraken M, Van der Schaaf T, De Jonge J, Rutte C. Defining near misses: towards a sharpened definition based on empirical data about error handling processes. Soc Sci Med. 2010;70(9):1301–8.
16. Hakimzada AF, Green RA, Sayan OR, Zhang J, Patel VL. The nature and occurrence of registration errors in the emergency department. Int J Med Inform. 2008;77(3):169–75.
17. Kubose TT, Patel VL, Jordan D. Dynamic adaptation to critical care medical environment: error recovery as cognitive activity. In: Proceedings of the 24th annual meeting of the Cognitive Science Society. Fairfax, Virginia; 2002. p. 43–4.
18. Sexton JB, Thomas EJ, Helmreich RL. Error, stress, and teamwork in medicine and aviation: cross sectional surveys. Br Med J. 2000;320(7237):745–9.
19. Rothschild JM, Hurley AC, Landrigan CP, Cronin JW, Martell-Waldrop K, Foskett C, et al. Recovery from medical errors: the critical care nursing safety net. Jt Comm J Qual Patient Saf. 2006;32(2):63–72.
20. Norman DA. The psychology of everyday things. New York: Basic Books; 1988.
21. Rasmussen J. The role of error in organizing behaviour. Ergonomics. 1990;33:377–85.
22. Blavier A, Rouy E, Nyssen A-S, de Keyser V. Prospective issues for error detection. Ergonomics. 2005;48(7):758–81.
23. Lighthall GK, Barr J, Howard SK, Gellar E, Sowb Y, Bertacini E, et al. Use of a fully simulated intensive care unit environment for critical event management training for internal medicine residents. Crit Care Med. 2003;31(10):2437–43.
24. Patel VL, Groen GJ. The general and specific nature of medical expertise: a critical look. In: Ericsson A, Smith J, editors. Towards a general theory of expertise: prospects and limits. Cambridge: Cambridge University Press; 1991. p. 93–125.
25. Patel VL, Arocha JF, Zhang J. Thinking and reasoning in medicine. In: Holyoak KJ, Morrison RG, editors. The Cambridge handbook of thinking and reasoning. New York: Cambridge University Press; 2005. p. 727–50.
26. Shetty P, Cohen T, Patel B, Patel VL. The cognitive basis of effective team performance: features of failure and success in simulated cardiac resuscitation. In: AMIA annual symposium proceedings. San Francisco, CA; 2009. p. 599–603.
27. Norman DA. Categorization of action slips. Psychol Rev. 1981;88(1):1–15.
28. Reason J. Human error. Cambridge: Cambridge University Press; 1990.
29. Zhang J, Patel VL, Johnson TR, Shortliffe EH. Toward a cognitive taxonomy of medical errors. In: AMIA annual symposium proceedings. San Antonio, TX; 2002. p. 934–8.
30. Allwood CM. Error detection process in statistical problem solving. Cognit Sci. 1984;8(4): 413–37.
31. Tallentire VR, Smith SE, Skinner J, Cameron HS. Exploring error in team-based acute care scenarios: an observational study from the United Kingdom. Acad Med. 2012;87(6):792–8.
32. Edmondson A. Learning from failure in health care: frequent opportunities, pervasive barriers. Qual Saf Health Care. 2004;13 Suppl 2:ii3–9.
33. Hutchins E. Cognition in the wild, vol. xviii. Cambridge: MIT Press; 1995. p. 381.
34. van Boxtel C, van der Linden J, Kanselaar G. Collaborative learning tasks and the elaboration of conceptual knowledge. Learn Instr. 2000;10(4):311–30.
35. Sexton JB, Helmreich RL. Analyzing cockpit communications: the links between language, performance, error, and workload. Hum Perf Extrem Environ. 2000;5(1):63–8.
36. Foushee HC, Helmreich RL. Group interaction and flight crew performance. In: Wiener EL, Nagel DC, editors. Human factors in aviation. San Diego: Academic Press; 1988. p. 189–277.
37. Teasley SD. The role of talk in childrens' peer collaborations. Dev Psychol. 1995;31:207–20.

38. Webb NM, Palincsar AS. Collaborative learning tasks and the elaboration of conceptual knowledge. In: Berliner DC, Calfee RC, editors. Handbook of educational psychology. New York: Simon & Schuster MacMillan; 1996.
39. Brown AL, Palincsar AS. Guided cooperative learning and individual knowledge acquisition. In: Resnick LB, editor. Knowing learning and instruction: essays in honor of Robert Glaser. Hillsdale: Lawrence Erlbaum; 1989. p. 395–451.
40. Westli HK, Johnsen BH, Eid J, Rasten I, Brattebo G. Teamwork skills, shared mental models, and performance in simulated trauma teams: an independent group design. Scand J Trauma Resusc Emerg Med. 2010;18:47.
41. Cook RI, Woods DD: Operating at the sharp end: The complexity of human error, in Bogner MS (ed): Human Error in Medicine. Hillsdale, NJ, Lawrence Erlbaum Associates, 1994. p. 225–310.
42. Amalberti R. The paradoxes of almost totally safe transportation systems. Saf Sci. 2001; 37(2–3):109–26.
43. Patel VL, Groen GJ, Norman GR. Reasoning and instruction in medical curricula. Cogn Instr. 1993;10(4):335–78.
44. Klein G, Pliske R, Crandall B, Woods DD. Problem detection. Cogn Technol Work. 2005;7(1): 14–28.
45. Kaushal R, Shojania KG, Bates DW. Effects of computerized physician order entry and clinical decision support systems on medication safety: a systematic review. Arch Intern Med. 2003;163:1409–16.
46. Kuperman GJ, Bobb A, Payne TH, Avery AJ, Gandhi TK, Burns G, et al. Medication-related clinical decision support in computerized provider order entry systems: a review. J Am Med Inform Assoc. 2007;14:29–40.
47. Pratt W, Reddy MC, McDonald DW, Tarczy-Hornoch P, Gennari JH. Incorporating ideas from computer-supported cooperative work. J Biomed Inform. 2004;37:128–37.
48. Xiao Y. Artifacts and collaborative work in healthcare: methodological, theoretical, and technological implications of the tangible. J Biomed Inform. 2005;38(1):26–33.

Chapter 5
Error Recovery in the Wilderness of ICU

Vimla L. Patel, Alisabeth L. Shine, and Khalid F. Almoosa

Introduction

Our previous investigations of error detection and correction in a laboratory setting (in-vitro) using error-embedded tasks show that individual physicians identified less than 50 % of the errors [1]. Experts corrected the errors as soon as they detected them and were better able to detect errors requiring integration of multiple elements in the case. Residents were more cautious in making decisions showing a slower error recovery pattern, and the detected errors were more procedural in nature with specific patient outcomes. In this study, error detection and correction are shown to be dependent on expertise, and on the nature of the everyday tasks of the clinicians, given that experts make top level decisions, while residents take care of patient-related problems on day-to-day basis.

Given that clinical decisions in healthcare are made in teams, this research was extended to a semi-naturalistic environment where clinical teams were given

V.L. Patel, PhD, DSc, FRSC (✉)
Center for Cognitive Studies in Medicine and Public Health,
New York Academy of Medicine, New York, NY 10029, USA

Department of Biomedical Informatics,
Columbia University, New York, NY 10032, USA

Department of Biomedical Informatics,
Arizona State University, Scottsdale, AZ 85259, USA
e-mail: vpatel@nyam.org

A.L. Shine, MA
Center for Cognitive Studies in Medicine and Public Health,
New York Academy of Medicine, New York, NY 10029, USA

K.F. Almoosa, MD, MS, FCCP
Transplant Surgery ICU, Memorial Hermann Hospital,
Texas Medical Center, Houston, TX 77030, USA

University of Texas Health Science Center, Houston, TX, USA

V.L. Patel et al. (eds.), *Cognitive Informatics in Health and Biomedicine*,
Health Informatics, DOI 10.1007/978-1-4471-5490-7_5, © Springer-Verlag London 2014

error-embedded cases during clinical rounds in a hospital critical care setting (Chap. 4). An attending physician presented two cases for the team to evaluate during rounds, following the error-embedded paradigm. Although the environment was naturalistic, the nature of the task was controlled, similar to the task in the laboratory condition. The study showed that more errors were identified and corrected during team interaction than in an individual condition, where team interaction facilitated error checks. However, as interaction continued, additional new errors were generated and some of which were not corrected, propagating to the level of patient care. Therefore, although the teams provided additional error checks, there was a danger of new errors going unchecked unless the team discussions were monitored.

Given the strengths and limitations of the in-vitro and semi-naturalistic studies, we decided to conduct a naturalistic (in-vivo) pilot study to investigate team decision-making and the nature of error management in a medical intensive care environment (MICU). We were opportunistic in that we used part of data that was being collected at the bedside for another purpose [2]. We used data from team interactions at the bedside that was recorded during three clinical rounds, and was analyzed using qualitative protocol analysis along with conversational analysis, including qualitative and descriptive analysis of transcript contents. The purpose of this study was to see the kinds of constraints the natural ICU environment imposed on error detection and correction, as compared to the other two experimental settings. Please note that the terms *error correction* and *error recovery* are used interchangeably in this manuscript.

Decision-Making in Naturalistic Environments

In contrast to the previous studies, in which experimental conditions were manipulated in order to investigate the process of error recovery, we discuss the paradigm of error recovery within the context of naturalistic decision-making [3]. This work is informed by the perspective that factors such as high workload, stress, fatigue and weak team coordination can contribute to human error [4], necessitating more complex explanations than provided by assigning blame for faulty decision making to a single negligent individual [5]. This perspective has shifted the priority of human error research from the study of error prevention to the study of error detection and correction [6]. In our view, the naturalistic study of the process of error detection and correction is complementary to the controlled and semi-naturalistic approaches we have presented in the previous chapters, as a means to reveal the contextual factors that influence error recovery in practice.

Current approaches in human error research in complex systems emphasize that the causes of cognitive errors that can be traced to the interaction between work context and problem solving [7]. A large body of error research has been reported in high-stress, high-risk domains such as aviation, firefighting, the military, space exploration, nuclear power, and oil and gas extraction – fields where errors would have disastrous consequences, and are exceedingly rare [8]. Researchers in the field of naturalistic decision-making (NDM), a discipline derived from cognitive science and decision-making research, have studied how experts in these complex real-world environments use their knowledge to make decisions. Decisions made in these environments can often be subject to time pressures, goal conflicts, dynamically changing conditions, and uncertain sources of information [9, 10]. As a result, decision makers in naturalistic situations tend to "satisfice," [11] or choose a solution adequate for achieving the goal at hand under the given constraints, even if it may not be the best of all possible solutions [8].

The following is a brief summary of key principles that served as a motivation for our study. Research by Gary Klein and colleagues in the military domain found that people rely on the synthesis of their prior experiences when judging new situations [3, 12]. This synthesis of knowledge from past experiences is also known as a schema, and it "leads to the anticipation of certain types of information…then directs…behavior to seek out certain types of information and provides a way of interpreting that information" [13]. Gary Klein refers to this reliance on past experiences, or schemas, as recognition-primed decision-making, where we develop schemas that are used to evaluate a situation in view to make decisions.

Klein and colleagues found four general factors that contribute to decision errors: (1) lack of relevant knowledge (i.e., not enough experience), (2) poor information (i.e., incomplete, ambiguous, or contradictory information) or accurate information which is difficult to interpret, (3) poor projection of consequences (i.e., underestimating risk, not anticipating particular consequences), and (4) goal conflicts (i.e., pressure to meet organizational and social goals taking priority over safety goals). Research in various domains and disciplines has confirmed that when operating under stress, people make more errors on a wide variety of tasks. This is because working memory is finite and overloading cognitive resources can lead to a less efficient performance.

Team Decision-Making in Domains Outside of Medicine

Teamwork is the process by which members of the team pursue, exchange, and synchronize information in order to decide the next steps [3]. Teamwork is important to ensure that the decisions made, and consequentially the task outcome, can be at their strongest. A study conducted by the U.S. Navy found that teams that are more effective showed more teamwork-related behaviors than less effective teams [14]. These more effective teams achieved higher scores on a technical evaluation than the less effective teams; scores on this evaluation were correlated to critical effective behaviors such as prompting other team members on what to do next, helping team members who were experiencing difficulty with the task, and making positive statements within the team. In this study, these specific behaviors were especially critical for helping other team members identify errors and make correct decisions.

Success of team decision-making has been attributed to a number of factors, including expertise of team members, nature of the task and the quality of team training [15]. Team macrocognition, or situation awareness, is another important aspect in the success of team decision-making, where macrocognitive processes appear to support collaborative team activity. For example, when a hostage situation arises and rescuing those captured requires an evacuation plan, the military forms a team of specialists with different levels of expertise and experience in the context of real field encounters. These experts, who possess knowledge of how decisions are made in the field, can organize that knowledge in the context of the situation and can formulate a plan for recovery steps [16].

Team Decision-Making in Medicine (ICU and ER)

The focus of decision-making in healthcare has shifted from individual care providers to teams of care providers. In healthcare, teams form for the purposes of providing patient care including morning rounds, consultations, and case conferences, where both the communication between team members and knowledge about team members influence the nature of decisions made by the team [17]. A crucial responsibility of the team in medical practice is to make accurate diagnoses and provide patient management plans that are consistent with the diagnoses. Effective teamwork can improve the likelihood of making accurate diagnosis and patient care plan. For example, in a medical emergency simulation study, Tschan et al. found that displaying more explicit reasoning and "talking to the room" enhanced the accuracy of diagnosis, while merely considering more information did not improve diagnoses [18]. In the natural environment, using these strategies to facilitate teamwork may contribute to correction of any errors that may be generated.

Two major factors that can substantially influence discussions on the nature of medical decisions have been identified: pre-discussing the distribution of problem-relevant information (e.g. [19]), and each team member's awareness of the other members' unique knowledge and talents (implicit knowledge). In a study on shared and unshared information in a three-person medical team, the shared information was immediately discussed during the team meetings, as predicted. It was also found that the team leaders repeated more clinical case information than the other team members, and over time the unshared information was repeated at an increasing rate [20]. This shows that leaders are important in fostering situation awareness between team members, where shared information is minimum.

In the ICU environment, the cognitive task is distributed across team members during decision making to reduce the cognitive load [21]. There is some shared decision making, but the rest is dependent on individual expertise of health professionals such as nurses, pharmacists, medical residents and the attending physicians (called "attendings" from now on).

In a pilot *in situ* study of expertise and team decision making by Kubose, Patel, and Jordan, the authors shadowed an attending, a resident, and a medical student in an ICU, and found that the attending detected the most errors [18] but also recovered from most errors [15]; the resident detected [13] and corrected [8] the second largest number of errors; and the student detected [8] and corrected [2] the fewest errors [22].

Most of the attending physician's decisions required expert knowledge, and the errors that were corrected were likely to have serious consequences, if unattended. The error corrected by the resident required domain knowledge as well as knowledge of some routine procedures. Student's errors corrected were mostly routine in nature. The fast pace of decision-making combined with a high level of confidence meant the mistakes were generated quickly and often. However, due to the attending's expert knowledge and ability to evaluate the situation, errors that were generated were also rapidly corrected.

Method

Study Site

The data were collected at a 16-bed "closed" adult medical intensive care unit (MICU) in a large teaching hospital in Texas that averaged over 33,000 admissions in 2010. The unit is considered "closed" as the MICU team holds the primary responsibility for the care of admitted patients [23]. The majority of admitted patients were older and from minority populations. Both paper and electronic charts were simultaneously maintained and used for patient care documentation in this unit at the time of the study.

Participants

Three clinician teams from the MICU were included in this study. Each team consisted of an attending physician, a clinical fellow, an outgoing resident, an outgoing intern, oncoming resident, oncoming intern, a respiratory therapist, a pharmacist, and patient's nurse. This is the typical composition of a clinical team participating in morning rounds.

The team on **Day 1** was composed of an attending physician, fellow, outgoing resident, outgoing intern, oncoming resident, oncoming intern, a respiratory therapist, a pharmacist, a patient's nurse and one medical student (Total participants = 10). The team on **Day 2** was composed of an attending physician, fellow, outgoing resident, outgoing intern, oncoming resident, oncoming intern, a respiratory therapist, a pharmacist, a patient's nurse and four medical students (Total participants = 13). Days 1 and 2 were consecutive day, and so, the attending, fellow, respiratory therapist, pharmacist are the same across these days. The oncoming resident and intern on Day 1 were the outgoing resident and intern on Day 2. The team on **Day 3** was a new team and included an attending physician, fellow, outgoing resident, outgoing intern, oncoming resident, oncoming intern, a respiratory therapist, a pharmacist, a patient's nurse and one medical student (Total participants = 10). A total of 26 individuals participated in the 3-day study. The team composition was reasonably consistent.

Data Collection: Morning Rounds in MICU

Data were collected during these morning rounds, where the daily patient assessment and management-planning sessions were done in the MICU. During these sessions, residents presented information on real patients at the bedside, and the clinical team discussed each patient's status, diagnosis, and management plan. Each round lasted approximately 5 h, and researchers spent 3 h per day for 3 days shadowing and observing clinician teams prior to the clinical Rounds. No instructions were given to the teams by the researchers. As mentioned earlier, the present study is the reuse of a subset of data collected as part of a larger research project [2]. Team interactions were audio-recorded and transcribed verbatim with all identifiers removed. A total of 9 h of audio-recordings of clinical rounds with 34 patients were used in our analysis. Our data-coding scheme was developed based on our laboratory-based studies, observations and from the review of the literature.

Data Coding

We used a mixed strategy to analyze the transcript data, performing a coding process using a priori codes from previous work and developing novel coding when necessary. This form of documentation enabled us to capture the nuances of interactions and speech content. As shown in our previous studies that analysis of data from audio recording, note taking, and shadowing of the physicians provide an in-depth account of the development of the clinical workflow in ICU and ER environments (e.g. [23, 24]).

In this research the audio recordings were transcribed verbatim, the transcripts were segmented into the smallest units of text, which retained semantic meaning, called "utterances" [25]. An utterance can be a single word, a phrase, or a complete sentence, as long as it is self-contained and easily understood as one unit. Breaking text down into small, meaningful units is a standard method of systematically compiling data in natural language dialogue [26].

Using ideas from the taxonomy developed by Apker et al. and modifying it using an open coding process, each clinically relevant utterance was coded for content (e.g., "management decision," "information interpretation," "information

Table 5.1 Case management coding categories for data analysis

Category	Description	Example
Information aggregation	Patient information aggregated by the presenter prior to its interpretation by the entire team; multiple instances of information aggregation possible depending on the number of ongoing medical issues in the case	"MICU day no 3, she was extubated yesterday. Her problems include altered mental status, hep C, alcoholic cirrhosis, alcoholic abuse, withdrawal, NSTGMI, GI bleed, thrombocytic leukemia, UTI stage 2 DQ ulcers."
Information interpretation	Patient information interpreted based on the evidence at hand	"Because of her size, I can pretty much guarantee to you, what's in there is probably a Bivona (Bivona® tracheostomy tube)"
Additional information	Patient information requested by individuals or teams at any stage of the discourse	"So, we're going to at least, uh, we gave her Lantus, yesterday, 10 mL?"
Management decision	Decisions made about the diagnosis or management plan of the patient	"We give erythromycin and we will discontinue that tomorrow and we will continue the rest of the antibiotics."
Information loss	1. Inaccurate recall: Recalled patient information that is inaccurate, where correct information is lost	1. Team member discusses patient having a history of diabetes, when the information available did not show this history
	2. Failure to follow up: Question posed by team member but never addressed in discourse	2. Team member asked if patient was passing urine but this question was never followed up
	3. Incomplete aggregation: All relevant information is not discussed because it was not considered necessary at the time	3. A case presenter omitted information, which was "relevant", for the purpose of summarizing
Inaccurate interpretation	Individual makes an assumption that isn't true; includes lack of knowledge	"…regular heart rate rhythm no murmurs…" when the patient had been in atrial fibrillation
Faulty decision-making	Most often a conceptual (not procedural) error in the process of decision-making in patient care	Admitting a patient to another unit from the ICU as an overflow when it is not permitted

aggregation") [27, 28]. Additionally, since errors in communication (including clinical content) are fundamental to our analysis, if an utterance contained or was related to an error, we categorized it as either "generated error," "corrected error," or "unresolved error." These terms are operationalized in Table 5.1. After coding 10 % of the transcripts, we expanded the taxonomy utilized by Apker and colleagues to reflect the specifics of ICU work and communication styles; the final coding taxonomy is included in Table 5.2. We provide a more detailed account of our data coding method and results in the following sections.

Table 5.2 Categories of coding for errors

Category	Description
Generated error	1. When the information uttered by a team member has something that is incorrect or doubtful; 2. Anything that is categorized as relevant information loss, inaccurate interpretation, or faulty decision-making
Unresolved error	1. When information is missing because it was not deemed relevant at the time and therefore was not collected 2. When a question or doubt goes unanswered and there is no way to tell what happened 3. When information is absent
Corrected error	1. When participants themselves or someone else corrects an error 2. When a mistake is detected and corrective actions are taken 3. When an incorrect interpretation or decision is corrected

Data Analysis: Descriptive Statistics

Descriptive statistics were used to describe the breakdown of utterances in different case management categories. Table 5.3 provides an example of team dialogue and how utterances were coded as unresolved errors, corrected errors, or statements not containing error. Chi-square tests were used to find significant deviations from expected distributions in the data.

Data Analysis: Qualitative

The transcripts were analyzed using (1) a method of discourse analysis, in particular, a version of team conversational analysis using *utterances* as units of speech examined, and (2) semantic network relationships, generated from these utterances or concepts used in the conversation by the team. To capture the temporal order of the conversation, the schematic structure of medical knowledge hierarchy from observations to findings was used [29]. The structure, by connecting observations (utterances) to findings (relevant observations) to facets (cluster of relevant findings) generate a path of decision flow, where the flow diagram was used to identify patterns of communication [30]. Observation types were further categorized into clinician and utterance types (error generated, error corrected, or neither).

Categories of Case Management

The data was first analyzed to determine if a common pattern of case management strategies found in our previous laboratory and semi-naturalistic studies could be identified in this team study. The seven components identified to form the basic structure of case management in an in-vivo setting are given in Table 5.1.

Table 5.3 An example of coding on a part of the team interaction transcript

Type of clinician	Transcript text	Case management category	Error type
Resident	Currently, her sodium is 134, her potassium is 2.9, chloride is 93, CO_2 is 25, BUN is 7, creatinine is 0.6 which is improving to 1.8, glucose is 138, calcium 8.2, phosphorus 60, mag 1.8,	Information aggregation	N/A
Resident	I am not sure if I requested it this morning…so…we have to check the orders and see.	Information loss	Unresolved error
Attending	And her K (potassium), do you know if you replaced her K this morning?	Additional information	N/A
Resident	I don't know.	Information loss	
Fellow	The K was at 80 this morning…no, it was at 145 this morning	Information aggregation	Corrected error
Resident	I haven't written them. I don't know if that is current.	Information loss	Corrected error
Resident	The thing is I just got the labs now…. yeah, she is at a total of 120 mg of plain and she is at 3.9, at first she got 40 mg and she dropped to 2.5, then she got 80 mg, then she was coming here and now she is 2.9.	Information aggregation	Corrected error
Attending	But, we don't know if that 2.9 was while she was getting the other K.	Wrong interpretation	Corrected error
Attending	I guess we wait one more day before we call…	Management decision	N/A

Figure 5.1 represents a framework for how case management categories relate to generation of error. The flow of case management categories towards management decision is presented in Fig. 5.1.

Categories of Error and Error Correction

Errors and error corrections were judged based on recognition of errors by the team and whether or not these errors were corrected. Errors were further detected for coding based on medical expertise from an uninvolved attending physician. If the team did not correct the error, the error was considered unresolved. Complete descriptions of generated errors, unresolved errors, and corrected errors can be found in Table 5.2. Errors were then connected in temporal order in the context of the topic discussed. Utterances relevant to the case that were neither errors nor corrections were marked as "not applicable."

Table 5.3 is an example from a transcript of one bed from the third day's interaction that illustrates the coding scheme. The case management categories that do not contain errors are patient information, additional information, information

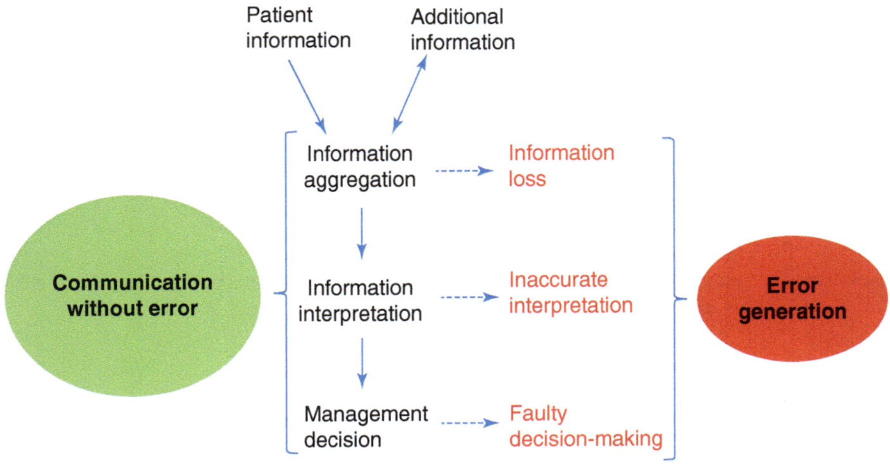

Fig. 5.1 Relationships between categories of case management and generation of errors

aggregation, information interpretation, and management decision. The categories that do contain errors are information loss, inaccurate interpretation, or faulty decision-making.

The teams have been collapsed in the following analyses to simplify the presentation of results. Additionally, since teams were made up of clinicians with different roles, to simplify presentation of data, the roles associated with the fewest utterances, including Case Manager, Intern, Nurse, Pharmacist, and Respiratory Technician, have been combined into the category "Other."

Our analysis shows that the team composition and communication at the bedside had following general characteristics: attendings dominated the conversation, producing 45.02 % of the interactions (as exemplified by utterances) in conversations during rounds. Residents were responsible for 21.60 % of the conversation, "other" clinicians for 13.27 %, and students for 10.07 %, and fellows for 10.04 % of the conversation. This pattern differed significantly from an even distribution of interaction among all clinicians on clinical rounds, $\chi^2(4)=497.04$, $p<.001$. This shows some hierarchy in team communication at the bedside during clinical rounds.

Errors Generated and Corrected

We first examined interactions in terms of errors generated and corrected. Overall, 74.40 % of the utterances made were case information that contained neither an error nor a correction, 11.42 % of which were not directly to the case, 8.40 % were errors, and 5.53 % were errors that were corrected.

Residents and Attending physicians were responsible for the greatest raw number of errors generated (75 and 74 raw errors, respectively, or 31.65 % and 31.22 %

Table 5.4 Number of errors generated (percentage of total utterances), corrected errors, and unresolved errors by all clinician types

	Generated errors	Corrected errors	Unresolved errors
Clinician type	# (%)	#	#
Attendings	74 (5.83)	41	33
Residents	75 (12.32)	54	21
Fellows	25 (8.93)	19	6
Students	27 (9.51)	20	7
Other clinicians	36 (9.63)	19	17
Total	237 (8.40)	153	84

of errors in the sample). Other Clinicians made 37 errors (15.19 %), students made 28 errors (11.39 %), and fellows made 25 errors (10.55 %).

When analyzed in comparison to the number of utterances produced by expertise, residents made the most errors (12.32 % of their total utterances), followed by other clinicians (9.63 %), students (9.51 %), and fellows (8.83 %). Attendings made the fewest errors (5.83 % of their total utterances).

Examination of the raw frequencies revealed that attendings made over half of all corrections (82, or 52.56 %), despite only one attending being present on each observed round, residents made 27 (17.31 %) corrections, other clinicians, 19 (12.18 %), fellows, 18 (11.54 %), and the students made 10 (6.41 %) corrections. When considered against the utterances produced by level of expertise, attendings had the largest percentage of corrections (6.46 % of their total utterances), followed very closely by fellows (6.36 %), other clinicians (5.08 %), residents (4.43 %), and students (3.52 %). Even though residents made the second highest number of corrections, because they produced so many utterances during the rounds, corrections accounted for a very low percentage of their total utterances. Number of errors generated (percentage of total utterances), corrected, and unresolved by all clinician types is given on Table 5.4.

In summary, errors accounted for a small proportion of the total number of interactions. In terms of raw numbers of errors, residents made the most errors, and attendings followed closely. Relative to the respective amount spoken, the proportion of utterances that were errors was greatest for residents, and smallest for attendings. This result is somewhat different from the Kubose and Patel study, where the expert made most errors as well as corrected most of them. However, this study was conducted in a different hospital cardio-thoracic IUC (in a busy urban setting) unlike our current study, where data was collected in general medical ICU.

Conversational Analysis: Utterance Categorization

Examining utterances at the level of case management categories shows that the three categories that contained errors included information loss (76.54 %

Table 5.5 Frequency and percentage of clinician errors by expertise

Error category	Clinician expertise				
	Attending	Resident	Fellow	Student	Other
Information loss	61 (82.43 %)	57 (76.0 %)	16 (64.0 %)	20 (71.43 %)	27 (75.0 %)
Inaccurate interpretation	3 (4.05 %)	12 (16.0 %)	6 (29.0 %)	5 (17.86 %)	6 (16.67 %)
Faulty decision-making	10 (13.51 %)	6 (8.0 %)	3 (12.0 %)	3 (10.71 %)	3 (8.33 %)

utterances), with wrong interpretation (13.17 % utterances), and faulty decision-making (10.29 % utterances).

Of the categories of conversation that contained errors, information loss was the largest. The task at the bedside is to make decisions about the patient management using the information at hand. This requires filtering out irrelevant information to make immediate decisions, and information loss at this point could indicate an editing process of the extra information that was not immediately necessary.

When all the categories under case management containing errors were analyzed, information loss constituted the largest category of error for all clinician types. Inaccurate interpretation made up the smallest percentage of attendings' errors, but made up a large proportion of the errors made by all other clinicians. Table 5.5 shows the frequency and percentage of clinician errors as a function of expertise. The role of the expert attending clinician becomes important in correcting inaccurate interpretation.

The temporal order of the case management categories relates to how errors are corrected or unresolved temporally and semantically. We provide two illustrated examples from segments of transcripts rather than a whole transcript of team conversation, in Fig. 5.2.

Decision Flow and the Correction of Errors

Figure 5.2 represents a sequence of conversation over time. This section of transcript from the first round, Bed 2, illustrates how errors are generated and are corrected in the course of team interaction. Table 5.3 contains the corresponding transcript to demonstrate the coding process. The objects with the light green fill were utterances said by the attending, those with the purple fill were said by the fellow, and those with the blue fill were said by resident. The utterances contained in the red hexagonal shapes are errors, those in ovals are corrections, and rectangular shapes represent other information important to the case that is neither an error nor a correction. The black arrows show temporal sequence of conversation while the red arrows show the backtracking from corrections to the errors that they corrected.

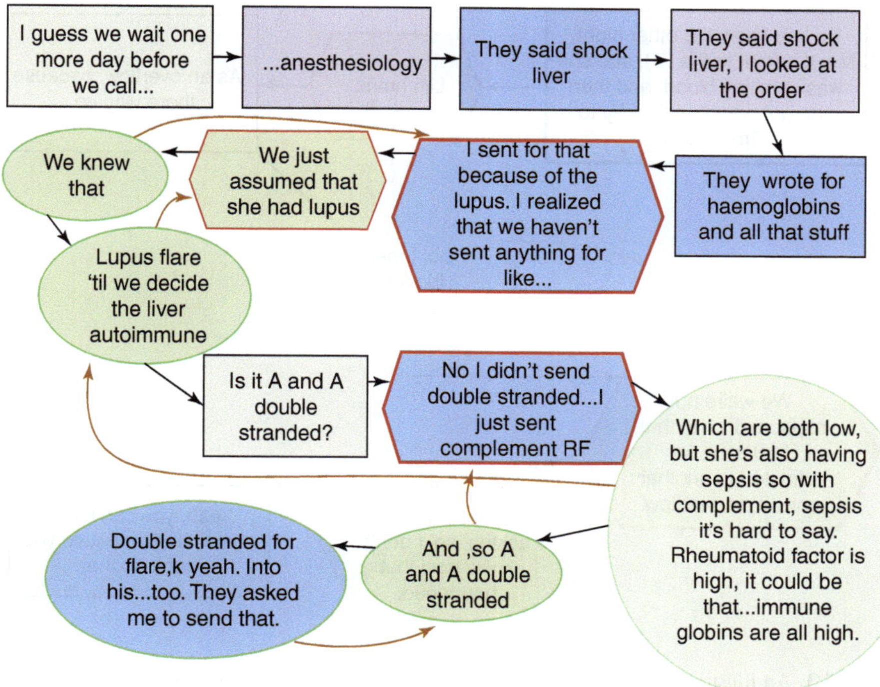

Fig. 5.2 An illustrative example of a decision flow diagram representing a segment of Team 1's interaction at the bedside of Bed 2 (See Table 5.3 for transcript)

An example of temporal events in a narrative text is given below:

Attending: So, is the Vanc ok? He is a little…yeah, you think we are going to over do it."

Interpretation asks if Vanc is at the right level

Resident: "When was it, yesterday?"

Interpretation asks when was Vanc given

Attending: "Ok. So if his urine output changes as his creatinine changes, we will re-check it again. Ok."

Interpretation: Will recheck Vanc if urine output changes

Although there is a temporal sequence to these utterances, there are also cognitive loopbacks from when the correction amends the error. One can see not only the flow of the conversation over time, but also the points in time when errors and corrections occurred and where the utterances refer to information that occurred earlier in the dialogue, illustrated by a backward directed flow. A similar pattern can be seen for Team 2, as shown in Fig. 5.3.

Figure 5.3 represents a sequence of utterances temporally as well as how errors are corrected from a section of transcript from the second round, Bed 4. The

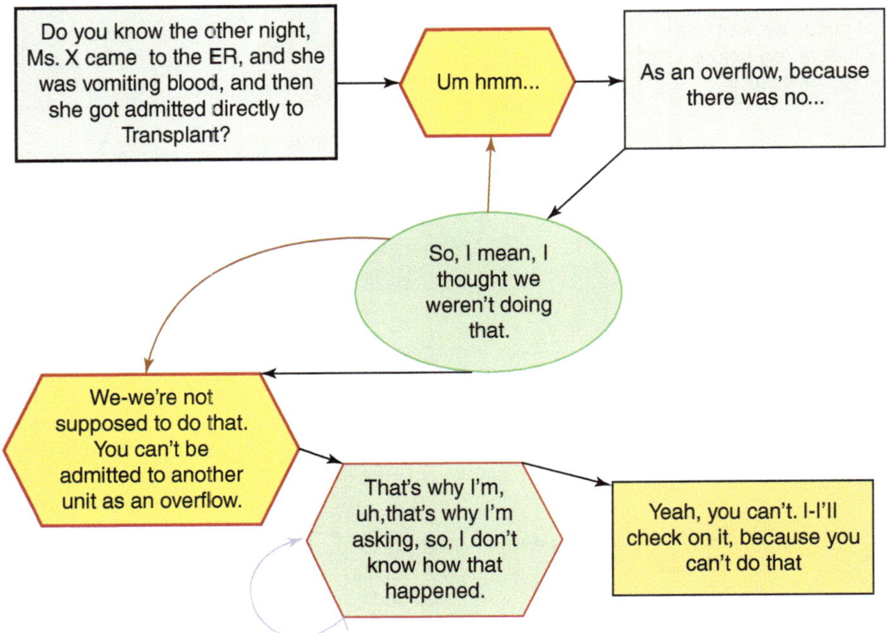

Fig. 5.3 An illustrative example of a decision flow diagram structure of a segment of Team 2's interaction at the bedside of Bed 4

transcript related to this figure is given on Table 5.6. The objects with the light green fill represent utterances made by the attending, while the nurse manager made those with the yellow fill. The utterances contained in the red hexagonal shapes are errors; those in ovals are corrections; rectangular shapes represent other information important to the case that is neither an error nor correction. The black arrows show temporal sequence while the red arrows show the backtracking from corrections to the errors that they corrected. The double-headed purple arrow represents an unresolved error.

As in Figs. 5.2 and 5.3 also shows the sequence of utterances as well cognitive loopback for a correction amending an error, or errors, but also shows an unresolved error and the possibility that it may propagate to patient care.

The example in Table 5.7 illustrates teamwork during clinical rounds. While the attending creates plans for the patient's care based on the underlying causes for their current condition, the resident and the fellow provide supporting information to assist in the attending's decision-making.

Relationship Between Error Correction and Error Propagation

Figure 5.2 represents a scenario where the error, or rather errors, was corrected to the point of what seems to be a resolution. This scenario involved errors surrounding the false assumed diagnosis of lupus, as well as sending for a test because of this

Table 5.6 Corresponding Clinical Round Transcript segment of Fig. 5.3

Type of clinician	Transcript text	Case management	Error type	Interpretation
Attending	Do you know the other night, Ms., Ms. ____ came to the ER, and she was vomiting blood, and then she got admitted directly to Transplant	Information aggregation	N/A	Asking nurse manager rhetorically if she knew of an issue with a patient
Nurse manager	Um hmm…	Faulty decision	Corrected error	Admitted patient directly as a transplant, can't do that
Attending	As an overflow, because, there was no…	Information aggregation	N/A	Letting nurse manager know the situation
Attending	So, I mean, I thought that, we weren't doing that, but.	Information aggregation	Corrected error	Corrects the notion that this procedure is allowed
Nurse manager	We-we're not supposed to do that. You can't be admitted to another unit as an overflow.	Faulty decision	Corrected error	Can't be admitted to another unit as overflow
Attending	That's why I'm, uh, that's why I'm asking, so, I don't know how that happened.	Information loss	Unresolved error	Doesn't know how that happened
Nurse manager	Yeah, you can't. I-I'll check on it, cause you can't do that.	Management decision	N/A	Agrees that this isn't correct and will check on the reason for this

assumed diagnosis, and the mistake of not sending out a particular test at all. The temporal order, or the path of the black arrows, shows the flow of information being given at each sequential slice of time, such as thinking the lupus test was not sent, then the assumption of lupus, and then the revelation of the team already knowing the test was sent. The cognitive loopbacks show how the corrections go back to rectify the errors made. For example, the team knowing the test was sent corrected the thinking that the lupus test was not sent. Sometimes two corrections will correct one error because of the semantics of the statements and the knowledge pieces that need to be put together. This can be clearly seen in the path of the red arrows.

In contrast, Fig. 5.3 represents a scenario where two errors are amended by one correction and one error is unresolved. The attending physician's utterance, "So I mean, I thought that, we weren't doing that," corrects both of the nurse manager's

Table 5.7 Clinical Round Transcript segment from Bed 5, Day 2

Type of clinician	Transcript text	Case management	Error type	Interpretation
Attending	Ok, we seem to have cultures yesterday. We still want him to get a perm cap, hopefully Monday if things start to defervesce on the weekend.	Management decision	N/A	Creates a plan for how to proceed given the patient's status
Attending	Because I am not sure he is really having renal recovery.	Information loss	Unresolved error	Does not know reason for current status
Attending	How much urine output do we have?	Additional information	N/A	Requests information
Resident	335	Information aggregation	N/A	Provides information
Fellow	345	Information aggregation	N/A	Provides information
Attending	355? 345? So, I mean that's something, but I am not sure.	Information loss	Unresolved error	Unclear results supporting the renal recovery hypothesis
Attending	Sure, I guess we'll just keep the foley then just to keep monitoring.	Management decision	N/A	Plans to continue monitoring condition
Attending	Ok, what is EUA yesterday?	Additional information	N/A	Requests information
Resident	I didn't write it down	Information loss	Unresolved error	Cannot provide information
Attending	His UA? We sent to UA for his fever.	Additional information	N/A	Attempts to clarify request
Fellow	…urine cultures are negative, blood cultures are negative, sputum cultures are negative	Information aggregation	N/A	Provides information

utterances, "Um hmm…" (In response to knowing that an error was made by sending a patient to an unit inappropriate for them) and "We-we're not supposed to do that. You can't be admitted to another unit as an overflow," because the nurse manager's utterances are of the same nature, since the nurse manager was either unaware or did not take appropriate actions to admit the patient to the proper unit. However, the error in which the attending did not know why the patient was admitted directly to the transplant unit was unresolved, since there was never a way to find out what really happened.

In summary, both Figs. 5.2 and 5.3 represent scenarios where errors are generated but then are corrected. However, in Fig. 5.3, the attending and the nurse manager attempt to resolve the misunderstanding, where the error remains unresolved.

Summary of Results and Discussion

In this section, we summarize our key findings from this pilot study.

The attending clinician spoke the most at the rounds, generated many errors, but also made the most corrections. This result is similar to the Kubose/Patel study of the ICU environment at another institution [22]. An expert's ability to correct or to recover from errors they generate in real world ICU appears to be more generic, as it reflects the findings from studies outside of medical domain.

Two-thirds of the errors generated were corrected during the three clinical rounds, leaving one-third unresolved. There were a few self-corrections of errors during patient round discussions, while most errors were corrected by more experienced members of the clinical team, especially the attending. This result is unlike the results from Kubose/Patel study, where most errors were self-corrected by the expert, although senior clinical team members did assist in error correction. The nature of Cardiothoracic ICU appears to demand a different nature of task and urgency than the medical ICU errors. The unresolved errors were picked up later in the discussion in the surgical unit, but we did not analyze the MICU rounds data any further to look at unsolved errors over time.

For all levels of expertise, information loss was the biggest category of errors. Large amounts of information has to be managed at the bedside such that relevant information is on focus for making quick decisions to manage the patient. Information loss is inevitable at this stage. However, any loss of information that is clinically relevant at the point of care at that moment can lead to adverse consequences for the patient. In the surgical ICU study, the focus was on the minimum amount of information that was necessary to deal with the patient at hand. This could relate to the nature of the patients in medical and surgical ICU.

There are many factors (e.g. time pressure, multitasking) that play a role in decision making in the naturalistic, complex working environment of the ICU, creating greater opportunities for the clinical team to generate errors, as compared to the semi-naturalistic conditions and lab-based studies. Patient management plans for one patient is completed before moving on to another patient, making sure that there are not too many problems left unresolved, leaving little time or lengthy discussion of any errors. They are quickly corrected, where possible. In the surgical ICU, the time pressure and multitasking are big factors, given that the unit has many technologies and the team uses these constantly during the clinical rounds. This is somewhat unlike the MICU environment.

In our previous research, individual clinicians allowed more errors in a sample case to propagate to the level of care than the teams in a semi-naturalistic study. In the current study, set in a naturalistic setting, errors were corrected at a ratio of 2 to

1. These errors were not exclusively patient management errors, of the sort embedded in our laboratory-based and semi-naturalistic examples. Rather, errors in information transfer and interpretation were more frequently encountered. The teams performed better in detecting and correcting errors, given the goal-directed nature of tasks in an ICU environment. It appears that the complex environment of critical care also helps in creating error checks, where people are on high alert.

Conclusions and Final Comments

The results from this pilot study in the MICU, together with the results from the earlier study by Kubose/Patel, add to our understanding of the nature of error generation and correction in the ICU in an in-vivo situation. The results of the pilot studies necessitate more careful systematic investigation of team interactions for decision-making in critical care and the pressures that push clinicians to make mistakes as well as to correct them. We will provide our final comments on the next steps in our investigations as well as some thought on the relationship between performance and learning in critical care.

Our earlier studies show that physicians' ability to detect errors in clinical problems in the intensive medical care domain is limited when tested individually in laboratory-based conditions (Chaps. 3 and 6). We extended this study to explore the mechanism of error detection and correction when working in teams, using (a) semi-naturalistic and (b) naturalistic empirical paradigms. The data were collected in a medical intensive care unit and were analyzed for the process of patient management and the frequency and nature of errors generated and corrected. The results show that the teams perform better than individuals, due to the advantages conferred by the distribution of cognitive tasks across multiple team members. Attendings and residents were found to generate more errors as well as recover from most of them in a real world setting. This was not the case in studies under other conditions.

However, in interpreting these results it is important to note the distinctions between this naturalistic work and our previous experiments that would limit the interpretation of our results. All of the errors embedded in the case scenarios used in our previous experiments were patient management errors (the subjects were asked to do evaluate the patient management), but most of the errors observed in practice were related to information loss related to direct patient care (because data had to be collected and aggregated). As discussed previously, attending physicians do not bear the burden of collecting and aggregating information. Rather, their clinician colleagues conduct this work.

Error detection and correction in a situation closer to complex real world practice appear to induce certain urgency for quick action resulting in rapid detection and correction. Here, complexity appears to put in some error checks. Furthermore, teams working at the bedside in real world optimize performance (finalizing decisions in very short period of time) with little room for explicating any mistakes and thus little learning from errors. There is a close relationship between competency in delivery of patient care and the need to minimize errors. This is juxtaposed with the competing demand for learning from errors, an essential part of the apprentice training process.

Errors in the healthcare environment can be fatal to a patient, and so the ultimate goal is to reduce or eliminate them. However, errors are also a necessary part of the learning process. During clinical rounds (also known as *teaching rounds* or *patient rounds*), the team is focused on patient management to provide competent patient care. Another purpose of these rounds is to mentor trainees and elaborate on the mistakes individuals or the teams make, in order to ensure that trainees are given the opportunity to learn. In the real world critical care environment, clinicians minimize learning and optimize performance when the goal is to focus on patient care. However, this is not true for situations in which the real world is simulated and there is no danger of harming the patient. This later condition provides the opportunity to make mistakes and learn from them without compromising patient safety. A combination of both mechanisms with a feedback loop is thus required, which promotes both competent patient care and learning opportunities.

Discussion Questions

1. The airline industry has been successful in managing human error to a large extent, but this is not true in the healthcare system. Discuss some of the challenges related to the management of human error faced by the healthcare system (namely, critical care) that are distinct from those encountered in the aviation context.
2. Studies on error detection and correction by health professionals show different results in naturalistic (in-vivo) and laboratory-based (in-vitro) environments. Discuss some of the factors that may contribute to these differences.
3. One needs to generate errors to learn from them and yet generation of errors, if not corrected, compromises patient safety. How might one reconcile these two positions?

References

1. Patel VL, Cohen T, Murarka T, Olsen J, Kagita S, Myneni S, et al. Recovery at the edge of error: debunking the myth of the infallible expert. J Biomed Inform. 2011;44(3):413–24.
2. Abraham J, Kannampallil T, Patel VL. Bridging gaps in handoffs: a continuity of care approach. J Biomed Inform. 2012;45(2):240–54.
3. Lipshitz R, Klein GA, Orasanu J, Salas E. Taking stock of naturalistic decision making. J Behav Decis Mak. 2001;14:331–52.
4. Reason J. Human error. Cambridge: Cambridge University Press; 1990.
5. Dekker S. The field guide to understanding human error. 2nd ed. Burlington: Ashgate Publishing; 2006.

6. Kontogiannis T, Malakis S. A proactive approach to human error detection and identification in aviation and air traffic control. Saf Sci. 2009;47(5):693–706.
7. Kontogiannis T. A framework for the analysis of cognitive reliability in complex systems: a recovery centered approach. Reliability Eng Syst Saf. 1998;58:233–48.
8. Orasanu J. Crew collaboration in space: a naturalistic decision-making perspective. Aviat Space Environ Med. 2005;76(6, Section II):B154–63.
9. Orasanu J, Martin L, editors. Errors in aviation decision making: a factor in accidents and incidents. Second workshop on human error, safety, and system development. Seattle, Washington; 1998.
10. Meso P, Troutt MD, Rudnicka J. A review of naturalistic decision making research with implications for knowledge management. J Knowl Manage. 2002;6(1):63–73.
11. Simon HA. Rational choice and the structure of the environment. In: Simon HA, editor. Models of man. New York: John Wiley; 1957.
12. Klein GA. Naturalistic decision making. Hum Factors. 2008;50(3):456–60.
13. Plant KL, Stanton NA. Why did the pilots shut down the wrong engine? Explaining errors in context using schema theory and the perceptual cycle model. Saf Sci. 2012;50(2):300–15.
14. Oser R, McCallum G, Salas E, Morgan BBJ. Toward a definition of teamwork: an analysis of critical team behaviors division HF; 1989. Contract no.: 89-004.
15. Paris CR, Salas E, Cannon-Bowers JA. Teamwork in multi-person systems: a review and analysis. Ergonomics. 2000;43(8):1052–75.
16. Fiore SM, Rosen MA, Smith-Jentsch KA, Salas E, Letsky M, Warner N. Toward an understanding of macrocognition in teams: predicting processes in complex collaborative contexts. J Hum Factors Ergon Soc. 2010;52(2):203–44.
17. Christensen C, Larson JR. Collaborative medical decision making. Med Decis Mak. 1993;13(4):339–46.
18. Tschan F, Semmer NK, Gurtner A, Bizzari L, Spychiger M, Breuer M, et al. Explicit reasoning, confirmation bias, and illusory transactive memory: a simulation study of group medical decision making. Small Group Res. 2009;40(3):271–300.
19. Abraham J, Nguyen VC, Almoosa KF, Patel B, Patel VL. Falling through the cracks: information breakdowns in critical care handoff communication. Washington, DC: American Medical Informatics Association (AMIA); 2011.
20. Larson JR, Christensen C, Abbott AS, Franz TM. Diagnosing groups: charting the flow of information in medical decision-making teams. J Pers Soc Psychol. 1996;71(2):315–30.
21. Patel VL, Kaufman DR, Magder SA. The acquisition of medical expertise in complex dynamic environments. In: Ericsson A, editor. The road to excellence: the acquisition of expert performance in the arts and sciences, sports and games. Hillsdale: Lawrence Erlbaum Publishers; 1996. p. 127–65.
22. Kubose TT, Patel VL, Jordan D, editors. Dynamic adaptation to critical care medical environment: error recovery as cognitive activity. In: Proceedings of the 2002 Cognitive Science Society. Fairfax, Virginia; 2002.
23. Abraham J, Kannampallil T, Patel B, Almoosa KF, Patel VL, editors. Ensuring patient safety in care transitions: an empirical evaluation of a handoff intervention tool. Chicago: Proceedings of AMIA 2012; 2012.
24. Laxmisan A, Hakimzada F, Sayan OR, Green RA, Zhang J, Patel VL. The multitasking clinician: decision-making and cognitive demand during and after team handoffs in emergency care. Int J Med Inform. 2007;76(11–12):801–11.
25. Patel VL, Arocha JF, Kaufman DR. Diagnostic reasoning and medical expertise. In: The psychology of learning and motivation: advances in research and theory, vol. 31. San Diego, CA Academic Press; 1994. p. 137–252.
26. George AL, McKeown TJ. Case studies and theories of organizational decision making. Adv Inf Process Org. 1985;2:21–58.
27. Owen WF. Interpretive themes in relational communication. Q J Speech. 1984;70:274–87.

28. Apker J, Mallak LA, Gibson SC. Communicating in the "gray zone:" perceptions of emergency physician-hospitalist handoff communication and patient safety. Acad Emerg Med. 2007;14:884–994.
29. Patel VL, Evans DA, Groen GJ. Biomedical knowledge and clinical reasoning. In: Evans DA, Patel VL, editors. Cognitive science in medicine: biomedical modeling. Cambridge: MIT Press; 1989. p. 53–112.
30. Patel VL, Kaufman DR, Allen VG, Shortliffe EH, Cimino JJ, Greenes RA. Toward a framework for computer-mediated collaborative design in medical informatics. Methods Inf Med. 1999;38:158–76.

Chapter 6
Training for Error Detection in Simulated Clinical Rounds

Elie Razzouk, Trevor Cohen, Khalid F. Almoosa, and Bela Patel

Introduction

In previous chapters, we have discussed experimental results that show that individual clinicians have difficulty detecting errors embedded in descriptions of clinical case scenarios, even when these errors are egregious in nature with life-threatening consequences for the hypothetical patient concerned. As one might anticipate on account of the additional attention and expertise they provide, teams of clinicians appear better equipped to perform this task than individuals. However,

---

Portions of this chapter, including Sections 2, 3, and 4, appeared in an article in the Proceedings of the 2012 Annual Symposium American Medical Informatics Association, Razzouk et al., *Approaching the Limits of Knowledge: The Influence of Priming on Error Detection in Simulated Clinical Rounds.*

E. Razzouk, MD, MS (✉)
Internal Medicine, Miller School of Medicine, University of Miami,
West Palm Beach, FL 33462, USA
e-mail: elierazzouk@yahoo.com

T. Cohen, MB ChB, PhD
School of Biomedical Informatics, University of Texas Health Science Center,
Houston, TX 77054, USA
e-mail: trevor.cohen@uth.tmc.edu

K.F. Almoosa, MD, MS, FCCP
Division of Critical Care Medicine, Memorial Hermann Hospital, Texas Medical Center,
Houston, TX 77030, USA

University of Texas Health Science Center, Houston, TX, USA
e-mail: khalid.f.almoosa@uth.tmc.edu

B. Patel, MD, DABSM, FCCP
University of Texas Health Science Center, Houston, TX, USA

Division of Critical Care Medicine, Memorial Hermann Hospital, Texas Medical Center,
Houston, TX 77030, USA

V.L. Patel et al. (eds.), *Cognitive Informatics in Health and Biomedicine*,
Health Informatics, DOI 10.1007/978-1-4471-5490-7_6, © Springer-Verlag London 2014

given that individual team members initiate the detection of error by teams, it remains desirable to enhance the performance of individual clinicians in this regard. In this chapter, we discuss a line of research that involves the use of simulated clinical rounds conducted in the context of a virtual world, a three-dimensional immersive computer-generated environment, for two purposes. Firstly, these simulated clinical rounds are used as a research tool, providing the means to evaluate error detection in conditions more closely approximating real-world rounds while maintaining experimental control. Subsequently, the same simulated rounds are embedded in an automated tutoring system focused specifically on error detection.

The Role of Clinical Rounds in Error Recovery

Clinical settings have been described as error prone complex systems where individuals' actions are interconnected and unpredictable. Within such environments, it is unrealistic to expect flawless performance, as some degree of error is to be anticipated on account of learning, conflicts and limited resources in the face of high demand [1]. Furthermore, research in highly complex fields other than medicine has shown that error recovery has a pronounced impact on safety [2]. However, relatively little is known about the processes that underlie error detection and recovery in medical settings.

Clinical rounds serve as a focal point for communication, decision-making, transition of care, and teaching. Frequent rounds remain an important part of the daily routine of clinical teams: on rounds different participants rapidly aggregate information from different sources to make clinical decisions [3]. Additionally, the lack of such rounds resulted in an increase in mortality, cardiac arrests, and other adverse events in specific settings [4]. Furthermore, rounds have been observed to be an important focal point for detection of, and recovery from medical errors [5]. Following lengthy ethnographic observations of an intensive care clinical team, Kubose, Patel, and colleagues determined that foci of high interactivity among physicians lead to higher incidence of error detection [6]. In particular, it was observed that a higher number of errors were detected in clinical rounds than in handovers, which involve fewer participants. Similarly, ethnographic observation revealed clinical rounds in a psychiatric emergency department (PED) to be a source of high-yield data for incidents of error recovery. Analysis of audio recordings of these rounds highlighted the importance of error recovery for overall patient safety and uncovered several errors with potentially harmful consequences [5]. Similar work done in other emergency departments demonstrated the role of communication and other strategies among nursing team members in detection and recovery from error [7]. Retrospective data obtained from an accident reporting system used in two hospitals in Belgium demonstrated the importance of standard checks in error detection [8].

In more recent work, also described in this volume, Patel and her colleagues employed a novel experimental paradigm using errors embedded in paper-based case scenarios to study error detection and recovery among experts and trainees [9].

Overall, error detection and recovery correlated poorly with years of experience. Additionally, no subject detected more than half of the embedded errors, regardless of level of expertise. If this laboratory-determined limit on error detection is an accurate reflection of the rate of detection "in the wild", the implications for patient safety are disturbing and urgent.

As acknowledged by the authors, this study had certain limitations. Firstly, the study design did not incorporate a method to discern whether failure to detect an error occurred on account of lack of knowledge, or for some other reason. A deeper understanding of the mechanisms that underlie failed error detection is required if we are to develop interventions to better equip current and future clinicians to detect and recover from potentially dangerous errors. In particular it is necessary to distinguish between a lack of the knowledge required to detect an error, and the failure to apply this knowledge, as these conditions suggest different intervention strategies. Moreover, information on rounds is generally presented verbally rather than as written text, and the presentation frequently involves input from several members of a clinical team. It is possible that the additional cognitive effort required to synthesize verbal information from multiple sources plays a role in the process of error recovery. Ideally, error recovery and detection would be studied in a setting that better approximates a clinical round, as it has been shown that error recovery frequently occurs in such settings.

The Virtual World as Research Instrument

This chapter documents a novel approach to the study of error detection and recovery in the context of clinical rounds using an immersive virtual world to approximate the information interchange that occurs on rounds, while retaining the control necessary to ensure the consistency of experimental conditions across subjects. A virtual world is a computer-based simulated environment, through which users can interact with scripted programs or with one another. Within a virtual world, users are embodied as avatars, virtual representations of themselves that they can direct to explore the environment and interact with it and other users. Virtual worlds are becoming increasingly popular in medical domains and are proving to be cost-effective and reliable training methods [10]. In some studies, virtual mentors have proven to be superior to traditional training and teaching methods [11]. The ability of virtual worlds to approximate real world settings has proved important for their role as training tools, and suggests a viable alternative for the study of error detection and recovery in a naturalistic setting without disturbing real-world clinical workflow. For our present purposes, virtual worlds provide the opportunity to maintain experimental control, such that all participants receive the same information in the same way, while providing a better approximation of a real-world clinical round than is provided by paper-based scenarios. The original purpose of our virtual world was to serve as a laboratory instrument through which we could present scripted scenarios in order to capture and study clinicians' cognitive and decision making processes.

Construction of a Virtual ICU

There are a variety of tools that can be used to build virtual worlds. Popular tools include Opensimulator (http://opensim.org) and Second Life (http://secondlife.com). Opensimulator (OpenSim) is an open source project that provides a host server for virtual worlds that can be accessed by a variety of clients. As is the case with the better-known SecondLife platform, it has the ability to support clients that allow for the visual exploration of three-dimensional virtual environments in real time. However, unlike SecondLife, the platform is open source and available for download. Users can maintain their own servers, and consequently do not need to pay fees for virtual real estate, or for the upload of graphics or sound files. The platform has attracted projects from companies such as Intel and IBM, which provide examples of the commercial prospects of virtual environments [13]. Scripting offers the ability to control and simulate events within virtual environments, and can be implemented in a variety of languages such as Linden Scripting Language (LSL), Opensim Scripting Language (OSSL), and C# using the OpenMetaverse library. OpenSim is supported by an active development community.

The environment simulating an Intensive Care Unit setting was developed using OpenSim due to the ease with which scripting languages can control this platform. Functions within the OpenMetaverse library were scripted using the C# programming language to gain control over characters representing the different participants in the multidisciplinary rounds. These functions allow us to control the timing with which and sequence in which recorded audio files are played. It is this strict control that allows us to successfully simulate a multidisciplinary round. The characters representing the various participants in the rounds include two residents, a nurse, a pharmacist, a respiratory therapist, a medical student, an attending physician, and a character representing the subject immersed in the round. There were several steps that were required to arrange and organize the rounds, depicted in Fig. 6.1. The first step was to build the world using OpenSim in-world building tools. Following that step, spoken dialog for each character on the round was recorded, and the audio files were partitioned into 10-s segments and uploaded to each character accordingly. The audio files were later organized using a C# program that calls the audio files at 10 s allowing for synchronization of the speaking roles performed by the various characters participating in the round. In addition to verbal interactions, characters communicated using gestures. In collaboration with a domain expert in non-verbal communication, customized gestures were developed using the animation tool qavimator (http://www.qavimator.org), and synchronized with the audio files using the C# script. These processes were not entirely straightforward and, as is often the case with bleeding edge open source code, we were occasionally surprised by unanticipated events such as the inexplicable disappearance of our characters' appendages, clothing or eyeballs during the development phase. However, we managed to resolve these problems prior to conducting our experiments. A screenshot of the resulting round is included in Fig. 6.2.

While not within the scope of this chapter, we note that the development of our rounds was informed by ethnographic data gathered in the course of other related

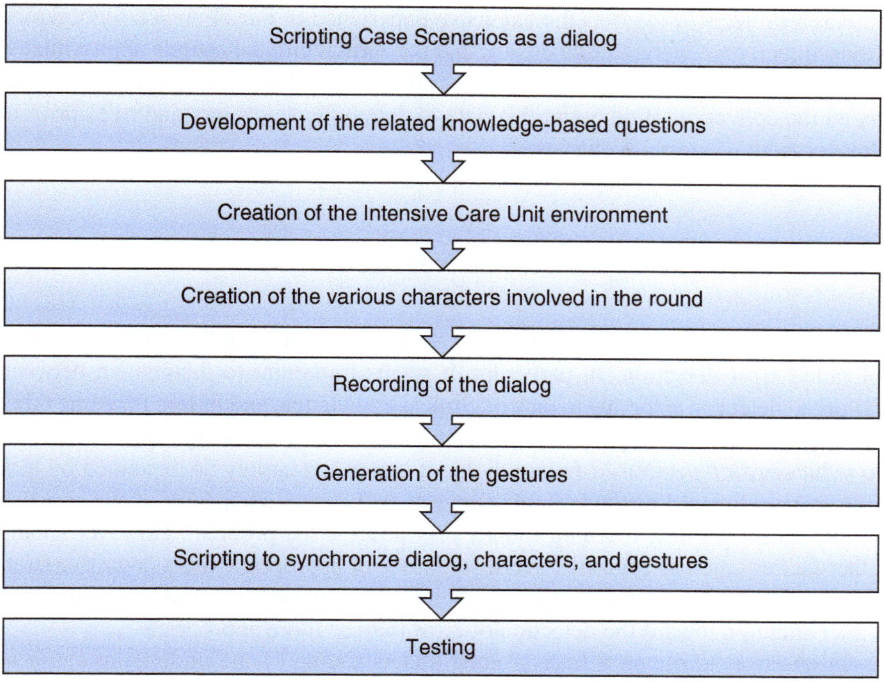

Fig. 6.1 Steps in the process of building virtual rounds

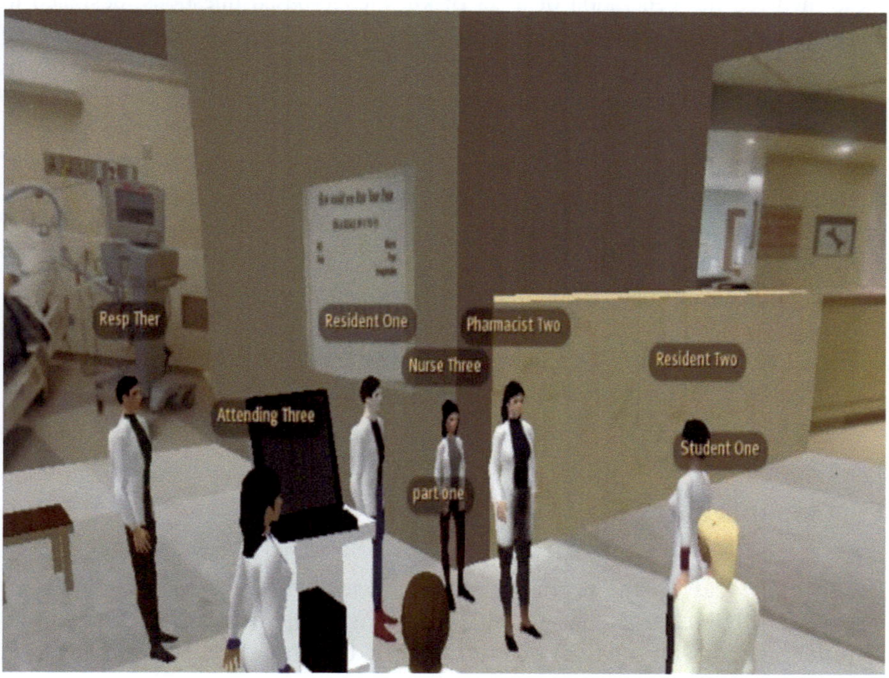

Fig. 6.2 A screenshot from the rounds within Opensim

research projects, as well as the extensive experience of our clinical collaborators. Consequently we were able to ensure that the virtual clinical rounds approximated actual clinical rounds. Without the availability of data of this sort, we would recommend the collection of ethnographic data to define the key actors and roles prior to development of virtual scenarios.

Failed Detection: Ignorance or Negligence?

An issue of importance related to error recovery has to do with the underlying cause of failed error detection. In particular, it seems important to distinguish between failure to detect an error due to lack of clinical knowledge, and failure for some other reason, as each of these possibilities has implications for the design of interventions to reduce error detection. If failure to detect errors can largely be explained by lack of relevant clinical knowledge, this suggests that didactic teaching of the sort that occurs during clinical teaching rounds may address the problem. However should other factors, such as cognitive overload or lack of appropriate meta-cognitive strategies play important roles, interventions that aim to preserve cognitive resources or direct attention toward the detection of error may be more appropriate.

In an effort to obtain a finer grained understanding of the underlying cause of failed error detection, we made two additions to our previous experimental protocol, in addition to moving from paper based cases to virtual clinical rounds. The first of these involved the generation of a set of knowledge-based questions, designed to elicit the clinical knowledge required to detect each of the errors embedded in the cases presented on the simulated rounds. So we would anticipate errors missed due to lack of knowledge being accompanied by an incorrect answer to the related question. In contrast, errors missed due to inattention or any other cause should have correctly answered related questions. In addition, in one of the two cases each participant was alerted to the presence of errors within the case, and explicitly asked to detect these errors. We refer to this process as *priming*, a term we use in the sense it which has been employed previously in medical education, where it refers to the process of orienting participants beforehand to the tasks and objectives they may have [14].

We anticipated that this combination of knowledge-based questions and priming would allow us to identify the extent to which participants were able to detect errors within the limits of their knowledge, with and without priming.

Participants and Case Construction

In order to focus on the processes of error detection in the Medical Intensive Care Unit (MICU), participants (N = 17) consisting of interns, residents, and fellows were recruited for the study. As part of the MICU team, all the subjects involved

Table 6.1 Examples of errors embedded in the case scenarios A and B

1. The coagulopathy (failure to form blood clots) was not corrected. This could have contributed to the bleeding that occurred in the case (Case B)
2. The gastrointestinal team did not come in earlier to do an esophagogastroduodenoscopy (Case B)
3. Paracentesis (a procedure through which fluid is removed from the abdominal cavity, often for the purpose of microbiological studies to detect infective organisms) should be done before or soon after antibiotics are started, so the antibiotics do not interfere with subsequent microbiological studies of the fluid (Case B)
4. Gentamycin is not the drug of choice for someone with renal insufficiency, as this drug is well known to have toxic effects on the kidneys (Case B)
5. The intravenous steroid dose is insufficient (Case A)
6. Dopamine was started instead of epinephrine (Case A)
7. No blood cultures were taken (Case A)
8. Gastrointestinal stress ulcer prophylaxis was not started (Case A)

were actively taking part in patient care, participating in clinical rounds, and making important management decisions. Two case scenarios were developed to represent typical ICU cases that trainees face over their month-long rotation at the medical intensive care unit. Our clinical collaborator and co-author, (KA), a practicing physician who is board-certified in internal medicine, pulmonary medicine, and critical care medicine, developed these scenarios and embedded errors with varying degrees of complexity and severity.

The main focus during the development of the cases was to maintain clinical plausibility. Therefore the number of errors included in each case was determined by the plausibility of the clinical scenario itself, and are not balanced across the cases. The first case scenario involved a patient with sepsis, and had six embedded errors, while the second involved a patient with a gastrointestinal bleed, and had 15 embedded errors. The study design, which will be discussed further in this section, compensates for these differences. Examples of errors embedded in case scenarios A and B are shown in Table 6.1.

After logging in to the world, subjects were taught to control their avatars, and given the opportunity to explore the virtual ICU. The subjects were then instructed to listen carefully to the first case presented (note taking was permitted), and subsequently asked to summarize this case and comment on the management. These responses were audio-recorded, for subsequent transcription and analysis. For the second case, the instructions were identical except that participants were explicitly told that the team responsible for the patient had committed a number of management errors. After each case, participants were asked to respond to a set of paper based questions that aimed to elicit the clinical knowledge required to detect each of the errors in the case concerned. Participants were assigned to two groups of approximately equal size. The first of these groups participated in the simulation of case A first, and then participated in the simulation of case B once primed. This order was reversed for the second group, which experienced case B first, before priming occurred.

Defining the Limits of Knowledge

In our evaluation of the results of this study, we were particularly interested in the extent to which participants reached their potential in the primed and unprimed state. A trainee cannot be expected to detect errors in cases in which their knowledge is lacking, and failed detection of this sort can only be addressed by imparting the knowledge required, which is the desired outcome of a training program. As trainees are not expected to have perfect knowledge, and trainees conduct much of clinical care at academic institutions, the finding that most trainees already operate at their full potential for error recovery would limit the opportunity for interventions to improving supervision. In contrast, the finding that priming improved error detection would raise the possibility of other interventions, as we will subsequently discuss.

To characterize the extent to which our participants detected errors within the limits of their clinical knowledge, we defined the detection ratio (DR) for a case as follows:

$$\mathrm{DR}(\mathrm{case}) = \frac{\text{errors detected}}{\text{correctly answered questions}}$$

We note that each error available for detection was related to exactly one knowledge-based question, and that it was the case throughout our data set that participants detected errors if and only if they also correctly answered the relevant knowledge-based question. There was no significant difference in detection ratio across the two cases. The results of these experiments are shown in Figs. 6.3, 6.4 and 6.5.

Figures 6.3 and 6.4 summarize both the detection of error, and the answering of knowledge based questions, for each group in each of the two experimental conditions (primed and unprimed). Error detection overall was limited, with subjects on average detecting 20.3 % of all embedded errors in case A, and 37.2 % of embedded errors in case B. As was the case with our previous paper-based studies [9], the low rates of error detection observed in the laboratory have alarming implications for patient safety. While teams in the context of a real-world clinical round appear collectively better equipped to detect errors than individuals in virtual clinical rounds (see the preceding chapter concerning these studies for further details), we note that similarly alarming rates of error detection have been observed in another context: one observational study of passenger airline flight crews during normal operations reported detection of less than half of all errors noted by expert observers [15].

The order of case presentation was reversed in each group, so the case seen prior to priming of Group 1 (Case A) was seen after priming by Group 2. This case appears to have been more difficult, as the average score for the knowledge-based questions for both groups was less than 50 % for this case. In contrast, for the case seen after priming by Group 1 (Case B), the average score on the knowledge-based

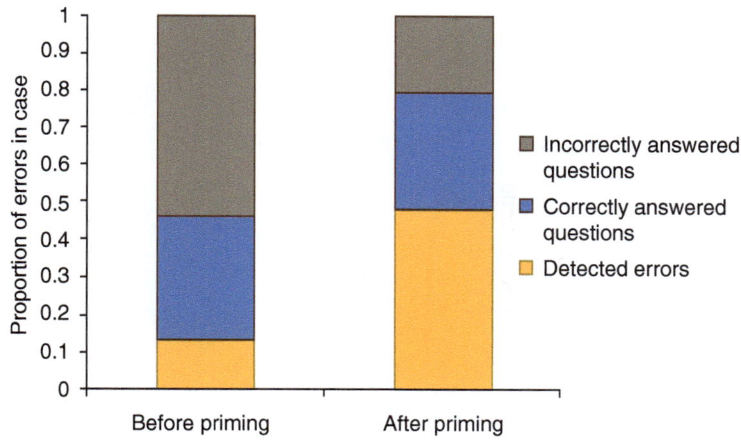

Fig. 6.3 Results for Group 1. The *lower* bar shows the proportion of total errors detected. The *middle* bar shows the proportion of questions that were correctly answered, and therefore represents the limits of the clinical knowledge of the participant concerned. Consequently, the proportion of the *middle* bar that is occupied by the *lower* bar represents the detection ratio

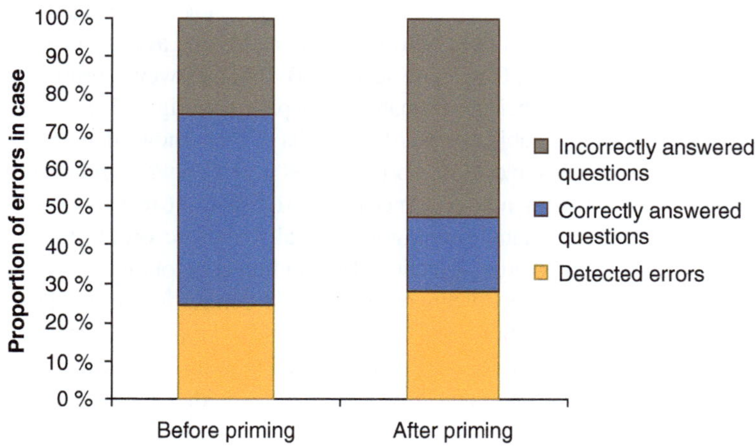

Fig. 6.4 Results for Group 2. The *lower* bar shows the proportion of total errors detected. The *middle* bar shows the proportion of questions that were correctly answered, and therefore represents the limits of the clinical knowledge of the participant concerned. Consequently, the proportion of the *middle* bar that is occupied by the *lower* bar represents the detection ratio

questions was greater than 70 % for both groups. This indicates that, on average, each group had similar knowledge resources. Figures 6.3 and 6.4 also show that the proportion of the errors that could have been detected that were detected (the DR, shown as the ratio between the lower (yellow) bar and the middle (blue) bar) was higher in both groups in the primed condition. This result is highlighted in Fig. 6.5, which shows the average detection ratio across all participants in the primed and unprimed condition.

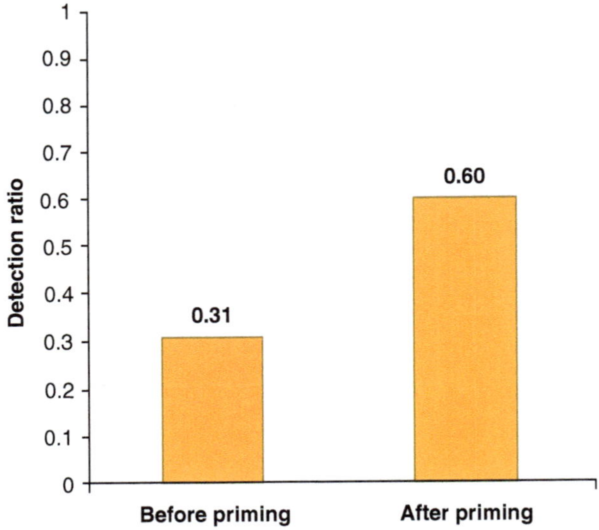

Fig. 6.5 Mean detection ratio with and without priming. The difference is statistically significant ($t(16)=5.1870, p<0.00001$)

Subjects cannot be expected to detect knowledge-based errors without possessing the prerequisite knowledge. As illustrated in Figs. 6.1 and 6.2, subjects' knowledge acts as a ceiling for their error detection rate. Across case scenarios, the average detection ratio was similar (Case scenario A: 0.44, Case scenario B: 0.47). However, priming subjects had a substantial effect on their performance as depicted in Fig. 6.5. Priming clearly shifted the performance of subjects toward the limits of their knowledge. Furthermore, the mean detection ratio of subjects after priming (DR = 59.9 %) was significantly higher than that of subjects who were not yet primed (DR = 31.1 %) ($t(16)=5.1870, p<0.0001$).

This suggests that clinicians listening to clinical rounds according to their usual practice exhibit sub-optimal error detection. This finding is encouraging, as it suggests a role for intervention. While we cannot pro-actively correct for all possible knowledge deficits, these results show that clinicians are capable of performance that is considerably better than their baseline, and suggest that it may be possible to develop training programs that shift error detection toward an individual's knowledge ceiling.

Training for Error Recovery

How then, might we design training programs that aim to enhance error detection and recovery in medicine? The notion of training for error recovery explicitly has been proposed in other domains. For example, Naikar and Saunders propose the training of domain-specific skills to promote error management in military pilots, by creating simulations of situations in which the boundaries of safe practice have been violated [16]. Their proposal involves the development of scenarios based on critical events that had occurred during a mission, such that pilots have the opportunity to practice recovery from error. Frese and his colleagues have developed and extensively evaluated a method of training called error management training (EMT),

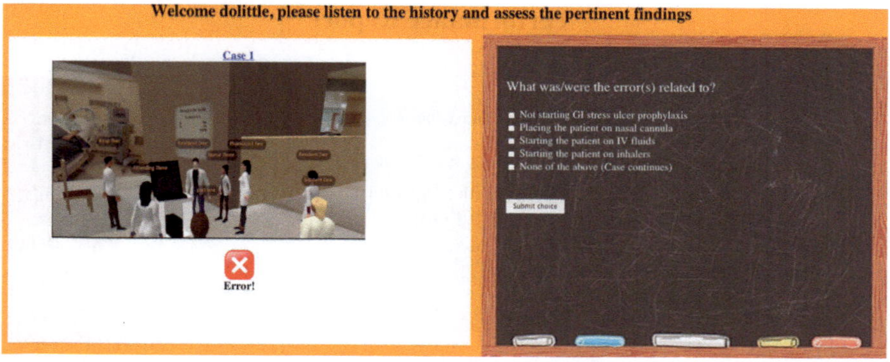

Fig. 6.6 Screenshot of the tutoring system's error detection component

which aims to leverage the learning opportunities identified by error commission to enhance learning outcomes [17]. During EMT, participants are explicitly encouraged to make errors during training. This approach was developed in the context of training software skills, where the consequences of error commission are less dire than in the case of real-world clinical management. Nonetheless, studies of post-training outcomes of EMT have shown advantages over traditional approaches to training with a positive relative effect on average across published studies [18]. However, the authors caution that further research is required to establish the extent to which these findings generalize to other tasks aside from the training of software skills. Within the surgical skills domain, Rogers and his colleagues have developed and evaluated a method of instruction that involves the generation of training videotapes illustrating commonly occurring technical errors [19]. Evaluation of this approach revealed a significant improvement in knot-tying skills for participants in training that included both correct and erroneous performance, over those trained with one of these modules only or none at all.

A Web-Based Tutoring System for Error Recovery in the ICU

In this section, we will describe the development of an automated tutoring system that aims to promote error recovery. The system is based on the two clinical scenarios that were utilized in our previous study. For educational purposes, these cases were altered slightly such that the some of the errors present in each scenario were more obvious. For example, in one error to do with the placement of an incorrectly sized endotracheal tube, the size of this tube was further reduced. The system was implemented with a web-based front end backed by a database that records the demographic details of participants. For research purposes, the front-end also provides the participants with a web-based consent form that has been approved for use by our local Institutional Review Board. In the section that follows, we will describe the system from the perspective of a user engaged in error detection training.

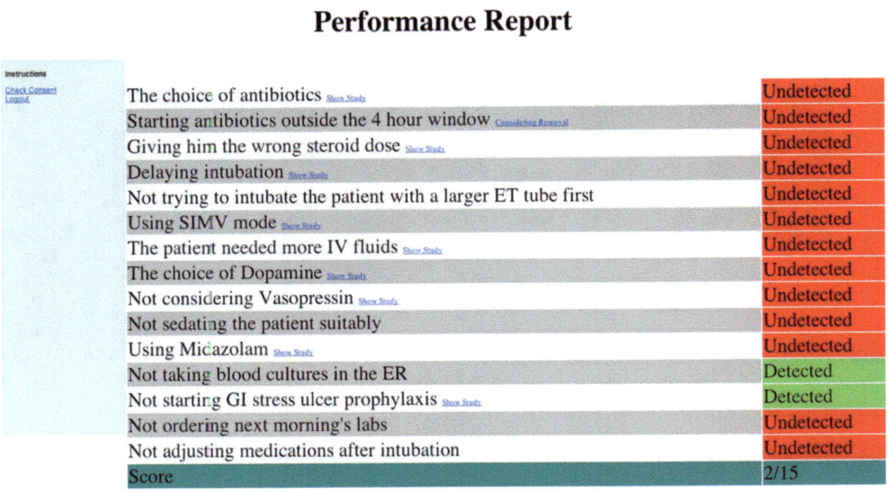

Performance Report

Instructions
Check Consent
Logout

The choice of antibiotics Show Study	Undetected
Starting antibiotics outside the 4 hour window Considering Removal	Undetected
Giving him the wrong steroid dose Show Study	Undetected
Delaying intubation Show Study	Undetected
Not trying to intubate the patient with a larger ET tube first	Undetected
Using SIMV mode Show Study	Undetected
The patient needed more IV fluids Show Study	Undetected
The choice of Dopamine Show Study	Undetected
Not considering Vasopressin Show Study	Undetected
Not sedating the patient suitably	Undetected
Using Midazolam Show Study	Undetected
Not taking blood cultures in the ER	Detected
Not starting GI stress ulcer prophylaxis Show Study	Detected
Not ordering next morning's labs	Undetected
Not adjusting medications after intubation	Undetected
Score	2/15

Fig. 6.7 Screenshot of the tutoring system's performance report

Participants log into the system through a web-based interface, and after completing a consent procedure are guided to the two cases. For each case, the interface allows them to observe the presentation of the case by members of the virtual clinical team, and they are encouraged to click the "Error!" button when they believe an error has been encountered Fig. 6.6. Upon clicking this button, they are presented with a set of potential errors to choose from, as well as the option of continuing to observe the clinical round without selecting an error. These choices are synchronized with the case presentation, such that choices relevant to the discussion immediately preceding clicking of the button are presented.

After completion of the case, participants are presented with a performance report, which provides links to evidence that supports the assertion that an error was committed where appropriate Fig. 6.7. At the time of this writing, research is underway to evaluate the extent that training with this tutoring system improves participants' ability to detect errors embedded in other case scenarios presented by attending physicians in the unit.

Summary and Implications

In this chapter, we have described a line of research involving the evaluation of trainees' ability to detect errors in virtual clinical rounds. Initially, these virtual rounds were used as a research instrument, to evaluate the detection of error in a controlled setting that is a better approximation of real world clinical rounds than the paper-based scenarios we have previously employed. An important finding from this research is that participants' ability to detect error, within the bounds of their clinical knowledge, was vastly improved when they were warned beforehand that errors would be present, which suggests the presence of untapped resources for error recovery. With the aim of realizing the potential improvements in patient safety that this implies, we developed a web-based automated tutoring system aimed specifically at error recovery.

Informatics Implications

A key finding presented in this chapter involves the role of directed attention in error recovery by clinicians. It is clear from the results presented that clinicians intentionally seeking errors approach the limits of their clinical knowledge when detecting errors embedded in clinical case scenarios, while clinicians listening to the presentation with some other goal in mind do not. This suggests that directing clinician attention toward the task of error detection may be beneficial for patient safety. While redirecting attention away from a clinically important task is not desirable, reducing the cognitive load of clinicians is a stated goal of many informatics implications. Once liberated, it may be possible to focus these newly available cognitive resources on the problem of error detection. Our tutoring application represents one attempt to do so. When evaluating it we will be testing the hypothesis that performance in error recovery, like other forms of skilled performance, may benefit from deliberate practice [20].

Discussion Questions

1. What other cognitive tasks might interfere with the ability of clinicians to detect errors embedded in clinical case scenarios?
2. What might be the consequences of focusing exclusively on error detection during the course of working clinical rounds?
3. Can skilled performance in error detection be developed through deliberate practice?
4. Aside from the use of automated tutoring systems, how might skilled performance in error detection be developed?

References

1. Rasmussen J. The role of error in organizing behaviour. Qual Saf Health Care. 2003;12(5): 377–85.
2. Amalberti R, Wioland LL. Human error in aviation. In: Soekkha H, editor. Aviation safety: human factors, system engineering, flight operations, economics, strategies, management. Utrecht: VSP; 1997. p. 91–108.
3. Irby DM. How attending physicians make instructional decisions when conducting teaching rounds. Acad Med. 1992;67(10):630–8.

4. Pronovost PJ, Jenckes MW, Dorman T, Garrett E, Breslow MJ, Rosenfeld BA, et al. Organizational characteristics of intensive care units related to outcomes of abdominal aortic surgery. JAMA. 1999;281(14):1310–7.
5. Cohen T, Blatter B, Almeida C, Patel VL. Reevaluating recovery: perceived violations and preemptive interventions on emergency psychiatry rounds. J Am Med Inform Assoc. 2007; 14(3):312–9.
6. Kubose TT, Patel VL, Jordan D. Dynamic adaptation to critical care medical environment: error recovery as cognitive activity. In: Proceedings of the 2002 Cognitive Science Society. Fairfax: Virginia; 2002. p. 43–4.
7. Henneman EA, Blank FSJ, Gawlinski A, Henneman PL. Strategies used by nurses to recover medical errors in an academic emergency department setting. Appl Nurs Res. 2006;19(2): 70–7.
8. Nyssen AS, Blavier A. Error detection: a study in anaesthesia. Ergonomics. 2006;49:517–25.
9. Patel VL, Cohen T, Murarka T, Olsen J, Kagita S, Myneni S, et al. Recovery at the edge of error: debunking the myth of the infallible expert. J Biomed Inform. 2010;44(3):413–24. PubMed PMID: 20869466.
10. Eagleson R, de Ribaupierre S, King S, Stroulia E. Medical education through virtual worlds: the HLTHSIM project. Stud Health Technol Inform. 2011;163:180–4.
11. Henderson BA, Kim JY, Golnik KC, Oetting TA, Lee AG, Volpe NJ, et al. Evaluation of the virtual mentor cataract training program. Ophthalmology. 2010;117(2):253–8.
12. Heidenreich C, Lye P, Simpson D, Lourich M. The search for effective and efficient ambulatory teaching methods through the literature. Pediatrics. 2000;105(1 Pt 3):231–7.
13. Prendinger H, Ullrich S, Nakasone A, Ishizuka M. MPML3D: scripting agents for the 3D internet. IEEE Trans Vis Comput Graph. 2010;17(5):655–68.
14. Grover M. Priming students for effective clinical teaching. Fam Med. 2002;34(6):419–20.
15. Thomas MJW. Predictors of threat and error management: identification of core nontechnical skills and implications for training systems design. Int J Aviat Psychol. 2004;14(2):207–31.
16. Naikar N, Saunders A. Crossing the boundaries of safe operation: an approach for training technical skills in error management. Cogn Technol Work. 2003;5(3):171–80.
17. Frese M, Brodbeck F, Heinbokel T, Mooser C, Schleiffenbaum E, Thiemann P. Errors in training computer skills: on the positive function of errors. Hum Comput Interact. 1991;6(1): 77–93.
18. Keith N, Frese M. Effectiveness of error management training: a meta-analysis. J Appl Psychol. 2008;93(1):59–69.
19. Rogers DA, Regehr G, MacDonald J. A role for error training in surgical technical skill instruction and evaluation. Am J Surg. 2002;183(3):242–5.
20. Anders K, Krampe RT, Tesch-Römer C. The role of deliberate practice in the acquisition of expert performance. Psychol Rev. 1993;100(3):363–406.

Chapter 7
Characterizing the Nature of Work and Forces for Decision Making in Emergency Care

Amy Franklin, David J. Robinson, and Jiajie Zhang

Introduction

Healthcare as a complex system [1] is exemplified in emergency medicine [2, 3]. Emergency Departments (EDs) are dynamic, adaptive, and self-organizing. Additionally, ED providers are faced with inherent unpredictability regarding the number and severity of patients, concurrent management of multiple individuals requiring timely responses, and a need to cope with limited resources all within a life-critical, interruption-laden environment [4]. The layered complexity of such units includes the functions of the work, the implementation of technology, the people, the activities and workflows jointly performed by the people and the technology, as well as the social, physical, cultural, and organizational environment in which the ED is embedded. Managing the cognitive, physical, spatial, and temporal resources in such systems is crucial for patient safety and quality of care. Understanding the interaction of the complexity of this work and the environment, particularly as it relates to decision-making, is a first step in engineering solutions to support physician efforts.

Section 3 is adapted from Franklin et al's (2011) paper Opportunistic decision making and complexity in emergency care, *Journal of Biomedical Informatics.* 44, 469–476.

A. Franklin, PhD (✉) • J. Zhang, PhD, MS, FACMI
School of Biomedical Informatics, University of Texas Health Science Center,
Houston, TX 77030, USA

National Center for Cognitive Informatics and Decision Making in Healthcare (NCCD),
Houston, TX 77030, USA
e-mail: amy.franklin@uth.tmc.edu

D.J. Robinson, MD, MS, FACEP
Department of Emergency Medicine, University of Texas Medical Center,
Houston, TX 77030, USA

V.L. Patel et al. (eds.), *Cognitive Informatics in Health and Biomedicine*,
Health Informatics, DOI 10.1007/978-1-4471-5490-7_7, © Springer-Verlag London 2014

The purpose of this chapter is to consider the complexity of emergency care at two levels: (1) methods for describing the functions of the emergency care work domain and the associated complexity and (2) the impact of specific workflows and environments on those functions. The ultimate goal of our efforts is to create health information technology to support the Emergency Department. We begin by creating a Work Domain Ontology or description of work. Then narrowing the focus of ED efforts to task transitions, we next describe decision-making patterns as physicians shift between activities finding use of local rules to govern action. Looking at specific implementations of different workflows and different physical layouts, we detail the impact of these factors on decision making. Finally, we conclude with future directions for Health Information Technology (HIT) interventions in complex healthcare scenarios.

Understanding Complexity Using a Work Domain Ontology (WDO)

In order to better reveal Emergency Department complexity, we need an abstract description of the clinical and cognitive work performed by clinicians, independent of how the setting is implemented with specific technology, artifacts, and environmental variables. The work domain ontology is a framework for this purpose [5–10].

A Work Domain Ontology (WDO) outlines the basic structure of the work that the system together with its human users will perform [6, 8, 9]. It is an explicit, abstract, implementation-independent description of that work. It describes the essential requirements independent of any technology systems, strategies, or work procedures. It tells us the inherent complexity of work; it separates work context (physical, organizational, computational, etc.) from the nature or functions of the work itself.

A WDO is composed of goals, operations (or actions), objects and the constraints that capture the functions of work. As an example, let's imagine a *goal* of treating a patient. One *action* or *operation* in treatment might be to prescribe a medication. Now, a prescription can be "written" in a number of different ways. A doctor can enter the order into a computer, write out the prescription on a pad, or make a call to the pharmacy. The underlying work domain for generating the prescription is the same across all of these means of creating it. In each case the *operation or action* is "prescribing a medication"; the *objects or required components* for this operation include patient name, medication name, dosage, frequency, duration, route, etc.; the *constraints* include the dependency relations between operations and objects (e.g., operation "write a medication prescription" and the objects "Metformin" and "500 mg"), between objects (e.g., the object "glucose level" and the object "Metformin"), and between operations (e.g., the operation "write a prescription"

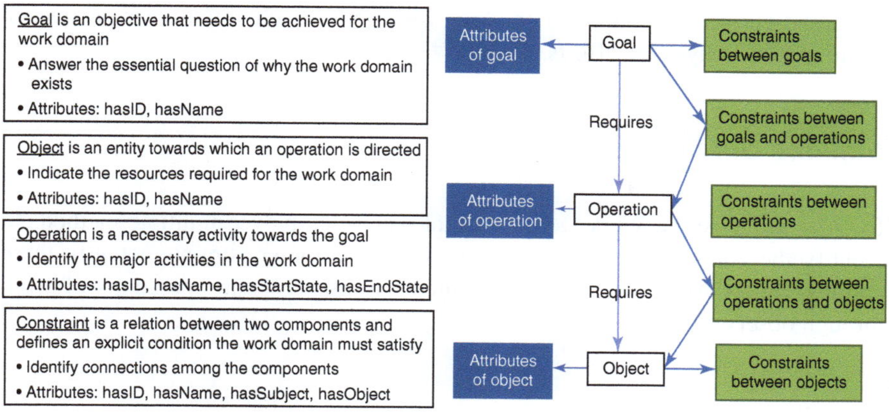

Fig. 7.1 Components of a work domain ontology

and the operation "modify allergy list"). The work domain is constant although the implementation varies if a computer or a prescription pad is used to generate the order.

Figure 7.1 shows the four components of WDO and their relations. The process of developing a WDO is similar to the process in ontology engineering, including defining the domain and the scope of the ontology, enumerating the goals, objects, operations, and constraints with various data collection methods (document analysis, observation, focus group, survey, etc.) and analysis methods (concept analysis, alignment, integration, etc.). The evaluation methods for ontology are also similar, including evaluation for different levels of granularity (e.g. lexical or concept level, semantic relations), fit for an application or with a context [10].

Partial Work Domain: A Single Perspective

We conducted a series of observations, interviews, and focus groups in order to develop a partial WDO for an emergency department. As this is a work in progress, we have completed the WDO from a single perspective of faculty physicians in a teaching hospital.

Faculty physicians at a teaching institution have at a minimum of three main and sometimes conflicting goals: (1) care of patients (individual patients and the totality of the unit), (2) management of resources and hospital administration, and (3) training and education of residents, fellows, and medical students. The tasks associated with each of these goals are a potentially many-to-many mapping (i.e. a single activity may answer any or all of the above goals). Our partial work domain includes only the faculty physicians' perspective. We anticipate many operations carry over to other perspectives or roles such as nurses, consultants, and trainees such as residents. The full work domain ontology will capture each of these perspectives in addition to the physician efforts.

Building Out the WDO

In order to create the Work Domain Ontology, we employed multiple methods to identify the goals, operations, objects of work and the constraints between these entities. Below we detail how we captured one aspect – the operations of work through observation.

Identifying Operations

Data were collected in a Level 1 Trauma Center in an Emergency Department of a large teaching hospital located in the Gulf Coast Region of the United States. This Emergency Department is separated into pediatric, medicine, and trauma units, with the trauma unit as the center of our study. We collected 55 hours of observation of attending physicians (three clinicians across two observations each) using pen and paper field recordings. The activities recorded included both ongoing activities (e.g. asking questions as part of medical history) as well as passive activities (e.g. observing a resident conducting a procedure). Think aloud data, for example "I am reviewing this chart", when provided by clinicians, created a pool of mental tasks. A total of 3,769 discrete activities were observed. Using the descriptive language from the field notes and grounded theory [11] to develop themes, these activities were distilled down to 125 individual tasks. These tasks such as *advising* (offering suggestions about the best course of action) and activities of direct patient care such as *performing procedures* were then implemented into our WDO as operations. The screenshot in Fig. 7.2 shows a sample 35 operations [12].

Refinement and Linking to UMLS

In addition to identifying the concepts observed during physician work, we also linked the activities (concepts) to the controlled vocabulary provided by the Unified Medical Language System (UMLS). Merging the UMLS concepts with our Emergency Department WDO required us to clearly identify our concepts and refine our understanding to match the contents of the UMLS meta-thesaurus. The intent of this integration was to clarify our WDO to a common terminology. Our method was to enter our initial terms for our ontology in the UMLS search query. When disparities were located, terms were either (1) reconciled by semantic type or (2) the search was split into several searches to create a combination of UMLS codes that incorporated our class properties.

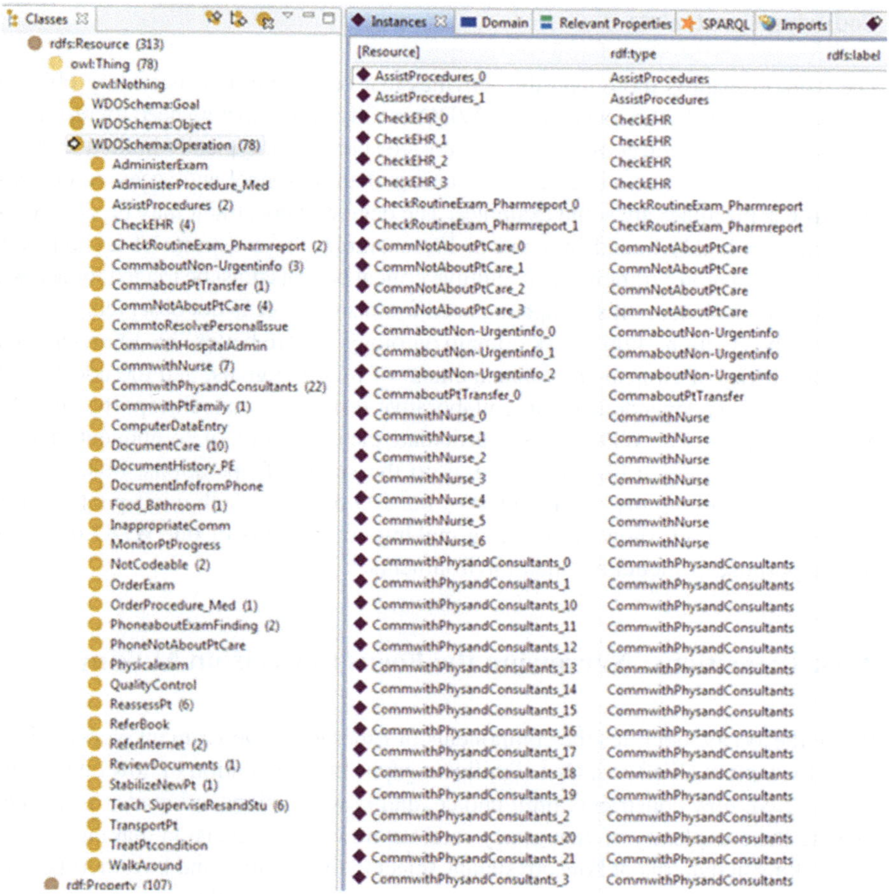

Fig. 7.2 A partial WDO of ED based on observed operations

Adding in Objects

In addition to the activities or operations, objects needed to be refined for specific emergency department work domain ontology. Objects can be broadly separated into (1) information and (2) resources, where (1) is any kind of information in the ED collected, starting with vital signs, as well as lab values and initial results of patients. Resources are personnel, workstations, and other artifacts in the ED. For example, a task such as communicating about a patient transfer requires not only the information regarding the patient (name, medical record number, current location) but also information regarding the receiving unit (new bed location, new physician name) as well as details regarding time and availability of position (e.g. whether transport has been ordered, whether the bed is currently available or pending). When possible, our objects were fit to the UMLS existing categories, however, additions were preserved.

Codifying Constraints

The work domain is more than the activities that occur and their necessary objects. Constraints must also be coded into the WDO, mainly the competing need for resources and the state of an object as available or not. Resources are typically limited to some extent in the ED. There are fewer workstations than personnel and access to devices such as CT machines are some examples. The degree of constraint may be viewed as subjective or highly bound by context. For example, the constraint of a single CT machine is felt more strongly when multiple critical patients must be triaged for access. In other circumstances, this competing need for this resource is not observed.

With the creation of this work domain ontology, we are better able to understand the complexity of clinical care, management of multiple goals, and the constraints in work such as dependencies on collaborative tasks (e.g. consult reports, compliance of patients). The WDO helps to articulate the interaction of components across efforts and provides a bigger picture as to the scope of operations, objects, and constraints. Additionally, the merging of our ED ontology with concepts from the UMLS terminology shows promise in making components of our WDO reusable for the purpose of modeling other environments.

Task Transitions: Narrowing the Focus to Decision Making

While the WDO identifies the components of Emergency Department work, it does not fully capture all efforts. One significant gap is the articulation of how operations are selected, how constraints limit choice, and how decisions are made. To further explore the complexity of emergency care, we now turn to decision making.

Looking at patterns of how physicians select their activities and how their behavior is governed by local rules are two aspects of complexity that emerge in such a non-deterministic environments.

Our approach to decision making is based on distributed cognition, which considers the ED as a system composed of individuals and technology situated in a complex physical, social, organizational environment that extends across space and time. Combining our method of categorizing physicians' behaviors with a cognitive, ecologically based Naturalistic Decision Making (NDM) [12] paradigm, we created a classification system that highlights the variability of the decisions made in this environment including across-task decisions that are not covered by existing models of medical decision making.

Decision Making

Current theories of decision making from classical models of risk and utility to contextual models of Naturalistic Decision Making (NDM) all emphasize the inherent factors of uncertainty and complexity in the medical decision process [13–15].

Task complexity, including that created by uncertainty and non-linearity, affects the efficiency of decision-making, as more complex tasks require more cognitive effort [16, 17]. However, much of the research on decision making and support systems has focused on the choices made during the care and treatment of a single patient. That is, these models revolve around a within-task choice often decisions in treatment or diagnostic reasoning. While this is a rich area for potential support with technology and a point in care with significant risk for error, physicians, particularly those in critical care environments such as Emergency Departments (EDs), also make many decisions *across* tasks (e.g. the selection of what to do next from multiple alternatives following a task). We extend the decision making model to consider selecting between potential activities.

Task Transition Decisions

From our previous work including the observations used to build the work domain ontology [18, 19], we began our exploration of decision making by reviewing canonical activities in the Emergency Department. Common tasks include patient assessment, observation, and communication. We analyzed these activities for the overarching goal for which each activity is conducted (e.g. care of patients, student teaching, etc.), the events surrounding each activity (e.g. patient arrival, x-rays complete), and the situational factors at that moment. Using these methods we determined that there are a number of task shifts in which a physician must select what their next action will be. The most clear cut selection of next task is the decision of *what to do following the completion of a goal.* However, the complexity of the ED rarely allows a physician to see a task (such as caring for a single patient) through from beginning to end without intervening activities. Therefore, the selection of between – task actions is a common occurrence that moves physicians from one activity to the next. Movement between the care of multiple patients is one example of a task transition decision.

Methodology

In our study of task transition decisions, the same faculty physicians from the Work Domain observations were again followed across multiple shifts. Data was collected for seven sessions across five physicians including two new additional doctors. The forty plus hours of observation provided rich data for the analysis of workflow processes and decision making. During the shadowing sessions, environmental elements in the ED were recorded, including the locations of the activities by physicians, the time, the participants engaged in the task (e.g. the other parties the physician might be speaking with, caring for, or interacting with), all observable antecedent events (e.g. being asked to attend to a patient, answer a call, responding to an alarm), and other ongoing activity in the ED (e.g. arrival of new patients, consulting physicians from other departments appearing in the ED, number of beds filled, etc.). In addition to shadowed observation, our methods included a 'think aloud' narration of the physician's activities in which the physicians were asked when possible to articulate their immediate goals [20]. However, given the demands of the ED, should a physician fail to provide this narrative no attempts were made to ask for clarification of the actions observed. Our observers did not interrupt or engage the physicians to prevent any potential harm or alteration in the functioning of the ED. Additionally, at patients' requests, observers waited outside treatment rooms limiting data collection for infrequent spans of time.

Categorizing the Decision Types

Decisions in the ED can be described at many levels of granularity. For example, there is the abstract level of patient care, viewing an image, generating a diagnosis, and levels all the way to a fine grain selection of picking an imaging technique (see Rosch [21], Smith and Medin [22] for discussions on categorization). Therefore, it is necessary to specify at what level of detail efforts should be concentrated and analysis should occur. Using the multi-stage iterative method described in the Hybrid Method to Classify Interruptions and Activities (HyMCIA) developed by Brixey and colleagues [19], we compared data collected across multiple observation sessions to clarify emerging categorizations and to redefine our protocols. From these activities, we adopted a flexible framework that allowed for categories to emerge both in data collection and analysis.

Categories of behavior emerged from our data such as a deciding on the next goal, moving between patients, switching between roles (physician as care giver versus physician as teacher), and coping with environmentally forced breaks in task (interruptions, delays, necessary communication). All of the aforementioned decisions are considered to be between task transition decisions (or choices in goal selection). Using this decision space, we then consider what types of decisions are made in these moments.

Results

Three main types of decisions emerged from our analyses. Physicians made planned decisions by following the logical progression of action such as moving into the next step in a protocol. For example in the care of a patient, planned decisions would include documentation following a patient exam. However, sequential activities along a planned course are often disrupted. While intervening activities may occur, a return to a plan is quite common. However, serial progression through a protocol is not required for a decision to be deemed planned. That is, although the

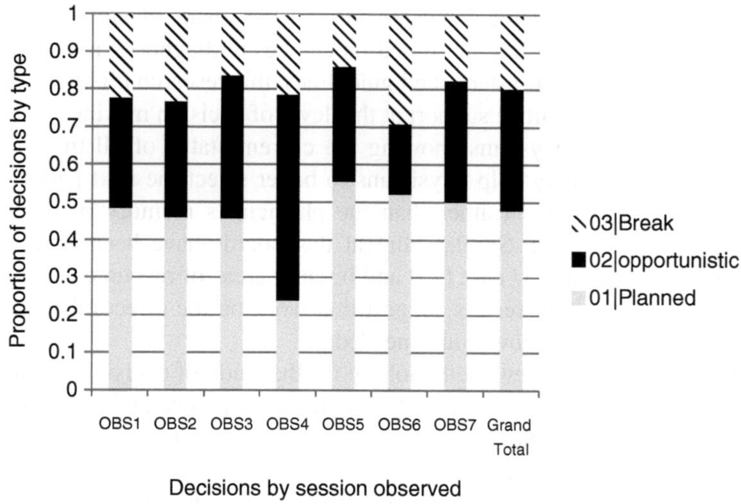

Fig. 7.3 Decision types observed

attending physician may have seen other patients since the initial exam of the patient, after reviewing the patient's x-rays the decision to then chart is considered a planned choice (or logical progression) in treating this patient.

A second type of decision that emerged from the data are opportunistic decisions. These decisions are a choice in action created through unanticipated circumstances such as proximity to another individual. For example, passing by a patient sitting in the hall is an opportunity to interact with that individual. It is through the unanticipated chance, the physician decided to interact with that patient rather than moving to the CT room (the intention articulated during his think aloud).

Breaks in task, our third decision type, are unanticipated choices forced upon a physician via an interruption, disruption or impediment to a task. The decision in these moments is to disrupt current activity to attend to a new requirement or demand. Breaks can be momentary such as the disruption of a pager going off (followed by a quick return to the previous activity) or may result in a complete change in task.

When we consider how often each type of decision is made in the course of a day's efforts, we find that on average 45 % (sd .14) of the physicians' decisions were planned, 34 % (sd .15) were opportunistic, and 21 % (sd .6) were produced by a break in task. The decision types for the seven sessions are displayed below in Fig. 7.3.

Through the exploration of task transition decisions, we can see that the choices made in the ER are most often (55 % opportunistic + break) created by the environment, rather than by conscious selection of the physician. While we might have anticipated a stronger adherence to protocol, response to local rules (e.g. responding to immediate needs rather than a global plan) is in line with our expectations of the Emergency Department as a complex system. Task transition decisions are not in most cases guided by protocol but are instead the result of situational factors. Further, as these decisions are not based on choices in diagnostic reasoning, treatment options or other well-established guidelines, this research highlights the need for new research on cognitive support at this level of decision making.

Dashboard displays systems showing the current status of all the patients in the emergency room may help physicians to better select the next patient to care for based on patient need (rather than the physician's memory of who needed assessment or proximity). Similar clinical dashboards have been developed for patient management in ICU care [23] and broader areas of resource allocation and project management. Our results suggest that work on the effect of opportunistic decision-making on workflow is also needed.

Here, we developed a new methodology for the study of decision making based on the distributed cognition framework that considers people and technology as an integrated system in complex physical, social, and organizational context. We identified three major types of decisions during task transitions and this taxonomy is important in understanding how physicians make decisions in the ED making. Next we look at the environmental factors influencing these choices.

Environmental Factors in Task-Transition Decisions

Beyond identifying decisions types based on the intent of the physician (next step in protocol = planned, respond to a break in task = disruption or interruption, or take advantage of an unexpected chance = opportunistic decision), we also must consider the role of the environmental or contextual factors that influence these decisions. Exploring the antecedents of task transitions decisions allows us to broaden each decision type. Next, we identified the contextual influences involved in physician choices.

Planned Decisions

Planned decisions follow the clinical pathway of treatment or the logical progression of care. Planned decisions can be influenced by the directions of a colleague (e.g. care plans handover over during shift change), determined by a set protocol (e.g. protocol for caring for a stroke patient), or may be routines determined by the preference of an individual (e.g. seeking out an ED wide update following the completion of documentation for each patient). We therefore broadly define planned decisions include the sources of influence:

Protocol/Logical Plan – next step in action series following common protocol or logical progression (e.g. following assessment there is creation of a treatment plan)

Preference – individual selection of next activity when no other outside forces influence the selection of the decision. This is a habitual choice or routine (e.g. completing walk around the unit to update situational awareness prior to charting)

External Forces – response to acknowledged/anticipated external forces that shape the selection of activity (e.g. being given patient priority during signout across shifts, following administrative policy etc.)

Break in Task

The catalyst for a break in task also comes from multiple sources. Physicians are often interrupted or disrupted during a task by needs of others including nurses, students, and patients. Interestingly enough, we have observed on a number of occasions, physicians interrupting themselves. Artifacts such as communication devices including phones, pagers, or alarms are also immediate sources of breaks in task. We classified breaks in task as having three main sources:

By organizational design – the physical layout of the workspace causes a disruption in work flow (e.g. chairs/beds/people impediment to ongoing activity)

Self – physician suspends an activity to perform another activity triggered by their own thought process (e.g. changing destination while walking down the hall) and captured through think aloud protocols

People or Artifacts – outside entity requires the suspension of current effort to perform task (e.g. needing to respond to an interruption for information, disruption caused by pager)

Opportunistic Decisions

Finally, opportunistic decisions arise from the conflation of several unforeseen events. This includes a doctor being in the right place to complete an unexpected act, someone having additional resources available to them (such as personnel) or having a bit of free time when blocked from completing a task. **Opportunistic Decisions** are choices in action created through unanticipated circumstances.

The three main sources of opportunity are proximity, time and resources. It is possible to have the right person, the right time, and the right resources simultaneously to allow for a decision/activity that otherwise would not have occurred.

In general, opportunities arise from:

Proximity – use of physical location in decision-making. Nearness makes desirable this course of action. Proximity is an opportunistic decision but not all opportunistic decisions require proximity. For example, a physician might select their next patient based on their proximity, but may also locate a piece of needed equipment when it is found unexpectedly on their way to complete a different task.

Time – often generated by artifact absence, lulls in workload or during necessary delays (e.g. time during an x-ray). For instance, in caring for a patient, a physician must step away from the bedside while x-rays are being taken. If the

Fig. 7.4 Relationship between factors and decision types

Environmental factor	Planned	Opportunistic	Break
Human	✦	✦✦	✦✦
Physical	✦	✦	✦
System	✦✦	✦	
Time	✦	✦	
Human • ✦ physical		✦	

✦✦ Single factor according for at least 70% of that decision type

physician uses these few minutes to check on the patient in the adjoining bed, this decision is considered an opportunity of time.

Resources – staff, materials, and other resources influencing decisions (e.g. additional attending physicians whose appearance alters the distribution of demands – Since you are here, I can now do another task.)

The Impact of the Environment on Decision Making

With multiple environmental factors are at play in each type of decision, we next considered the frequency of occurrence for each sub-type of task transition decision [24]. To do this, we created a matrix of the decision types and our categories of environmental influences. Using this grid, we determined the most frequent environmental factor(s) for each decision type (e.g. medical devices as related to breaks in task.) We then determined the most frequent type(s) of decision for each factor (e.g. opportunistic decisions relationship with factors such as time.) The next step was to survey the grid created by the factors and decisions and to isolate those cells that contained both the most frequent factors and the most frequent types accounting here for at least 70 % of the data. (If a single factor did not account for 70 % of the data, the next most common factor was included. This allows for multiple decision types/multiple factors to be considered the predominant influence). From this we determined that certain factors co-occur consistently with particular types of decisions. In Fig. 7.4 below, we illustrate this by indicating which factors were found for each decision type. The larger ◆ shape indicates the most prevalent environmental factor for each decision type.

As can be seen in the table, some decision types were affected by more than one category of environmental factors. Breaks in task are influenced by other individuals in the ED (e.g. residents, nurses, patients) and physical factors such as medical devices. However, for opportunistic decisions, there is also a combination of factors that robustly co-occur. Opportunistic decisions are influenced by time, proximity and by other individuals in the environment, and a combination of location and personnel is also common. That is, opportunities arise when the right person is located in a place that engenders an unexpected interaction. For example, as an attending physician is walking towards an exam room to care for a patient, he sees a resident looking at images at a PACS station. Stopping to talk with this resident about the images for another patient takes advantage of the opportunity presented by both the presence of the resident and proximity to the PACS station. It is the combination of these two factors that creates the opportunity. Therefore we have created a combined factor that incorporates both aspects.

Understanding the role of environment on each kind of decision has implications for the interventions created. If the goal is to increase adherence to protocol through a decrease in interruptions, it is necessary to understand the source of these interruptions. Similarly, to capitalize on opportunistic decisions, we much explore the impact of proximity on decision making.

Implementation Effects

The WDO created for the emergency department is implementation independent, meaning the tasks, objects and constraints are not influenced by the current installation of the EHR system or the staff working on a particular day. Task-transition decisions, on the other hand, are shaped by situational factors. Looking at a different implementation of work in our original hospital site allows us to tease apart how physical and workflow changes impact decision-making.

In a natural experiment, the same Trauma 1 hospital from the initial studies elected to implement a significant workflow change moving to a model that is known as "split-flow". The goal of split flow is to alter wait times and improve process flow by separating out the very ill and less acute patients at a different point in care (i.e., triage). This model splits the flow of patients into two categories: (1) those needing expedited treatment that proceeds in a typical fashion and (2) less serious patients are tested, treated and monitored in a results pending space. These less acute patients progress directly from the triage space to the results pending waiting room without being treated in the main section of the emergency department. This reduces the overall patient through put in the back unit, reduces wait to treatment for those patients and alters the physical space. Figure 7.5 below indicates this new physical layout.

When this change was implemented in the department under study, a dedicated triage physician was not assigned. Rather doctors, including residents, working in the ED cared for and now monitored patients across a larger space. This space includes no line of sight between spaces (i.e. you cannot see between the units of the ED into the results pending room.) This change in workflow moves the physicians through a different series of room disrupting previous behavior patterns.

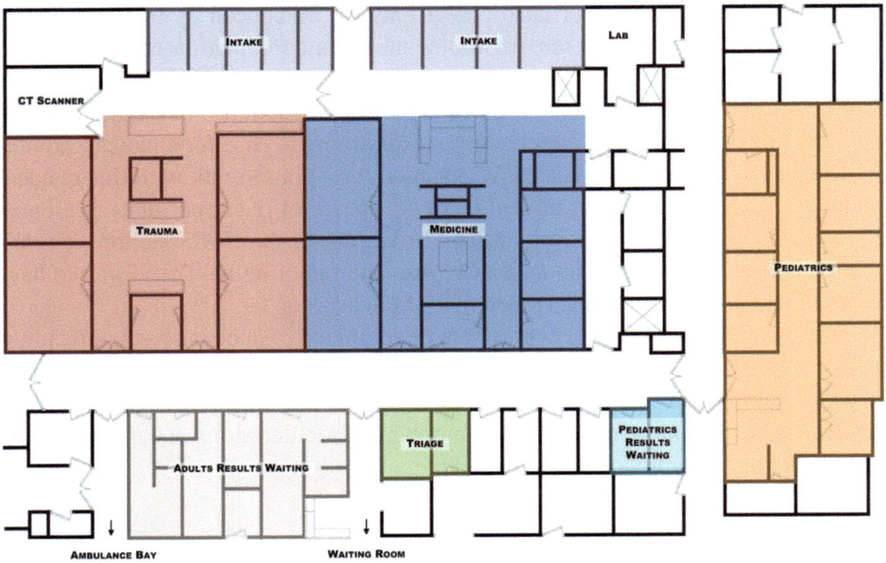

Fig. 7.5 Split flow layout of the hospital

While the change in workflow is significant, it is not expected to alter the WDO created for the Emergency Department. The patients in this flow receive the same treatment, have the same constraints, and the same care is required as in the previous sample – only the implementation has changed. Looking at task transition decisions we can now begin to explore the impact of implementation on complexity.

Decreasing Opportunities

Opportunistic decisions in the original study were determined by factors such as proximity. We predicted that such opportunities would decrease with the workflow change. Both the alteration to work and the change to the physical layout were hypothesized to negatively impact the ability of faculty physicians to make such choices by decreasing line of sight (e.g. could see the potential opportunities) and altering movement patterns as predictable routines were hypothesized to support opportunistic task transitions.

Methods

The same five attending physicians from the above study were shadowed. We compared 20 hours of their behavior in the initial workflow studies to 20 hours of post "split-flow" efforts. Paired T-tests were used compare performance across these points.

Results

While we had anticipated a decrease in the circumstances leading to opportunistic decisions (e.g. proximity), such decisions increased in each session after the layout change with 16 % growth on average ($p<.02$). We believe that this may have occurred as the new physical layout required the physicians to move through larger ED spaces. Such movement may have resulted in more opportunities taken. Further, the split-flow may have increased communication needs (e.g. monitoring of unseen patients) that may have driven additional opportunistic choices of catching conversations when possible. The limitations of our study, including small rates of think aloud data, do not allow us to conclusively determine what in fact caused this shift. However, these results do indicate a change in previously seen patterns with a different implementation of workflow and physical layout.

To further continue the study of the impact of implementation on decision making, we conducted another study following our group of clinicians – this time in a different hospital system.

Implementation 2

At our second site, many factors have changed. While still located at a teaching institution in the same major metropolitan area, the second hospital is a county hospital servicing a different clientele (e.g., fewer trauma cases, etc.). Additionally, a different EHR is implemented at this site, the physical layout is different and the work flow includes smaller pods within a unit limiting overall patients per provider. So the question is how well does the WDO generalize and how well will our task transition decisions hold up at a new site?

Replication Methods

In this iteration of the study, seven faculty physicians were shadowed at the second hospital site for a total of twelve four hour sessions observations (48 hours total). As with the previous study, the physicians were observed as they went about their daily work. Attention to task transitions was again the focus of the efforts.

Although this site differed in terms of physical layouts, EHR system and to some degree the severity of patients presenting (e.g. fewer trauma patients), we see a similar pattern to previous findings. As shown in Fig. 7.6, task transition patterns (depicted with averages across physicians observed more than once) are roughly equivalent to previous findings. Opportunistic decisions are 28 % (sd .026) of the task transitions made at this new site. Planned decisions account for 48 % (sd .0356) of choices and breaks in task influence 23 % (sd .0347) of the decisions made.

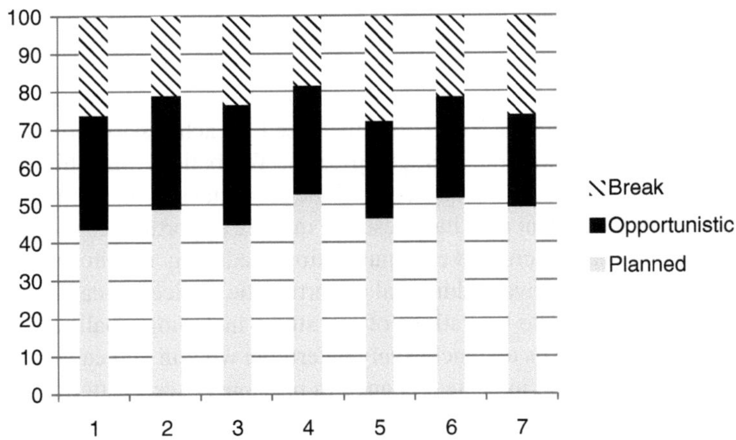

Fig. 7.6 Decision making at second site implementation 2

So while we see some variation, such as a decrease in opportunistic decisions from 90 to 28 %, this it is not significant change in performance. Contrary to our previous findings within a single site, the impact of workflow and physical layout (i.e., split-flow) had a greater effect in the first hospital site than in this different hospital site.

The potential reasons for this are many. Perhaps the change within a single department with set expectations is different than the set of expectations that play out in another hospital. Perhaps a mix of more acute (trauma cases) in conjunction with less severe (results pending) patients leads to different mental and physical work. What these results show us is that the work of emergency care and the decisions required to complete this care result from the interplay of the functions of work and the ways in which that work is expressed.

Summary

Our studies show that approximately half of the times ED physicians follow plans or protocols to make their decisions on task transitions and the rest of the times they make the decisions based on situational factors. This finding is observed at two separate hospitals with different physical layouts and different EHR systems.

This finding is based on the observations of operations and actions which are guided and coded by the Work Domain Ontology. A Work Domain Ontology, even in a partial state, proved vital in understanding the work and the complexity of the work in this domain from the influence introduced by the implementation of workflows within the system. Topics for future studies include detailed analyses of workflow dynamics and how information technology affect the dynamics in terms of care quality, patient safety, and efficiency of care delivery.

Health Information Technology Solutions

ED clinicians perform life-critical tasks that require acquisition, processing, transmission, distribution, integration, search, and archiving of significant amount of data in a distributed team environment in a timely manner. Monitoring the constantly changing information environment, responding to unpredictably occurring issues, collaborating and communicating with other people in the system as issues arise are all tasks required as part of patient care. Rather than focusing on a single task at a time, ED clinicians are forced to switch between multiple tasks and usually multiple patients. And many of these switching decisions are based on unplanned, unorganized, and unpredictable environmental factors. ED clinicians are constantly under information overload, multitasking, time pressure, and information requests.

Information visualization, if designed properly with human-centered principles, can make use of people's powerful visual system to efficiently process information that otherwise requires a lot more cognitive effort. The human visual system is powerful because it can process information in parallel, automatically, and unconsciously, and it can bypass the bottleneck of human working memory that is limited in capacity. Visualization is an important tool for healthcare due to the vast amount of data that have to be processed by the clinicians.

Information dashboards have become important business intelligence tools for many industries. However, the tracking board and other dashboard type of displays designed for the ED in EHR systems have significant challenge. The electronic ED whiteboard developed by Aronsky and colleagues [25] is an important step towards good visualization for the ED, which is an advanced version of the physical whiteboards with carefully selected advanced functionality. HIT solutions such as dashboards, information push systems and even smart phone technology are all potential means of supporting decision making through greater situation awareness. Managing the complexity of the ED environment through HIT supports aims to achieve better individual performance, better team communication, and better clinical outcome important to patient safety and care quality.

Discussion Questions

1. Given the impact of environmental factors on performance, prior to changes in workflow or physical layout in a hospital system what kind of potential impact studies might you recommend?
2. Emergency Room clinicians are faced with high information demands in an ever-changing environment. What are some training considerations with the implementation of health information technology (HIT) solutions?

References

1. Plsek P, Greenhalgh T. The challenge of complexity in health care. BMJ. 2001;323:625–8.
2. Smith M, Feied C. The emergency department as a complex system. 1999. Available at: http://nesciorg/projects/yaneer/emergencydept.ex.pdf.
3. Nugus P, Carroll K, Hewett DG, Short A, Forero R, Braithwaite J. Integrated care in the emergency department: a complex adaptive systems perspective. Soc Sci Med. 2010;71(11): 1997–2004.
4. Croskerry P, Cosby K, Schenkel S, Wears R. Patient safety in emergency medicine. Philadelphia/London: Wolters Kluwer; 2009.
5. Butler KA, Zhang J, editors. Design models for interactive problem-solving: context & ontology, representation & routines. In: SIGCHI conference on human factors in computing systems. Atlanta; 2009.
6. Butler K, Zhang J, Esposito C, Bahrami A, Hebron R, Kieras D. Work-centered design: a case study of a mixed initiative scheduler. In: Proceedings of CHI. California, USA: San Jose; 2007. p. 747–56.
7. Butler K, Zhang J, Hunt A, Huffer B, Muehleisen J. Ontology models for interaction design. Proceedings of the SIGCHI conference on human factors in computing systems. Atlanta: ACM; 2010.
8. Zhang J, Butler K, editors. UFuRT: A work-centered framework and process for design and evaluation of information systems. In: Proceedings of HCI International. Presented at: HCI International. Beijing, China; 2007.
9. Zhang J, Walji M. TURF: toward a unified framework of EHR usability. J Biomed Inform. 2011;44(6):1056–67.
10. Brank J, Grobelnik M, Mladenić D. A survey of ontology evaluation techniques. SIKDD 2005 at multiconference IS 2005; Oct 17 2005. Ljubljana.
11. Glaser B, Strauss A. The discovery of grounded theory. New York: Aldine Publishing; 1967. Klein GA, Orasanu J, Calderwood R, Zambok CE, editors. Decision making in action: models and methods. Norwood: Ablex Publishing Corporation; 1993.
12. Zhu M. Formalizing a conceptual framework of work domain knowledge [PhD]. Houston: University of Texas Health Science Center at Houston; 2010.
13. Beach LR, Lipshitz R. Why classical decision theory is an inappropriate standard for evaluating and aiding most human decision making. In: Klein GA, Oransanu J, Calderwood R, Zsambok CE, editors. Decision making in action: models and methods. Norwood: Alex; 1993. p. 21–35.
14. Klein GA, Orasanu J, Calderwood R, Zsambok CE, editors. Decision making in action: models and methods. Norwood: Ablex; 1993.
15. Beach LR, Lipshitz R. Why classical decision theory is an inappropriate standard for evaluating and aiding most human decision making. In: Klein GA, Oransanu J, Calderwood R, Zsambok CE, editors. Decision making in action: models and methods. Norwood: Ablex Publishing; 1993. p. 21–35.
16. Bystrom KJK. Task complexity affects information seeking and use. Inf Process Manag. 1995;31:191–213.
17. Chinburapa VLL, Brucks M, Draugalis JL, Bootman JL, Puto CP. Physician prescribing decisions: the effects of situational involvement and task complexity on information acquisition and decision making. Soc Sci Med. 1993;36:1473–82.
18. Zhang J, Patel VL, Johnson TR, Shortliffe EH. A cognitive taxonomy of medical errors. J Biomed Inform. 2004;37:193–204.
19. Brixey JJ RD, Johnson CW, Johnson TR, Turley JP, Patel V, Zhang J. Towards a hybrid method to categorize interruptions and activities in healthcare. Int J Med Inform. 2007;76(11–12): 812–20.
20. Newall A, Simon HA. Human problem solving. Englewood Cliffs: Prentice-Hall; 1972.

21. Rosch E. Principles of categorization. In: Rosch E, Lloyd B, editors. Cognition and categorization. Hillsdale: Erlbaum; 1978.
22. Smith E, Medin D. Categories and concepts. Cambridge: Harvard University Press; 1981.
23. Koch SH, Weir C, Westenskow D, Gondan M, Agutter J, Harr M, Liu D, Gorges M, Staggers N. Evaluation of the effect of information integration in displays for ICU nurses on situation awareness and task completion time: A prospective randomized controlled study. Int J Med Inform. 2013;82(8):665–75.
24. Liu Y. The Impact of Environmental Factors on Physician Decision Making in Emergency Department, Master's Thesis, unpublished, University of Texas HSCH, 2010.
25. Aronsky D et al. Supporting patient care in the emergency department with a computerized whiteboard system. J Am Med Inform Assoc. 2008;15:184–94.

Chapter 8
Adaptive Behaviors in Complex Clinical Environments

Mithra Vankipuram, Vafa Ghaemmaghami, and Vimla L. Patel

Introduction

In an ideal scenario, hospital systems would deliver care in a timely manner to a large number of patients with a variety of diseases. There would be no hospital-acquired infections, staff-related oversights or prescription errors that result in complications. As patients, we would want to be treated in such an institution. Insurance companies, a principal (financial) driving force in the healthcare industry, would prefer that their customers visit hospitals where reduced complications result in

Portions of this chapter has been adapted from (a) an open access article in the proceedings of the 2012 annual symposium American Medical Informatics Association, Vankipuram et al., Adaptive Behaviors of Experts in Following Standard Protocol in Trauma Management: Implications for Developing Flexible Guidelines, and (b) Kahol et al., Deviations from protocol in a complex trauma environment: errors or innovations? *Journal of Biomedical Informatics*, 44(3), 425–31.
The description of research methods and results for this chapter has been adapted from (a) Kahol K, et al. Deviations from protocol in a complex trauma environment: errors or innovations? *Journal of Biomedical Informatics*. 44(3): 425–31.

M. Vankipuram, MS, PhD (✉)
HP Labs, Hewlett-Packard (HP), Palo Alto, CA 94304, USA
e-mail: vankipuram.mithra@gmail.com

V. Ghaemmaghami, MD, FACS
Trauma Division, Department of Surgery, Banner Good Samaritan Hospital,
Phoenix, AZ 85006, USA

University of Arizona College of Medicine, Phoenix, AZ USA

V.L. Patel, PhD, DSc, FRSC
Center for Cognitive Studies in Medicine and Public Health,
New York Academy of Medicine, New York, NY 10029, USA

Department of Biomedical Informatics, Columbia University, New York, NY 10032, USA

Department of Biomedical Informatics, Arizona State University, Scottsdale, AZ 85259, USA

V.L. Patel et al. (eds.), *Cognitive Informatics in Health and Biomedicine*,
Health Informatics, DOI 10.1007/978-1-4471-5490-7_8, © Springer-Verlag London 2014

shorter hospital stays and lower overall costs due to better outcomes. From the clinicians' point of view, working in a safe and efficient system increases their reputation and work morale. Such an institution would attract a large volume of patients. This will result in greater reimbursement, which would make a strong case for improving quality of care from a business perspective as well. Although not all the features described may be practicably achievable, quality of care is a fundamental concept that is critical to building a safe, cost-effective and sustainable healthcare system.

Unlike other domains such as aviation and nuclear power [1], medicine continues to rely on individual error-free performance as opposed to designing systems around principles of safety [2]. In order to build safer systems, understanding the cognitive mechanisms that drive errors and other adaptive deviations in complex systems is needed. The Institute of Medicine (IOM) released a number of reports that have increased the public awareness about quality in healthcare and patient safety. The 2000 report "To Err Is Human" [3] drew attention to the vulnerability of the healthcare system to medical errors. This report estimated that in the United States (US) alone, 44,000–98,000 lives were lost annually due to preventable medical errors. These figures were based on injury rates estimated by two key studies that performed retrospective reviews of medical records [4]. The significance of this statistic lies in the fact that it is more likely to be an under-estimate. Chart review processes catch only errors reported in the hospital setting, which is only a small part of the care continuum [5]. Leape compared the reported figures to "three fully loaded jumbo jets crashing every-other day" [6]. In any field other than healthcare, such a high error rate would be unacceptable. This report made a number of recommendations for reducing errors. These included setting national goals for patient safety, developing evidence-based knowledge, understanding the cause of errors and encouraging voluntary error reporting. A 2001 IOM report, "Crossing the Quality Chasm" [7], provided broad recommendations for the future of healthcare, stating that systems should aim to be "safe, effective, patient-centered, timely, efficient and equitable". Together, these two IOM reports have largely served to draw attention to the critical task of error prevention, enlist the support of stakeholders, and had impact on practices in all levels of care [8].

Following these reports, a variety of interventions have been implemented at various healthcare centers across the United States. These interventions include incorporation of computer-based provider order entry (CPOE) systems, protocol adoption and team training, to name a few [8]. There is evidence of small but significant improvement in patient safety at various institutions. Fewer patients die from medication errors [9], and infection rates have been reduced due to the use of protocols and checklists for specific procedures [10, 11]. Despite evidence of some improvement, health systems nation-wide did not show an anticipated (and necessary) overall level of progress in improving patient safety (IOM recommended reducing errors by 50 % within 5 years) [5, 8]. A more recent report on Patient Safety and Health Information Technology (HIT) (IOM report, 2010) summarized that there was not enough evidence that HIT made positive difference, based on the current literature. One of the reasons for the lack of sufficient improvement is that

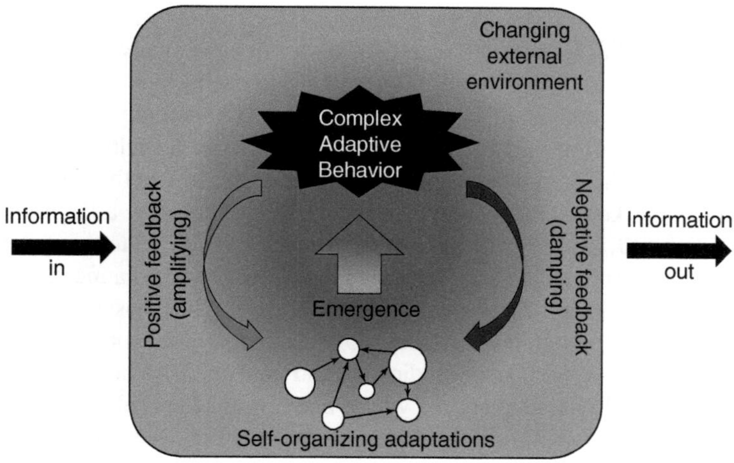

Fig. 8.1 Overview of complex adaptive systems

errors are often not caused by individual clinicians or practices, but are the result of some fundamental systemic problems. Leape and Berwick [8], in their assessment of barriers to quality improvement, suggested that system complexity compounded by professional fragmentation and a hierarchical authority structure, may dissuade the creation of a culture of individual accountability and coordinated teamwork, both attributes of a safe and robust system. Therefore, in order to understand the root cause of errors, researchers would first need to investigate how clinicians behave and interact within the complex healthcare system.

Clinical environments, such as emergency departments (ED), intensive care units (ICU) including trauma critical care are complex and dynamic, where complexity is defined by non-linearity, continuous interaction with the external environment, self-organization through emergence of new entities such as teams (Cohen and Patel, Chap. 2; Kannampallil et al., Chap. 19). Changes in staff involved in the care process (due to shift changes, rotations, or departure/new hires) continually alter team dynamics, as they adapt to new situations. This is exuberated by the volume and variety of patients that enter the ER and ICUs. In addition, the plethora of technology and equipment used in these units create unforeseen demands on clinicians to multitask in a nonlinear fashion. These characteristics make the clinical environments to be categorized as complex adaptive systems.

Healthcare as a Complex Adaptive System

Recent research has approached the study of social systems, such as clinical environments, using a theory based on complex adaptive systems (depicted in Fig. 8.1) [12]. Plesk and Greenhalgh define complex systems as "*a collection of individual agents with freedom to act in ways that are not always predictable, and whose actions are interconnected so that one agent's actions, change the context for other agents*" [13, 14]. Such systems typically involve a dynamic network of entities acting simultaneously, while continuously reacting to each other's actions [15, 16]. Complex systems are adaptive, unpredictable, and inherently non-linear [17]. Inconsistencies, tension, and anxiety are by-products of such environments [14, 18].

Figure 8.1, an illustration adapted from "Complexity: Life at the Edge of Chaos" [19], depicts the key elements of a complex system. Typically, a large amount of information is utilized and generated by the system. In addition to the systems having an environment in which information and knowledge are dynamically changing, the overall behavior of such systems is also affected by the positive and negative feedback received through interactions among the individuals working in these systems. In order to cope with an unpredictable and dynamic environment, individuals tend to develop ad-hoc adaptations, which may eventually evolve into strategies. This "emergence" of stable strategies makes up the overall behavior of a complex adaptive system.

In addition to the challenges faced by clinicians, the very nature of complex environments makes studying interactions in these systems difficult as well. This is primarily due to a disassociation between the non-linear nature of the environment and the tools available to analyze cognitive and workflow processes, which are most often linear (Kannampallil et al., this volume). The tools currently used for analyzing processes in these environments include qualitative methods such as ethnographic observation, use of think aloud protocols, shadowing of individual clinicians, surveys and questionnaires [20]. The data collected by these methods can be used to model segments of the clinical workflow centered on a particular individual and his or her activities [21]. Although the workflow documented in this manner captures many aspects of the overall system behavior, the presence of dense and interrelated interactions between various entities often makes operations in complex environments intractable. For example, observations are usually gathered from a single individual's point of view. A single observer may not be able to capture information on communication, movement and decision making, occurring at an instant of time. Theoretically, by increasing the number of observers it is possible to capture most of the information about the activities in the environment from several perspectives. However, based on informal interviews conducted with clinicians, more than two observers are considered disruptive to the clinical workflow. With such constraints imposed on data collection in complex environments, there is a need for an unobtrusive alternative that can augment existing methods of data collection, and help piece together a more complete description of system behaviors; both from individual and team perspectives.

Assessment of Behaviors in Complex Systems

In complex environments, adaptations ("deviations" from standards) and the resultant emergent behaviors provide insight into the processes that shape the system. In order to understand the root cause for errors in these systems, researchers would first need to examine the cognitive basis of these adaptive mechanisms. Protocols and guidelines have proven to be very useful in understanding complex tasks by dividing them into simpler observable units. Typically, protocols and guidelines suggest a sequence of atomic tasks and define a criterion for success. Checklists, a tool that has proven to be very effective in the management and control of processes in some complex environments (especially those structured by rigid protocols, as opposed to flexible guidelines) [22–24], are then utilized to assess clinician performance by examining the adherence to a protocol.

Much of the research assessing behaviors in complex systems follows this paradigm [25–27]. In these studies, deviations from protocols and guidelines are considered to be errors. The IOM, in fact, defines errors as "*…a deviation from that (protocol, procedure) which is generally held to be acceptable*" [28]. Although this definition of an error as a deviation is valid, the converse need not necessarily be true. In other words, while clearly all errors are deviations, not all deviations are errors. In fact, it is possible that a deviation from a protocol may be an innovation designed to maximize patient safety or an adaptation to enable the clinician to simply cope with the environment.

An example of complex social system that is similar to a clinical environment is aviation. Both pilots and clinicians operate in environments where teams interact with numerous technology and the risks originate from a number of sources in the environment. Errors, in these environments, occur due to a number of reasons; most of which are related to human error [29]. In contrast to medicine, however, errors in aviation often involve the loss of massive number of lives. A number of mechanisms have been adopted to minimize errors in aviation, focusing primarily on the task of error management in complex situations [30].

Crew resource management (CRM) [31], a major safety training in aviation, focuses on error training individuals in the countermeasures of human performance limiters (stress and fatigue). These counter measures include encouraging behaviors such as leadership, continuous monitoring, briefings, decision-making and dynamic modification of plans. In addition to CRM, simulation allows pilots to practice dealing with error management and receive feedback about the performance in dealing with complexity [29]. In addition to technical training, the domain of aviation has recognized the need to train both individuals and teams in dealing with complex error-prone situations, situations where plans may need to be altered dynamically to tailor the solution to the problem at hand.

An example of such an adaptive situation is the emergency landing of US Airways flight 1549 (on January 15, 2009) in the Hudson River is very well known. It involved a situation in which the airplane lost engine power shortly after takeoff. In this case, the flight captain used his own judgment and followed some protocols, while departing from others [32] and managed to land the heavy plane safely in the river. In emergency situations, the US Airways protocol calls for the first officer to take control of the flight, so that the captain can focus on making time-critical decisions. In this case, however, the captain quickly assessed the situation and deviated from the protocol. He took control of the plane instead and left his first officer to go through the checklist for restarting the engines. The decision was made because he felt that he was the more experienced pilot (and consequently had a better chances of landing the flight safely), while his first officer was more familiar with the specifics of the aircraft and would be able to go through the checklists more efficiently. The plane was in the river before the first officer completed the first page of the three-page checklist. This is an example where deviations from protocols (a dynamic alteration in action plan) resulted in a positive outcome.

A lesser known example from aviation is that of Air France flight 447 that disappeared over the Atlantic on June 1, 2009. The analysis of the black box (published in December, 2011) revealed a disturbing finding [33]. The pilots encountered a storm and had to disengage from auto pilot. This was not an unusual situation. The captain then left the helm to junior co-pilots for a routine break. Fifteen minutes later, the plane crashed killing the 228 people on board. The situation called for the junior pilots to coordinate their efforts in order to pass through the storm. However, the more inexperienced pilot of the two was overcome by the intensity of the situation and reverted to a protocol that was no longer applicable. By the time the captain returned to the cockpit, it was too late to prevent the crash.

> While (the first officer's) behavior is irrational, it is not inexplicable. Intense psychological stress tends to shut down the part of the brain responsible for innovative, creative thought. Instead, we tend to revert to the familiar and the well-rehearsed …It's not surprising, then, that amid the frightening disorientation of the thunderstorm, (the first officer) reverted to flying the plane as if it had been close to the ground (normal conditions), even though this response was totally ill-suited to the situation [33].

This example highlights the fact that complexity, in some cases, cannot be controlled by protocols and standards. Individuals operating in such environments may be required to step outside the boundaries of "standard solutions" in order to solve time-critical problems. Based on safety mechanisms implemented in aviation it is evident that there is a need for research in medicine that examines the adaptive behavior of experts in order to improve the existing criteria for evaluation of performance in complex clinical environments. This chapter describes research in assessing the behavior of teams of clinicians in trauma critical care, a prototypical example of a complex healthcare environment.

Trauma Critical Care

In critical care settings, teams of professionals who care for patients typically involve clinicians with varying backgrounds and expertise, working in a collaborative manner. A patient may interact with as many as fifty different employees (including nurses, physicians and technicians), during a typical 4-day stay at a hospital [34]. These teams are characterized by their dynamic social structures [35]. In response to an equally dynamic and unpredictable environment, the individuals in the team are required to adapt to varying task demands and coordinate their efforts to carry out activities necessary for task completion [36].

The accepted method for systematic treatment of patients in trauma critical care is the Advanced Trauma Life Support (ATLS) guideline [37], developed by the American College of Surgeons (ACS). It is mandatory that this protocol be followed in every Level 1 trauma center for accreditation purposes. Research has shown that the ATLS protocol is effective in improving the quality of care in trauma centers across the United States [38]. The tasks and goals for "Initial Survey and Management" of the patient, as prescribed by the ATLS guideline, are summarized in Table 8.1. These tasks and goals are common to both physicians and nurses working as a team to provide care to the trauma patient. The guideline to be followed can be divided into three sections: (1) primary survey and resuscitation, (2) secondary survey and examination, and (3) definitive care and transfer. In the primary survey, all immediate, life-threatening conditions are mitigated. Once the patient's vital signs stabilize, a thorough head-to-toe examination can be performed. Information obtained from examinations (and diagnostic tests) allows the trauma team leader to make decisions relating to the care of the patient. In addition to providing a methodical way to treat patients, the ATLS guideline serves to establish a common vocabulary for multi-disciplinary trauma teams to function effectively.

Trauma team structures are fluid. The teams converge dynamically when a patient arrives and aid in rapid identification and treatment of life-threatening conditions. They are responsible for: (1) assessment of the patient upon arrival, (2) resuscitation and management of critical conditions, and (3) diagnosis and transfer of the patient to the appropriate facility. The core team typically includes the attending surgeon, residents, an anesthesiologist, and nurses. Supporting members include a respiratory therapist, pharmacist and an X-ray technician.

While team formation may be dynamic, the roles and responsibilities of individuals within the team are well defined. The trauma *team leader* supervises the trauma care, making major decisions and delegating work to other members of the trauma team. The trauma lead may be assisted by a resident physician. The *assisting physician* performs hands-on evaluation and treatment. The *primary trauma nurse* is responsible for the immediate care of the patient. He or she may be assisted by a *nurse recorder* who documents events in trauma workflow sheets. The structure of the core team is often dynamic. Roles of the team leader and assisting physician may shift between residents and the attending trauma surgeon. In teaching hospitals, attending surgeons mostly play the role of a guide overseeing residents serving as the trauma leader.

Much like a complex adaptive system, trauma critical care units have a large amount of information available to the team. This information evolves as new observations are made, tests are analyzed and consults are obtained. Trauma teams receive information from a variety of sources including pre-arrival patient information, trauma workflow sheets, the patient vital signs monitor, x-ray images, computerized tomography (CT) scans, diagnostic tools to analyze blood and urine samples, and information shared by other care providers [39].

Although team members follow the same guideline for treating the patient, the boundaries of an individual's role (within the team) impact the types of information processed and utilized by each team member. For example, x-rays and CT scans are

Table 8.1 Key steps in initial assessment and management ATLS protocol

(A) Primary survey assessment of ABCDE's	1. Airway with cervical spine protection 2. Breathing 3. Circulation with control for external hemorrhage 4. Disability with brief neurological evaluation 5. Exposure/Environment
(B) Resuscitation	1. Oxygenation and ventilation 2. Shock management and delivery of fluids 3. Management of life-threatening problems
(C) Adjuncts to primary survey and resuscitation	1. Monitoring (a) Arterial blood gas analysis and ventilator rate (b) End-tidal carbon dioxide (c) Electrocardiograph (d) Pulse oximetry (e) Blood pressure 2. Urinary and gastric catheters 3. X-rays and diagnostic studies (a) Chest (b) Pelvis (c) C-Spine (d) Diagnostic peritoneal lavage or abdominal ultrasonography
(D) Secondary survey, total patient evaluation: physical examination and history	1. Head and skull 2. Maxillofacial 3. Neck 4. Chest 5. Abdomen 6. Perineum/Rectum/Vagina 7. Musculoskeletal 8. Complete neurologic examination 9. Tube and fingers in every orifice
(E) Adjuncts to the secondary survey	1. Computerized Tomography 2. Contrast X-ray studies 3. Extremity X-rays 4. Endoscopy and ultrasonography
(F) Definitive care	Based on the diagnosis, patient treated in trauma care (if applicable)
(G) Transfer	Based on the type of care needed, patient may be transferred (to the operating room or intensive care unit) or be discharged from the facility

always assessed by the trauma leader, which forms the basis for decisions about treatment and definitive care of the patient. In such conditions, one of the main challenges faced by teams is decision making with evolving information. Often the complete medical history of the patient may not be available when critical decisions have to be made. Trauma teams may be required to adapt they decision making as more information emerges.

Trauma Scenario Walkthrough: Certain key steps are performed (in quasi-sequential order) to evaluate every patient admitted to a trauma unit, regardless of

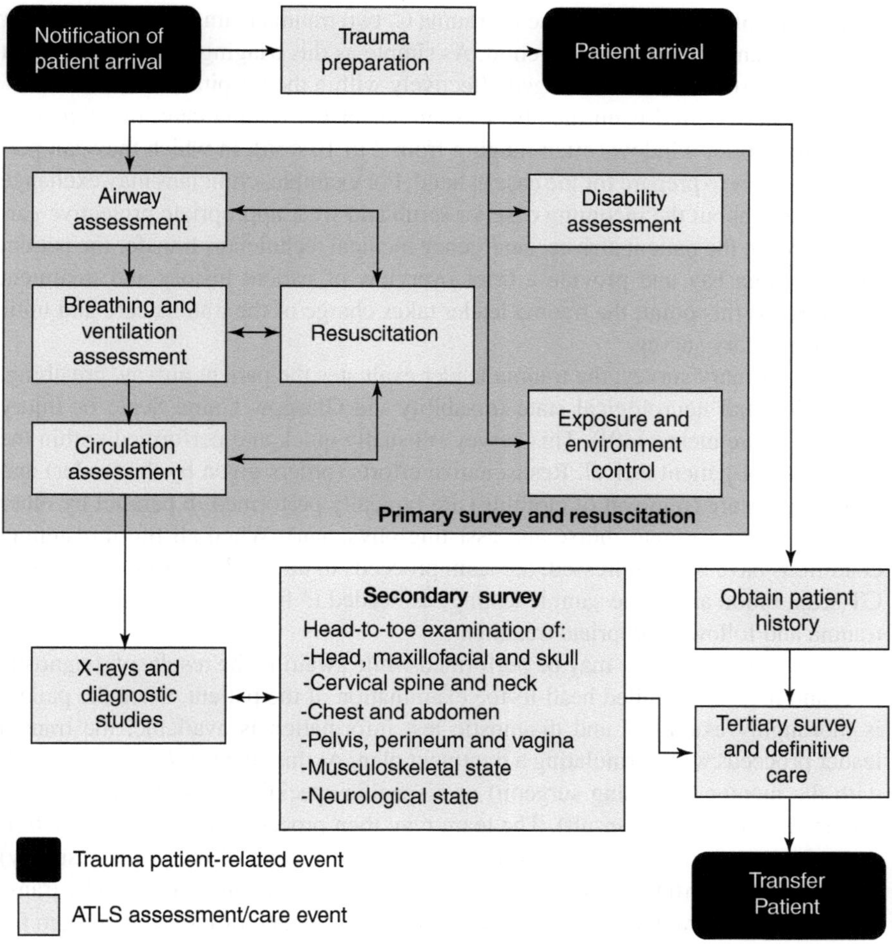

Fig. 8.2 Trauma scenario walkthrough: typical workflow observed in trauma care

the type of trauma involved. The workflow in trauma care can broadly be divided into (1) primary survey and resuscitation, (2) secondary survey, and, (3) tertiary survey and definitive care. Our descriptions of the scenario described is based on workflow observed on site at a Level-1 trauma center as well as on the existing literature on ATLS guideline implementation [37] (Fig. 8.2).

A trauma care scenario begins with an announcement of trauma arrival with an associated acuity or case type indicator. This indicator is usually specific to the trauma care site. With respect to a representative venue, Banner Good Samaritan Hospital (Phoenix, AZ), trauma cases that may require an anesthesiologist are classified as "trauma A". Cases with lower severity are classified as "trauma B". There may be other classifiers that are independent of severity. For example, any case involving a pregnant woman is classified as "trauma C". Based on the trauma severity or type indicator, care provider teams assemble in configurations predetermined for the type of trauma. In the case of trauma C, two trauma teams assemble; one for the mother and the other for the child. As simple as this triaging scheme may be, it allows for resources to be managed effectively within the hospital.

Once the required team members assemble for the trauma care, the clinicians may have a brief window (often ranging from 2 to 10 min), in which they can perform activities to prepare for the case at hand. For example, clinicians may exchange information about the incoming case, or scrub and wear appropriate protective garments. When the patient arrives, emergency medical technicians transfer the patient to the trauma bay and provide a brief overview of patient history and treatment provided. At this point, the trauma leader takes charge of the trauma care and initiates the primary survey.

In the primary survey, the trauma leader evaluates the patient airway, breathing, circulation and neurological state (disability via Glasgow Coma Scale or Injury Severity Score metric [40]). This survey is usually quick and performed within the first 2 min of patient arrival. Resuscitative efforts (orders given by the leader) and patient exposure (removal of clothing) are typically performed in parallel by other team members (primary nurse and assisting physician). When all life threatening conditions have been addressed, the team proceeds to utilize diagnostic tests (x-ray, CT scan, blood and urine sample testing) as needed to further diagnose the patient trauma and follow appropriate treatment.

The secondary survey may be performed while awaiting the results of diagnostic tests and involves detailed head-to-toe examination of the patient. Once the patient is thoroughly examined and diagnostic test information is available, the trauma leader proceeds with formulating a treatment plan. At this stage, he/she may consult with the mentor (attending surgeon) or a specific specialty consult (for example, orthopedic or plastics consult). The team may then proceed with providing definitive care (management of conditions not treated at the end of the primary survey) and conducting tertiary surveys, if required. When the patient is ready to be transferred out of the trauma unit, the patient may be discharged or moved to a room for monitoring and extended treatment by a consult.

The ATLS standard described (and tabulated in Table 8.1) is a *guideline* as opposed to being a fixed protocol. A guideline is defined as "*a statement or other indication of policy or procedure by which to determine a course of action*" [41]. In contrast, a protocol is "*a precise and detailed plan … for a regimen of diagnosis or therapy*" [42]. Since trauma care is a complex system that is inherently dynamic and unpredictable, providing clinicians with a rigid protocol would limit their ability to adapt to the situations at hand. A guideline, on the other hand, does not inherently penalize a clinician for not performing a particular step in order. This allows clinicians to adapt the guideline to suit the dynamic needs and requirements of the team.

For the purpose of this research, the ATLS guideline is considered to be a set of minimum specifications. The guideline provides general direction for the team and describes role boundaries, resources and constraints [43, 44]. The implementation of such a guideline, as opposed to detailed protocols, can result in the emergence of innovative and complex behaviors [45]. The key challenge here is to ensure that the deviations or novel adaptations made by the team members do not contradict the purpose of the guideline and consequently compromise patient safety.

A Preliminary Classifications of Deviations from Standards in Trauma Care

In order to cope with the complexity of a typical trauma environment, clinicians tend to develop ad-hoc adaptations to function in an effective manner. It is these adaptations or "deviations" from expected behavior that provide insight into the processes that shape the overall behavior of the complex system. Deviations can be defined as steps performed that are not on an accepted pre-defined standard. In our research, we adopted the ATLS guidelines as the standard from which deviations were identified [37]. We developed a preliminary classification of deviations based on field observations of ten cases conducted in a Level-1 trauma unit at Banner Good Samaritan Medical Center [46]. Our hypothesis for this study was (1) that deviations do occur, and (2) while some deviations may be errors, other deviations may be innovations (that emerge out of complex adaptive systems).

The field observations for this work were conducted in Banner Good Samaritan's trauma unit, one of six Level-1 trauma centers in the Phoenix metropolitan area. Approximately 3,000 patients are treated annually in this 5-bed unit. The trauma center has dedicated hospital resources for the management of trauma patients throughout all aspects of care, including initial evaluation and resuscitation, acute care and rehabilitation. In addition, the trauma unit collaborates with surgeons from neurosurgery, cardiothoracic, vascular, orthopedic, plastics, ophthalmology, urology and internal medicine departments to provide the required care for incoming patients. The trauma team (present during every shift) includes 1 trauma resident, 2 trauma nurses, 1 trauma attending, 1 anesthesiologist, one to two junior residents, one to two medical students, and radiology and lab technicians. Trauma nurses supporting the trauma leader are experienced registered nurses (RNs) with 5–10 years of critical care experience.

The study was approved by the Institutional Review Board and the informed consents were obtained from the participants on each encounter. Field observations were gathered by one researcher over a period of 3 months from December 2009 to February 2010. Trauma cases that occurred between 9 am and 9 pm (Monday through Thursday) were observed. The researcher logged observations simultaneously as the trauma team treated the patient. All observations were gathered unobtrusively. Clarifications about the events that occurred were obtained from clinicians between trauma events. Within the time period specified, a total of ten trauma cases were observed with seven attending trauma surgeons (experts), seven junior trauma residents (novices in the first and second year of residency training) and seven senior residents (in the third and fourth year of residency training). The trauma cases were of two types; trauma A and trauma B (trauma A refers to high criticality cases that require the presence of an anesthesiologist, while trauma B cases are those cases that are classified as low criticality). Out of the ten cases observed, eight cases were trauma B cases and two were trauma A.

The ATLS standard for Initial Assessment and Management was utilized to assess these cases for deviations. Irrespective of the types of the cases, all steps of the Initial Assessment and Management are required to be followed by the core trauma team. This allows for a valid comparison between the ten trauma cases. The deviations identified were broadly classified as errors, innovations, and proactive and reactive deviations. While errors were defined as deviations that potentially impact patients and their treatment outcome *negatively*, innovations may be thought of as deviations from the protocol that may *positively* affect the patient's outcome. In addition to errors and innovations, there were some deviations that did not directly impact patient outcomes but rather were actions demanded by the dynamic nature of the complex environments. Deviations performed in reaction to patient-specific actions or condition changes were classified as reactive deviations. On the other hand, steps taken to improve the efficiency of the trauma care by anticipating future needs were classified as proactive deviations. Using this analytic framework, individual (or unit) deviations identified using ATLS protocol for "Initial Assessment and Management" (detailed in Table 8.1), were classified to answer the following questions:

1. How often do the trauma team members deviate from standard practice?
2. When clinicians deviate, what are the types of deviations made?
3. How do these types of deviations vary with the experience (level and type) of the members of the clinical team?

The analysis of the data was performed by one researcher in collaboration with an expert trauma clinician (an attending). The data set was then analyzed using statistical means and interpreted to answer the questions outlined in the previous section. Independent group *t*-test was used to find the differences between numbers and types of deviations in trauma A and trauma B cases. A p-value of $p<0.05$ was accepted as statistically significant.

Mean Deviations per Trauma Case: The results are presented as mean (μ) ± standard deviation (σ). Figure 8.3 depicts the mean deviations that occurred in the ten trauma cases for: (1) trauma A and trauma B (9.1 ± 2.14), (2) trauma A (14 ± 1.41), and (3) trauma B cases (7.5 ± 2.79). The mean numbers of deviations in trauma A cases were higher compared to the mean deviations in trauma B cases. Typically, trauma A cases involve unstable and unpredictable patients. Consequently, the trauma team makes a relatively larger number of deviations to adapt to the dynamic situation at hand.

Deviation Distribution and Trauma Severity: Fig. 8.4 shows the distributions of (1) errors (trauma A: $\mu = 1.5 \pm 1.06$, trauma B: $\mu = 2.63 \pm 1.1$), (2) innovations (trauma A: $\mu = 0.5 \pm 0.35$, trauma B: $\mu = 0.75 \pm 0.7$), (3) proactive deviations (trauma A: $\mu = 0.5 \pm 0.35$, trauma B: $\mu = 0.38 \pm 0.37$), and (4) reactive deviations (trauma A: $\mu = 11.5 \pm 1.06$, trauma B: $\mu = 4.13 \pm 1.15$). From Fig. 8.4, it can be seen that errors make up a small percentage (26.38 %) of the total deviations in the ten trauma cases. This is an important result from these observations, since it points to the limitations

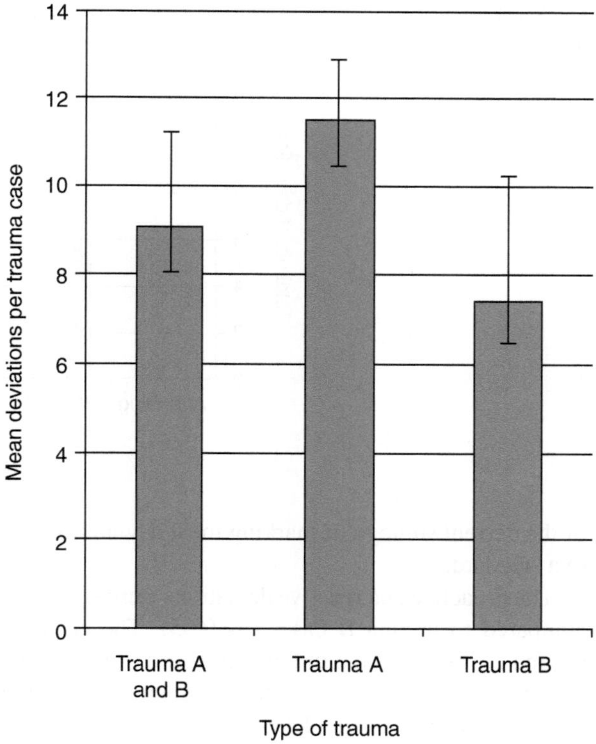

Fig. 8.3 Mean deviations per trauma case

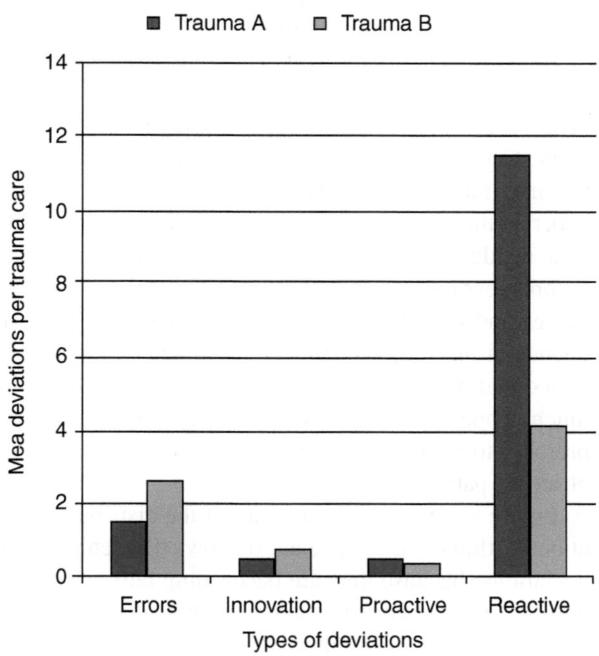

Fig. 8.4 Deviation distribution in two trauma settings

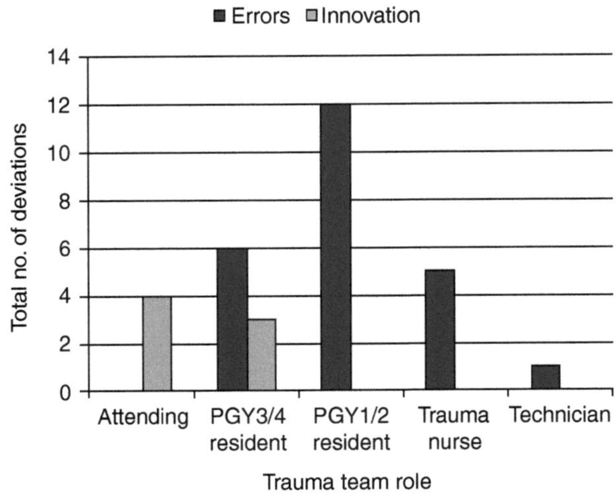

Fig. 8.5 Error and innovation as a function of expertise

of the current strategy of marking most deviations as errors in assuring compliance to a standard.

The proactive and reactive deviations were significantly higher in trauma A when compared to trauma B cases ($p<0.05$). The critical condition of the patients in trauma A cases and the individual nature of the problem cause the trauma team to deviate often in order to manage the unique situation at hand. The analysis also showed that most of the deviations were reactive in nature, in both trauma A and trauma B cases. This can be attributed to the dynamic nature of the critical care environment. Clinicians are required to react quickly to the changes to ensure efficient operation in trauma care.

Deviation Distribution and Clinician Expertise: Fig. 8.5 depicts the total number of errors and innovations made by core team members in the ten trauma cases observed. In this study, the experts made no errors as defined in the analytic framework. Care givers with lesser expertise (from the third and fourth year resident to the first and second year residents), made fewer innovations, when compared to the experts (attending trauma surgeons). While intermediate clinicians (third and fourth year residents) made more errors compared to the attendings, novices (first and second year residents) made more errors than any other group of clinicians. Trauma nurses and technicians show little evidence of innovation. Although this low frequency of innovation cannot be attributed to a lack of experience, it can be hypothesized that within the confines of their roles in interacting with a patient, there is not much scope for innovation. Nurses and technicians are trained to follow a strict protocol to support the trauma team, and that training may be responsible for the observed patterns.

Figure 8.6 provides a snapshot of the distribution of proactive and reactive deviations within the trauma team. It shows that senior residents make the most reactive deviations (because they are performing bulk of the tasks), followed by the trauma nurses. Junior residents who generally assist but may lead a few trauma cases also made a significant number of reactive deviations. These observations show that

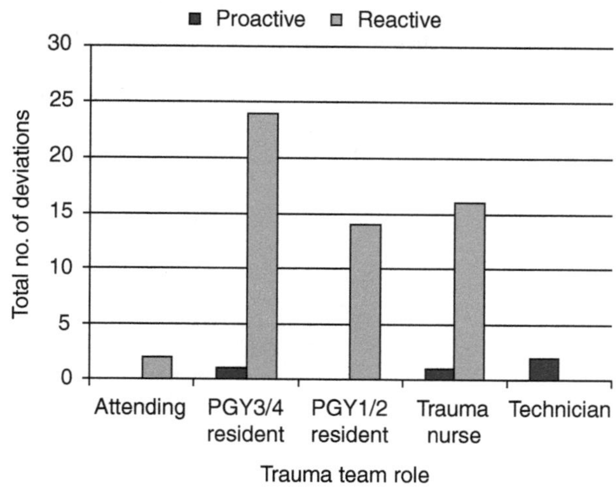

Fig. 8.6 Proactive and reactive deviations as a function of expertise

leadership role and associated tasks may be connected to generating deviations to the protocol.

This study provides supportive evidence for the claim that deviations do occur in critical care environments and not all deviations are errors. Deviations from the standard can be important innovations and are tied to complex decision making and judgment calls at the point of care. The results from this study show that expertise of the caregivers and criticality of a patient's condition influence the number and type of deviations from standard practice. Although this research was a novel approach for assessing protocols and guidelines, there were not enough subjects studied to enable tests of significance. In addition, errors and innovations were defined in terms of patient outcome. The causal effect between deviations and specific patient outcomes may be difficult to track in critical care environments. For this reason, there is a necessity to define deviations in relation to protocols and guidelines instead. This will also enable definitions to be more generalizable to other critical care environments.

Deviations from Standards and Expert Cognition and Team Decision Making

From a cognitive perspective, error, innovation and effectiveness in carrying out a protocol is intimately linked with expertise of the clinicians. This was partially established in our preliminary analysis of deviations in ten trauma cases. Our findings are consistent with previous studies that looked at the relationship between task difficulty and expertise [47]. Patel et al. found that experts were able to use a well-developed knowledge base and superior strategies in clinical reasoning. Furthermore, Patel and Groen [48] showed that in medicine, experts tend to follow a top-down reasoning strategy wherein reasoning from a hypothesis is done to account for the

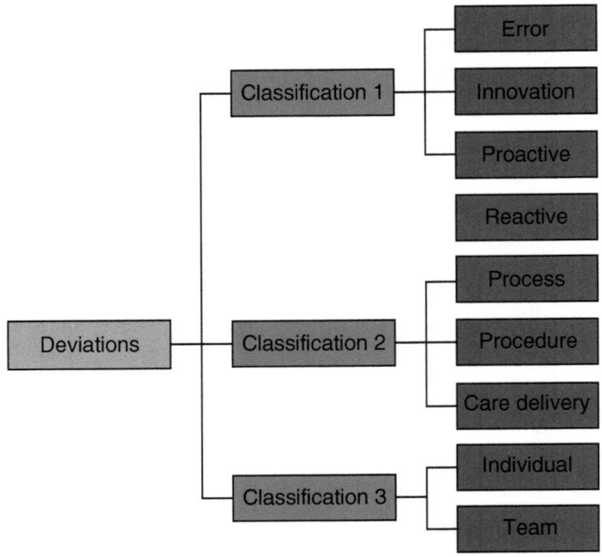

Fig. 8.7 Extended classification of deviations in trauma care

case data. It has been shown that this methodology when combined with experience-driven cognitive constructs results in experts making fewer errors compared to novices. It is plausible that when experts do deviate, the deviations are more likely to be innovations. While our preliminary results alluded to this hypothesis being true, we needed more concrete definitions for the types of deviations to provide a consistent and replicable methodology or qualitative analysis of deviations in the domain.

Extended Framework for Deviations from Standard Practice

Figure 8.7 depicts the hierarchy for an extended classification of deviations [49]. In previous research [46], deviations were classified as (1) errors, (2) innovations, and (3) proactive and (4) reactive deviations. Further examination showed that deviations could also be classified by how they affected the trauma care (Classification 2), and how many members were involved in the decision making (Classification 3). In this section, the previous classification of deviations is revisited (providing more concrete definitions for the ideations of error and innovation) and an extended classification is presented.

Classification Schema 1 – Deviations as Errors: An error is defined as a deviation from the standard, if it: (1) violated a prescribed order of activities with a negative impact on workflow, (2) resulted (directly or indirectly) in compromising patient care, or (3) resulted in an activity being repeated due to failure in execution or a loss of information.

An example of an error that violates order of activities is a resident completing the secondary survey prior to ordering chest and pelvis x-rays. Due to the change in order, obtaining the x-rays for diagnosis was delayed. As the deviation caused a delay in receiving information critical to treating the patient in a timely manner, it can be classified as an error.

A junior resident attempting to remove the spine board before the patient's spine was cleared (confirmed not to be injured) is also an error. In this case, the deviation directly compromises patient care and can consequently be classified as an error.

Another form of error is one of implementation; a lab technician needing to redraw a sample for blood work when additional tests were ordered. In this case, the lab technician had discarded previous samples obtained. A lack of communication within the team resulted in this deviation. While not as severe as the previous error, the repetition of a task by a team member due to a failure in communication can be considered to be an error.

Classification Schema 1 – Deviations as Innovations: Innovations are defined as deviations that potentially benefit the individual, team or patient by bringing novelty to the situation at hand [50]. We now present a few scenarios that describe situations when innovations occurred.

A patient required a translator in order to communicate with the resident. The team was unable to find a translator. The attending asked the trauma nurse to see if the patient's family could help. The patient's sibling was able to come into trauma facility and act as a translator. This allowed the resident to continue with his examination, leading to successful assessment and treatment of the patient. The standard protocol of seeking an in-house translator was violated. A novel step (that resulted in a positive outcome) was introduced in the workflow, which qualifies as an innovative deviation.

In another case, a patient was nervous about the damage done to his face due to an accident. In order to calm the patient, the nurse provided him with a small mirror so that he could assess the damage for himself. The patient then relaxed. For such a case, the guideline provides no instruction on how to deal with a difficult patient. The clinician deviated by introducing an action outside the scope defined by the guideline to successfully care for the patient.

The resident examined a patient's leg injury (in fewer than 15 s), and ordered an x-ray of the extremity along with chest and abdomen x-rays. By introducing a brief examination of the injury site, the resident was able to anticipate a future need and advance a step in the standard. The results were relayed back to the team more promptly than if the prescribed order of steps had been followed. The introduction of a novel step that resulted in a positive outcome on the workflow was considered to be an innovation.

Classification Schema 1 – Proactive Deviations: A proactive deviation occurs when (1) an activity is performed (without compromising patient care) in anticipation of a future requirement (or lack thereof) when treating a patient or (2) an activity (which may be out of the bounds of an individual's role in the trauma team) is performed in order to correct or prevent error occurrence.

A radiology technician setting up the x-ray sensor board for a chest x-ray prior to the trauma arrival is an example of a proactive deviation. It is considered to be proactive as the step was taken in anticipation of patient whose trauma type was conveyed to the team. A trauma nurse calling the radiology unit to let the unit know that the technician would not be required as the scans had already been taken in the previous facility is also a proactive deviation on the part of the nurse. Finally, a trauma nurse reminding a junior resident that c-spine results have to be received prior to removal of the spine board is an example of a proactive deviation that is performed to prevent an error.

Classification Schema 1 – Reactive Deviations: Reactive deviations occur when an activity is performed in reaction to an unanticipated event or change in patient condition, diagnostic process or treatment plans. Examples of reactive deviations found in this study include the team reacting to a patient who was violently reacting to pain. This patient needed to be held down by the trauma team in order to complete the primary survey and intubate the patient. Ordering additional tests due to inconclusive results from tests at hand is also an example of a reactive deviation. Finally, on-the-fly deviations made to treatment plan based on specific requests made by patients can be considered reactive. In one case, the patient requested plastics consult as he was concerned about his facial injuries. The treatment plan had to be altered to accommodate the patient's request and this deviation was marked as a reactive one.

While in this study, errors, innovations, proactive and reactive deviations are treated as mutually exclusive, in reality there may exist an overlap between these categories. While further investigation is required is assess of the schema should be modified to examine inter-relationships between the categories, for this exploratory study the categories are treated as mutually exclusive groups.

In addition to classify deviations by the impact they may have on workflow, deviations may also be classified by how they impact the steps of the trauma standard. Based on the granularity of the step deviated from and the type of activity performed, deviations may also be classified as (1) process-related, (2) procedure-related, or (3) care delivery-related deviations.

Classification Schema 2 – Process-related Deviations: Deviations that may be related to how the guideline is implemented are classified as process-related deviations. Examples of process-related deviations include log roll not being performed correctly or an x-ray being ordered after the secondary survey. In both examples, clinicians deviated from the recommended method for guideline implementation.

Classification Schema 2 – Procedure-related Deviations: In contrast to process-related deviations, procedure-related deviations deal with how a specific step in the guideline is performed. An example of a procedure-related deviation is a clinician making an error in stapling a wound. The key difference between process- and procedure-related deviations lies in the granularity of unit activities in trauma care. Changes in order or presence/absence of activities are considered as a process-related deviation, whereas changes made to the unit activity itself are procedure-related.

Classification Schema 2 – Care Delivery-related Deviations: Any deviation dealing with the care provided to the patient (not specified in guidelines) is classified as a care delivery deviation. These deviations include a nurse providing a mirror to a patient concerned by facial injuries or providing medications for a patient in pain. Whereas procedure related deviations typically involve medical interventions, care delivery-related deviations involve activities performed that support the trauma team and patient.

Finally, deviations may be differentiated by the number of trauma team members involved in the decision making process that ultimately resulted in the occurrence of the deviation. Deviations may be classified as (1) individual, or (2) team deviations.

Classification Schema 3 – Individual Deviations: Deviations initiated by a single clinician are classified as individual deviations. Examples of individual deviations include a resident making an error in a procedure, or an attending suggested a novel methodology for a step in the protocol or a trauma leader proactively performing certain steps in the protocol. In each of these cases the deviations were initiated by a decision made by a single individual.

Classification Schema 3 – Team Deviations: Whereas an individual may initiate many deviations, some deviations occur at the team level. Such deviations involve more than one clinician participating in the event. For example, a resident may decide on an alternate course of treatment based on a discussion with his attending or the team. Such a deviation is classified as a team deviation. Tables 8.2, 8.3 and 8.4 summarize the terminology involved in classifying deviations as described in this section.

Table 8.2 Summary of classification schema 1

Error	Related to standard practice: Task order violatio Task omission Task repetition due to communication or execution failure Impact on workflow: **NEGATIVE** Causes delays Compromises patient care
Innovation	Related to standard practice: Novel task addition Impact on workflow: **POSITIVE** Improves workflow efficiency Improves quality of patient care
Proactive	Related to standard practice: Task advancement Error prevention Out of role expectations Impact on workflow: **NUETRAL** No observable impact on workflow or patient care
Reactive	Related to standard practice: Common task addition in response to random event Impact on workflow: **NUETRAL** No observable impact on workflow or patient care

Table 8.3 Summary of classification schema 2

Process	Related to standard practice: Deviations (including task order change, omission and addition) that related to how the standard is implemented
Procedure	Related to standard practice: Deviations (including tasks repeated due to execution failure) that related to medical interventions provided to the patient
Care Delivery	Related to standard practice: Deviations related to supportive care interventions provided to the patient

Table 8.4 Summary of classification schema 3

Individual	Initiated by decision making process of a single clinician in the team
Team	Initiated collaboratively by two or more clinicians in the team

It should be noted that the three types of classification schema are treated as independent of one another. A team deviation can be an error or an innovation, for example. Such a classification allows researchers to examine the context of various types of deviations. This can further the understanding of various factors that contribute to deviations.

In our next study, the following themes were explored; (1) various types of deviations that occur in trauma care, (2) how they relate to expertise, and, (3) whether they were initiated by an individual or by a team. Field observations were conducted by one researcher from September 2010 to December 2010 at Banner Good Samaritan's Level-1 trauma unit. A total of 20 trauma cases were observed. This, added to the ten trauma cases previously observed, resulted in a total of 30 cases with 15 cases being led by fourth or fifth year (senior) residents and 15 cases led by second or third year (junior) residents. Out of the 30 cases, 6 cases were categorized as trauma A (patient in critical condition) and 23 cases as trauma B (moderate criticality of patient). One case was classified as trauma C as it involved a pregnant woman. As patient identifiers such as Glasgow coma scale (GCS) and injury severity score (ISS) were not captured (the protocol involved shadowing clinicians alone), the classification of the trauma is used as a proxy to assess severity of the incoming patient.

The trauma cases were observed by one researcher using the A(×4) model [51]. This model requires contextual observations (snapshots) to be captured by highlighting four key parameters, namely, actors, activities, atmosphere and artifacts. Observations captured in this manner provide rich contextual descriptions of the situation, which is required for analysis of deviations.

Each time-stamped observation was compared to the corresponding step in the ATLS guideline [37] in order to determine (1) if a deviation had occurred, (2) the type of the deviation and (3) if the deviation resulted from individual or team-level processes. The data were analyzed iteratively until the number and type of deviations stabilized. The analysis methodology is similar to the methods described in the preliminary analysis of deviations [46]. As before, the study was approved by the Institutional Review Board and the informed consents were obtained from the participants on each encounter.

Table 8.5 Chi-square p-values of pair-wise relationships between variables

Variables	Leader	Role	Phase	Class1	Class2	Class3
Leader	–	**<0.0001**	0.2975	**0.0150**	**0.0258**	0.8469
Role	**<0.0001**	–	**<0.0001**	**<0.0001**	**0.0174**	0.8129
Phase	0.2975	**<0.0001**	–	**<0.0001**	**<0.0001**	0.0648
Class1	**0.0150**	**<0.0001**	**<0.0001**	–	**0.0002**	0.0720
Class2	**0.0258**	**0.0174**	**<0.0001**	**0.0002**	–	0.7919
Class3	0.8469	0.8129	0.0648	0.0720	0.7919	–

A total of 165 deviations were identified from the 30 trauma cases observed. Of these deviations, four were found to be related to auxiliary activities in trauma care. The activities corresponding to these deviations included (1) attendings teaching residents specifics of trauma care, and (2) clinicians gathering evidence in trauma cases that resulted from criminal activities. These deviations are unrelated to trauma team expertise or guideline implementation. Consequently they were omitted from the analysis.

The 161 remaining deviations are described categorically using the variables (1) training of the resident leading trauma care (Variable – Leader), (2) role played by clinician initiating the deviation in the trauma team (Variable – Role), (3) phase of the trauma standard at which the deviation took place (Variable – Phase), (4) deviation type based on classification schema 1 (Variable – Class1), (5) deviation type based on classification schema 2 (Variable – Class2), and (6) deviation type based on classification schema 3 (Variable – Class3). The severity of the trauma case was not considered as a variable as a disproportionate number of trauma B cases were observed compared to trauma A during the duration of the study. For each pair of variables, Chi-square analysis was performed to tease out relationships that may exist. Table 8.5 summarizes the results of pair-wise relationship tests conducted for the variables described. Significant relationships (p-value <0.05) are indicated by bold font.

From Table 8.5 it is seen that (1) expertise of the trauma leader, (2) the phase in which the deviation occurs, and (3) the role played by the clinician have significant relationships with types of deviations made. There is also an indication of a strong association between classification schema 1 and schema 2. It should be noted that near-significant relationships are found between classification schema 3 and schemas 1 and 2. This indicates a possible relationship that may need additional data to verify its validity. In the following sections, the individual significant relationships are further characterized.

Deviations and Expertise of Trauma Leader: Although no significant difference was found in the frequency of deviations, the types of deviations made were found to be related to the experience level of the clinician leading the trauma. Chi-square analysis between team leader and deviations classified using schema 1 showed significant relationship between these variables (Chi-sq = 10.4608, df = 3, p = 0.0150). Figure 8.8 depicts the relationship between the experience level of the trauma leader and errors, innovations, proactive and reactive deviations.

Trauma cases led by senior residents had more proactive deviations and innovations compared to cases led by a junior resident. Errors and reactive deviations were

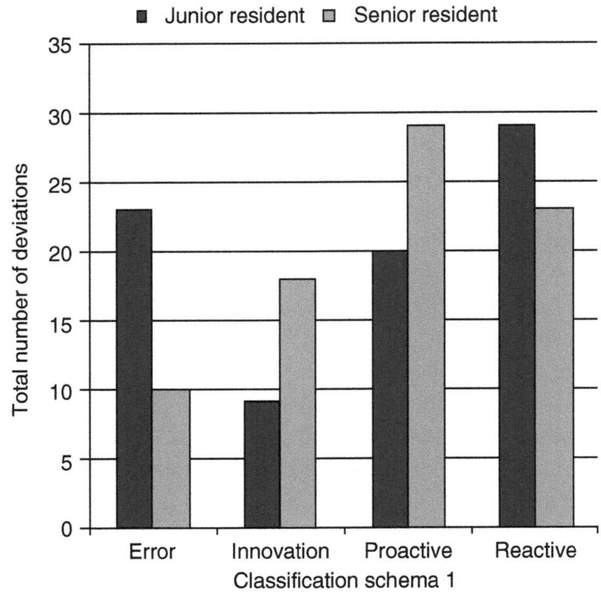

Fig. 8.8 Deviations (classification schema 1) and expertise of trauma leader

found to be greater in cases led by junior residents. These finding suggests that (1) trauma leaders with more experience are able to adapt (making innovations) to the dynamic environment while minimizing errors, and (2) experience enables leaders to guide a more proactive trauma team. Thus, it can be hypothesized that the proactive nature of expert trauma leaders enables them to anticipate future needs and possible errors, thereby minimizing resource wastage and unnecessary negative impact on patient outcomes.

A significant relationship was also found between the experience level of the team leader and deviations classified using schema 2 (Chi-sq = 7.3179, df = 2, p = 0.0258). Figure 8.9 depicts the relationship between leader expertise and process-, procedure-, and care delivery-related deviations. Cases led by junior residents had fewer care delivery-related deviations and more procedure-related deviations compared to cases led by a senior resident. Junior residents focused more on specific procedures. This is indicative of their level of training. Senior residents have mastered procedures, and can focus on developing other skills, such as communication. The number of process-related deviations was found to be similar for the two groups.

Finally, Fig. 8.10 depicts the significant relationship (Chi-sq = 83.7175, df = 4, p = <0.0001) between role of the clinician in the trauma team (junior resident, senior resident, attending, nurse and technician) and expertise of trauma leader. Whereas the statistics indicate a strong association between the variables, this could largely be attributed to the importance of the trauma leader handing a case. As seen in Fig. 8.10, most deviations are made by the leader. Consequently, it is difficult to draw conclusions about flexibility of leadership based on the data available. However, it can be seen that the attending plays a larger role in cases led by a junior resident. This is expected in a teaching setting.

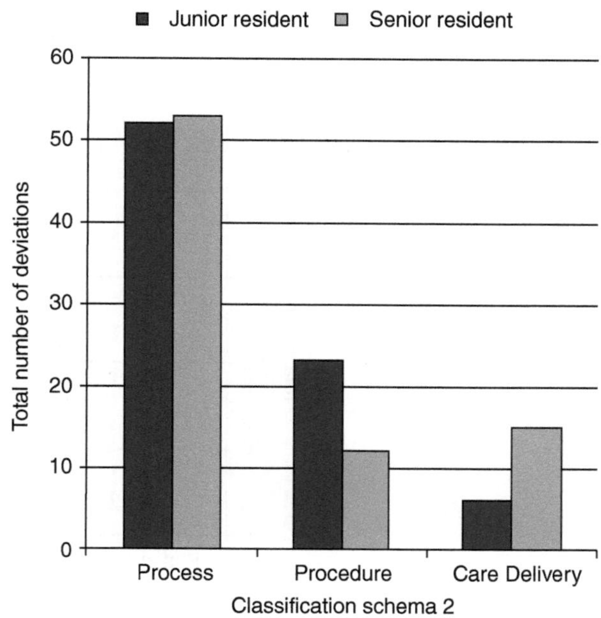

Fig. 8.9 Deviations (classification schema 2) and expertise of trauma leader

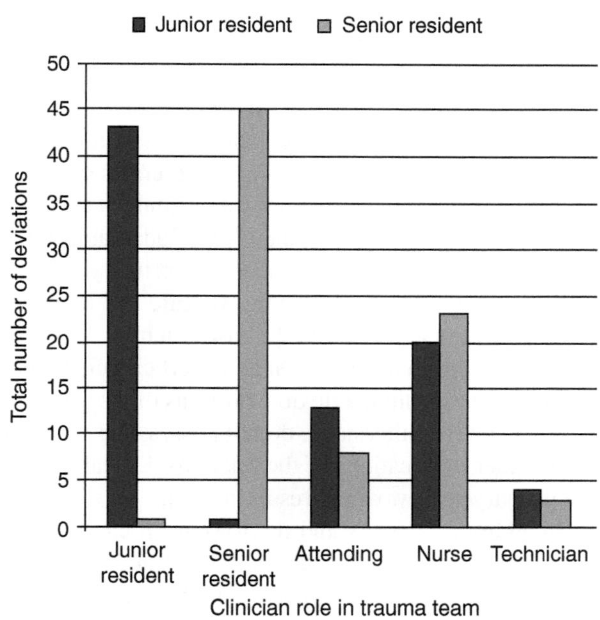

Fig. 8.10 Deviations (clinician role) and expertise of trauma leader

Deviations and Phases of Trauma Standard Protocol: Fig. 8.11 shows total number of deviations identified at each key stage in the trauma management standard (Phase 1: Trauma Preparation, Primary Survey and Resuscitation, Phase 2: X-ray and Diagnostic Studies, Phase 3: Secondary Survey, Phase 4: Tertiary Survey and

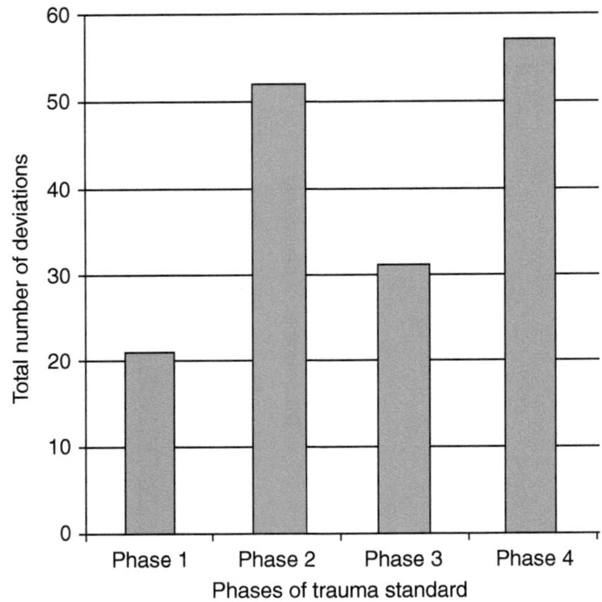

Fig. 8.11 Total number of deviations in phases of trauma standard

Definitive Care). A greater number of deviations were found to occur in the phases following trauma preparation and primary survey and resuscitation (Percentage of deviations in Phase 1: 13.04 %, Phases 2–4: 86.96 %).

Using chi-square analysis, a significant relationship was found between the phase in the standard and deviations classified using schema 1 (Chi-sq = 44.255, df = 9, $p < 0.0001$). As seen in Fig. 8.12, errors occur throughout the various stages of the trauma care, whereas innovations only occur once the primary survey is completed. This is indicative of the level of adaptability the guideline allows for in the earlier stages of trauma treatment. The primary survey is protocol-driven, whereas the secondary survey and definitive care are more flexible, allowing the trauma team to deviate and adapt to the case at hand.

The key difference between an expert clinician and a novice is that expert clinicians deviate within the flexible portions of the guidelines, resulting in innovations. Novices, on the other hand, do not possess the necessary knowledge to understand the broader implications of their actions. Deviations made in critical steps, such as the primary survey, would result in error.

In addition to errors and innovations, it can be seen that more proactive deviations occur in the earlier stages of the trauma standard, while reactive deviations occur in the tertiary survey and definitive care stages. This is expected. As more information becomes available to the team, decisions about care of the patient may be altered in a reactionary manner. Figure 8.13 shows the relationship between phase of the trauma standard to deviations classified using schema 2 (Chi-sq = 40.0974, df = 6, $p < 0.0001$).

The total number of process-related deviations is higher when x-ray and diagnostic tests are ordered (27.95 % in Phase 2). This indicates that certain steps in trauma

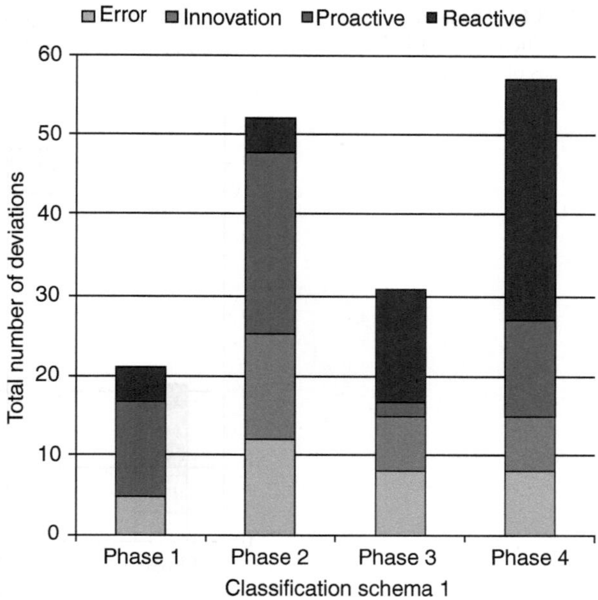

Fig. 8.12 Deviations (classification schema 1) and phases of trauma standard

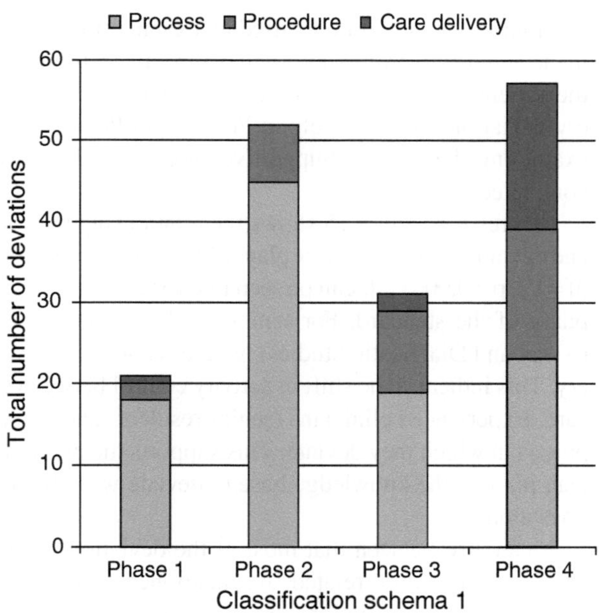

Fig. 8.13 Deviations (classification schema 2) and phases of trauma standard

treatment may be more adaptable than others. Identifying such critical steps and monitoring the deviations that occur could provide more information that will help direct guideline updates. In addition to the differences in process related deviations, it is interesting to note that procedural deviations linearly increase as trauma care proceeds through the various phases. This is expected, because the initial phases of

Fig. 8.14 Deviations (classified by role) and phases of trauma standard

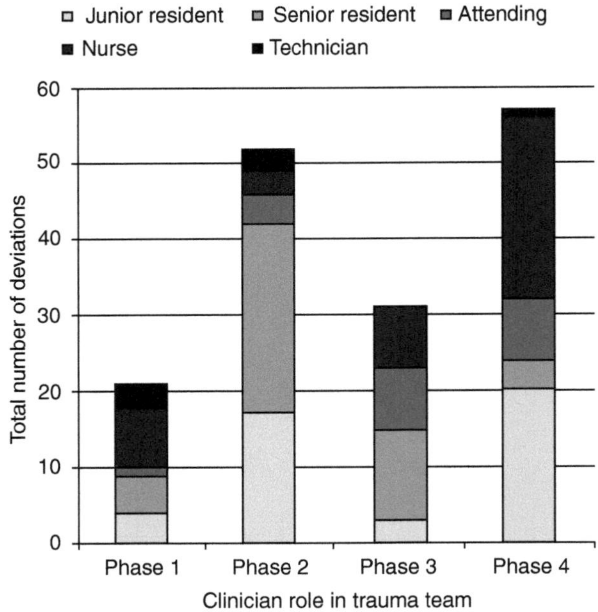

the trauma care are more focused on examination of the patient. Once a diagnosis is made and results from x-rays and diagnostic tests are obtained, interventions to treat the patient trauma are performed. It should also be noted that supportive care delivery deviations occur largely in Phase 4. In Phases 1–3, the focus of the team is in examining the patient. Supportive case is usually provided after these phases are completed.

Figures 8.14 and 8.15 shows the relationship between phase of trauma standard and deviations classified role played by clinician in the trauma team (Chi-sq = 51.3650, df = 12, $p < 0.0001$). It can be seen that for each role deviations are biased in a certain phase of the standard. For senior residents, most deviations are made in Phase 2 (X-ray and Diagnostic Studies), whereas nurses make most deviations in care delivery. This indicates the shift in activity control between clinicians involved in trauma care. Experienced clinicians (senior residents and nurses) also show restraint in the phases in which they deviate. This supports the previous statement that expert clinician possess the knowledge base to deviate with the flexible portions of the guidelines alone.

It can also be seen that most of the deviations performed by residents are process- and procedure-related. As mentioned earlier and corroborated by Fig. 8.16, junior residents' deviations are more biased towards procedures. It is not unusual that deviations made by nurses are predominately care delivery-related. Trauma teams have well-defined role boundaries. This enables teams to function effectively in chaotic situations.

Expertise is critical to formation of adaptive teams in trauma critical care. The results show that trauma leaders with more experience are able to adapt to the dynamic environment while minimizing errors. Novices, on the other hand, are

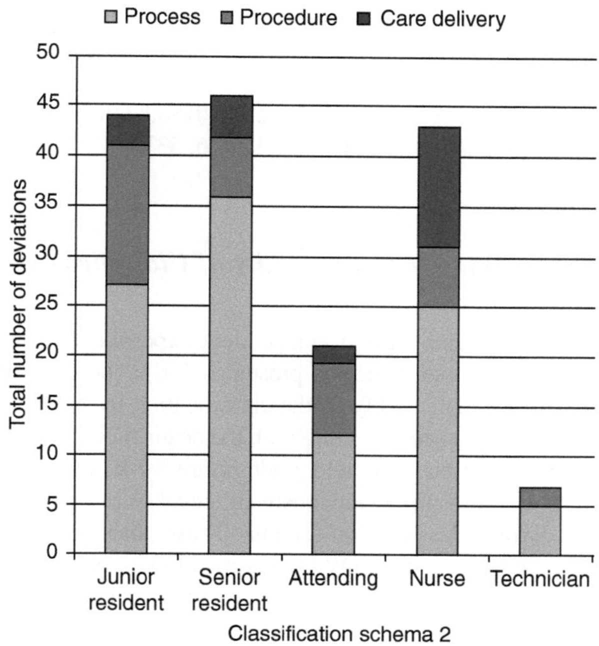

Fig. 8.15 Deviations (classification schema 1) and clinician role

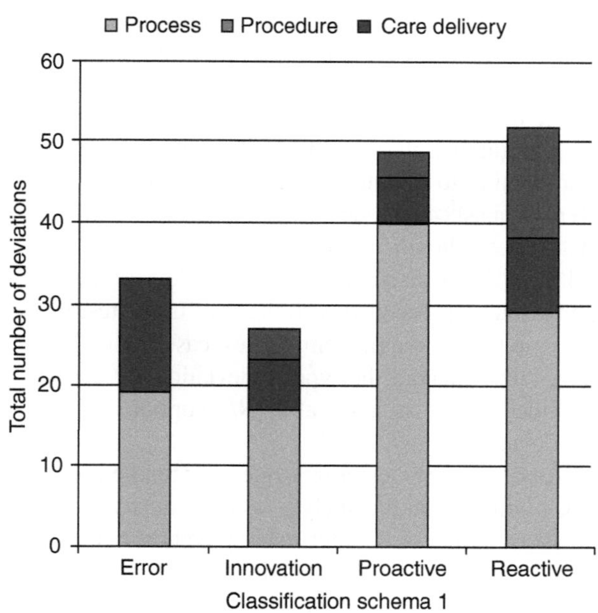

Fig. 8.16 Deviations (classification schema 2) and clinician role

preoccupied by procedural aspects of trauma care and fail to achieve the necessary levels of communication needed to facilitate team innovations. Another key difference between experts and novices lies in their ability to recover from errors and unexpected events. Patel and colleagues [52] showed that experts' knowledge is adapted to recognize familiar patterns of stimuli. However, their heuristic reasoning from the pattern recognition strategy may not be effective in some complex situations [47]. Experts may make errors, but are adept at correcting them before negative consequences occur. Novices on the other hand fail to perceive the consequences of their decisions until it is too late [6, 53].

Evaluating Generalizability of Classification Schemas

We also conducted two independent experiments to assess the generalizability of the classification schemas presented [50]. The experiments were designed to (1) assess the replicability of the classification by independent raters, and (2) concordance of their rating/coding with the original classification. The results of the experiments described will help guide future work in this domain.

The observations previously collected were de-identified and utilized to develop the current classification schema. These observations were used in the experiment to assess the replicability of classification by other raters. This study was approved by the Institutional Review Boards of Arizona State University and Banner Good Samaritan Medical Center. Fifteen trauma cases were randomly chosen from the existing pool of 30 trauma cases. Deviations from five of these cases were used for training two raters. The deviations in the remaining ten cases served as the test set. The raters chosen for this experiment had prior clinical environments experience (having spent 30–60 h observing clinicians). Raters with experience were chosen due to the contextual nature of the task.

The training phases consisted of a PowerPoint® slideshow that provided a brief introduction to trauma critical care and the various classification schemas. Raters were then asked to code each deviation in the training set (a total of 17 deviations). After every classification, the answers from the current classification were present followed by a discussion about the deviation. Upon completion of the training phase, raters proceeded with the test. In the test phase, raters were presented with deviations from the randomized test cases (a total of 38 deviations). For each deviation, raters marked the type of deviation for classification 1, 2 and 3. They were provided with a not applicable (N/A) option, if they were unsure of how to classify the deviation.

Among the 38 deviations, one rater marked N/A for one deviation. This sample was omitted from the analysis as an anomaly. Following the coding, the data were analyzed to assess (1) inter-rater agreement between the two raters, and (2) concordance with existing classification though a similar agreement measure. A simple Cohen's Kappa statistic was used for the analysis. As the classification schema is not ordered, all categories were given the same weight (one).

There are a number of guidelines available for interpreting Kappa statistics. For example, Fleiss's [53] guidelines consider Kappa >0.75 as excellent, 0.40–0.75 as fair to good, and <0.40 as poor agreement. Landis and Koch [55], on the other hand present a more granulated scale for measuring agreement. They consider Kappa

Table 8.6 Kappa statistics for test between rater A and rater B

Classification	Kappa	95 % lower conf. limit	95 % upper conf. limit
Schema 1	0.7743	0.6125	0.9361
Schema 2	0.7632	0.5079	1.0000
Schema 3	0.5355	0.1344	0.9366

Table 8.7 Kappa statistics for test between rater A and original classification

Classification	Kappa	95 % lower conf. limit	95 % upper conf. limit
Schema 1	0.8879	0.7689	1.0000
Schema 2	0.7000	0.4629	0.9371
Schema 3	1.0000	1.0000	1.0000

values of 0.81–1.00 as almost perfect agreement, 0.61–0.81 as substantial, 0.41–0.6 as moderate, 0.21–0.40 as fair, 0.0–0.20 as slight agreement and <0 as poor agreement. Since the nature of the classification task is subjective, the scale proposed by Landis and Koch [55] is used to interpret the results of the Kappa tests performed. In the following section the results of this experiment are presented.

Inter-rater Agreement for Classification Schemas: For each of the classification schemas (1: Error, Innovation, Proactive, and Reactive; 2: Process, Procedure, and Care Delivery, and 3: Individual and Team), the rating or classification provided by the two raters was analyzed using Cohen's Kappa. Table 8.6 summarizes the statistics for the inter-rater reliability test between Rater A and Rater B.

There was substantial agreement for classification 1 and 2. However, there is moderate agreement for classification schema 3. One reason for this result could be the lack of sufficient examples of team deviations in the current data set. Another reason could be the difficulty in defining what constitutes a team deviation in trauma care. Take, for example, the case where the log roll step in trauma care is missed. One could argue that the trauma leader is responsible for how trauma care is conducted. Hence is it an individual error. On the other hand, there were a number of other team members who could have prevented the error. In that sense it could be a team error. Such a difficulty could be resolved by studying individual and team interactions further in trauma care.

The results of the inter-rater reliability test are promising. For classification schemas 1 and 2, the relatively high Kappa score indicates that the classification schema can be used by independent raters.

Concordance with Original Classification: Tables 8.7 and 8.8 show the results of tests conducted between (1) Rater A and the original classification, and (2) Rater B and the original classification. Rater A had very high (almost perfect) agreement with the original classification in all three schemas. Such high levels of agreement are unexpected. Rater B, on the other hand had substantial agreement for schema 1 and moderate agreement for schema 2 and 3.

These results indicate the natural differences between raters. The high agreement with rater A and moderate to substantial agreement with rater B validates the categories developed to assess deviations. Combined with the results of agreement

Table 8.8 Kappa statistics for test between Rater B and original classification

Classification	Kappa	95 % lower conf. limit	95 % upper conf. limit
Schema 1	0.7729	0.6090	0.9367
Schema 2	0.5068	0.2252	0.7885
Schema 3	0.5355	0.1344	0.9366

between Rater A and Rater B, this indicates that the classification schema is replicable and can be effectively used by other researchers.

This work attempts to provide definitions and structure to a subjective form of analysis. Classifying deviations using the methodology described (based purely on observations) is difficult since there may not be enough contextual information to make a concrete decision. Video recording of trauma cases or using data gathered using the hybrid framework described in this section will enable capture of all the activities that take place in trauma care. This will especially be useful in cases where it is difficult to identify the clinicians involved in initiating the chain of events that resulted in a particular deviation.

The key limitation of the study to assess generalizability of the classification schema is that raters obtain their contextual information from tertiary observations. The process of immersing oneself in an environment provides information about several nuances of behavior that may be completely missed in written observations. Reproducing the study with data from the hybrid framework or video recording of trauma cases will provide the raters with all the information they would need to make a classification. It is also possible that the Kappa scores will improve even further if raters were provided with comprehensive data.

Classifying deviations to understand cognitive decision making processes is a very subjective process. One example from the test set is an attending asking a nurse if there is a tuberculosis protocol to follow, after it was discovered that the patient may be infected. The classification schema stated that it was a proactive deviation. Rater A marked it as an innovation and Rater B marked it as a reactive deviation. All three cases can be argued. It is a proactive deviation, since the attending went out of the bounds of his role in requesting the information (possibly in anticipation of steps to follow). It can be considered to be reactive, since it is a common task addition in reaction to the patient being infected (a random event). If thought of as a novel task addition that greatly improves patient and team safety, then it is an innovation. These arguments are based on (1) what the rater finds is accepted, or common behavior, and (2) what they perceive the impact of the deviation might be. Prior to classification and analysis, researcher will need to develop a rubric for addressing these two factors.

Summary

Protocols and standards are important for ensuring process consistency and patient safety in healthcare. While it has been shown that linear systems and processes are aided by protocol and checklist deployment, most critical care environments are characterized by non-linear interactions and dynamic emergent behavior [14]. In such environments, clinicians need to make dynamic adjustments to protocols and guidelines, in order to adapt to the operational conditions and to achieve high accuracy and efficiency. The analysis of 30 trauma cases in this work showed that an average of 5.37 deviations occur during each case. Therefore, complex systems similar to trauma critical care *cannot be treated as a zero-tolerance environment.* While protocols and guidelines serve to control complexity and errors through standardization, the importance of adapting standards safely to adjust to the environments needs to be recognized by clinicians and researchers alike.

Protocols and standards are based on observations and evidence gathered from practices. New information and novel findings from practice need to be incorporated into the guidelines and protocols. So how do such novel ideas get generated from practice? When regular or standard patterns do not fit or match the current problem, possible alternative ideas get generated. This is the process of innovation, and innovation is not possible without deviations. As practitioners gain experience in the execution of a task, their performance become increasingly smooth and efficient. While developing proficiency with attention-demanding complex tasks, some component skills become automatic, so that conscious processing can be devoted to reasoning and reflective thought with minimal interference in the overall performance. A great deal of experts' knowledge is finely tuned and highly automated enabling them to execute a set of procedures in an efficient manner. Yet they can perform such tasks in a highly adaptive manner which is sensitive to shifting contexts. The findings from this research showed that expert clinicians (senior residents and attending surgeons), do make errors. However, they are able to correct errors made before they result in a critical failure. The analysis of deviations also showed that the expertise of the trauma team leader impacted the types of deviations made. Expert teams were more innovative, compared to teams led by a novice resident. Not only are these finding consistent with emerging knowledge about medical errors and expertise [53], it also indicates that *expertise is critical to the formation of adaptive clinical teams.*

There is a strong need for informatics tools that will enable novices to adapt to the trauma environment in following certain standards, allowing for fewer errors. The classification of deviations could allow for a scientific framework for modification of protocols and enable protocol developers to leverage a data-driven approach to modifications. Currently available tools such as checklists and protocols need to allow for note takers to mark and document deviations, errors and innovation. In protocol-driven environments, checklists have been found to be a valuable tool in minimizing error rates. However, since experts' deviations are important for education and practice, these checklists would have to be flexible enough to be automatically updated. For a dynamic environment like trauma, these checklists when implemented would need to be adaptable as well. In order to develop such a tool, one would need to know the general decision process in trauma and the various types of deviations that may occur. Using the classification of deviations presented in this work, it may be possible to create such a checklist; one that is customized to the expertise and the role of the individuals in a trauma team.

In addition to supporting dynamic checklists, the classification schema can also enable the development of simulators driven by real-world data that provide training to maximize innovation and minimize error occurrence. Such an educational tool will be critical in developing decision making skills of residents and care givers. It would allow for a comprehensive evaluation of the skills of the caregivers as well as a means to train teams for not only adherence to a protocol but enabling recognition of circumstances where innovation is needed. The classification schema developed is generic and can be utilized to study deviations in other environments where similar complexity is experienced. Such environments include emergency departments and intensive care units.

The recognition of deviations utilizing a schema that classifies deviations as errors, innovations and procedural deviations can significantly alter compliance procedures and provide an overall adaptive framework to modification of existing protocols. For example, if deviations are consistently seen on a particular step in a protocol, then that step may have to be re-analyzed. Similarly if innovations are continuously seen and replicated in multiple sites, then it could be incorporated into the next version of a protocol. Therefore, the analysis of deviations as described in this work can help guide efforts to update existing protocols and guidelines in meeting the requirements of complex adaptive systems.

Implications for Informatics and Cognition

Clinicians deviate from protocols when managing patients. The studies discussed in this section show that clinical teams in critical care environments make a significant number of deviations per case, and that not all deviations are errors. The study of these deviations can provide new insight into how teams operate in complex environments and what distinguishes experts from novices. The results are in coherence with existing literature on exploring the cognitive basis of clinical expertise. It can be hypothesized that existence of retrieval structures in experts and top-down information processing allows for time-critical thinking that supports innovation by experts. This is supplemented by the information filtering that the retrieval structures support. On the other hand, novices are driven by bottom-up reasoning mechanisms and, without retrieval structures and filtering, are overwhelmed by the data and often make errors. Although only further experimentation can investigate this hypothesis, the observations clearly point to the plausibility of such mechanisms.

An analysis of deviations can enable the building of models of expertise and workflow that can be then used to design the next generation of effective interventions. Interventions could be standardized communication tools, and uses of information technology that supports innovations by effective presentation of information and cognitive decision support through educational efforts such as simulations. Simulations offer an exciting means of teaching clinical care givers to learn how to effectively innovate in complex environments. The Accreditation

Council of Graduate Medical Education recognizes simulation as an effective means of promoting critical thinking, professionalism and clinical knowledge [56]. It is generally seen only as an effective means of promoting standardization and adherence to a protocol [57]. This study, however, shows that simulation should be used for teaching clinical care givers the nuances of errors and innovations. Simulation offers a safe environment to achieve such goals. Simulations that are not just a means of achieving standardization but also help develop certain knowledge structure fairly quickly (through practice that would make any deviations safer) can be developed.

The results presented in this chapter suggest that there is a strong link between innovations, errors and expertise. Expert care givers deviate from the protocol almost as often as novices but make significantly more innovations. This seems to suggest that expert have a strong mental model of how and when to innovate and can employ their knowledge and application abilities to innovate on the fly. Such innovations and recognizing them should be an important part of clinical practice as it helps is redesigning protocols and procedures.

The next steps for this research include studies to explore in detail the underlying mechanisms of expertise and innovations in trauma. The methodologies described by Arocha and Patel [58] will be employed for these studies. Focusing on semantic analysis as a means of studying the innovations process in experts and novices will greatly add to the conclusions of this work. Semantic analysis will yield important insights into how information is assimilated and processed by clinical care givers. This would be crucial in understanding how to develop novel protocols and standards. For example, given the seriality of information as it passes from working memory to long term memory [59], one may include markers within the case description that may invoke the correct knowledge structures in long-term memory that support creativity. Continuation of this research will enable testing such interventions (including simulations mentioned above) and evaluating the same.

Discussion Questions

1. There exist a tension between following standards for protocol use and deviating from such standards. What is the precise nature of such tension and what are some of the key issues being discussed.
2. What is the relationship between development expertise and deviation from the standard?
3. Protocols and guidelines (flight control, for example) are used in many other domains to provide efficient and safe services. Describe one other such domain and identify similarities and differences with the clinical domain in terms of use of protocol?
4. What are some of the challenges in using protocols and guidelines for safe medical practices?

References

1. Reason J. Human error. Cambridge: Cambridge University Press; 1990.
2. Leape LL, Woods DD, Hatlie MJ, Kizer KW, Schroeder SA, Lundberg GD. Promoting patient safety by preventing medical error. JAMA. 1998;280(16):1444–7.
3. Institute of Medicine (IOM), U.S. Committee on Quality of Health Care in America. In: Kohn LT, Corrigan JM, Donaldson MS, editors. Errors in Health Care: A leading Cause of Death and Injury. Washington, D.C.: The National Academies Press; 2000.
4. American Hospital Association. Hospital statistics. Chicago: American Hospital Association; 1999.
5. Consumers Union. To err is human – to delay is deadly. Yonkers: Consumers Union; 2009.
6. Leape LL. Preventing fatal medical errors. Editorial, New York Times. 1999 December 1.
7. Institute of Medicine (IOM), U.S. Committee on Quality of Health Care in America. Crossing the quality chasm: a new health system for the 21st century. Washington, D.C: National Academy Press; 2001.
8. Leape LL, Berwick DM. Five years after to err is human: what have we learned? JAMA. 2005;293(19):2384–90.
9. Kelly JJ, Sweigard KW, Shields K, Schneider D, John M. Eisenberg patient safety awards. Safety, effectiveness, and efficiency: a web-based virtual anticoagulation clinic. Jt Comm J Qual Patient Saf. 2003;29(12):646–51.
10. Whittington J, Cohen H. OSF healthcare's journey in patient safety. Qual Manag Health Care. 2004;13(1):53–9.
11. Pronovost P, Needham D, Berenholtz S, Sinopoli D, Chu H, Cosgrove S, et al. An intervention to decrease catheter-related bloodstream infections in the ICU. N Engl J Med. 2006; 355(26):2725–32.
12. Goldspink C. Modelling social systems as complex: towards a social simulation meta-model. J Artif Soc Soc Simul. 2000;3(2):Available at: http://jasss.soc.surrey.ac.uk/3/2/1.html. Last Accessed on 20 Apr 2012.
13. Plsek PE. Some emerging principles for managers of complex adaptive systems (CAS), (Working Paper). 1997. Available at: http://www.directedcreativity.com/pages/ComplexityWP.html. Last Accessed on 25 Sep 2013.
14. Plsek PE, Greenhalgh T. The challenge of complexity in health care. Br Med J. 2001; 323:625–8.
15. Waldrop WM. Complexity: the emerging science at the edge of order and chaos. New York: Simon and Schuster; 1992.
16. Holland J. Hidden order: how adaptation builds complexity. New York: Addison-Wesley; 1995.
17. Lorenz EN. Danz J, Danz J, editors. What else is chaos? In: The essence of chaos. Seattle: CRC Press; 1995.
18. Sibthorpe B, Glasgow N, Longstaff D. Complex adaptive systems: a different way of thinking about health care systems. Australian Primary Health Care Research Institute, Canberra, Australia. 2004.
19. Lewin R. Complexity: life at the. Edge of Chaos: University Of Chicago Press; 2000.
20. Horsky J, Gutnik L, Patel VL, editors. Technology for emergency care: cognitive and workflow considerations. AMIA Annu Symp Proc. 2006;344–8.
21. Malhotra S, Jordan D, Shortliffe E, Patel VL. Workflow modeling in critical care: piecing together your own puzzle. J Biomed Inform. 2007;40(2):81–92.
22. Gilmour D, Woodwards S. The surgical safety checklist: legacy and next step. J Perioper Pract. 2010;20(3):78.
23. Duane TM, Brown H, Borchers CT, Wolfe LG, Malhotra AK, Aboutanos MB, et al. A central venous line protocol decreases bloodstream infections and length of stay in a trauma intensive care unit population. Ann Surg. 2009;75(12):1166–70.
24. Semel ME, Resch S, Haynes AB, Funk LM, Bader A, Berry WR, et al. Adopting a surgical safety checklist could save money and improve the quality of care in U.S. Hospitals. Health Aff. 2010;29(9):1593–9.

25. Donchin Y, Gopher D, Olin M, Badihi Y, Biesky M, Sprung C, et al. A look into the nature and causes of human errors in the intensive care unit. Qual Saf Health Care. 2003;12(2):143–7.
26. Weingart SN, Wilson RM, Gibberd RW, Harrison B. Epidemiology of medical error. Br Med J. 2000;320:774–7.
27. Rothschild JM, Landrigan CP, Cronin JW, Kaushal R, Lockley SW, Burdick E, et al. The critical care safety study: the incidence and nature of adverse events and serious medical errors in intensive care. Crit Care Med. 2005;33(8):1694–700.
28. Brennan TA. The institute of medicine report on medical errors–could it do harm? N Engl J Med. 2000;342(15):1123–5.
29. Helmreich RL, Foushee HC. Why crew resource management? empirical and theoretical bases of human factors training in aviation. In: Wiener E, Kanki B, Helmreich R, editors. Cockpit resource management. San Diego: Academic Press; 1993. p. 3–45.
30. Helmreich RL. On error management: lessons from aviation. Br Med J. 2000;320(7237):781–5.
31. Helmreich RL, Merritt AC, Wilhelm JA. The evolution of crew resource management in commercial aviation. Int J Aviat Psychol. 1999;9:19–32.
32. Langewiesche W. Fly by wire: the geese, the glide, the miracle on the Hudson. New York: Farrar, Straus and Giroux; 2009. p. 208.
33. Wise J. What really happened aboard Air France 447. Pop Mech. 2011;6:2011.
34. Hughes RG. Patient safety and quality: an evidence-based handbook for nurses. Agency for Healthcare Research and Quality: Rockville; 2008.
35. Laxmisan A, Hakimzada F, Sayan OR, Green RA, Zhang J, Patel VL. The multitasking clinician: decision-making and cognitive demand during and after team handoffs in emergency care. Int J Med Inform. 2006;76(11–12):801–11.
36. Salas E, Dickinson TL, Converse SA, Tannenbaum SI. Toward and understanding of team performance and training. In: Swezey RW, Salas E, editors. Teams: their training and performance. Norwood: Ablex Pub. Corp; 1992. p. 3–29.
37. American College of Surgeons. Advanced trauma life support for doctors. 7th ed. Chicago: American College of Surgeons; 2004.
38. Collicott PE, Hughes I. Training in advanced trauma life support. JAMA. 1980; 243(11):1156–9.
39. Sarcevic A, Burd RS. What's the story? Information needs of trauma teams. AMIA Annu Symp Proc. 2008:641–5.
40. Pal J. The value of the Glasgow coma scale and injury severity score: predicting outcome in multiple trauma patients with head injury. J Trauma. 1989;29(6):746–8.
41. National Assocation of EMS Physicians. Emergency medical dispatching. Prehosp Disaster Med. 1989;4(2):163–6.
42. American Society for Testing and Materials. Standard practice for emergency medical dispatch. Philadelphia: Annual Book of ASTM Standards; 1990.
43. Burns JP. Complexity science and leadership in healthcare. J Nurs Adm. 2001;31(10):474–82.
44. Zimmerman BJ, Lindberg C, Plsek PE. Edgeware: insights from complexity science for health care leaders. Irving: VHA Publishing; 1998.
45. Plsek PE, Wilson T. Complexity, leadership, and management in healthcare organisations. BMJ. 2001;323(7315):746–9.
46. Kahol K, Vankipuram M, Patel VL, Smith ML. Deviations from protocol in a complex trauma environment: errors or innovations? J Biomed Inform. 2011;44(3):425–31.
47. Patel VL, Groen GJ, Arocha JF. Medical expertise as a function of task difficulty. Mem Cogn. 1990;18(4):394–406.
48. Groen GJ, Patel VL. Medical problem-solving: some questionable assumptions. Med Educ. 1985;19:95–100.
49. Vankipuram M. Understanding adaptive behaviors in complex clinical environments. Scottsdale: Arizona State University; 2012.
50. West MA, Wallace M. Innovation in health care teams. Eur J Soc Psychol. 1991;21(4):303–15.
51. Anderson L, Rothstein P, editors. Creativity and innovation: consumer research and scenario building. Urbana: Advances in Consumer Research; 2004.

52. Patel VL, Cohen T, Murarka T, Olsen J, Kagita S, Myneni S, et al. Recovery at the edge of error: debunking the myth of the infallible expert. J Biomed Inform. 2011;44(3):413–24.
53. Patel VL, Arocha JF, Kaufman DR. Diagnostic reasoning and medical expertise. In: Psychology of learning and motivation: advances in research and theory, vol. 31. San Diego: Academic press; 1994. p. 187–252.
54. Fleiss JL. Statistical methods for rates and proportions. 2nd ed. New York: John Wiley; 1981.
55. Landis JR, Koch GG. The measurement of observer agreement for categorical data. Biometrics. 1977;33:159–74.
56. Accreditation Council for Graduate Medical Education. ACGME competencies: suggested best methods for evaluation 2000. Available from: http://www.acgme.org/Outcome/assess/ToolTable.pdf. Cited 20 Dec 2007.
57. Smith CC, Huang GC, Newman LR, Clardy PF, Feller-Kopman D, Cho M, et al. Simulation training and its effect on long-term resident performance in central venous catheterization. Simul Healthc. 2010;5(3):146–51. doi:10.1097/SIH.0b013e3181dd9672.
58. Arocha JF, Wang D, Patel VL. Identifying reasoning strategies in medical decision making: a methodological guide. J Biomed Inform. 2005;38(2):154–71.
59. Groen GJ, Patel VL. The relationship between comprehension and reasoning in medical expertise. In: Chi M, Glaser R, Farr M, editors. The nature of expertise. Hillsdale: Erlbaum; 1988. p. 287–310.

Chapter 9
Standard Solutions for Complex Settings: The Idiosyncrasies of a Weaning Protocol Use in Practice

Sahiti Myneni, Trevor Cohen, Khalid F. Almoosa, and Vimla L. Patel

Healthcare Standardization

Patient safety efforts in health domain are oftentimes compared with other safety-critical and high-reliability domains including aviation, banking, and nuclear plants. In these industries, standardization of practices is seen as a viable strategy to mitigate error and improve safety [1]. Along similar lines, extensive efforts were made in medical domain to engineer high-safety processes by standardizing care delivery procedures and reducing practice variation. While standardization of procedures is based on the best scientific evidence available for a particular clinical problem at hand, it is also supposed to allow for practice of individual medicine to address patient-specific issues. Studies examining the impact of standardization reported improvements in quality of care – better clinical

S. Myneni, MSE (✉)
School of Biomedical Informatics, University of Texas Health Science Center, Houston, TX 77054, USA
e-mail: sahiti.myneni@uth.tmc.edu

T. Cohen, MB ChB, PhD
University of Texas Health Science Center, Houston, TX, USA

K.F. Almoosa, MD, MS, FCCP
University of Texas Health Science Center, Houston, TX, USA

Transplant Surgery ICU, Memorial Hermann Hospital, Texas Medical Center, Houston, TX 77030, USA

V.L. Patel, PhD, DSc, FRSC
Center for Cognitive Studies in Medicine and Public Health, New York Academy of Medicine, New York, NY 10029, USA

Department of Biomedical Informatics, Columbia University, New York, NY 10032, USA

Department of Biomedical Informatics, Arizona State University, Scottsdale, AZ 85259, USA

V.L. Patel et al. (eds.), *Cognitive Informatics in Health and Biomedicine*, Health Informatics, DOI 10.1007/978-1-4471-5490-7_9,

outcomes and reductions in infection transmissions. At the same time, standardization has also been shown to reduce healthcare expenditures [2].

Several hospital processes have been standardized using a variety of clinical decision support tools and techniques such as checklists, protocols, and Computerized Provider Order Entry (CPOE) systems [3–9]. These tools add structure and predictability to highly complex tasks in critical care, which has been proven effective in aviation. Such structured workflow removes unnecessary variation and improves the overall performance of the unit. A combination of these standardization techniques have been used to improve four important critical care processes- ventilator management, ventilator weaning, sedation and analgesia [10–12]. This chapter provides the assessment of a weaning protocol that aims to standardize the weaning process of critically-ill mechanically-ventilated patients. The objective of the assessment is to understand the socio-technical factors that affect the optimal use of the protocol. Detailed description of the weaning protocol is provided in section "Weaning protocol use in a medical intensive care unit" of this chapter. In section "Barriers to effective use of standardized clinical decision support", we examine the performance-related issues encountered with standardized decision support systems including weaning protocols reported in the existing literature. The remaining sections of the chapter focuses on three studies we conducted to evaluate the particular weaning protocol (described in section "Weaning protocol use in a medical intensive care unit") in a complex critical care setting. The central theme of the chapter is to provide a methodology that facilitates the consideration of complex systems' characteristics into the design, evaluation, and implementation phases of standardization tools in critical care.

Weaning Protocol Use in a Medical Intensive Care Unit

Mechanical Ventilation (MV) is a lifesaving procedure, however, prolonged ventilation carries numerous life threatening complications including increased mortality, ventilator-associated pneumonia, and airway trauma [13]. On the other hand, premature discontinuation of MV can result in unsuccessful extubation, requiring re-intubation [14]. Therefore, it is important to discontinue mechanical ventilation at the earliest possible and optimal time. Recent published literature suggests that daily screening of respiratory function in mechanically ventilated patients, followed by a sedation holiday and Spontaneous Breathing Trial (SBT) can result in a reduction of ventilator days, lower ICU costs and fewer related complications [10, 15]. The weaning protocol evaluated as part of the studies described in this chapter is currently used in a Medical Intensive Care Unit (MICU) and is primarily led by Respiratory Therapists (RTs). The objective of the weaning protocol is to provide adequate clinical decision support to clinicians and facilitate early, safe and evidence-based liberation from the ventilator. The decision support characteristics of the weaning protocol under study are discussed in detail in [16].

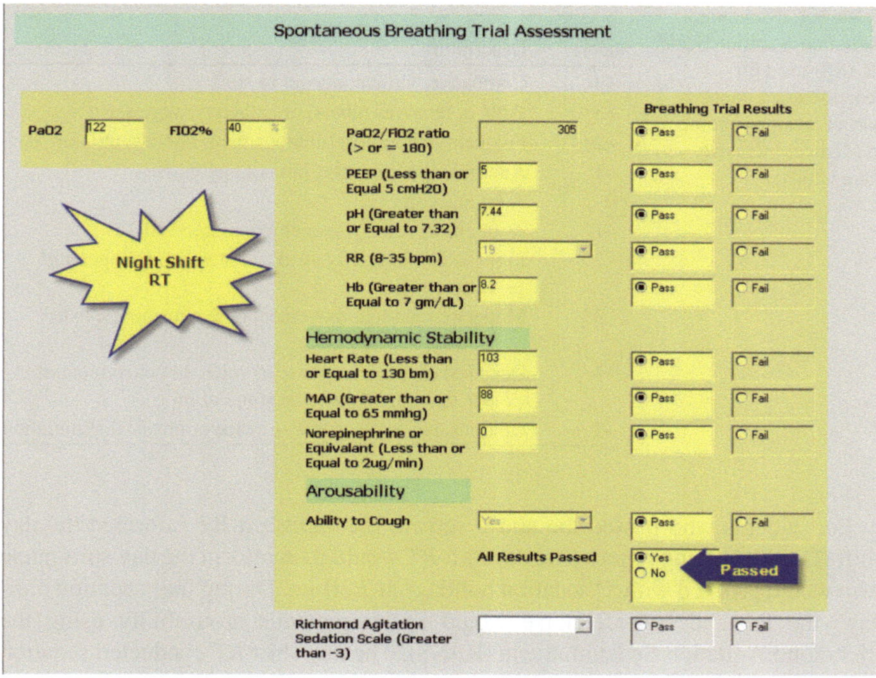

Fig. 9.1 Sample illustration of the Computerized Weaning Protocol (CWP) Form

The workflow of the Respiratory Therapist (RT) led weaning protocol is as follows. The protocol involves four major steps- (a) Data collection: Patient-related data collected by RTs (night shift and day shift) as part of the protocol's requirements were recorded in the Electronic Health Record (EHR), (b) Screening for SBT eligibility: All mechanically-ventilated patients were screened daily to determine their eligibility and readiness for a Spontaneous Breathing Trial (SBT) by the night shift RT starting at 4 am every day. Physiological data (e.g. hemodynamic stability, respiratory rate, positive end-expiratory pressure, fractional concentration of inspired oxygen) were collected at this point and fed into the EHR. The inbuilt Computerized Weaning Protocol (CWP) module uses these data to automatically assess the patient's eligibility for SBT and provides the clinicians with the results (Pass/Fail, see Fig. 9.1) provides an illustration of the protocol data entry. The RT manually entered the weaning mechanics data into the text boxes seen in the figure and the subsequent results (Pass/Fail) seen in Fig. 9.1 were generated by the system based on the values entered in the corresponding data fields. The CWP provided guidance to the RT in every step (cuff leak checks, ventilator mode selection) using checklists and simple data entry. All data related to weaning mechanics (e.g. tidal volume, rapid shallow breathing index) were collected using CWP module. If the patient failed any part of the SBT screen, then it was considered that the patient did not meet criteria required to proceed to the actual SBT. The patient will be re-screened again the next day.

Table 9.1 Richmond Agitation Sedation Scale (RASS) used for sedation assessment as part of weaning protocol in Medical Intensive Care Unit

RASS score	Description
+4	Combative, violent, danger to staff
+3	Pulls or removes tube(s) or catheters; aggressive
+2	Frequent nonpurposeful movement, fights ventilator
+1	Anxious, apprehensive, but not aggressive
0	Alert and calm
−1	Awakens to voice(eye opening/contact) >10 s
−2	Light sedation, briefly awakens to voice(eye opening/contact) <10 s
−3	Moderate sedation, movement or eye opening. No eye contact
−4	Deep sedation, no response to voice, but movement or eye opening to physical stimulation
−5	Unarousable, no response to voice or physical stimulation

For patients who passed the above screen, the nightshift RT informed the day shift RT when giving report. The dayshift RT would then inform the day shift nurse who would proceed with a "sedation holiday" at 7:30 am. During the "sedation holiday" the RT and bedside nurse would assess patient's arousability using the Richmond Agitation Sedation Scale (RASS). The day shift RT conducted sedation assessment using Richmond Agitation Sedation Scale (RASS) to determine if the patient's eligibility to be included in the SBT (see Table 9.1). If a patient had a RASS score > −3, the RT indicated that the patient passed the sedation assessment and proceeded with the trial by placing the patient on the appropriate trial ventilator settings. The RT would remain at the patient's bedside for the first 5 min of the trial to assess tolerance to the SBT settings, then remained in the unit for the duration of the trial and continued to monitor the patient. For patients who failed the sedation assessment, the protocol was deemed complete and these patients would be re-screened for SBT readiness the next day. The aggregated data were then presented to the attending physician and the clinical team for the final decision on ventilation during daily morning multi-disciplinary team rounds.

Barriers to Effective Use of Standardized Clinical Decision Support

A Clinical decision support system (CDSS), which encompasses a variety of interventions including computerized alerts, electronic clinical guidelines providing clinicians with just-in-time evidence-based support [17, 18], thereby enabling safe and efficient care delivery [19]. Often used in critical care units to mitigating life-threatening complications associated with mechanical ventilation is CWP, a form of decision support to ensure early and safe extubations. An overview of various weaning protocols (WPs) that are in use currently by various health institutions can be found in [20–25]. With growing emphasis on digitizing health care, Health Information Technology (HIT) is a frequent component of these protocols and other standardization efforts. Automation and technology are seen as two major carriers of these policies. Introduction of new workflow procedures and/or modification of existing practices are often the primary consequences of these efforts.

Several studies identified problems with efficient implementation and safe use of CWP. Most of these problems are socio-technical found within the protocol (e.g. software errors, underlying logic errors) and distributed across the clinicians' understanding of the protocol [26–29]. Understanding complex interdependencies commonly observed in the critical care environment is essential in order to improvise the sub-optimal implementation practices of weaning protocols [30, 31]. Clinician adherence and compliance to the newly established guidelines is also cited as a major challenge that needs to be addressed in order for our health systems to fully benefit from any CDSS [32]. Therefore, detailed understanding of all the involved components (e.g. care setting, support algorithm, user impression) is incumbent to maximize the benefits and minimize the losses that may be caused by ineffective implementation and/or unintended consequences [33, 34]. It has been suggested that such assessments should take the context and complexity of CDS environment into account for high yield in quality improvement [35, 36], and that failure to assess the environment prior to implementation of an intervention can have harmful unintended consequences [37, 38]. Several studies have documented the rise of medical errors as a result of unintended consequences of the standardization tools [37, 39–44]. Failure to understand the dynamics of complex adaptive environments such as critical care can be one reason for the emergence of these unintended adverse consequences. Most protocols and checklists have been created with a high-level objective such as improving a clinical outcome or process. However, such a clinical process is a conglomeration of multiple low-level processes that in turn involves a multitude of actors, tools, and events. In other words, the patterns found in complex adaptive systems at higher levels emerge from localized interactions and selection processes acting at lower levels [45]. Therefore, it is essential to carefully understand the localized interactions of standardization strategies to successfully anticipate and address the emergence of high-level patterns. This chapter introduces a new method that analyzes localized interactions to explain high-level risks in a complex setting. We explain the findings derived from a set of evaluation studies of a CWP, which is under use in a MICU.

Evaluation of the Standardization Tools

For evaluation of risks posed by a given standardization strategy or protocol, a variety of retrospective and proactive safety engineering approaches have been used in health care. The Department of Veterans Affairs had adapted the classic failure mode and effect analysis (FMEA) approach for use in medical domain [46, 47], thus setting stage for a series of methodological adaptions of risk assessment frameworks. In addition to FMEA, a variety of risk management methods have been tested- root cause analysis, fault tree analysis, cause and effect diagram, hazard operability study, probability tree method, man- machine systems analysis, and probabilistic risk assessment to name a few [48–50]. With the phenomenal growth of electronics and computer technologies in the past decade, the socio-technical underpinnings of the workflow and technical infrastructure have become quite complex in almost every safety-critical area including healthcare [41]. To keep up with growing complexity, risk analysis methods have also been transitioned from being linear approaches to non-linear models attempting to understand the local patterns to understand global effects. In this chapter, we present and demonstrate the use of a non-linear risk assessment methodology to analyze the safety issues concerning the use of the previously described protocol in the context of weaning mechanically-ventilated patients in a critical care unit. Functional Resonance Accident Method (FRAM) motivated by complex systems research was chosen given its proven applicability to intractable environments such as manufacturing plants and financial markets [51, 52]. FRAM is a systemic method originally developed for the analysis and prediction of adverse events in the aviation industry. Motivated by complex systems research, the method considers local variations within the protocol, related actors, and events, thus accounting for the complexity of MICU environment.

Functional Resonance Accident Method

Functional Resonance Accident Method provides a way to describe how multiple individual functions and conditions can combine to produce an adverse outcome accounting for the interactions and interdependencies within complex settings and offering us insights into the how and why of a particular event chain [53]. FRAM is based on the following four major principles [51]:

1. The principle of equivalence of successes and failures: FRAM adheres to the resilience engineering view that failures represent the flip side of the adaptations necessary to cope with real-world complexity [54]. Success depends on the ability of teams and individuals to anticipate risks and critical situations, to recognize them in time, and to take appropriate action.
2. The principle of approximate adjustments: Since the conditions of work never completely match what has been specified, individuals must adjust their performance so that they can succeed under the existing conditions.
3. The principle of emergence: The variability of normal performance is rarely large enough to be the cause of an ineffective activity in itself or even to constitute a risk. But the local variability from multiple functions may combine in unexpected ways, leading to consequences that are disproportionally large producing a non-linear effect at global scale.
4. The principle of functional resonance. The variability of a number of functions may resonate, i.e., reinforce each other and thereby cause the variability of one function to exceed normal limits. The consequences may spread through tight couplings rather than via identifiable and enumerable cause-effect links.

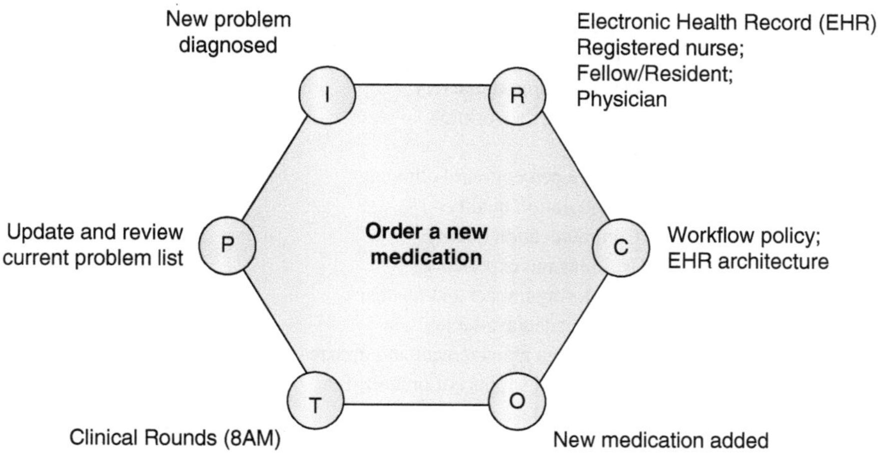

Fig. 9.2 A FRAM module describing a function (*I*-Input, *O*-Output, *T*-Time, *R*-Resource, *C*-Constraint, *P*-Precondition)

The steps to apply FRAM for evaluation of the effective use of standardized CDSS tools ((in this context, a CWP) are as follows. In step 1, we identify and characterize essential functions that are being accomplished using the standardized CDSS. All functions required to complete a decision support activity are specified in this step. Each function is separately identified, but not pre-arranged in any way. A function may, for instance, be to update the medication list of a patient. Each function is modeled using six parameters: Input, Output, Time, Resource, Precondition, and Control (see Fig. 9.2).

Input (I): that which the function transforms or that which starts the function, Output (O): that which is the result of the function, either an entity or a state change, Preconditions (P): conditions that must exist before a function can be executed, Resources (R): that which the function needs or consumes to produce the output, Time (T): temporal constraints affecting the function (with regard to starting time, finishing time, or duration) and Control (C): how the function is monitored or controlled

In Step 2, we describe the potential variability of the functions. For this purpose we adopted previously established practices to assess the common performance conditions (CPCs) outlined in (1) Hollnagel's cognitive reliability and error analysis method (CREAM) [55], and (2) Ten Commandments for effective use of CDSS [56]. A list of CPCs from both the above sources was presented to an expert physician, who chose the final list with 12 CPCs (Table 9.2) that captures the working conditions in MICU. Then, in Step 3 we identify functional resonance and potential variability. The functions identified in Step 1 may be coupled via their parameters. For example, the pre-condition of a function may be the output of another function, which in turn may be an input a third function. Similarly same functional parameter can serve an input to another function, or provide a resource, fulfill a pre-condition, or enforce a control. Couplings between functions can be identified by analyzing commonly related parameters. These couplings may then be combined with the results of Step 2, the characterization of variability, to specify how

Table 9.2 Variability checklist for context-dependent evaluation of clinical decision support

Conditions for effective clinical decision support	Rating scale
On-time support delivery	*Adequate*
Fit into user's workflow	*Inadequate*
Usability	*Unpredictable*
Positive perception of clinicians	
Collaboration quality	
Communication quality	
Training and experience	
Monitoring impact and feedback	
Time needed/available	
Knowledge management and update	
Quality and support of organization	
Operational support	

the variability of one function may have an impact on the variability of another by categorizing them into (1) Human, (2) Technology, and (3) Organization. In order to gain deeper understanding of this functional classification, please refer to [57]. Functional dependencies can spread variability across the activity beyond the normal boundaries, pushing the outcome into a danger/suboptimal zone and result in an adverse or unfavorable event. Finally in Step 3, we propose variability monitoring and attenuating interventions. Understanding the nature, cause, effect, and propagation of variability in CDSS is essential to contain the inefficiencies and improve performance.

Now, let us demonstrate the way this method can be used to evaluate standardization tools. The next sections of this chapter attempts to dissect and present how FRAM has been used to evaluate the weaning protocol previously described in section "Weaning protocol use in a medical intensive care unit".

Study 1 – Application of FRAM to Evaluate the Use of the Weaning Protocol

The clinical version of FRAM was adopted to identify the risk factors creating barriers to effective use of the CWP in the MICU. A FRAM-based normative model of the CWP was created following a sequence of steps . The first step in FRAM was to identify essential functions of an activity. Five essential steps in the CWP were identified using multiple methods (observations, review of hospital manuals, semi-structured interviews) as follows: (1) patient inclusion, (2) SBT screening assessment, (3) sedation assessment using RASS score (see Table 9.1), (4) SBT, and (5) decision making: extubation. As shown in Table 9.3, each of these functions was modeled using six parameters -input (I), output (O), resource (R), time (T), precondition (P), and control (C).

Table 9.3 Essential functions of the computerized weaning protocol

Function	Input	Output	Resource	Time	Control	Pre-condition
Function 1: patient inclusion	Ventilator settings; protocol order	SBT screening assessment order	EHR; day RT; fellow		MICU weaning policy	Patient exclusion criteria
Function 2: SBT screening assessment	SBT screening assessment order	Eligible/ineligible for SBT; respiratory mechanics	EHR; night RT	4 AM	MICU weaning policy	Patient exclusion criteria; Protocol order
Function 3: sedation assessment (RASS Score)		Arousability score	EHR; day RT; RN	7:30 AM	MICU weaning policy; RASS	Sedation holiday; eligible for SBT
Function 4: spontaneous breathing trial (SBT)	Ventilator settings	Pass/Fail SBT	day RT; EHR		MICU weaning policy	Eligible/ineligible for SBT; arousability score > −2
Function 5: decision making: extubation	Ventilator settings	Patient extubation	RN; day RT; Physician; Fellow; Residents; EHR	8 AM	Clinical objectives; MICU weaning policy	Pass/Fail SBT; arousability > −2

Table 9.4 FRAM based variability checklist for weaning protocol

Conditions for effective clinical decision support	Rating
On-time delivery of decision support	Unpredictable
Fit into user's workflow	Adequate
Usability and understanding	*Inadequate*
Positive perception of clinicians	*Inadequate*
Collaboration quality	Unpredictable
Communication quality	Unpredictable
Training and experience	*Inadequate*
Monitoring impact and feedback	*Inadequate*
Time needed/available	Unpredictable
Knowledge management and update	*Inadequate*
Quality and support of organization	Adequate
Operational support	Adequate

In Step 2, using the CPC-based checklist, the variability of the CWP functions was assessed (see Table 9.4). Different factors were considered to assess the variability of the protocol and it was found that on-time support delivery, collaboration and communication quality, and the time needed to complete the CWP in order to standardize the weaning process in the MICU were unpredictable. The factors were rated by domain experts- physician and RT. Cohen's Kappa measure was used to determine inter-rater reliability. The raters had a reliability of 0.855 ($p<0.001$) with only one disagreement in "positive perception of clinicians" category. The disagreement has been resolved by asking two additional raters to assign a rating for that particular condition, and the final rating was the one that has most agreement. It was clear from Table 9.4 that multiple factors were given inadequate and unpredictable rating. This highlights the possibility that the CWP under evaluation may be subjected to variability by several sources, which are possibly inter-dependent.

The local dependencies and global networks of the CWP components were also analyzed. We identified and analyzed possible ways in which these variability sources might resonate and affect the performance of the protocol [16]. Next, we describe the functional dependencies of one of the CWP functions- the "Sedation assessment (RASS Score)".

Sedation assessment (RASS Score) is function 3 of the CWP. The control for this function is the use of RASS to determine the arousability of a patient (see Fig. 9.3). The output of function 3 is a precondition for functions 4 and 5. Once the functional dependencies such as this were all identified, the functions were reexamined using the list of previously determined CPCs by mapping the functions to three categories into human, technology, and organization. From this analysis, it was found that the sedation assessment is primarily dependent on the human resource applying RASS to assess the sedation level of a patient and the immediate variability sources were traced to usability and understanding, training and experience, both of which are rated inadequate by domain experts. For instance, consider a hypothetical case where a clinician assigns a wrong score to a patient because of inadequate understanding of the sedation assessment scale. At that point, the patient would be ineligible to

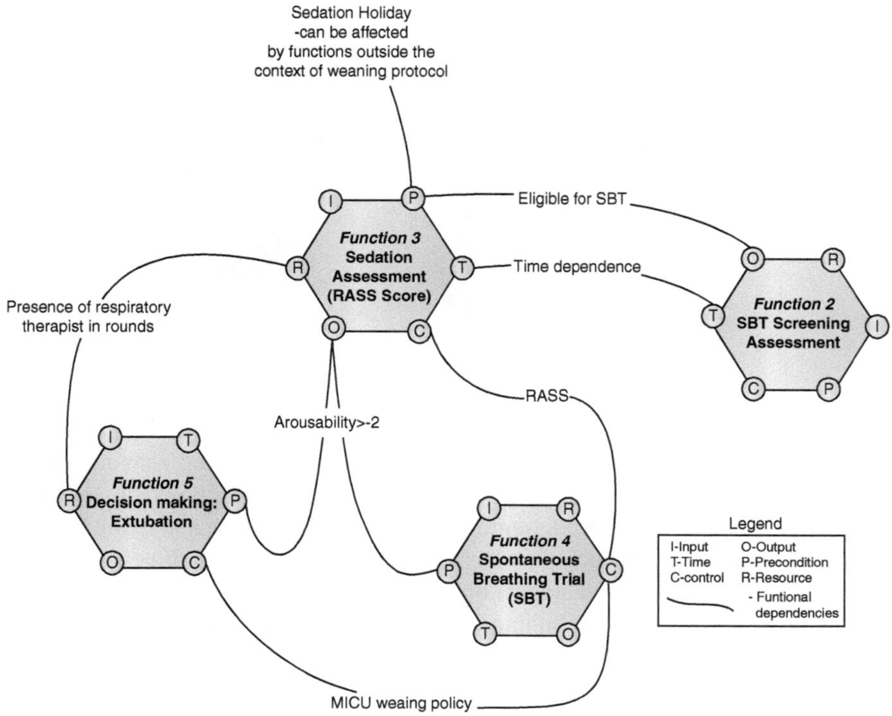

Fig. 9.3 Functional dependencies of Function 3- Sedation Assessment (RASS Score)

proceed to function 4, and therefore cannot be timely extubated. From this example, it was evident that inadequate understanding of protocol mechanisms (such as RASS) might pose risks to the effective use of CWP. However, such discrepancies in score assignment could be resolved during case discussions. Given the expert rating that the communication among clinicians is unreliable, this safety net might not be trustworthy enough. Other variability sources affecting optimal use of the CWP were identified to be: a) misinterpretation of the sedation scale, b) lack of RTs presence in the daily rounds, c) communication breakdown among clinicians, d) problems of on-time support delivery, e) clinicians' negative perception of the protocol.

Finally in Step 4 we propose variability monitoring interventions to mitigate the risks posed by the standardization of the weaning process in MICU. Reinforced clinician education on the new policies and guidelines, facilitating improved communication, and disseminating the impact of the newly introduced workflow practices can help minimize the unintended variability in the CWP functions. Examples of immediate short-term and long-term intervention strategies include-

Training and Education: Design a training module for clinicians to fill existing knowledge gaps and conceptual misunderstandings. Such a refresher module should be developed based on multi-disciplinary input from clinicians involved in the daily use of the CWP. Efforts need to be channeled to identify and address confusing aspects in the protocol's procedures.

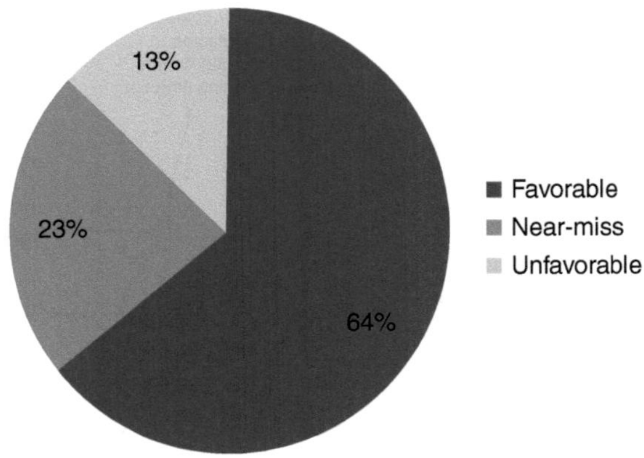

Fig. 9.4 Classification of the outcomes from 65 weaning sessions

Feedback and Impact Monitoring System: Research and development of a virtual platform that establishes a communication channel among clinicians soliciting feedback on CWP operations, disseminating quality metrics relevant to the CWP to all the involved clinicans such that they stay motivated to adhere to new workflow practices that make a positive impact on the care setting and culture.

Before we can set out and implement the above stated interventions, it is important for us to validate the finding derived using FRAM. To our knowledge, the use of FRAM as a risk assessment method in critical care medicine is the first attempt of its kind, and we are not aware of any published work that employed FRAM to evaluate the standardization tools such as the weaning protocol. Henceforth, we carried out a second study to validate our findings.

Study 2: Validation of the FRAM Method for Use in Critical Care

The objective of this study was to validate that the use of FRAM as an evaluation method to identify the risks posed by the standardization tools such as the computerized weaning protocol. As part of the study, a trained researcher conducted ethnographic study by unobtrusively observing clinicians as they conducted weaning sessions using the CWP. A total of 65 weaning sessions were observed and these data were coded into three categories- favorable, unfavorable, and near-miss. As shown in Fig. 9.4, 45 (69 %) of the 65 sessions were favorable, 16(25 %) fell under near-miss category, while the remaining four (6 %) were unfavorable [58]. A weaning session was classified as *favorable* if a mechanically-ventilated (MV) patient passes night-RT assessment AND sedation assessment AND spontaneous breathing trial, and then he/she is extubated (OR) if a MV patient fails night RT assessment OR sedation assessment OR spontaneous breathing trial), and then he/she is not extubated. (OR) if a MV patient passes night RT assessment AND sedation assessment AND spontaneous breathing trial, and then he/she is not extubated because of airway management issues or other clinical objectives. A weaning session was classified as *unfavorable* if a MV patient passes night RT assessment AND sedation assessment AND spontaneous breathing trial, and then he/she is not extubated (OR) if a MV patient fails night RT assessment OR sedation assessment OR spontaneous breathing trial, and then the patient is extubated and is again re-intubate (OR) a physician makes a decision on extubation with no or erroneous data from the protocol. Unfavorable sessions can be a result of functional coupling among locally variable components. A weaning session was coded as a *near-miss* event if the variations of the individual components at local level did not couple with one another causing an unfavorable outcome.

Major problems identified with the CWP in the shadowing sessions were related to misinterpretation of sedation scores, issues with on-time delivery support, inadequate communication and collaboration among clinicians, and insufficient feedback of protocol's impact on quality of care delivery in MICU. Detailed explanations of some important observations made in this study with respect to CWP use in the critical care unit are described below.

Misinterpretation of sedation scale was observed in seven of these sessions. The sedation scale was misinterpreted, which subsequently led to erroneous extubation and re-intubated, and therefore placing the patient at unnecessary risk and preventable harm from inadequate respiratory support. Reason for the wrongly assigned sedation scores is that the RTs misinterpreted the word "sedation" in the RASS scale as referring to the prescription sedative, instead of an assessment of the physical arousable state of the patient, there by indicating that knowledge issues with the protocol mechanisms posed problems to the effective use of the CWP. There were five instances during which the SBT was prolonged for more than 150 min, where the protocol-based time limit was 30–120 min. The RTs placed the patients on minimal ventilator support subjecting patients to higher levels of discomfort. Such practice was potentially life-threatening for patients with airway management issues. Problems with on-time data delivery were also observed which limited the just-in-time application of the weaning protocol. During two sessions, the physician had to make a decision without considering the CWP data because of data collection delay caused by ICU crowding and resource allocation to another critically ill patient. Lack of compliance by clinicians to the protocol procedure was also found to be a risk factor. Adherence issues were as a result of some physicians who did not trust the protocol, although the protocol is evidence-based, and henceforth, disregarded RT's data.

In summary, our findings from this evaluation study were in agreement with the results from Study 1. The FRAM based analysis positively predicted 81 % of the variability sources that resonated to cause near-misses and unfavorable outcomes observed as part of Study 2. The two studies described so far enabled us to identify the risk sources proactively and retrospectively. While the findings were intuitive enough to develop remedial solutions, the sources of the risks were not quite clear. These risks might have stemmed because of multiple reasons- (a) knowledge-related deficiencies, (b) lack of cognitive support such as reminders, and (c) ignorance or workarounds. In the next section of the chapter, we describe the findings of a study that attempted to look at knowledge structures of individual clinicians

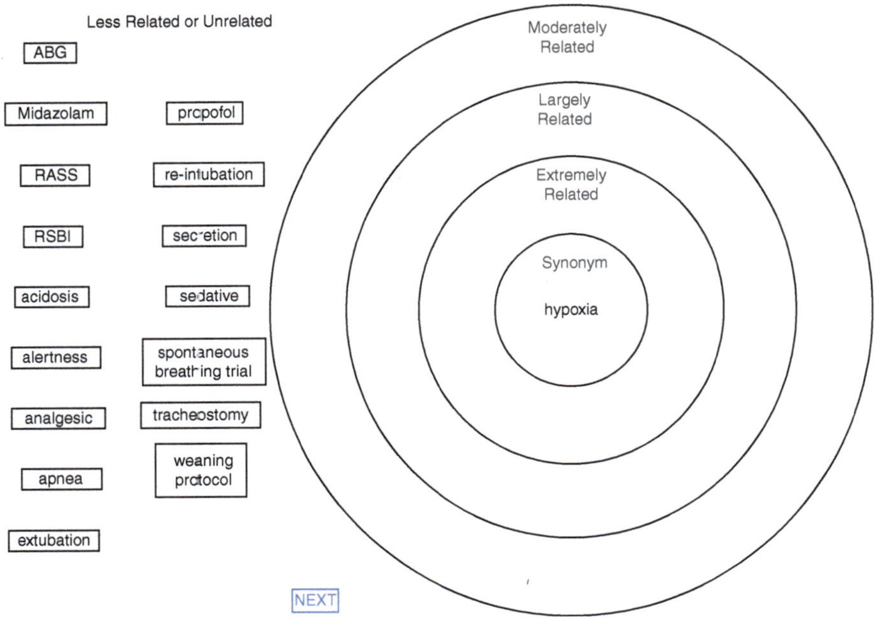

Fig. 9.5 Target – a concept-mapping tool to assess knowledge structures

to identify knowledge-related risk sources, which in turn can be addressed by deploying effective training interventions.

Study 3: Tracing the Knowledge Gaps to Improve Standardization Tools

In the previous sections, we have learned that conceptual knowledge gaps can sometimes lead to underutilization of the standardization tools. Such knowledge-related shortcomings can be remedied by having a strong training regimen in place to bolster important clinical concepts so as to enhance patient safety. In this study, we used a concept-mapping methodology to analyze knowledge-structures of the clinicians. Cognitive psychologists have long used memory organization and inference patterns to understand the specialized knowledge structures of an individual. One way to gain insight into memory organization is by using conceptual proximity data, often derived from pairwise estimates of conceptual relatedness provided by participants. Concepts related to one another are nearer, and those that are not related are farther. To elicit these data, we used a concept-mapping tool called "Target", which gives us an estimate of how subjects relate several concepts related to specialized content, thereby letting us explore their knowledge structures. Target (shown in Fig. 9.5) is based on Pathfinder network scaling [59, 60] which can be used to assess learning of an individual by examine their knowledge structures. A Pathfinder

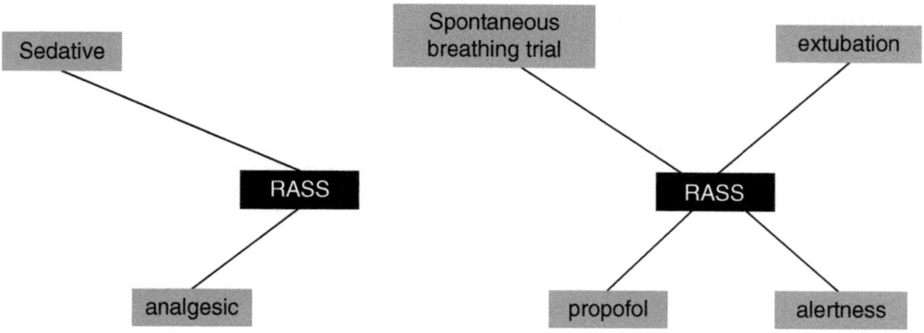

Fig. 9.6 Conceptual gaps- In the image on the left, RASS is not connected to alertness or SBT- (the RT contributing the proximity ratings that underlie the image on the left also assigned an incorrect RASS score during an observed clinical encounter)

network is derived from proximities for pairs of concepts with a pattern of relationships [59]. In the Pathfinder network, the concepts correspond to the nodes of the generated network, and the links in the network are determined by the patterns of proximities. Pathfinder eliminates links in the network where a shorter path between the nodes concerned can be found through some other node, thereby revealing the most significant links in the network based on local patterns of proximity.

We asked eight MICU clinicians (RTs and physicians) to use Target to rate the distance between concepts related to the CWP. A total of 17 concepts are used for the purpose of this study. Each clinician was required to drag concepts related to the concept in the center of the target from a location on the left. Each concentric circle represents a degree of relatedness, ranging from moderate to extremely related, to the concept in the center. Each concept is at the center of the target once before the completion of the task.

Based on the proximity data captured using Target, knowledge structures of the clinicians (with respect to the CWP) were created using Pathfinder. Based on these structures, we were able to trace the risk sources and conclude if they originated because of knowledge deficiencies. For instance, see Fig. 9.6, it shows the knowledge structure of two RTs for RASS concept alone. As you can see, one of the RTs related RASS to sedative and analgesic alone (see structure on left in Fig. 9.6), while the correct representation of RASS should include alertness as well (see structure on right in Fig. 9.6).

When mapped to shadowing data collected as part of Study 2 (described in section "Study 2: Validation of the FRAM Method for Use in Critical Care" of the chapter), this RT also gave wrong RASS score to the patient thus leading to failed extubation. Similar pattern was observed in case of the two other RTs who assigned faulty RASS scores. Using this knowledge elicitation methodology, we conclusively determined that incorrect RASS scoring occurred on account of knowledge deficiencies. The aforementioned technique can be used for the formulation of new training strategies by identifying and remedying the knowledge deficiencies, and therefore improving the effectiveness of the existing standardized solutions such as the CWP.

Summary and Discussion

Standardization solutions including clinical decision support aids such as computerized weaning protocols (CWPs) aim to reduce medical errors by standardizing care process. Health Information Technology (HIT) plays a major role in these efforts. However, the dynamic nature of critical care environments demands context-specific and complexity -inclusive assessment of these support tools for optimal results. In this chapter, we describe three studies that focus on the safety assessment of a Computerized Weaning Protocol (CWP) which has been used to standardize the weaning process of mechanically-ventilated critically-ill patients. The factors posing risk to effective use of CWP included misinterpretation of CWP's sedation assessment scale, communication and collaboration breakdowns, problems with on-time support delivery, and negative perception of the protocol among clinicians. The identified risk factors are socio-technical in nature: inherent to the protocol and externalized in the environment, in addition to trust and understanding. These factors have led to sub-optimal protocol outcomes that are classified into near-misses and adverse events, which constituted almost 34 % of protocol outcomes. Some of the potential risks, such as clinicians' negative perception, protocol misinterpretation, and inadequate collaborative practices identified using FRAM are consistent with the results from previous research [15, 21, 26, 28]. These risks might have stemmed because of multiple reasons- a) knowledge- related deficiencies, b) lack of cognitive support such as reminders, and c) ignorance or workarounds. Variability monitoring interventions to mitigate the risks posed by the standardization of the weaning process in MICU can range from clinician education, improved communication, and impact demonstration. Multi-disciplinary collaborative input from clinicians involved in the daily use of the CWP needs to be considered in view to identify and address confusing aspects in the protocol's procedures. Tools that provide unique, unambiguous, and multifaceted perspective of clinical processes to all the involved stakeholders in a health institution is essential to optimally exploit the advantages of standardization with minimal disruptions. Methods such as FRAM show strong potential for assessment of critical care safety and standardization interventions by providing a holistic view of complex processes. Adoption of a non-linear risk assessment methodology based on resilience engineering concepts is a valuable approach to address dynamic, non-deterministic nature of critical care environment. FRAM when complemented with common performance conditions representing critical care context can help us determine local variability risk sources leading to sub-optimal use of standardization tools at global scale [16]. However, it is important to note that not all variability of a system is risky in nature. Deviations from normal working conditions might sometimes be an act of resilience and positive adaption to an unanticipated or emerging event [54]. Once the individual risk sources are identified, it is essential to understand their triggers to develop remedies. Such deeper understanding of the risk factors related to the effective use of the decision support can enable us to optimize the standardization solutions by minimizing unintended consequences and maximizing end user acceptance.

Implications for Biomedical Informatics

Health Information Technology (HIT) solutions form the basis for standardization efforts in this era of digital medicine. Without proactive safety improvement approaches, the same interventions designed to improve patient safety can in fact lead to medical errors. The growing complexity of health care environment mandates methods that can tend to intractability of the system. This chapter provides an account of three studies that focus on the safety assessment of a computerized weaning protocol. The first two studies describe the application and validation of a novel risk assessment method that accounts for complexity in critical care. Lastly, the third study provides the readers with an objective method that enables researchers and applied health professionals to devise a refinement plan to enhance the effectiveness of the existing HIT interventions such as the weaning protocol. While HIT systems such as the weaning protocol discussed in this chapter are essential for improvement of patient safety and to reduce medical errors, these "safety nets" require continuous assessment and refinement in order for them to reach optimal working conditions in a complex environment like critical care. Ways to improve the performance of such standardization tools are context-specific and can range from education and motivation to workflow re-engineering. In addition, it is also essential to consider the aspects of cognitive risk management employed by clinicians during error detection and recovery during intervention design [61]. This understanding can inform the design of HIT systems that support the workflow in critical care. This chapter provides a methodological foundation for biomedical informaticians in terms of design, evaluation, and improvisation of HIT-based standardization tools in complex critical care settings. The method also facilitates health professions to predict and mitigate the unintended consequences of these omnipresent HIT based standardization strategies in the real- world health care environment.

Discussion Questions

1. Consider you are appointed to design a new HIT-based standardization solution for an intensive care unit. How do you approach your job assignment? Provide a brief overview of your standardization strategy and evaluate it. Describe its pros and cons bearing in mind that your new improvements can also lead to unintended consequences.
2. Describe a real-life standardization practice or event that you think has made a major positive or negative impact on health care delivery. If the impact is positive, what do you think the benefits might have been in terms of efficiency, quality improvement, and patient safety? If the impact of the standardization effort is negative, what would you do to improve?

References

1. Bion J, Heffner J. Challenges in the care of the acutely ill. Lancet. 2004;363(9413):970–7.
2. Rozich JD, Howard RJ, Justeson JM, Macken PD, Lindsay MF, Resar RK. Standardization as a mechanism to improve safety in health care. Joint Commission Journal on Quality and Patient Safety. 2004;30(1):5–14.
3. Boord JB, Sharifi M, Greevy RA, Griffin MR, Lee VK, Webb TA, et al. Computer-based insulin infusion protocol improves glycemia control over manual protocol. Journal of the American Medical Informatics Association. 2007;14(3):278–87.
4. Gross PA, Bates DW. A pragmatic approach to implementing best practices for clinical decision support systems in computerized provider order entry systems. Journal of the American Medical Informatics Association. 2007;14(1):25–8.
5. Holcomb BW, Wheeler AP, Ely EW. New ways to reduce unnecessary variation and improve outcomes in the intensive care unit. Current opinion in critical care. 2001;7(4):304–11.
6. Meade MO, Ely EW. Protocols to improve the care of critically ill pediatric and adult patients. JAMA: the journal of the American Medical Association. 2002;288(20):2601–3.
7. Morris AH. Treatment algorithms and protocolized care. Current opinion in critical care. 2003;9(3):236–40.
8. Winters BD, Gurses AP, Lehmann H, Sexton JB, Rampersad CJ, Pronovost PJ. Clinical review: checklists-translating evidence into practice. Crit Care. 2009;13(6):210.
9. Wood KA, Angus DC. Reducing variation and standardizing practice in the intensive care unit. Current opinion in critical care. 2001;7(4):281–3.
10. Girard TD, Kress JP, Fuchs BD, Thomason JWW, Schweickert WD, Pun BT, et al. Efficacy and safety of a paired sedation and ventilator weaning protocol for mechanically ventilated patients in intensive care (Awakening and Breathing Controlled trial): a randomised controlled trial. The Lancet. 2008;371(9607):126–34.
11. Hasibeder WR. Does standardization of critical care work? Current opinion in critical care. 2010;16(5):493–8.
12. Zed PJ, Abu-Laban RB, Chan W, Harrison DW. Efficacy, safety and patient satisfaction of propofol for procedural sedation and analgesia in the emergency department: a prospective study. CJEM. 2007;9(6):421.
13. Burns SM. Making weaning easier. Pathways and protocols that work. Critical care nursing clinics of North America. 1999;11(4):465.
14. MacIntyre NR. Evidence-based guidelines for weaning and discontinuing ventilatory support: a collective task force facilitated by the American College of Chest Physicians; the American Association for Respiratory Care; and the American College of Critical Care Medicine. CHEST Journal. 2001;120(6_suppl):375S–96.
15. Ely EW, Meade MO, Haponik EF, Kollef MH, Cook DJ, Guyatt GH, et al. Mechanical ventilator weaning protocols driven by nonphysician health-care professionals: evidence-based clinical practice guidelines. CHEST Journal. 2001;120(6_suppl):454S–63.
16. Myneni S, McGinnis D, Almoosa K, Cohen T, Patel B, Patel V. Effective use of clinical decision support in critical care: using risk assessment framework for evaluation of a computerized weaning protocol. Annals of Information Systems: Special issue on Healthcare Informatics. 2013. (Accepted in press)
17. Osheroff J, Pifer E, Teich J, Sittig D, Jenders R. Improving outcomes with clinical decision support. Chicago: HIMSS; 2005.
18. Osheroff JA, Teich JM, Middleton B, Steen EB, Wright A, Detmer DE. A roadmap for national action on clinical decision support. Journal of the American medical informatics association. 2007;14(2):141–5.
19. Kawamoto K, Houlihan CA, Balas EA, Lobach DF. Improving clinical practice using clinical decision support systems: a systematic review of trials to identify features critical to success. BMJ. 2005;330(7494):765.

20. Brochard L, Rauss A, Benito S, Conti G, Mancebo J, Rekik N, et al. Comparison of three methods of gradual withdrawal from ventilatory support during weaning from mechanical ventilation. American Journal of Respiratory and Critical Care Medicine. 1994;150(4):896–903.
21. Burns KEA, Meade MO, Lessard MR, Keenan SP, Lellouche F. Wean earlier and automatically with New technology (the WEAN study): a protocol of a multicentre, pilot randomized controlled trial. Trials. 2009;10(1):81.
22. Esen F, Denkel T, Telci L, Kesecioglu J, Tütüncü A, Akpir K, et al. Comparison of pressure support ventilation (PSV) and intermittent mandatory ventilation (IMV) during weaning in patients with acute respiratory failure. Advances in experimental medicine and biology. 1992;317:371.
23. Esteban A, Frutos F, Tobin MJ, Alía I, Solsona JF, Valverdu V, et al. A comparison of four methods of weaning patients from mechanical ventilation. New England Journal of Medicine. 1995;332(6):345–50.
24. Lellouche F, Mancebo J, Roesler J, Jolliet P, Schortgen F, Cabello M, et al. Computer-driven ventilation reduces duration of weaning: a multicenter randomized controlled study. Intensive Care Med. 2004;30:S69.
25. Rose L, Presneill JJ, Johnston L, Cade JF. A randomised, controlled trial of conventional versus automated weaning from mechanical ventilation using SmartCare™/PS. Intensive care medicine. 2008;34(10):1788–95.
26. Ely EW, Bennett PA, Bowton DL, Murphy SM, Florance AM, Haponik EF. Large scale implementation of a respiratory therapist–driven protocol for ventilator weaning. American journal of respiratory and critical care medicine. 1999;159(2):439–46.
27. McLean SE, Jensen LA, Schroeder DG, Gibney NRT, Skjodt NM. Improving adherence to a mechanical ventilation weaning protocol for critically ill adults: outcomes after an implementation program. American Journal of Critical Care. 2006;15(3):299–309.
28. Randolph AG, Clemmer TP, East TD, Kinder AT, Orme JF, Wallace CJ, et al. Evaluation of compliance with a computerized protocol: weaning from mechanical ventilator support using pressure support. Computer methods and programs in biomedicine. 1998;57(3):201–15.
29. Vitacca M, Clini E, Porta R, Ambrosino N. Preliminary results on nursing workload in a dedicated weaning center. Intensive care medicine. 2000;26(6):796–9.
30. Amalberti R. The paradoxes of almost totally safe transportation systems. Safety Science. 2001;37(2):109–26.
31. Hollnagel E. The changing nature of risk. Ergonomics Australia Journal. 2008;22(1–2):33–46.
32. Cabana MD, Rand CS, Powe NR, Wu AW, Wilson MH, Abboud PAC, et al. Why don't physicians follow clinical practice guidelines? JAMA: the journal of the American Medical Association. 1999;282(15):1458–65.
33. Friedman CP. "Smallball" evaluation: a prescription for studying community-based information interventions. Journal of the Medical Library Association. 2005;93(4 Suppl):S43.
34. Kaplan B. Evaluating informatics applications—clinical decision support systems literature review. International journal of medical informatics. 2001;64(1):15–37.
35. Sinuff T, Cook D, Giacomini M, Heyland D, Dodek P. Facilitating clinician adherence to guidelines in the intensive care unit: a multicenter, qualitative study. Critical care medicine. 2007;35(9):2083–9.
36. Weiss CH, Amaral LA. Moving the science of quality improvement in critical care medicine forward. American Journal of Respiratory and Critical Care Medicine. 2011;184(3):383–4.
37. Ash JS, Sittig DF, Campbell EM, Guappone KP, Dykstra RH, editors. Some unintended consequences of clinical decision support systems. In: AMIA Annual Symposium Proceedings Washington, DC: American Medical Informatics Association; 2007.
38. Patel VL, Cohen T. New perspectives on error in critical care. Current opinion in critical care. 2008;14(4):456–9.
39. Ash JS, Berg M, Coiera E. Some unintended consequences of information technology in health care: the nature of patient care information system-related errors. Journal of the American Medical Informatics Association. 2004;11(2):104–12.

40. Ash JS, Sittig DF, Dykstra R, Campbell E, Guappone K. The unintended consequences of computerized provider order entry: findings from a mixed methods exploration. International journal of medical informatics. 2009;78:S69–76.
41. Ash JS, Sittig DF, Poon EG, Guappone K, Campbell E, Dykstra RH. The extent and importance of unintended consequences related to computerized provider order entry. Journal of the American Medical Informatics Association. 2007;14(4):415–23.
42. Campbell EM, Sittig DF, Ash JS, Guappone KP, Dykstra RH. Types of unintended consequences related to computerized provider order entry. Journal of the American Medical Informatics Association. 2006;13(5):547–56.
43. Harrison MI, Koppel R, Bar-Lev S. Unintended consequences of information technologies in health care—an interactive sociotechnical analysis. Journal of the American Medical Informatics Association. 2007;14(5):542–9.
44. Koppel R, Metlay JP, Cohen A, Abaluck B, Localio AR, Kimmel SE, et al. Role of computerized physician order entry systems in facilitating medication errors. JAMA. 2005;293(10): 1197–203.
45. Levin SA. Ecosystems and the biosphere as complex adaptive systems. Ecosystems. 1998;1(5):431–6.
46. DeRosier J, Stalhandske E, Bagian JP, Nudell T. Using health care failure mode and effect analysis: the VA national center for patient safety's prospective risk analysis system. Joint Commission Journal on Quality and Patient Safety. 2002;28(5):248–67.
47. Spath PL. Using failure mode and effects analysis to improve patient safety. AORN journal. 2003;78(1):15–37.
48. Shojania KG, Duncan BW, McDonald KM, Wachter RM, Markowitz AJ. Making health care safer: a critical analysis of patient safety practices. Rockville: Agency for Healthcare Research and Quality; 2001.
49. Vincent C, Neale G, Woloshynowych M. Adverse events in British hospitals: preliminary retrospective record review. BMJ. 2001;322(7285):517–9.
50. Vincent C, Taylor-Adams S, Stanhope N. Framework for analysing risk and safety in clinical medicine. BMJ. 1998;316(7138):1154.
51. Hollnagel E, Pruchnicki S, Woltjer R, Etcher S, editors. Analysis of Comair flight 5191 with the functional resonance accident model. In: Proceedings of the 8th International Symposium of the Australian Aviation Psychology Association; Sydney, Australia; 2008.
52. Sundström GA, Hollnagel E. The importance of functional interdependencies in financial services systems. Resilience engineering in practice. Aldershot: Ashgate; 2010.
53. Herrera IA, Woltjer R. Comparing a multi-linear (STEP) and systemic (FRAM) method for accident analysis. Reliability Engineering & System Safety. 2010;95(12):1269–75.
54. Hollnagel E, Woods DD, Leveson N. Resilience engineering: concepts and precepts. Aldershot: Ashgate Publishing Company; 2006.
55. Hollnagel E. Cognitive reliability and error analysis method (CREAM). Oxford/New York: Elsevier Science; 1998.
56. Bates DW, Kuperman GJ, Wang S, Gandhi T, Kittler A, Volk L, et al. Ten commandments for effective clinical decision support: making the practice of evidence-based medicine a reality. Journal of the American Medical Informatics Association. 2003;10(6):523–30.
57. Hollnagel E. Barriers and accident prevention. Aldershot: Ashgate Pub Limited; 2004.
58. Myneni S, McGinnis D, Almoosa K, Cohen T, Patel B, Patel V. 553: Socio-technical barriers to effective use of a weaning protocol in a medical intensive care unit. Critical Care Medicine. 2011;39(12):153.
59. Schvaneveldt RW. Pathfinder associative networks: studies in knowledge organization. Norwood: Westport, CT, US: Ablex Pub. Corp; 1990.
60. Tossell CC, Smith BA, Schvaneveldt RW, editors. The Influence of Rating Method on Knowledge Structures. Proceedings of the Human Factors and Ergonomics Society Annual Meeting. San Antonio, TX: SAGE Publications; 2009.
61. Morel G, Amalberti R, Chauvin C. Articulating the differences between safety and resilience: the decision-making process of professional sea-fishing skippers. Human Factors: The Journal of the Human Factors and Ergonomics Society. 2008;50(1):1–16.

Chapter 10
Enhancing Medical Decision Making When Caring for the Critically Ill: The Role of Cognitive Heuristics and Biases

Velma L. Payne and Vimla L. Patel

Introduction

The foundations of human judgment and decision theory have influenced studies on decision making for decades in various domains. A specific area of human judgment is decision-making under conditions of uncertainty. Medicine is an example of decision-making under conditions of uncertainty where doctors constantly make decisions with incomplete information, knowledge gaps and sometimes with inaccurate information. These conditions are exacerbated in critical care environments (Emergency Departments (ED) and Intensive Care Units (ICU)) which are complex in nature with information intensive, time sensitive, highly stressful, non-deterministic, interruption-laden, and life-critical [1]. Caring for critically ill patients within these situations often requires clinicians to make life-and-death decisions within a few seconds while relying on large quantities of questionable information. In order to make these decisions in a timely manner, the clinician must

---

The audio recordings used in this study were collected as part of a larger research project; in addition to recordings, researchers conducted general observation and clinician shadowing. Further information can be found in Abraham, Kannampallil, & Patel, 2012.

V.L. Payne, PhD, MS (BMI), MBA, MS (CIS) (✉)
Houston Veterans Affairs, Health Services Research and Development Center of Excellence, Houston, TX 77030, USA

School of Biomedical Informatics, University of Texas Health Science Center, Houston, TX 77054, USA
e-mail: vl.payne@comcast.net

V.L. Patel, PhD, DSc, FRSC
Center for Cognitive Studies in Medicine and Public Health, New York Academy of Medicine, New York, NY 10029, USA

Department of Biomedical Informatics, Columbia University, New York, NY 10032, USA

Department of Biomedical Informatics, Arizona State University, Scottsdale, AZ 85259, USA

V.L. Patel et al. (eds.), *Cognitive Informatics in Health and Biomedicine*, Health Informatics, DOI 10.1007/978-1-4471-5490-7_10, © Springer-Verlag London 2014

reduce the large quantity of data to a manageable dimension and quickly determine what information is critical to handle the current situation [2]. Studies have shown that individuals often deal with such situations by using cognitive heuristics, or mental shortcuts [1, 2]. Even though the use of heuristics can lead to appropriate judgments, inappropriate heuristic use can result in severe and systematic errors [3–5]. In medicine, such errors include incorrect or delayed diagnosis, and inappropriate or delayed treatment, all of which can result in adverse medical events and patient harm. Due to the severe consequences of medical errors, it is imperative to minimize inappropriate use of cognitive heuristics by developing techniques to identify cognitive heuristic use.

The purpose of this chapter is to describe a theoretical framework, with associated methods that characterize physicians' use of cognitive heuristics and biases when caring for critically ill patients. Given that heuristics can be very beneficial and result in sound judgments, where as biases can (but do not always) result in flawed judgment [3–5], the framework we developed enables identification of specific actions associated with heuristic and bias use leading to sound decisions, as well as actions leading to flawed judgment. Identification of these events can facilitate the development of computer-based modules that can detect when clinical reasoning is deviating toward flawed judgment, and suggest reasoning strategies to nudge the clinician to sound judgment. These computer modules can be incorporated into biomedical informatics tools to enhance decision-making at the point-of-care. Development of such automated error detection and correction systems are critical for the management of medical errors and enhancing patient safety.

This chapter begins with a review of the literature on theories of decision-making and cognitive heuristics and biases. We then discuss how heuristics and biases are used in medicine and how they can impact clinical reasoning. Next we describe the methods we used to develop and validate a theoretical framework. Our methods include a pilot study where we ascertained physicians' view of heuristics and biases they use in their daily practice, a proof-of-concept study based in naturalistic data from the ICU, supplemented with a thorough review of the heuristic and bias literature. Following the presentation of our methods, we discuss our critical care cognitive heuristic and bias framework in detail. Finally, we discuss the implications of the framework, suggest ways it can be used in the real world to minimize flawed judgment and enhance patient safety.

Background

Theories of Decision-Making

When individuals make decisions they choose a course of action from a set of alternatives with the aim of achieving a goal [6]. There are two primary categories of decision theory including Normative Decision Theory and Descriptive Decision

Theory. Normative decision theories propose the manner in which people *should* make decisions in order to optimize an outcome, whereas descriptive decision theories depict how individuals *actually* make decisions. Normative Decision Theories utilize axiomatic mathematical models of human behavior that include probability theories such as Bayesian Theory; and utility theories such as the Expected Utility Theory [7–9]. Normative decision theories assume an ideal decision maker, who is fully informed and rational, is able to process information with perfect accuracy, resulting in an optimal decision [10]. Since individuals are unable to process information with perfect accuracy, and people do not behave in ways consistent with axiomatic rules, a related area of decision-making came into being that describes how people actually make decisions. Descriptive Decision Theories describe the manner that individuals have been *observed* making decisions. These theories or models include the Satisficing Model [11], Conjunctive/Disjunctive Model [12], Recognition Primed Decision Model [13], the Mental Model Theory [14], and the Dual Process Theory [15].

A concept that applies to normative and descriptive decision theories is *rationality*. In general, it is thought that individuals are *rational decision makers,* in that people make choices to maximize utility or self-benefit. Rational behavior is characterized by an individual who has a "well-organized and stable system of preferences and a skill in computation that enables him to calculate, for the alternative courses of action, which alternative will permit him to reach the highest attainable point on his preference scale" [16]. Rational decision-making is nearly impossible due to the limitations of humans and circumstances humans must face. According to Simon, "rationality denotes a style of behavior that is appropriate to the achievement of given goals, within the limits imposed by given circumstances and constraints" [17]. As a result of studying these limitations, Herbert Simon developed the concept of Bounded Rationality [18] which theorizes that in decision-making, rationality of individuals is limited by three things: (1) available information; (2) cognitive limitations of the mind; and (3) the finite amount of time available to make decisions. When making decisions, we do not always have the information necessary to make the optimal decision. We are limited in formulating and solving complex problems due to our ability to receive, store, retrieve and transmit information. We also find ourselves in time-critical situations that restrict our ability to assess, comprehend and process information in order to make optimal decisions. Such constraints result in humans using heuristics rather than using a strict rigid rule to arrive at a decision.

In summary, this section discussed theories of decision-making across many domains (not specific to medicine). Normative theories of decision-making propose humans are able to arrive at the optimal decision given they have the ability to execute axiomatic mathematical computations during the decision-making process. Descriptive decision theories assert humans do not have the ability to quickly execute these computations, and that decisions are actually made much differently than the normative theories propose. Descriptive theories propose people tend to arrive at a decision when primed by knowledge readily accessible within their memory, and when people arrive at a solution (decision) that is satisfactory, they discontinue problem-solving process

[11, 13]. Experts discontinue the problem-solving process quickly, while novices continue problem solving for an extended period. Within both paradigms of decision-making, people are bounded by the limitations imposed by constraints such as cognitive limitations and circumstances such as time constraints. It is these factors that induce the use of mental short cuts to assist in the decision-making process. The normative and descriptive theories also can be applied within the domain of medical decision-making. For a more detailed discussion of the paradigms of cognition in medical decision-making, reference Patel, Kaufman and Arocha [19]. Decision-making techniques specific to the diagnostic process are detailed in (reference section "The Diagnostic Process and the Use and Impact of Heuristics and Biases in Medicine").

Heuristic and Bias Theoretical Foundation

A cognitive heuristic is a mental shortcut applied to make complex tasks simpler. Kahneman and Tversky spent nearly three decades studying how people make judgments under conditions of uncertainty. Based on empirical studies they found (1) people rely on a limited number of heuristic principles to reduce complex tasks of probabilistic assessment and prediction to simpler judgmental operations; (2) people rely on heuristics when confronted with a complicated judgment or decision; and (3) people use heuristics during problem solving to speed up the process of finding a solution where an exhaustive search is impractical [3, 10, 18, 20]. Use of heuristics are unconscious to the decision-maker, and are largely due to our cognitive and environmental limitations; i.e. the cognitive limitations of short-term memory and memory retrieval, and environmental limitations such as the finite amount of time one has to make a decision, and the need to assess a large amount of information within a short period of time. Use of heuristics can result in a close approximation to the optimal decision suggested by normative theories, can be very efficient, and result in appropriate judgments [5]. However, when not used properly they can also lead to severe and systematic errors, or cognitive bias, which are departures from the normative rational theory [5, 21]. It should be noted that inappropriate use of heuristics and use of biases do not necessarily result in errors or flawed judgment, but such use can result in these events.

Although best known as the work of Kahneman and Tversky, the cognitive heuristic and bias paradigm has also been studied by other researchers including the ABC Research Group headed by Gerd Gigerenzer who takes a disparate approach to heuristic-based reasoning. According to Gigerenzer, other researchers have promoted only one side of heuristics, i.e. heuristics are bad and result in biased judgment [22]. Gigerenzer focuses on the benefits of heuristics and promotes the advantages associated with heuristic use. The approach to heuristic-based reasoning, according to Gigerenzer, is the 'Fast and Frugal' strategy that enables decision makers to make good decisions with limited information. The two attributes of this strategy are *fast* and *frugal*, where (1) fast involves utilizing a minimum amount of time, knowledge and computation; and (2) frugal involves searching a subset of the available information rather than the entire database. Gigerenzer proposes that both of these attributes are exploited within one's environmental structure to yield adaptive decisions [22]. Fast and frugal heuristics limit the decision makers' need to search for information using easily computable stopping rules, and allows them to make choices with easily computable decision rules [23]. This type of reasoning can be used to solve problems of sequential search through options, or to select a choice between simultaneous options that require searching for cues, features or consequences within each option. Gigerenzer and his colleagues consider the 'Fast and Frugal' heuristic paradigm a descriptive decision theory in that it captures how people make decisions within the real-world under constraints of limited time, knowledge and computational power [22]. Gigerenzer's approach does not go unchallenged. A criticism of the fast and frugal strategy is that its simplicity might result in highly inaccurate decisions, compared to complex statistical classification methods that process and combine all available predictors [24].

Given that healthcare is complex with different settings sometimes requiring complicated judgments to be made in an expedient manner (the same conditions in which people commonly use heuristics), a better understanding of the role of heuristics and biases within medicine will enable us to develop and integrate resilient health information technology within these settings.

The Diagnostic Process and the Use and Impact of Heuristics and Biases in Medicine

There have been a number of empirical studies that have shown physicians use of heuristics and biases while gathering and interpreting information during the diagnostic process [4, 19, 25–28]. The diagnostic process includes assessing clinical data in order to generate a hypothesis of the patient's diagnosis (differential diagnosis), followed by reviewing additional data and/or performing a course of action (such as carrying out a procedure or running a medial test) in order to narrow the differential to a more specific list of diseases (rule-in or rule-out specific diseases). Once a diagnosis has been established, action is taken to treat the patient.

During hypothesis generation when a diagnosis or a differential diagnosis is generated, physicians are susceptible to biases based on *Representativeness* and *Availability*. *Representativeness* is used to determine how closely a patient's findings resemble the prototypical manifestations of diseases [29]. Use of such pattern-recognition methods can lead to errors when the physician does not consider atypical representations [29]. *Availability* occurs when a diagnosis is triggered by recent cases similar to the current case. If a diagnosis is made based on cases recently assessed, but there are attributes in current case that do not correspond with the disease, a diagnostic error could occur. A misdiagnosis can also occur if the physician assumes this patient cannot possibly have the same diagnosis as the last three patients they have seen (*Gambler's Fallacy*) [29]. A number of cognitive biases such as *Confirmation Bias*, *Search Satisficing*, *Premature Closure* and *Overconfidence* bias can prompt clinicians to make errors when pruning, selecting and/or validating a diagnosis [29]. *Search Satisficing,* or calling off a search once something is found, may occur when a physician arrives at an initial diagnostic hypothesis based on the review of only a portion of the clinical data available, and does not review additional clinical data once their initial diagnosis has been specified. *Premature Closure* is when a physician accepts a diagnosis before it has been fully verified. *Confirmation Bias* is the tendency to look for confirming evidence to support a diagnosis rather than look for disconfirming evidence to refute it even when the latter is persuasive and definitive [29]. When a physician does not review additional data or order additional tests because they are confident in their diagnosis, they may be committing the *Overconfidence* bias, which is a "tendency to act on incomplete information, intuitions or hunches; or when too much faith is placed in an opinion instead of carefully gathered evidence" [29].

When selecting a course of action to treat the patient, the *Omission Bias* and *Outcome Bias* can adversely influence treatment decisions if the physician focuses too heavily on what could happen, rather than what is most likely to happen once a treatment or therapy is initiated [30]. Physicians can underutilize preventive interventions in order to avoid having a direct role in bad outcomes [30–32]. Death by natural causes can be viewed as better than death by prescription [3]. *Outcome bias* is when a physician places too much emphasis on patient outcomes, and does not consider the rationale and evidence underlying medical decisions [3, 33]. Other heuristics physicians use in the therapeutic process include *Extrapolation*, which is when outcomes are generalized to the general populations not included in clinical trials and/or research studies; and that the extrapolation is done inconsistently. For example, the outcome of a study to test moderate antihypertensive treatment study in men was extrapolated to women (who were not study participants) [22, 34].

Based on empirical studies, Elstein and Chapman describe decision biases they believe are used within medicine including biases occurring when judging the likelihood of events such as potential diagnoses and treatment outcomes; and biases occurring when determining preferences and evaluations of outcome utility when choosing a treatment or patient management plan [35]. Heuristics and biases that can occur when judging the likelihood of events include *Support Theory*, the *Unpacking Principle*, *Outcome Bias* and *Confirmation Bias*. *Support Theory* is a descriptive theory that posits an *unpacking principle* that states providing a more detailed description of an event increase its judged probability [36]. For example, when given a clinical scenario to diagnose, one group of subjects were given three options to choose from – the patient has gastroenteritis, ectopic pregnancy or 'none of the above'; whereas another group of subjects were given five diagnoses including gastroenteritis, ectopic pregnancy, appendicitis, pyelonephritis, pelvic inflammatory disease, and 'none of the above' [37]. For each group, the probability for all options should total 100 %. The percentage assigned to the 'none of the above' option in the short-list group should equal the total for the appendicitis, pyelonephritis, pelvic inflammatory disease, and 'none of the above' options in the long-list group since the 'none of the above' option in the short-list includes the other diseases specified in the long-list condition. The study outcome showed that the probability assigned to the 'none of the above' option in the short-list group was 50 %; whereas the sum of the probabilities assigned to the appendicitis, pyelonephritis, pelvic inflammatory disease, and 'none of the above' options in the long-list group was 69 %. Unpacking the 'none of the above' option by specifying particular diseases (appendicitis, pyelonephritis, pelvic inflammatory disease) resulted in an increase in the probability of the additional diseases [37]. Inflating the probability of a diagnosis can result in misdiagnosis and incorrect and/or delayed treatment. Another bias that occurs when judging the likelihood of events is the *Outcome Bias,* which is when decisions are evaluated more favorably if they result in a good outcome rather than a poor outcome. An impact of this bias is that a clinician may not attempt a treatment for fear of it producing an unfavorable outcome, when there is no evidence that the poor outcome will occur in the patient being treated. *Confirmation Bias* is another bias in this category. This is when the decision maker searches for evidence to support an initial hypothesis, and ignores evidence that refutes the hypothesis. Implications of this bias in clinical practice is unnecessary tests may be ordered that are do not contribute to revising an initial hypothesis; having additional data that does not refute a hypothesis does not necessarily increase the accuracy of that diagnosis.

The second decision bias Elstein believes occurs in medicine is determining preferences and evaluations of outcome utility including *Framing Effects*, *Attraction Effect*, *Sunk Cost Bias* and *Omission Bias*. The *Framing Effect* is when the less risky outcome is preferred when the same situation is presented differently. In a classical study conducted by Kahneman and Tversky, two groups of health officials were presented with the same scenario of an outbreak of the Asian flu that was expected to kill 600 people [38]. One group of health officials was presented with a plan that would save lives; the other group was presented with the same plan that was framed in terms of lives lost. The lives saved scenario indicated that the plan to combat the outbreak would save 200 lives for sure, with a one-third probability that all 600 people would be saved. The lives lost scenario indicated that 400 people would die for sure, with a two-thirds probability that all 600 people would die. The health officials preferred the plan framed in accordance with lives saved [38]. If present, the framing effect could have implications in clinical practice in that a treatment that may have a better outcome may not be selected simply because it was presented in a manner that implied the outcome would be more detrimental. Another effect that impacts a decision-maker within clinical practice is the *Attraction Effect* that occurs when adding decision alternatives. The addition of choice options, much like the framing of a situation should not have an effect on the choice made; however studies have shown that factors that should have no effect on the decision does have an effect. Redelmeier and Shafir conducted a study where they presented two groups of family physicians with a case of a patient that had osteoarthritis of the hip and a set of management plans to treat the condition [17]. One group of physicians was presented with two plans (refer to orthopedist and do not start any new medication; refer to orthopedist and start ibuprofen); the other group was presented with three plans (refer to orthopedist and do not start any new medication; refer to orthopedist and start ibuprofen; refer to orthopedist and start Piroxicam). In the group that was presented with two options, 53 % of the physicians selected option one (refer to orthopedist and do not start any new medication). In the group where three options were presented, 72 % chose the first option. The addition of alternative three increased the preference for alternative one; this is called the *Attraction Effect* [39]. The third choice (commonly referred to as a decoy) is seldom chosen, but it does influence the choice between the other two "attracting market share to the option that is superior in every way to the decoy" [35]. The *Sunk Cost Bias* is "when a decision maker continues to invest resources in a previously selected action or plan even after it is perceived to be suboptimal" [35]. There have been few empirical studies investigating this bias in medical decision-making. One study investigated the bias during the patient management process by asking residents in Internal Medicine and Family Practice to review four scenarios (one medical scenario and three non-medical scenarios) and decide if the current management strategy should be continued or discontinued. The residents were more likely to stay with the original plan if a high level of resources had already been invested; however, this effect was most evident in the non-medical scenarios. This study demonstrates that there is some evidence that physicians avoid the sunken cost fallacy in their own area of expertise, and that choosing the most effective treatment overrode the sunken cost fallacy in the medical domain [35, 40, 41]. *Omission Bias* is another bias in this category. This bias is when the decision maker feels an omission, or doing nothing, is a better alternative than an action that leads to a harmful outcome. In medicine, this bias is commonly occurs when a physician chooses not to treat a patient (they opt to do nothing) in order to avoid feeling guilty about committing an act that may bring harm to the patient. This finding has been confirmed by empirical studies that have shown "decision makers saw omissions that led to harmful outcomes as less immoral or less bad than acts that led to the same outcomes" [7, 35, 42].

Most of the empirical studies have investigated heuristic and bias use during the diagnostic process, but a small proportion has studied their use throughout the therapeutic process. Other researchers have investigated heuristic and bias use by looking at specific cognitive processes associated with the diagnostic process, i.e. when judging the likelihood of events and when determining outcome utilities. We know that heuristics and biases play a role in the hypothesis generation, pruning a differential diagnosis, validation of a specific diagnosis, as well as establishing a therapeutic course of action (i.e., patient management plan) [22, 29–34]. Our work extends prior research in that we investigate the use of heuristics and biases in both the diagnostic and therapeutic processes in a very specific medical setting – hospital critical care units – where the fast paced environment should induce clinicians to rely on cognitive short-cuts and rules-of-thumb. The manner that heuristics and biases are utilized within hospital emergency departments and intensive care units has not been formally studied. Our work is novel in that we assessed data throughout the entire patient care process and we used naturalistic (real-world) clinical reasoning data. An understanding of the role and impact of heuristics and biases in these environments is required in order to design healthcare information technology systems that enable clinicians to attend to pertinent information (and not become bogged down with irrelevant information), and expedite the decision-making process without compromising the quality of healthcare. This provides the theoretical foundations for our methods.

Methods

Data Collection

We based our critical care heuristic and bias framework on three sources of data including: (a) Review of the heuristic and bias literature; (b) Data from a pilot study conducted to ascertain physicians' view on heuristics and biases they utilize; and (c) Data from a proof-of-concept study performed to obtain naturalistic clinical reasoning data from critical care settings. We chose to carry out these particular studies in a sequential manner so as to progressively explore the use of heuristics and biases in a broad domain then narrowing our investigation to a very specific domain. We started by exploring published literature for how heuristics and biases are used during decision-making in psychology – heuristics and bias' domain of origin. We then searched the literature specifically looking for heuristic and bias use in medicine and medical decision-making. Since a large proportion of studies in the literature were based on empirical studies conducted in a laboratory, we wanted to obtain data on heuristic and bias use within real world naturalistic settings. We asked critical care clinicians to provide their perception on the prevalence of heuristics and biases in the ER and ICU (pilot study). We then immersed ourselves into the ICU to observe team interaction and decision-making sessions (proof-of-concept study). We chose this environment as we felt this highly dynamic environment would induce clinicians to use mental short cuts in order to keep pace with the quickly changing and fast paced environment. Conducting these different studies allowed us to build our framework on a solid foundation of rich data from a variety of sources. Procedures of data collection for each source are described below.

Literature Review

We performed a heuristic and bias **literature review** from multiple domains including psychology and medicine. Our primary focus was on empirical studies assessing heuristic and bias use during the diagnostic and therapeutic processes. We also reviewed literature that documents the opinion of experts on heuristic and bias use in medicine.

Clinicians' View of Heuristic Use (Pilot Study)

We conducted a **pilot study** ascertaining critical care attending physicians' perception of how frequently they use various heuristics and biases during clinical reasoning. We developed a semi-structured questionnaire that contained a definition and clinical example of 37 heuristics and biases [9]. The definitions were drawn from the literature; clinical examples were created with the assistance of physicians. Practicing critical care physicians were contacted via email and asked to rate the prevalence of heuristic and bias use in clinical practice (on a scale of 1–5, where 1 was the least prevalent and 5 was the most prevalent). Attending physicians from various regions of the United States practicing in ER and ICU settings participated in the study.

Naturalistic Clinical Reasoning (Proof-of-Concept Study)

The data was collected during morning rounds at a 16-bed adult Medical Intensive Care Unit (ICU) at large teaching hospital in Houston. A clinician team from the Medical ICU was included in the study. The team consisted of an attending physician, a clinical fellow, residents, trainees-interns, medical students, nurses and ancillary staff. The clinicians conduct the daily patient assessment and management-planning sessions in the MICU. During these sessions, residents presented information on real patients at the bedside, and clinical teams discussed each patient's status, diagnosis, and management plan. Each morning round lasted approximately 5 h, and researchers spent 3 h per day for 3 days shadowing and observing clinician teams. Clinical team interactions were audio-recorded and transcribed verbatim with all identifiers removed. We used data collected over two morning round sessions. Several months later we conducted a second observation session where we shadowed clinicians 3 h a day for three non-consecutive days. The clinical team observed during this session was a different clinical team than those observed in the first session. A total of 24 h of observations was available for analysis. Table 10.1 provides details the sessions. Data from the first observation, along with data from the literature, was used to develop our framework. Data from the second observation was used to validate and enhance the framework.

Data Analysis

Clinicians' View of Heuristic Use (Pilot Study)

We analyzed the data from the *pilot-study* by calculating the mean perceived heuristic and bias prevalence provided all study participants. Then the data was also analyzed by comparing participant groups, i.e. comparisons were drawn between ER and ICU physicians.

Naturalistic Clinical Reasoning (Proof-of-Concept Study)

We then analyzed the data from the proof-of-concept study by performing an in-depth coding process employing the Grounded Theory Method [43]. Using 10 % of

Table 10.1 Clinical observation sessions

	Session duration	Session attendees	Session description	Session purpose
Session 1	5 days – 3 h per day 15 h of observation Same team observed all 5 days	Nurse Intern physicians Resident physicians Attending physician	Clinical team discussed patient status, diagnosis and treatment plan	Framework development
Session 2	3 days – 3 h per day 9 h of observation Same team observed all 3 days Different clinical team than team observed in Session 1	Nurse Intern physicians Resident physicians Attending physician	Clinical team discussed patient status, diagnosis and treatment plan	Framework validation

the transcripts we analyzed the data inductively, reading and rereading transcripts in order to extract relevant text. Themes present in the transcripts were identified and text was grouped according to the emerging themes. Themes included clinicians making decisions on patients' diagnosis and treatment plan, information used to arrive at a decision and clinicians performing actions associated with standard clinical practice. Once themes were identified, we explored the data by breaking the transcripts into sentences, and sentences into small parts, each part representing a single thought, decision or action. Once single purpose phrases were identified, we assigned a code to each phrase. Once this was process was established, we coded and analyzed the remaining transcripts. We maintained consistency of applying codes so that it would be possible to group codes and determine in where in the patient care process the decision or action was occurring (categories). We located axes between the codes and categories and developed the theoretical framework of heuristics and biases use within critical care settings. A further description of the themes and codes produced are listed below. Table 10.2 is an example of a coded transcript.

Decisions Made – A decision was defined as reaching a conclusion after consideration of available clinical data. If possible, a decision was identified as decisions relating to arriving at a diagnosis or a decision regarding the patients' treatment plan. A decision does not necessarily result in an action being taken; there are times when a conclusion has been reached but no action is performed. The decision to not medicate the patient (Table 10.2) is a decision that was made while caring for the patient.

Information Leading to Decision – This is the information that led the clinical team to make a decision or arrive at a conclusion. The information leading to the decision to not medicate the patient (Table 10.2) is that the patient came out of the seizures on her own.

Actions Associated with Standard Clinical Practice – We identified actions associated with standard clinical practice. Standard clinical practice was defined as thought processes, practices or procedures commonly used when caring for patients.

Table 10.2 Example of a coded transcript

Clinician	Transcription text	Process description	Coder's notes
R3 resident	Bed 4 is a 57 year old, African American female	Presenting information	Patient has two issues: vomiting blood, seizure
	Came in for, I quote, "I was throwing up blood"	Chief complaint	
	She presented to the ER on the twelfth complaining of throwing up dark red blood with clots in the morning	History of present illness	
	She reports having felt weak, dizzy, nauseated with blurring vision	History of present illness	
	She called EMS that took her to Hermann ER where she had two episodes of Hematemesis and Atonic Clonic Seizure each lasting about 20 s. She came out of the seizure on her own.	History of present illness	
	No meds were given to her	Decision 1 – do not medicate patient	Information leading to Decision 1 – patient came out of seizure on own
R3 resident	She doesn't have a history of seizures – They (ER clinicians) just attributed it to Hypervolemia	Decision 2 – identify the cause of symptom of hypervolemia	Information leading to Decision 2 – no history of seizure, patient vomiting blood
A1 attending physician	What diseases are associated with the symptom of seizures?	Seeking information	Cognitive heuristic of *Representativeness* – judgment based on how closely an instance (patient symptoms) represents the disease model
R3 resident	Um, Epilepsy for one. Not sure of other diseases	Associating patient symptom with disease model	
R3 resident	She got a head CT just in case	Decision 3 – perform procedure to identify problem	Information Leading to Decision 3 – no history of seizure
	Head CT was negative	CT	Standard clinical practice – identify reason for symptom and/or rule-out hypothesis (disease) by conducting test or procedure
		Decision made by ER clinicians	Standard clinical practice – head CT is a common test used to determine or confirm the reason for a seizure

Table 10.2 (continued)

Clinician	Transcription text	Process description	Coder's notes
R3 resident	So, her vitals in the ER, Pulse 110, BP 86/71, Respiration is 18	Presenting information Vital signs	
R3 resident	She got 4 units of **blood** in the ER, after her Hemoglobin was nearer to 5.9	Decision 4 – perform procedure to stabilize patient Give patient blood	Information leading to Decision 4 – lab result (Hemoglobin) Standard clinical practice – perform procedure if lab value is below the normal level
		Decision made by ER clinicians	Standard clinical practice – give blood if Hemoglobin is below certain level
R3 resident	She was then sent to the Transplant ICU, as a MICU overflow	Decision 5 – transfer patient Transport from ER to transplant ICU	Information leading to Decision 5 – Patient condition (stable enough to move)
R3 resident	In the ICU, GI was consulted	Decision 6 – seek clinical consult	Information leading to Decision 6 – patient signs and symptoms
R3 resident	She underwent an Emergent Upper GI Endoscopy	Decision 7 – perform procedure to identify problem	Information leading to Decision 7 – patient condition and signs/symptoms
	Procedure showed a Duodenal Bulb Ulcer on the anterior wall with active arterial bleed	Emergency upper GI endoscopy Decision made by GI consult team Problem identified	Standard clinical practice – perform procedure to rule-out GI condition

For example, a common technique used when diagnosing a problem is to rule-in and rule-out diseases (diagnoses) by conducting a test or performing a procedure. An example of a standard clinical practice is to perform a head CT for a patient having seizures. An example of a therapeutic standard clinical practice was to give blood when the patient's Hemoglobin was below a specific level.

Use of Heuristic or Bias – Once the above items were coded, we reviewed the coded transcripts to identify heuristics and biases used while caring for critically ill patients. To accomplish this we mapped events that took place during the critical care process to the definition of heuristics and biases (as documented in the literature). An example of use of the cognitive heuristic *Representativeness* is shown in Table 10.2 where the attending physician and resident discuss what diseases are associated with (representative of) a seizure. An example (not shown in the tables) of actions corresponding with the *Anchoring* heuristic (locking on an initial diagnosis early in the diagnostic process) and *Confirmation Bias* (seeking information that supports an initial diagnosis and overlooking critical data that refutes the initial diagnosis) is if a clinician diagnoses a patient with chest pain with a Myocardial

Infarction, but they ignore evidence indicating the patient is not within the population that commonly suffers from a heart attack (a patient that is 25 years of age) and that the patient is of a Type A personality with a very stressful job (all symptoms that may correspond to stress or a panic attack). Once heuristics and biases were identified we determined where in the critical care process the heuristic or bias was used. We identified the heuristics and biases used during the needs assessment, hypothesis generation, hypothesis testing, establishing or revising a treatment (management) plan and monitoring the patient.

Methods for Framework Development and Validation

Our overall goal was to identify heuristic and bias use within critical care settings. For each step of the critical care process, we identified heuristics and biases commonly used; then through consultation with experienced critical care clinicians, we identified associated reasoning errors and patient outcomes. To frame our analysis, we started by identifying the heuristics and biases used in medicine in general, then assessed the real-world critical care environment to ascertain heuristics and biases used specifically in critical care. Once we developed the framework, we validated it with data from real-world decision-making sessions within an intensive care unit.

Heuristics & Biases Used in Medicine

The first step of developing the framework was to compose a list of the heuristics and biases used when physicians diagnose a patient and determine their treatment plan, regardless of where the diagnosis and treatment occurs. Based on our literature review and pilot study, we found that physicians commonly use *Representativeness, Anchoring and Adjustment, Availability, Confirmation Bias, Premature Closure, Search Satisficing, Omission and Outcome Bias, and Over Confidence* when diagnosing and treating patients.

Heuristics & Biases Used in Critical Care Settings

Steps Within the Critical Care Process

We consulted with two board-certified attending physicians that specialize in critical care to determine the steps that commonly occur in critical care settings. We reviewed the coded transcripts from the proof-of-concept study with these consultants to determine if the processes involved in caring for critically ill patients were evident in the data. During this process we looked for key actions that were consistent when caring for multiple patients. We grouped the events into logical steps, identifying a high-level category and low-level steps that comprise each category.

Heuristic and Bias Use Within Critical Care Process

Once we determined the steps that commonly occur within the critical care environment, we analyzed the data collected during observations (coded transcripts) of the proof-of-concept study to determine what heuristics and biases are used within each step of the critical care process.

Reasoning Errors and Patient Outcomes

Based on our literature review and data from our pilot and proof-of-concept studies we had extensive discussions with the board-certified critical care attending physicians, to comprise a list of potential reasoning errors and patient outcomes associated with inappropriate use of heuristics within each step of the critical care process.

Framework Validation

We validated the framework using real-world data collected during a second observation session from the proof-of-concept study (reference section "Data collection" for a description of the observation sessions). We coded and analyzed the data from the second observation in the same manner as we processed data from the first observation. We then determined if the framework adequately reflected heuristics/biases physicians use in critical care. The worksheet shown in Table 10.3 was used to document our findings of the framework validation. Where applicable, we

Table 10.3 Framework validation worksheet

Framework development Based on proof-of-concept observation session 1 (OS1)	***Framework validation*** Based on proof-of-concept observation session 2 (OS2)	***Comparison results***
Critical patient care steps (OS1)	Critical patient care steps (OS2)	No additional steps. Steps in OS1 correspond with steps in OS2
Step 1 ….	Step 1 ….	
Step 2 ….	Step 2 ….	
etc.	etc.	
Heuristics/Biases (OS1)	Heuristics/Biases (OS2)	Already in framework
Representativeness	Availability	New heuristic (add)
Availability	Search satisficing	
etc.	etc.	

modified the framework as necessary, adding additional heuristics and biases that were apparent from the second observation session.

Results

Literature Review

The results of our literature review are detailed in the Background of this chapter. We have provided an overview of various theories of decision-making (reference section "Theories of Decision-Making"), described the theoretical foundation of heuristics and biases (reference section "Heuristic and Bias Theoretical Foundation"), detailed the use and impact of heuristic and biases throughout the diagnostic process (reference section "The Diagnostic Process and the Use and Impact of Heuristics and Biases in Medicine") and explained how heuristics and biases are used in critical care settings (reference section "Naturalistic clinical reasoning (proof-of-concept study)").

Clinicians' View of Heuristic Use (Pilot Study)

The top five perceived heuristics and biases are detailed in Table 10.4 [9]. Physicians practicing in the ICU perceive *Confirmation Bias* to be most prevalent, followed by the *Availability*, *Planning Fallacy*, *In-group Bias* and *Deformation Professionelle*. Emergency room attending physicians perceive *Clustering Illusion*, *Deformation Professionelle*, *Illusory Correlation*, *Disconfirmation Bias*, and *Availability* to be most prevalent. Across both groups, attending physicians perceived *Availability*, *Deformation Professionelle*, *In-group Bias*, *Planning Fallacy*, and *Anchoring & Adjustment* are most prevalent in critical care settings.

Table 10.4 Most prevalent heuristics and biases used in critical care

Care setting	Heuristic/bias	Mean ± SD
ICU	*Confirmation Bias*	4.25 ± 0.89
	Availability	4.23 ± 0.99
	Planning Fallacy	4.00 ± 1.31
	In-group Bias	3.75 ± 1.28
	Deformation Professionelle	3.75 ± 1.75
ER	*Anchoring & Adjustment*	3.56 ± 1.13
	Deformation Professionelle	3.44 ± 1.33
	Disconfirmation Bias	3.33 ± 1.00
	Illusory Correlation	3.33 ± 1.32
	Availability	3.22 ± 1.56
Overall	*Availability*	3.45 ± 1.31
	Deformation Professionelle	3.45 ± 1.57
	In-group Bias	3.45 ± 1.14
	Planning Fallacy	3.29 ± 1.14
	Anchoring & Adjustment	3.26 ± 1.44

Table 10.5 Least prevalent heuristics and biases used in critical care

Care setting	Heuristic/bias	Mean ± SD
ICU	*Value-Induced Bias*	2.25 ± 1.28
	Texas Sharpshooter Fallacy	2.00 ± 0.83
	Clustering Illusion	1.88 ± 1.07
	Illusory Correlation	1.75 ± 0.71
	Gambler's Fallacy	1.63 ± 0.74
ER	*Overconfidence Effect*	2.11 ± 1.05
	Confirmation Bias	2.11 ± 1.17
	Hindsight Bias	1.11 ± 1.27
	Retrospective Bias	2.11 ± 1.54
	Representativeness	2.00 ± 0.53
Overall	*Neglect of Prior Base Rates*	2.33 ± 1.21
	Selection Bias	2.33 ± 1.21
	Texas Sharpshooter Fallacy	2.17 ± 1.17
	Value-Induced Bias	1.67 ± 0.52
	Illusory Correlation	1.50 ± 0.55

The heuristics and biases ER and ICU attending physicians feel are least prevalent are listed in Table 10.5. ICU attending physicians perceive the *Value-Induced Bias*, *Texas Sharpshooter Fallacy*, *Clustering Illusion*, *Illusory Correlation* and *Gambler's Fallacy* to be least prevalent. ER attending physicians perceive and *Overconfidence Effect*, *Confirmation Bias*, *Hindsight Bias*, *Retrospective Bias* and *Representativeness* to be least prevalent in their setting. Across both groups attending physicians feel *Neglect of Prior Base Rates*, *Selection Bias*, *Texas Sharpshooter Fallacy*, *Value-Induced Bias* and *Illusory Correlation* to be least prevalent.

Naturalistic Clinical Reasoning (Proof-of-Concept Study)

Identifying heuristic and bias use within the real world by examining transcripts of team discussion and decision-making sessions was not as straightforward as techniques used to assess data from the pilot study. From the transcripts of the 15 h of team clinical reasoning sessions we used to develop our framework (Session 1), we found evidence of *Anchoring & Adjustment*, *Confirmation Bias*, *Availability*, *Search Satisficing*, *Deformation Professional* and *In-group Bias* (reference Table 10.6). From the transcripts of the 9 h of clinical reasoning sessions used to validate the framework (Session 2), we found evidence of *Deformation Professional*, *In-group Bias*, *Representativeness* and *Confirmation Bias* (reference Table 10.6).

Critical Care Heuristics and Bias Framework

Our critical care heuristic and bias framework is illustrated in Fig. 10.1. This diagram depicts the steps associated with caring for a critically ill patient (top row). The middle of the diagram shows the heuristics and biases associated with each of

Table 10.6 Heuristics and biases used in team clinical reasoning sessions

Session	Heuristics/biases	Frequency of use
1	*Anchoring & Adjustment*	7
	Confirmation Bias	7
	Search Satisficing	7
	Availability	2
	Deformation Professional	4
	In-group Bias	3
2	*Deformation Professional*	2
	In-group Bias	1
	Representativeness	1
	Anchoring & Adjustment	3
	Confirmation Bias	3

the critical patient care steps based on data from all three data sources utilized in this research (literature review, pilot study and proof-of-concept study). The bottom of the diagram reflects potential reasoning errors and patient outcomes associated with each of the patient care categories; this data is based on the opinion of our expert critical care physicians. The heuristics, biases, reasoning errors and patient outcomes specified in Fig. 10.1 are not a comprehensive list of items that can occur during the critical care process; they are examples of items identified in this study. The definition of each heuristic and bias listed in Fig. 10.1 can be found in Table 10.7.

Steps in Critical Patient Care

Based on the data from our proof-of-concept study and consultation with expert critical care physicians, we identified three main steps of the critical care process: *Immediate Need Assessment*; *Address Problem* and *Patient Management*. The steps presented are a snapshot of a part of critical care process that has been simplified for the purpose of this chapter. It should be noted that even though these steps are presented as linear steps, rarely do they happen linearly as the critical care setting is an ever changing, dynamic setting where actions are dependent on critical changes of a patient's condition. Table 10.8 contains a description of steps within each of these categories that take place when a patient is in a critical care setting such as the ICU. Critical care physicians are often times dealing with a patient in a life-and-death situation. In such situations, stabilizing the patient as quickly as possible is necessary. Therefore, the first steps of the critical care process are to identify the immediate need of the patient and determine what is required in order to stabilize the patient. After the patient is stabilized, the clinical team identifies the problem associated with the patient's chief complaint. This step consists of comprising a list of possible hypotheses or diagnoses (differential diagnosis), and determining if a hypothesis is accurate (testing the hypothesis by running test, performing procedures, etc.). When the problem (diagnosis) has been identified, an action is

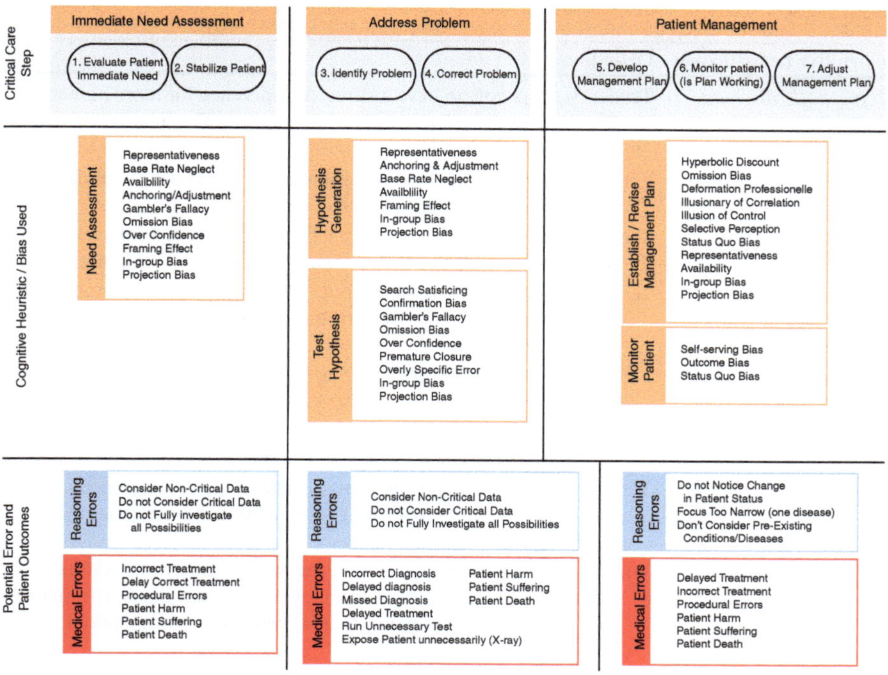

Fig. 10.1 Critical care heuristic and bias framework

Table 10.7 Definition of heuristics and biases

Cognitive heuristic/bias	Definition [9, 27]
Anchoring and adjustment	The insufficient adjustment up or down from an original starting value, or anchor. Tendency to fixate on specified features of a presentation too early in the diagnostic (or therapeutic) process, and to base the likelihood of a particular event on information available at the outset.
Availability	Tendency for things to be judged more frequent if they come readily to mind. Things that are common will be readily recalled. Availability is a heuristic in which decision maker assess the frequency of a class, or the probability of an event, by the ease with which instances or occurrences can be brought to mind.
Base rate neglect	Failing to adequately take into account the prevalence of a particular disease within a particular patient population.
Commission bias	Tendency toward action rather than inaction.
Confirmation bias	Tendency to look for confirming evidence to support a hypothesis, rather than look for disconfirming evidence to refute it.
Deformation professional	Tendency to look at things according to the conventions of one's own profession, forgetting any broader point of view.
Framing effect	Presenting the same information in different formats can alter one's decision; using too narrow of an approach or description of the situation or issue.
Gambler's fallacy	Tendency to believe a sequence that has repeatedly appeared cannot continue. The belief that a series of independent trials with the same outcome will soon be followed by an opposite outcome.

(continued)

Table 10.7 (continued)

Cognitive heuristic/bias	Definition [9, 27]
Hyperbolic discount	Tendency for people to have a stronger preference for more immediate payoffs relative to later payoffs, the closer to the present both payoffs are.
Illusionary correlation	Phenomenon of seeing the relationship one expects in a set of data even when no such relationship exists.
Illusion of control	Tendency for people to overestimate their ability to control events (they control outcomes) that they demonstrably have no influence over.
Hyperbolic discount	Tendency for people to have a stronger preference for more immediate payoffs relative to later payoffs, the closer to the present both payoffs are.
In-group bias	People tend to have positive views of and give preferential treatment to who they perceive to be members of their own group.
Omission bias	Tendency toward inaction, or reluctance to treat, due to fear of being held directly responsible for the outcome.
Outcome bias	Tendency to judge the decision being made by its likely outcome. People tend to prefer decisions that lead to good outcomes than those that lead to bad ones.
Overconfidence bias	When someone's subjective confidence in their judgments is reliably greater than their objective accuracy. Placing too much trust in one's own opinions without having sufficient evidence to support a decision.
Overly specific error	When a correct diagnosis is eliminated even though the clinical findings are consistent with the diagnosis. This error can be ascribed to the clinician's overly specific expectations for the disease.
Premature closure	Tendency to apply closure to the problem-solving process prior to examination and/or investigation of all evidence. When a diagnosis (or treatment) is accepted before it is fully verified.
Projection bias	A psychological defense mechanism where a person sub-consciously denies his/her own attributes, thoughts and emotions, which are ascribed to outsiders. Projection involves imagining or projecting the belief that others originate those feelings. Example – blaming another person for your own failure – you avoid the discomfort of consciously admitting personal faults by keeping the feelings unconscious and by redirecting them to another person.
Representativeness	Basing a decision about whether or not something belongs to a particular category by how well it matches the characteristics of members of that category. Something is the same thing if they both have the same characteristics. Representativeness is the judgment of probabilities by the degree to which A is representative of B (the degree A represents B)
Search satisficing	Tendency to call off a search once something is found. Once a diagnosis/treatment has been found, do not look any further for evidence to determine if that is the proper diagnosis/treatment.
Selective perception	Interpreting information in a way that is congruent with our existing values and beliefs. Tendency for expectations to affect perception.
Self-serving bias	When people attribute their successes to internal or personal factors but attribute failures to situational factors beyond their control. Taking credit for successes but denying responsibility for failure.
Status quo bias	People prefer things remain the same, or that things change as little as possible; tendency for people to like things to stay relatively the same.

Table 10.8 Critically ill patient care process

Step	Process	Description
1	**Immediate need assessment**	
	(a) Evaluate patient's immediate need	Determine the patient's state and action required to stabilize patient
	(b) Stabilize patient	Perform actions necessary to stabilize the patient
2	**Address problem**	
	(a) Identify problem	Identify cause of the patient's chief complaint
	Hypothesis generation	Compose a list of possible diagnoses (differential)
	Test hypothesis	Determine if hypothesis is valid
	(b) Treat problem	Perform steps necessary to correct the problem
3	**Patient management**	
	(a) Develop patient management plan	Determine actions necessary to return patient to their normal state of health
	(b) Monitor patient/determine if management plan is working	Monitor patient to ensure patient's health is improving
	(c) Adjust management plan	Revise management plan if required

performed to alleviate the problem (treat patient). After the patient's problem has been addressed, a management plan is developed to bring the patient to an optimal state. The patient is then monitored to ensure the plan is sufficient and the patient improves. If the patient is not improving, the management plan is adjusted. Steps 6 and 7 are repeated until the patient's health has reached the state where they can be moved out of the critical care environment. These steps are in accordance with the data collected for this study and are not necessarily the steps carried out in every hospital ICU.

Heuristics and Biases Used Within Critical Care

Based on the data from our literature review, heuristics and biases critical care physicians indicate they use (pilot study), and data from our real-world observations (proof-of-concept study), we determined that within each step of the critical patient care process several heuristics and biases are prevalent. First we present the descriptive statistics of heuristics and biases critical care physicians use (based on the opinion of critical care providers and observation of team decision making within critical care settings), then we describe where in the care process these heuristics and biases are used.

During the immediate need assessment phase, a number of cognitive heuristics and biases are used. A clinician may base their diagnosis or management plan on similar patients they have recently seen (*Availability*), or on diseases or treatments common for a set of symptoms (*Representativeness*). If the clinician locks on to a diagnosis early in the assessment process (*Anchoring*), seek evidence to support that diagnosis and ignore data that refutes the diagnosis, they are committing *Confirmation Bias*. If a diagnosis is made without considering the incidence and prevalence rates within the population of the patient, they are committing *Base Rate Neglect*. If a diagnosis or treatment is not selected because several prior patients have had the same outcome, *Gambler's Fallacy* is being used. If a clinician arrives at a diagnosis quickly, without performing diagnostic tests to confirm their decision, they may be *Over Confident*. If the clinician resorts to inaction out of fear of being held responsible for harming the patient, they are committing *Omission Bias*. Cognitive heuristics and biases are prevalent when teams of clinicians are collaborating on a patient's case. *In-group Bias* can occur when preferential treatment is given to those within your own group. For example, a physician may consider the views of a physician as more accurate than the view of a nurse that has considerable knowledge of the patient. *Projection Bias*, the tendency to assume others in your group share the same thoughts, beliefs, values and opinions as you, is another bias that can occur within a team decision-making environment.

Many of the same cognitive heuristics and biases apply during the addressing the problem stage of critical patient care. When assessing the patient's symptoms, commonly a clinician will quickly begin to generate a list of possible diagnoses (hypotheses). During this *hypothesis generation* step physicians may compare the patient's signs and symptoms to a mental disease model (*Representativeness*), or compare the patient to a recent patient they cared for (*Availability*). Neglecting to take into account disease rates for a specific population (*Base Rate Neglect*), preferring the opinion of those in your alliance (*In-Group Bias*) and/or assuming others share your views (*Projection Bias*) are potential flaws when hypothesizing about the patient's diagnosis. Once a hypothesis has been generated, physicians look for clinical information to either confirm or refute the hypothesis (test the hypothesis). As they seek information to test the hypothesis, several heuristics and biases such as *Over Confidence*, *Premature Closure*, *Confirmation Bias* and *Gambler's Fallacy* may be used.

A different set of heuristics and biases are commonly used during the construction and monitoring of the patient management plan. The heuristics used in this phase include *Hyperbolic Discount,* which is the tendency for people to prefer immediate payoffs relative to later payoffs; *Omission Bias,* which is when inaction is selected over action to avoid being held accountable for bring the patient harm; *Illusory Correlation*, which is when a relationship is inaccurately perceived (i.e., if an assumption is made that a particular event is the cause of the patient's condition when that event is not connected to the condition); *Selective Perception*, when a clinician's expectation affects their perception. Other heuristics used in the patient management phase is *Representativeness*, *Availability* and *Status Quo Bias* which are based on the premise that what works for others will also work in the present situation. Common team-based heuristics that may be used include *In-group Bias*, *Projection Bias*, *Deformation Professionelle* (looking at things according to the conventions of one's own profession, forgetting any broader point of view) and *Illusion of Control* (the tendency for one to believe they can control or influence outcomes in which they cannot control). Once the management plan has been established, the patient is monitored to ensure the plan is resolving the issue.

Heuristics that are commonly used once the management plan has been established are *Self-serving Bias,* which is the tendency to claim more responsibility for successes than failures; and *Outcome Bias* which is the tendency to judge a decision by its eventual outcome instead of based on the quality of the decision at the time the decision was made.

Reasoning Errors and Patient Outcomes

Based on our findings from the heuristic and bias literature review, data from our pilot and proof-of-concept studies, and the opinion of critical care specialists practicing in our study site, we identified potential reasoning errors that can lead to flawed judgment, which, in turn, can lead to negative patient outcomes.

In the immediate need assessment phase, common potential reasoning errors resulting from inappropriate use of heuristics and/or use of biases include neglecting base rate information for the patient population, considering data that is not critical, ignoring data that is critical, inaccurate mapping of the current patient's situation to disease models and/or prior patient's situations, not considering all the possible diagnoses which involves not reviewing additional clinical data or not ordering additional tests once a diagnosis has been reached. As a result of these reasoning errors, patients could receive incorrect treatment and/or a delay of the proper treatment, both of which may lead to patient outcomes of elongated or undue suffering and/or death.

In the address the problem phase of the critical patient care process, potential reasoning errors include not considering data critical to making the correct diagnosis, considering data that is not associated with the correct diagnosis, and not fully investigating all the diagnostic possibilities. These reasoning errors may result in completely missing a diagnosis, incorrectly diagnosing a patient, or a delay in diagnosing a patient. These could lead to not treating a patient, incorrectly treating a patient and/or a delay in treatment.

In the patient management phase, common reasoning errors include not noticing a change in the patient; and having too narrow of a focus, which may occur if the patient is only being monitored for the problem they had when entering the critical care unit, and not recognizing that a preexisting condition of the patient is at a less than optimal state or is impacting their current state. These errors could result in a missed, incorrect or delayed diagnosis and/or treatment; all which can cause patient harm, suffering and/or death.

Discussion

The objective of this research was to develop a framework to characterize the ***use*** and ***impact*** of cognitive heuristics and biases in complex hospital critical care environments such as emergency rooms and intensive care units. Our framework details heuristics and biases used at each step of the critical patient care process from the time the patient enters critical care, through transition to a non-critical state (including assessing the patient's immediate needs and stabilizing their condition, identifying and treating problems contributing to the patient's illness, and developing and monitoring a treatment and management plan). The framework includes heuristics and biases used by individual clinicians making independent decisions and teams of clinicians collaborating on the optimal plan for a patient. In addition, the framework specifies potential reasoning errors and patient outcomes that may occur as a result of inappropriate heuristic use. We developed and validated the framework with real-world clinical decision-making data, a through review of the literature, and physicians' view of the heuristics and biases they use in their clinical practice.

The findings of our real-world clinical observations indicate that multiple heuristics and biases are used throughout the entire critical patient care process. The majority of the heuristics and biases, reasoning errors and patient outcomes associated with 'Assessing the Immediate Need' of the patient are also used during the 'Addressing the Problem' phase. It is not surprising that similar heuristics and biases are used during these steps since similar cognitive processes occur; in that clinicians are assessing the patient's symptoms and clinical data to determine factors contributing to their illness, and ruling in and out applicable diseases. Heuristics and biases used during these steps of patient care are commonly based on specific reasoning strategies such as comprising a differential diagnosis and then narrowing down the diagnosis to a specific disease (*Anchoring and Adjustment*); basing a diagnosis on past events such as patients the clinician has recently seen (*Availability, Gambler's Fallacy*); and comparison of the patient's signs and symptoms to disease mental models and disease prevalence rates acquired throughout their career (*Representativeness, Base Rate Neglect*). Flaws in clinical reasoning during the 'Addressing the Problem' step (*Premature Closure*, *Confirmation Bias*) may be due to the critical nature of the patient and the urgency to determine what is causing the patient to be so ill. Once a clinician has formulated a list of hypotheses (differential diagnosis), they 'Test the Hypotheses' by gathering additional clinical data by running tests and/or performing procedures. Our findings indicate that during this step biases are commonly used (*Search Satisficing, Confirmation Bias, Outcome Bias* and *Overconfidence Bias*). Since hypotheses are tested after the patient has been stabilized, clinicians have the opportunity (and time) to more thoroughly assess the patient's illness by running tests and/or procedures. Therefore, it is somewhat surprising that biases are so common when validating the hypotheses.

Our findings also indicate that a unique set of heuristics and biases are used when developing the patient's treatment and management plan and when monitoring the patient once the treatment plan has been put into action. Heuristics and biases used in these steps are commonly action and/or payoff based. For example, *Hyperbolic Discount* (tendency for people to have a stronger preference for more immediate payoffs relative to later payoffs) and *Omission Bias* (tendency toward inaction, or reluctance to treat, due to fear of being held directly responsible for the outcome) are prevalent during the therapeutic stages of patient care. A unique set of reasoning errors occurs when establishing a patient treatment management plan. These potential errors can occur when the focus (or framing) of the problem is not accurate. For example, the clinician may be focusing on treating a specific problem (such as the patient's chief complaint) instead of realizing that a pre-existing condition may be contributing to the problem and/or impacted by a specified treatment (a drug that fixes one problem may negatively impact another problem). Given that critical care clinicians commonly deal with patients of co-morbidities, it is surprising that such reasoning errors are prevalent. It would be expected that critical care physicians would be more inclined to assess the interaction of a treatment on multiple problems.

Our findings confirm and extend findings of prior research associated with clinicians' use of heuristics and biases. The critical patient care process we identified from observations in hospital intensive care settings are similar to the steps in the diagnostic and treatment processes identified within the literature [4, 19, 25–28, 32, 35]. The heuristics and biases we identified in the 'Immediate Need Assessment' and 'Address Problem' steps are similar to the heuristics/biases identified in the hypothesis generation and the pruning, selecting and/or validating a diagnosis steps as documented in the literature (reference section "The diagnostic process and the use and impact of heuristics and biases in medicine") [29]. The heuristics/biases we identified in the 'Patient Management' step are similar to those documented in the literature when clinicians select a course of action [29, 32, 35]. Our research extends prior research in that we assessed heuristic and bias use within a specialized area of the hospital that cares for patients with critical life-threatening issues. Limited empirical research exists to assess heuristic and bias use during the therapeutic phase of patient care; our research includes a detailed analysis of this phase of patient care in conjunction with the diagnostic phase. In addition, we assessed heuristics and biases used by a single clinician making a stand-alone decision, as well as a team of clinicians engaged in team decision-making. We not only identified heuristic and bias use within medicine, we also identified potential reasoning errors and patient outcomes associate with such use. A significant contribution of our research, not found in prior research, is that our framework was developed and validated using *real-world clinical decision-making data by multiple teams of clinicians*. The majority of research studies assessing heuristics and biases have been laboratory-based. Assessing heuristic and bias use within real-world environments, especially in a specialized area such as critical care, provide researchers and the healthcare community with a firm insight on the benefit of heuristic use and how such use can enhance patient care, as well as how inappropriate heuristic/bias use can be detrimental to patients.

Limitations to this research include the generalizability of these findings given the framework was, in-part, based on observations of two clinical teams practicing within the same intensive care unit at the same institution. Even though we followed each clinical team for several days, team interaction was comparable from day-to-day. However, there were differences in team interactions between the two teams, which provides more generalizability than if we had observed only one clinical team. Another limitation to our study was that only one research scientist coded and analyzed the decision-making session transcripts. The results may have differed had multiple researchers coded and analyzed the data. We feel basing the framework on a thorough review of the literature and data collected from multiple studies provides a solid framework to understand decision-making within critical care settings.

Our framework depicts the heuristics, biases, potential reasoning errors and patient outcomes associated with the patient care process occurring in critical care settings. Given that patient care within critical care settings requires clinicians to make life-and-death decisions within a few seconds when assessing large quantities of information, this setting is ripe for heuristic and bias use. Heuristic use can be a powerful reasoning strategy within such an environment. However, when heuristic and bias use results in flawed reasoning, the outcome can be detrimental. As healthcare progresses, it is crucial to incorporate tools into critical care environments that enhance clinical reasoning and enable clinicians to use strategies such as heuristics in a manner that will produce unassailable judgments. The potential exists for technology to play a role in enhancing clinicians' clinical reasoning, reduce adverse patient outcomes, and improve patient care.

Summary

Critical care settings such as hospital emergency departments and intensive care units are complex environments that are stressful, time sensitive and interruption laden, where clinicians, influenced by factors such as extended work hours and sleep-deprivation, make life critical decisions. Within such dynamic environments, decision-making requires the use of cognitive heuristics, or mental short cuts, in order to sustain the required pace. It is crucial to understand the use and impact of cognitive heuristics and their associated biases by clinicians on patient care within critical care. The objective of this chapter is to describe a theoretical framework with associated methods, designed to characterize the use of cognitive heuristics and biases in critical care. This framework was developed and enhanced by an in-depth coding and analysis of real-world clinical decision-making data collected through an ethnographical study, a study ascertaining physicians' perspectives of heuristics they use in their daily practice, supplemented by a review of literature on empirical studies assessing use of heuristics and biases. We show that application of the framework can facilitate identification of specific actions associated with heuristics and biases that result in better decisions, and actions with the potential for patient harm. Identification of these actions will permit generation of procedures that can be incorporated into computer-based medical systems to detect reasoning processes leading to flawed judgment, and signal clinicians to alternatives that could lead to unassailable judgments. The development of automated detection and correction systems is critical to the advancement of health information technology within healthcare, the reduction of medical errors and enhancing patient safety.

Implications for Biomedical Informatics

The application of our framework facilitates identification of specific actions associated with heuristic and bias use. These actions can serve as the basis for the development of modules that can be incorporated into computer-based health information tools to recognize when clinicians' reasoning strategies may lead to flawed judgment, and provide alternative reasoning strategies to enhance clinical reasoning and the patient care process. Our goal is to develop and incorporate such ***auto-detection and correction tools*** at the point-of-care in order to reduce medical errors such as missed or incorrect diagnosis and incorrect or delayed treatment. To our knowledge, such a system does not exist at the point-of-care. Incorporating health information technology within critical care settings has the potential to greatly enhance medical decision-making and enhance patient care of the critically ill.

Conclusion

Caring for the critically ill requires clinicians to quickly assess and act upon a large amount of information, as time does not permit an exhaustive search process. The use of cognitive heuristics can be a valuable tool, and provide a means for clinicians to accelerate the process of assessing the immediate need of the patient, identifying the correct diagnosis, and establishing a management plan that will reduce the patient's pain and suffering.

Our framework characterizes and identifies cognitive heuristics and biases used during this patient care process within critical care settings. It spans the entire patient care process from diagnosing the patient to establishing and monitoring the patient management plan. Our model was validated against data collected from real-world decision-making sessions within an ICU of a large academic hospital. Use of this framework will result in the identification of specific actions and events that lead to flawed judgment within critical care settings. Based on this, computer-based tools can be developed to detect specific actions that lead to flawed judgment and prompt clinicians to consider alternative reasoning strategies that will result in sound judgment, ultimately resulting in enhanced patient care, and a reduction of adverse patient outcomes.

Discussion Questions

1. Select three of the various types of biases described in this papers, and think of an example each from (a) everyday experience, and (b) health care domain. How do these biases influence judgment and decisions?
2. What are the key aspects in the dispute in Kahneman & Tversky and Gigerenzer's theories on the use of heuristics and biases in decision-making?

3. Describe how the framework in this chapter can inform the development of biomedical informatics tools to enhance clinical decision-making.
4. Define Heuristics. Rule based Expert Systems are sometimes called heuristic system. Explain.

References

1. Franklin A, Liua Y, Li Z, Nguyen V, Johnson RR, Robinson D, et al. Opportunistic decision making and complexity in emergency care. J Biomed Inform. 2011;44(3):469–76.
2. Patel VL, Evans DA, Kaufman DR. Cognitive framework for doctor-patient interaction. In: Evans DA, Patel VL, editors. Cognitive science in medicine: biomedical modeling. Cambridge, MA: MIT Press; 1989. p. 253–308.
3. Tversky A, Kahneman D. Judgment under uncertainty: heuristics and biases. Science. 1974;185:1124–31.
4. Patel VL, Zhang J, Yoskowitz NA, Green RA, Sayan OR. Translational cognition for decision support in critical care environments: a review. J Biomed Inform. 2008;41(3):413–31.
5. Patel VL, Cohen T, Murarka T, Olsen J, Kagita S, Myneni S, et al. Recovery at the edge of error: debunking the myth of the infallible expert. J Biomed Inform. 2011;44(3):413–24. PubMed PMID: 20869466.
6. McDonald CJ. Medical heuristics: the silent adjudicators of clinical practice. Ann Intern Med. 1996;124:56–62.
7. Simon HA. Rational choice and the structure of the environment. In: Simon HA, editor. Models of man. New York: John Wiley; 1957.
8. Richards M, Wierzbicki M. Anchoring effects in clinical like judgments. J Clin Psychol. 1990;46:358–65.
9. Dragotoniu A, Robinson D, Patel B, Patel VL. Perceptions of cognitive biases in decision making by critical care clinicians and lay persons. unpublished work.
10. Slovic P. Thinking. In: Osherson D, Smith E, editors. An invitation to cognitive science. Cambridge, MA: MIT Press; 1990.
11. Redelmeier DA, Koehler DJ, Liberman V, Tversky A. Probability judgment in medicine: discounting unspecified possibilities. Med Decis Making. 1995;15:227–30.
12. Edwards W. The theory of decision making. Psychol Bull. 1954;51:380–417.
13. Kahneman D, Tversky A. On the psychology of prediction. Psychol Rev. 1973;80:237–51.
14. Johnson-Laird P. Mental models and deduction. Trends Cogn Sci. 2001;5:434–43.
15. Evans JSB. In two minds: dual-process accounts of reasoning. Trends Cogn Sci. 2003;7:454–9.
16. Redelmeier DA, Ferris L, Tu J, Hux J, Schull M. Problems for clinical judgment: introducing cognitive psychology as one more basic science. CMAJ. 2001;164:358–60.
17. Redelmeier DA, Shafir E. Medical decision-making in situations that offer multiple alternatives. JAMA. 1995;271:302–5.
18. Simon HA. Theories of bounded rationality. In: McGuire C, Radner R, editors. Decision and Organization. Amsterdam: North-Holland Publishing Company; 1972. p. 161–76.
19. Patel VL, Kaufman DR, Arocha JF. Emerging paradigms of cognition in medical decision making. J Biomed Inform. 2002;35:52–75.
20. Hershberger P, Part H, Markert R, Cohen S, Finger W. Development of a test of cognitive bias in medical decision-making. Acad Med. 1994;69:839–42.
21. Gilovich T, Griffin D. Heuristics and biases: then and now. In: Gilovich T, Kahneman D, editors. Heuristics and biases: the psychology of intuitive judgment. New York: Cambridge University Press; 2005.
22. Gigerenzer G, Todd P, Group AR. Simple heuristics that make us smart. New York: Oxford University Press; 1999.

23. Friedlander M, Stockman S. Anchoring and publicity effects in clinical judgment. J Clin Psychol. 1983;39:637–44.
24. Kahneman D, Tversky A. On the reality of cognitive illusions: a reply to Gigerenzer's critique. Psychol Rev. 1996;103:582–91.
25. Kassirer J, Kopelman R. Learning clinical reasoning. Baltimore: Lippincott Williams and Wilkins; 1991.
26. Plous S. Heuristics and biases. In: The psychology of judgment and decision-making. New York: McGraw-Hill; 1993.
27. Croskerry P. Achieving quality in clinical decision-making: cognitive strategies and detection of bias. Acad Emerg Med. 2002;9:1184–204.
28. Pines J. Profiles in patient safety: confirmation bias in emergency medicine. Acad Emerg Med. 2006;13:90–4.
29. Croskerry P. The importance of cognitive errors in diagnosis and strategies to minimize them. Acad Med. 2003;78(8):775–80. PubMed PMID: 12915363.
30. Huber J, Payne JW, Puto C. Adding asymmetrically dominated alternatives: violations of regularity and the similarity hypothesis. J Consum Res. 1982;9:90–8.
31. Ellis M, Robbins E, Schult D, Ladany N, Banker J. Anchoring errors in clinical judgments: type I error, adjustment or mitigation? J Couns Psychol. 1990;37:343–51.
32. Elstein A. Heuristics and biases: selected errors in clinical reasoning. Acad Med. 1999;74:791–4.
33. Graber M, Gordon R, Franklin N. Reducing diagnostic errors in medicine: what is the goal? Acad Med. 2002;77:981–92.
34. Kempainen R, Migeon M, Wolf F. Understanding our mistakes: a primer on errors in clinical reasoning. Med Teach. 2003;25:177–81.
35. Chapman GB, Elstein AS. Cognitive processes and biases in medical decision-making. In: Chapman GB, Sonnenberg FS, editors. Decision-making in health care: theory, psychology, and applications Cambridge. Cambridge/New York: Cambridge University Press; 2000. p. 183–210.
36. Sternberg RJ, Sternberg K. Cognitive psychology. Belmont: Wadsworth Cengage Learning; 2009.
37. Poses R, Anthony M. Availability, wishful thinking, and physicians' diagnostic judgments for patients with suspected bacteremia. Med Decis Making. 1991;11:159–68.
38. Spranca M, Minsk E, Baaron J. Omission and commission in judgment and choice. J Exp Soc Psychol. 1991;27:76–105.
39. Gruppen L, Margolin J, Wisdom K, Grum C. Outcome bias and cognitive dissonance in evaluating treatment decisions. Acad Med. 1994;69:S57–9.
40. Chapman GB, Bornstein BH, Elmer AC. The sunk cost fallacy in medical management decisions. Med Decis Making. 1996;16:452.
41. Bornstein BH, Elmer AC, Chapman GB. Is there a sunk cost effect in medical treatment decisions? Soc Sci Med. 1999;49:215–22.
42. Baaron J, Ritov I. Reference points and omission bias. Organ Behav Hum Decis Process. 1994;59:475–98.
43. Birks M, Mills J. Grounded theory, a practical guide. Thousand Oaks: Sage Publications; 2011.

Part II
Communication

Chapter 11
Communication and Complexity: Negotiating Transitions in Critical Care

David R. Kaufman, Joanna Abraham, and Lena Mamykina

Introduction

There is considerable truth to the old adage that successful conversation will take you very far. Of course, the proposition is more complex when applied to the healthcare system. Hospital institutions are complex structures that use a multilayered approach and employ multiple modes of communication in caring for patients including paging systems, telephones, e-mail, fax, and face-to-face interactions [1]. It is reasonable to propose that electronic health records constitute another medium of communication although a decidedly less than optimal one at this point in time. However, the patient care process in ICU relies heavily on face-to-face verbal exchange [2]. It has been reported that clinicians devote 50—60 % of clinical time to talk in ICU settings.

In an influential paper, Coiera [3] developed a concept of the communication space which is argued to be instrumental in all facets of patient care. This space is said to be enormous in terms of the total information transactions and clinician time. However, it is also a source of significant morbidity and mortality. In one review, communication issues were implicated in nearly 70 % of all sentinel events in hospitals and health care institutions in the United States [4]. In addition, about

D.R. Kaufman, PhD (✉)
Department of Biomedical Informatics, Arizona State University, Scottsdale, AZ 85259, USA
e-mail: david.kaufman.1@asu.edu

J. Abraham, PhD
Department of Biomedical and Health Information Sciences, College of Applied Health Sciences, University of Illinois, 1919 West Taylor Street, Chicago, IL, USA
e-mail: abrahamj@uic.edu

L. Mamykina, PhD
Department of Biomedical Informatics, Columbia University, New York, NY 10032, USA

V.L. Patel et al. (eds.), *Cognitive Informatics in Health and Biomedicine*, Health Informatics, DOI 10.1007/978-1-4471-5490-7_11,

50 % of all adverse events detected in a study of primary care physicians were associated with communication difficulties [5]. According to Coiera [3], the clinical communication space is interruption-driven and has poor communication systems and poor practices. He argues that informaticians need to rethink their approach to facilitating communication and careful scrutiny and observational studies are warranted. On the flip side, a positive link exists between communication, teamwork and patient outcomes in the ICU [6]. Wheelan [7] conducted a study of close to 400 care providers in 17 ICUs and found that that mortality rates were lower in ICUs that had higher stages of group development, had more structured and organized teams, had more trusting team members and were less dependent.

The chapter presents an argument for a systems-centered approach to the study of handoff as a transition in critical care. It also serves to discuss the four chapters in this section of the book and how they employ a systems-centered approach in endeavoring to understanding or change the process of handoff. The subsequent section considers theoretical issues in the development of common ground and shared understanding. In our view, this remains the most vexing problem for researchers investigating clinical communication. The final section revisits handoff in the context of some of the issues discussed in the earlier sections of this chapter.

Handoff Communication and Complexity

The chapters in this volume consider the fact that the ICU is a dynamic, high velocity, high stress environment with complex temporal patterns and unfolding of events that are highly interdependent [8]. The ICU exemplifies a complex and safety-critical environment with a range of subsystems, tasks, organizational and physical characteristics, and tools and technologies [9]. Each of these components plays a distinct and critical role toward patient care. However, successful outcomes in this environment are not only predicated on the individual performance of each component but also on the successful synergy among them [9]. Efforts to understand or intervene in the ICU environment needs to consider both the individual components of the ICU work system as well as the complex interactions among them.

Carayon et al. [10] propose a theoretical framework referred to as the Balance Theory Model that makes a clear and compelling case for acknowledging complex interactions. According to the model, an ICU work system can be characterized by five elements: including an *individual* in an ICU (e.g., attending, fellow, resident, nurse, and patient) with their physical characteristics, psychological characteristics, education, skill level, experience and motivation affecting their performance. This individual performs a range of *tasks* that have different physical, mental, temporal demands on the individual (e.g., inserting a central line, handing off patients, ordering medications). Different *tools and technologies* (e.g., computerized provider order entry (CPOE) system, a paper-based checklist) enable individuals to perform these tasks. These tasks are executed in the ICU's *physical environment* that has its own characteristics (e.g., spatial layout, presence of nursing station(s), noise level) under specific *organizational conditions* (e.g., hospital and local policies, level of teamwork, labor relations, connection to the broader community) [10].

There are two central issues that emerge from this framework. The first is that it is possible to study performance and plan interventions based on robust and multi-faceted models that endeavor to capture a significant slice of the complexity. The other issue is that if we factor 4 or 5 elements into a plan or designed intervention, the permutations are enormous. Any research program must endeavor to capture the commonalities that underlie performance; however the challenge is also to appreciate that there is enormous variation and that is a central part of the methodological challenge. Drews and Durso [11] conceptualize healthcare as a socio-natural system, and analogously argue that it will benefit from "interventions that are informed by sophisticated models run in enriched, realistic contexts that acknowledge the variety of stakeholders and that produce results that are assessed and evaluated against a long-term, global perspective that goes beyond the keyhole perspective currently taken".

The studies in this volume employ a wide range of methods across laboratory, semi-naturalistic and naturalistic environments. However, they eschew a reductionist approach that decomposes a problem into approximately linear elements; an approach common to experimental psychology and other behavioral sciences. According to Rouse [12], the approach of hierarchical decomposition has worked well for designing automobiles, laptops, cell phones and a host of other devices, but falls short as a means to study or to intervene in complex adaptive systems such as the ICU. Complex adaptive systems are said to have the following properties [12]: They are nonlinear and dynamic and do not typically reach fixed-equilibrium points. As a consequence, system behaviors may appear to be random or chaotic. They are composed of independent agents "whose behavior is based on physical, psychological, or social rules rather than the demands of system dynamics". Since agents' needs are not homogenous, their goals and behaviors are likely to clash some of the time. As agents experiment and gain experience, they learn and change their behaviors accordingly. As a consequence, overall system behavior intrinsically changes over time, and adaptation and learning lead to self-organization. Behavior patterns emerge naturally rather than being designed into the system [12]. Emergent system behaviors may be unpredictable and uncontrollable, though they may be influenced by internal and external mediators such as electronic tools.

Given the immense complexity of ICU environments, how can we possibly conduct meaningful studies of related phenomena without a reductionist strategy A systems-oriented approach helps us render the problem as tractable. Systems thinking views human activity as occurring within a community of practice, facilities, representational tools, reasoning, and perceptual-motor coordination [13, 14]. It also involves studying phenomena in a holistic way – understanding the causal dependencies and emergent processes among the elements that comprise the whole system situated in an environment (or part of a larger context). For example, a phenomenon may reflect a cell situated within an organism or a set of practitioners within a larger community of practitioners. In the introduction chapter, we make reference to the figure-ground strategy in which our phenomena of interest or our specific analytic foci is positioned within a broader context. The strategy enables a researcher to closely scrutinize a phenomenon of interest without decoupling it from a broader context. The context is attenuated (or faintly visible), but can be brought to the foreground to give meaning or offer another dimension to the phenomena of interest. We can also invert the figure and bring the background to foreground and shift our foci.

The four chapters in this section present in-depth analyses of different facets of transitions in care with a particular focus on handoff. They embrace a systems-centered focus that rejects a facile examination of handoff as a discrete event involving the mere transmission of information. The chapters support a naturalistic approach that incorporates a range of methods including observations, interviews and the analysis of artifacts. The analytic foci or subject of interest can be conceptualized as sets of concentric zones with the phenomena of interest placed in the center and other phenomena relegated to more peripheral zones. Of course, something that at first may appear to be more peripheral can prove to be instrumental. For example, in the study conducted by Collins and colleagues (Chap. 15), the initial focus was on cross disciplinary communication and artifacts were collected as a secondary source or contextual data. As the story unfolded, it was apparent that the documents revealed an important and somewhat surprising facet of interdisciplinary practices, namely that there is substantial overlap in their content, much of it being disciplinary specific. It was also revealing how these artifacts coordinated work and served as communication tools.

The system-centered approach to clinical communication cautions against the treatment of events as single slices in time and places a premium on the temporal properties of events–in other words, situating them in a broader time frame. For example, patients have a certain trajectory beginning with their admission to a particular unit and a pre-history of health-related events that preceded the admission (possibly including prior admissions). Abraham and colleagues (Chap. 12) situates handoff in the context of workflow and carefully scrutinizes the time periods that precede and follow the handoff event. The approach characterizes the interdependencies between the various tasks that constitute the workflow and serves to surface a range of contextual factors that mediate quality of care. It also serves to identify and diagnoses sources of communication breakdowns and clinical errors. The work by Mamykina and colleagues (Chap. 14) similarly situates handoff within a particular patient trajectory but with a particular focus on the development of shared understanding in a clinical team across days. The chapter also serves to quantify shared understanding in terms of shared mental models and characterize how they evolve over time in response to other mitigating factors.

The distributed view of cognition represents a shift in the study of cognition from being the exclusive property of the individual to being "stretched" across groups and material artifacts [15]. In the distributed approach, cognition is viewed as a process of coordinating distributed internal (i.e., knowledge) and external representations (e.g., visual displays, documents). The distributed view is co-extensive with a system-centered approach that situates a cognitive or communication task in a broader context. A particular focus, and the focal point of the research discussed by Collins and colleagues, is on how the tools such as artifacts or electronic health records serve to mediate cognition [16]. It also informs the intervention study carried out by Abraham et al. (Chap. 13). In a pre-post design, the authors compared.

the efficacy of two paper-based document tools for supporting handoffs: SOAP note and HAND-IT (Handoff Intervention Tool). The objective was to introduce a document format that adhered more closely to their lived clinical to reduce communication complexity and reduce transition errors. In keeping with the hypothesis, use of the HAND-IT tool resulted in fewer transition breakdowns. It may have also led to better learning outcomes for less-experienced clinicians when compared to the current (SOAP) tool.

In Pursuit of Common Ground

Common ground is an essential element in all forms of conversation and coordinated work whether the participants are two jazz musicians engaging in an improvised duet, two chess players, designers of next generation health information system or nurses involved in patient handoff. There is a certain level of synchronization, coordination and adjustments made in response to the other participant [17]. This entails a vast amount of shared information, mutual knowledge, common beliefs and shared assumptions. Grounding is the process of establishing and re-establishing the common ground that is essential to any communication. Of course, understanding is invariably imperfect. The criterion for grounding is critically dependent on the situation [18]. For example, we may reasonably anticipate that the grounding criterion would be much stricter for physicians engaged in handoff as compared to acquaintances talking about baseball.

Pre-emptive grounding refers to the process when individuals share knowledge prior to a specific conversational task, in view to use it at some point in the future [1]. There are costs associated with grounding and participants may elect to bear the grounding cost ahead of time. Of course, the risk is that their effort may be wasted. In a handoff context, two clinicians may choose to review an acutely ill patient's chart an hour or two prior to handoff. This could be a good strategy given that the task time is very limited and the problem is of sufficient complexity to warrant the grounding effort. In highly grounded conversations, for example between two nurses who know each other well and know the patient being exchanged, the conversation can be very succinct. Indeed, this is consistent with many of our observations. On the other hand, a newcomer to the unit who may be less familiar with protocol and the patient population would necessitate additional efforts to achieve common ground. The principle of least collaborative effort suggests that participants try to minimize their collaborative effort—the work that both do from the initiation of each contribution to its mutual acceptance [17]. In other words, interlocutors tend to do the minimum to establish common ground.

In intensive care settings, handoffs are most likely to be conducted face-to-face. But in other settings, the communication may take place using a range of modalities including telephone conversations, email and exchanges of paper documents. Clark and Brennan [17] characterize constraints on grounding for different media. For example, face-to-face is the only media that enables copresence (i.e., A and B share the same physical environment), visibility and simultaneity (A and B can send and receive at once/synchronously). Email, on the other hand, lacks those properties, but offers reviewability. If a communication is complex, an individual can take the time needed to review the information, whereas in face-to-face the physical message (the sound) is ephemeral and there is no affordance of reviewability. Considerations of these constraints are important in light of a technology that may serve to augment or even replace some face-to-face handoffs.

Common ground is a construct of considerable importance in communication-related disciplines and is crucial to understanding computer-mediated communication. The dominant view, as espoused by Clark and colleagues, characterizes common ground as a specialized type of mental representation that interlocutors bring to the table. Communication is conceptualized as transfers-between minds which treats intentions and goals as pre-existing psychological entities that are later somehow formulated in language and evidenced in the encounter. A more recent socio-cognitive view rejects the communication as a transfer of information; rather, establishing common ground is viewed as involving a trial and error process in which shared understanding is co-constructed by participants. It can be conceptualized as a non-summative and "emergent interactional achievement" rather than as overlapping knowledge or the sum of pooled knowledge [20]. The socio-cognitive approach underscores that common ground is a dynamic construct that is "mutually constructed by interlocutors" throughout the communicative process [19].

Kecskes' [20, 21] developed a dynamic model of meaning theory which identify two components of common ground: *core common ground*, which is composed of common sense, cultural sense, and formal sense, and derives from the interlocutors' shared knowledge of prior experience, and *emergent common ground*, which is composed of shared sense and current sense, and primarily derives from the interlocutors' individual knowledge of prior and/or current experience that is pertinent to the current situation. The construction of common ground is a dynamic process as opposed to the static process of transfer that is implicit in the prior models. Common ground is constituted by the convergence of the mental representation of shared knowledge that is activated, shared knowledge sought, and rapport as well as knowledge that we create in the communicative process. In terms of the handoff process, this raises the status of the receiver to the co-creator of common ground and it suggests that mutual understanding is an emergent property not equivalent to the intersection or even union of relevant or pooled knowledge.

Handoff Redux

Handoffs are invariably situated in complex contexts [22]. Although there are common elements and general principles that might result in a more productive process, the key to success is in developing a detailed understanding of how those principles will play out in each specific context. This is a science of particulars rather than one committed to the pursuit of universal truths—at least that seems to be the case for the foreseeable future. According to Wears et al. [22], an unspoken assumption about handoffs is that variation is bad and that standardization is good in virtually any circumstance. Although an extended treatment of the standardization issue is beyond the scope of this chapter, it is fair to say that the evidence presented in this volume and elsewhere mitigates against any facile approach to standardization, for example, one that equates the quality of handoff with the accuracy of information transfer according to specific content inclusion criteria. Of course accuracy is very important, but the mere transmission of information is not synonymous with the development of a shared understanding. In addition, handoff serves a range of functions in the coordination of tasks and the facilitation of teamwork [4].

There are numerous studies and reports that indicate that handoffs are fraught with errors [23] and that communication failures are a leading cause of medical errors and adverse events in healthcare [24]. Although these problems are beyond dispute, observational studies of handoffs have found that handoffs sometimes serve to correct a course of events that was misdirected and could have otherwise resulted in tragedy had it continued [22]. Handoffs are critical communication events that serve a range of positive functions. According to Wears and colleagues[22], conceptualizing handoffs as sources of rescue has important implications for intervention, since one common approach to "the handoff problem" is to reduce its frequency, for example, by extending shifts closer to their limits. Such a strategy may reduce hazards related to miscommunication, but could increase risks related to premature closure and would forgo the opportunity for recovery in such cases. In addition, handoff serves to initiate a shared process related to the synthesis of events, data, and information that have accumulated as isolated fragments over time [22]. It also serves to increase reflection and offers the opportunity for error detection and course correction.

It is always tempting to trot out the hoary cliché that "more research is needed". In fact, there are volumes of published research on handoff. What is needed most is a coherent framework that serves to synthesize the bodies of work and begins to fashion theoretically motivated and empirically – grounded solutions as evidenced in the chapters discussed in this review. In fact the works of Cohen and Hiligoss [4] as well as that of Wears, Perry and Paterson [22] have begun to develop such a synthesis. The work in the four chapters serves to accentuate a system-oriented approach to handoff. They also serve to highlight the importance of document-mediated cognition on the communication process. It is reasonable to argue that attaining common ground is at the heart of handoff. Yet the problem is complex and remains poorly understood. Perhaps, the cliché of more research needed has some enduring value in this context after all.

References

1. Alvarez G, Coiera E. Interdisciplinary communication: an uncharted source of medical error? J Crit Care. 2006;21(3):236–42.
2. Munir SK, Kay S. Simplifying the complexity surrounding ICU work processes–identifying the scope for information management in ICU settings. Int J Med Inform. 2005;74(7–8):643–56. PubMed PMID: 16023407.
3. Coiera E. When conversation is better than computation. JAMA. 2000;7(3):277–86.

4. Cohen MD, Hilligoss PB. The published literature on handoffs in hospitals: deficiencies identified in an extensive review. Qual Saf Health Care. 2010;19(6):493–7.
5. Bhasale AL, Miller GC, Reid SE, Britt HC. Analysing potential harm in Australian general practice: an incident-monitoring study. Med J Aust. 1998;169(2):73–6. PubMed PMID: 9700340.
6. Manser T. Teamwork and patient safety in dynamic domains of healthcare: a review of the literature. Acta Anaesthesiol Scand. 2009;53(2):143–51. PubMed PMID: 19032571.
7. Wheelan SA, Burchill CN, Tilin F. The link between teamwork and patients' outcomes in intensive care units. Am J Crit Care. 2003;12(6):527–34. PubMed PMID: 14619358.
8. Patel VL, Kaufman DR, Magder S. The road to excellence: the acquisition of expert performance in the arts and sciences, sports and games. In: Ericsson A, editor. The acquisition of medical expertise in complex dynamic decision-making environments. Hillsdale: Erlbaum; 1996. p. 127–65.
9. Ayse PG, Bradford DW, Priyadarshini RP, Pascale C, Peter JP. Human factors and ergonomics in intensive care units. In: Handbook of human factors and ergonomics in health care and patient safety. 2nd ed. Boca Raton (Florida): CRC Press; 2011. p. 693–708.
10. Carayon P, Smith MJ. Work organization and ergonomics. Appl Ergon. 2000;31(6):649–62. PubMed PMID: 11132049.
11. Durso FT, Drews F. Health care, aviation, and ecosystems: a socio-natural systems perspective. Curr Dir Psychol Sci. 2010;19:71–5.
12. Rouse WB. Health care as a complex adaptive system: implications for design and management. Bridge. 2008;38(1):17.
13. Lave J. Cognition in practice: mind, mathematics and culture in everyday life. Cambridge: Cambridge University Press; 1988.
14. Clancey WJ. Scientific antecedents of situated cognition. In: Cambridge handbook of situated cognition. New York: Cambridge University Press; 2008. p. 11–34.
15. Hutchins E. Cognition in the wild. Cambridge, MA: MIT Press; 1995. xviii, 381.
16. Horsky J, Kuperman GJ, Patel VL. Comprehensive analysis of a medication dosing error related to CPOE: a case report. JAMA. 2005;12:377–82.
17. Clark HH, Brennan SE. Grounding in communication. Perspect Soc Shar Cogn. 1991;13(1991): 127–49.
18. Clark HH, Schaefer EF. Contributing to discourse. Cogn Sci. 1989;13(2):259–94.
19. Kecskes I, Zhang F. Activating, seeking, and creating common ground: a socio-cognitive approach. Pragmat Cogn. 2009;17(2):331–55.
20. Kecskes I. Dueling contexts: a dynamic model of meaning. J Pragmat. 2008;40(3):385–406.
21. Kecskes I. The paradox of communication-socio-cognitive approach to pragmatics. Pragmat Soc. 2010;1(1):50–73.
22. Robert LW, Shawna JP, Emily SP. Handoffs and transitions of care. In: Handbook of human factors and ergonomics in health care and patient safety. 2nd ed. Boca Raton (Florida): CRC Press; 2011. p. 163–72.
23. Mistry KP, Jaggers J, Lodge AJ, Alton M, Mericle JM, Frush KS, et al. Using Six Sigma methodology to improve handoff communication in high-risk patients. 2008. 10 July 2011. Available from: http://www.ahrq.gov/downloads/pub/advances2/vol3/Advances-Mistry_114.pdf
24. Sutcliffe K, Lewton E, Rosenthal M. Communication failures: an insidious contributor to medical mishaps. Acad Med. 2004;79(2/February):186–94. PubMed PMID: doi:10.1097/00001888-200402000-00019

Chapter 12
Falling Through the Cracks: Investigation of Care Continuity in Critical Care Handoffs

Joanna Abraham and Khalid F. Almoosa

Conceptualizing Handoffs

A handoff, in lay terms, refers to the act or instance of handing or transferring something to another person (to complete/to do). For instance, you hand the baton off to the next runner in a relay race. Handoffs are an everyday yet essential process in high-reliability, safety-critical settings that operate around the clock, such as between shifts at space shuttle mission controls [1, 2], nuclear power plants [3], railroad dispatch centers [4] and hospitals [5]. Regardless of the type of setting, a well-executed handoff process helps to maintain the continuity of work across shifts and between workers.

In hospital settings, handoffs refer to the transfer of care from one clinician to the next and involve a transfer of information, responsibility and authority for patient care [6–8]. While this definition assumes a more passive role of the oncoming clinician, the Joint Commission emphasized the importance of interactivity and active participation by oncoming clinicians by re-conceptualizing the handoff as a "contemporaneous, interactive process of passing patient specific information

---

Portions of this chapter has been adapted from Abraham et al. Bridging gaps in handoffs: A continuity of care based approach, *Journal of Biomedical Informatics*, 45(2), 240–54, with permissions from Elsevier.

J. Abraham, PhD (✉)
Department of Biomedical and Health Information Sciences,
College of Applied Health Sciences, University of Illinois,
1919 West Taylor Street, Chicago, IL, USA
e-mail: abrahamj@uic.edu

K.F. Almoosa, MD, MS, FCCP
University of Texas Health Science Center, Houston, TX, USA

Transplant Surgery ICU, Memorial Hermann Hospital, Texas Medical Center,
Houston, TX 77030, USA

V.L. Patel et al. (eds.), *Cognitive Informatics in Health and Biomedicine*,
Health Informatics, DOI 10.1007/978-1-4471-5490-7_12, © Springer-Verlag London 2014

from one caregiver to another for the purpose of ensuring the continuity and safety of patient care"[9].

In this context, a handoff is also referred to as handover [10], sign-out [11], transition in care [12], bedside reporting [6], and transfer of accountability [13].

Handoffs are recognized as a critical clinical and organizational process. They occur at all levels of hospital work, from an individual level (e.g. between nurses during shift reports [14] to an organizational level (e.g. between hospitals during patient transfers [15]). Irrespective of the levels, handoffs can be categorized based on certain healthcare work characteristics such as number of participants involved in the handoff process (individual or group), profession of participants involved in the handoff process (similar or different professions), and mode of interaction (synchronous or asynchronous).

Individual handoff refers to the transfer of care from an outgoing care provider to an oncoming care provider. The transfer of care from an outgoing nurse to an oncoming nurse during shift changes is an example of individual handoff. Group handoff is defined as the transfer of care from an outgoing care provider to a group/team of care providers. The transfer of care from outgoing resident to patient care team during morning rounds is an example of group handoff.

Intra-professional handoff refers to the transfer of care between care providers belonging to the same profession. For example, transfer of care between residents belonging to critical care medicine is a case of intra-professional handoff. In contrast, inter-professional handoff refers to the transfer of care between care providers belonging to different professions. Transfer of care between sending physician in internal medicine service and receiving physician in surgical service is a case of inter-professional handoff.

Synchronous handoff refers to a simultaneous transfer of care between providers. For example, a face-to-face transfer of care between outgoing ED resident and oncoming emergency resident is an example of synchronous handoff. Asynchronous handoff refers to the transfer of care between care providers that take place at different times. An audio-taped handoff (on a voicemail system) between a sending physician in internal medicine service and a receiving physician in surgical service is an example of asynchronous handoff.

Handoffs have been a fairly recent topic of interest for researchers and hospital quality performance and improvement personnel. Despite their important role in ensuring the continuity of patient care activities and patient safety [6, 16], handoffs are often considered complex and error-prone [17–21]. Next, we highlight the ubiquity and relevance of handoff problems.

Communication failures have been cited as the leading cause of a range of medical errors and adverse events (nearly 70 %) in healthcare [22]. Almost half of these communication errors occurred during handoffs between care providers [9]. Several anecdotal reports, empirical studies and systematic and integrative reviews on handoff research have illustrated the ubiquity and relevance of clinician handoffs in hospitals [8, 23–26].

Background

In this section, we describe prior research on handoffs with specific emphasis on the theoretical framings of handoffs. We also highlight the prior studies on handoffs, including the methods supporting their investigation, the barriers they present to effective patient care, and the proposed solutions.

Theoretical Framings on Handoffs

Handoff, by the very nature of its definition is conceptualized primarily as an information transfer activity. In addition to this function of information transfer that is explained by the information processing, researchers have identified six other theoretical perspectives and goals for handoffs. For the purposes of understanding these theoretical framings of handoffs, we have borrowed these definitions from [26–28]. They include: stereotypical narratives that allows for the creation of a narrative and highlight the deviations in activities; social interaction that affords the co-construction of meaning through shared mental models; and resilience that supports the cross-checking of assumptions with a fresh perspective; accountability that supports the transfer of responsibility and authority; distributed cognition, that emphasizes how cognition is distributed across human minds, external cognitive artifacts, and groups of people; and cultural norms that focuses on how group values and norms are maintained over time.

In addition to these seven framings, Arora et al. [29] proposed a conceptual competency-based framework grounded in theories from social science research that provides insights on how handoffs can be improved. The two theories are the costs of coordination and the agency theory. Based on a case study of handoffs, the authors found that handoff resulted in (a) increased coordination costs due to communication failures and uncertainty in decision-making and (b) agency problems due to shift-work mentality, lack of responsibility and other cross-coverage issues. The competency-based framework emphasizes that handoff communication and professionalism issues can be alleviated by providing formal education on handoff communication and by focusing on a "shared responsibility" model of handoffs, respectively.

From our review of the research [26], we found that the majority of prior studies (explained below) have analyzed handoffs from an information processing and distributed cognition perspective.

Prior Studies on Handoffs

In general, handoff studies mostly focused on understanding the content, structure and order of "communication" during handoffs. For example, Manias et al. [30]

considered ways in which intra-departmental nursing handover involved a complex network of communication that impacts nursing interactions. The critical ethnographic study upon which the paper is based involved a research participant group of six nurses who worked in one critical care unit. The nursing handover took on many forms and served different purposes. At the start of a shift, the nurse coordinator of the previous shift presented a 'global' handover of all patients to oncoming nurses. Nurses then proceeded to the bedside handover, where the intention changed from one that involved a broad overview of patients, to one that concentrated on a patient's individual needs. Data analysis identified five practices for consideration: the global handover serving the needs of nurse coordinators, the examination, the tyranny of tidiness, the tyranny of busyness, and the need to create a sense of finality. By challenging nurses' understanding of these practices, they can become more sensitive to other nurses' needs, thus promoting the handover process as a site for collaborative and supportive communication.

A prominent example of a formal inter-departmental handoff occurs during patient report between sending and receiving nurses when a patient is being transferred between departments. For example, Crocker [31] described a study that traces the patient's journey from emergency admission to inpatient unit, including a brief period of stay in a high-dependency unit, and finally to discharge. By highlighting this journey, the author identified a number of critical events that could impact effective management of medicines, such as omission of an antibiotic, late administration of IV drugs and safety of prescribing process. Adverse events and near misses were found when tracing the patient journey. For instance, oxygen was prescribed in the medical notes but not on the drug card. To reduce such adverse events, the author argued that nurses need to pay more attention to improve safety in medication management.

Studies on Handoff Barriers

A vast majority of handoff studies have focused on the evaluation of barriers, resulting from communication and information-related bottlenecks. For example, Apker et al., [32] examined handoff communication between ED and hospitalist physicians. From the interview data analysis, they highlighted that handoffs are characterized as a "gray zone" filled with information ambiguity. They also identified three types of information ambiguity during inter-service handoffs: ambiguity of patient diagnosis, ambiguity of patient disposition, and ambiguity of patient boarding. After an examination of the barriers in the gray zone, they argued that the two main barriers consisted of communication challenges that arise due to incomplete information, missing information and incorrect information flow, and information expectation challenges that arise due to disagreements resulting from the differing and conflicting worldviews of the two services.

Arora et al. [33] described the mediating role of "sign-out" in transfer of care for hospitalized patients between inpatient physicians. Using the insights gathered from interns in a general medicine unit on adverse events that occurred due to suboptimal sign-outs in the preceding shift, the authors identified 25 discrete events resulting from handoff communication breakdowns during earlier sign-out. Based on these events, the two main handoff communication challenges identified were content omissions either related to medications, treatments, tests, consults or active medical problems, and failure-prone communication processes due to the lack of face-to-face communication, double sign-outs (night floats), and illegible/unclear notes.

Smith et al. [34] examined how anesthetists transfer information and responsibility to nurses. The authors observed 45 handovers that took place either in the operating room, the recovery room or in the corridor, and conducted interviews with 17 anesthetists and 15 recovery nurses. The authors highlighted that handovers took place among other activities, and context played an important role in handoffs. The length and content of handoffs between the anesthetists varied depending on the complexity of the patient's condition and surgical operation. The handoffs were audit points where care providers reviewed what had been done, checked that everything was in order and put everything in place to prepare the patient for transfer to the ward. The authors found that the transfer of information during inter-professional handoffs did not automatically guarantee a transfer of responsibility from the anesthetists to the recovery room nurses. Some responsibilities were transferred, some were delegated, and others were retained by anesthetists. Therefore, the authors argued that a standardized approach to handoffs might not be effective in improving inter-professional handoff practices due to the informality in handoffs and cultural factors underlying handoff behavior.

Another study highlighted five attributes of resident handoffs that contributed to care-related problems. First, handoffs were truncated or omitted due to work demands. Second, ongoing diagnostic or care activities carried through a shift change were at a risk for getting dropped or unfinished. Third, the oncoming physician lacked confidence in the outgoing's physician judgment. Next, cross-coverage issues increased information loss and lack of familiarity with patients. Finally, coordination issues and lack of sense of the patient care provider affected handoffs [35].

In addition to the studies on physician handoff barriers, nursing handoff challenges have also been an area of research scrutiny. Berkenstadt et al. [36] examined nursing shift handoffs in a critical care unit. The authors analyzed a patient case event using a risk management perspective right after the event was recorded on the incident reporting system. From the incident reporting system, deviations from institutional protocols were identified. Some of the deviations and problems included missing documentation of insulin dose, nursing handoff not taking place near the patient's bed, lack of institutional protocols, lack of training on handoff skills, and interpersonal issues among nurses in the department.

Furthermore, researchers have highlighted that the contextual characteristics of a critical care environment, such as presence of interruptions, time-pressures, and information uncertainty, can have an effect on the quality of handoffs. For instance, Laxmisan et al., [37] examined information flow in an emergency department with a particular focus on interruptions, multitasking, and handoffs during shift changes. The authors reported that the majority of information transfers occurred during shift changes. The process of handoffs varied significantly depending on the oncoming and outgoing physicians. For instance, handoffs occurred in different locations such as "sit-down" rounds and "walk" rounds. Additionally, Kowalsky et al., [38] found that communication content and form were influenced by patient condition uncertainty.

Some of the consequences related to ineffective handoff incidents included delays in treatment and ordering of tests [39], incongruence in patient data [40], and increased patient length of stay [41].

The subsequent section will highlight some of the key solutions proposed and adopted in various healthcare settings to address these challenges and their related consequences.

Studies on Handoff Solutions

To address the handoff failures, the Joint Commission's National Patient Safety Goal 2E requires hospitals to incorporate a *standardized* approach to handoff communication, including an opportunity to ask and respond to questions of oncoming providers. Collaborative efforts by researchers and hospital administrators have resulted in several handoff mechanisms, both in terms of design of tools (e.g., checklists [42, 43], templates [44–47], EMR-integrated tools [48–51]), processes (e.g., support for read/hear-back technique [52], face-to-face interactions [7, 53, 54] and interactive questioning [5, 55]).

Additionally, several studies have suggested the incorporation of training and standard operating protocols (SOP) to maintain the quality of handoffs in different ways, for instance, the identification of communication skills needed for effective handoffs, and also incorporation of interactive simulation exercises [38, 56].

Furthermore, evidence-based guidelines for effective handoffs have been identified; for instance, Alvarado et al. [13] reported four guiding principles for the transfer of accountability (TOA) process that can improve standardization of the handoff process. First, a safety checklist to review key patient safety issues, identify errors and limit patient harm. Second, an opportunity to clarify information. Next, reliance on memory should be minimized. And finally, one person should be aware of the entire unit and its patients. Based on their evaluation, the authors found that the TOA guidelines improved effectiveness and coordination of communication among nurses at shift changes.

Research Motivation

Handoffs continue to remain an ongoing safety threat despite these studies. This can be attributed to three reasons. *First*, the research focus has been primarily on understanding the nature of "communication" behavior during handoffs [30, 57]. Researchers have adopted a handoff-centered approach to studying communication activity between clinicians. While these data collection and analytical methods are useful for understanding the types of breakdowns in communication *during* handoffs, they were inadequate for evaluating the outcomes of handoff communication [8], which we believe is often dependent on clinician activities that precede and follow the formal communication activity.

Second, although prior research provides a strong foundation for understanding the problems associated with the handoff communication activity, there is still very limited knowledge on the nature of these handoff barriers [58]. In other words, it remains unclear what challenges impact the continuity of care, and what sources of the information breakdowns lead to transition errors.

Third, there are currently no universally adopted "gold" standards for handoff communication [23]. As a result, very seldom are these handoff strategies and solutions followed [59]. The solutions are "conceptually limiting" [60]; some are structured and exhaustive (for e.g., [42]), while others are ambiguous and open-ended in nature (for e.g., [61]). Additionally, conclusive links between the various handoff solutions and reduction in medical errors and adverse events have not yet been established [57].

Due to these challenges, hospitals are still very apprehensive about adopting these solutions. We believe that the limited adoption of such standardized practices for handoffs could be partially traced to a lack of proper understanding of the nature of handoffs, the challenges faced during handoffs, and their root contributors.

To address this, we need to understand what we are trying to fix, as suggested by communication experts [62]. First we need to identify where the problems occur and why the solutions cannot be implemented or even standardized within hospitals. This calls for a deeper examination and analysis of the current handoff process in hospitals, which in turn requires a methodological approach predicated on a continuity of care model in order to effectively capture all handoff-related activities within the context of the overall clinical workflow.

Case Study: Investigation of Handoffs in Critical Care[1]

To understand the handoff process, a study was conducted in a medical intensive care unit (MICU) at a large academic hospital.

Study Setting

The medical intensive care unit (MICU) is a 16-bed unit located in a large teaching hospital within the Texas medical center with an average of 55,000 emergency department (ED) visits per year. The MICU in this hospital is a "closed" ICU, where

[1] This section (including figures and tables) has been adapted with permission from Abraham et al. Bridging gaps in handoffs: A continuity of care based approach, *Journal of Biomedical Informatics*, 45(2), 240–54.

Table 12.1 Medical Intensive Care Unit (MICU) team member roles and responsibilities

MICU roles	Patient-care responsibilities
Attending Physician	Intensivist head of the MICU team and is in charge of all patient-care decisions.
Clinical Fellow	Intensivist in training and makes major decisions in the absence of the attending, and keeps the attending informed of patients' status and also supervises all residents and students for daily duties, including patient care and procedures.
Medical Resident	Post-graduate physician in their second or third year of internal medicine residency training and is in charge of patient-care activities in the MICU, and works under the direction and supervision of the attending physician.
Medical Intern	A physician in their first year of residency training and is in charge of care activities for patients in the MICU, and works under the direction and supervision of the attending physician and the resident.
Pharmacist	Monitors drug therapy; reviews medication regimen and provides other medication recommendations.
Respiratory Therapist	Evaluates and performs therapeutic treatment and diagnostic procedures for patients with respiratory or other cardiopulmonary disorders

the MICU team is primarily responsible for the care of patients admitted to the unit. Before the start of this study, the first author attended an MICU training session for new residents and interns rotating in the unit in order to learn more about the roles and responsibilities of the MICU team and become familiar with the unit's policies and protocols. Our research team also provided an overview to the MICU staff about our prior research on patient safety, our expertise in conducting fieldwork in hospital settings, and our efforts to ensure confidentiality of data. The institutional review board (IRB) approved the study.

Participants

Participants included *patient-care teams* that were on-call (i.e., on service) and actively involved in continuity of care activities in the MICU.

These care teams were comprised of an attending physician, a clinical fellow, residents, interns, a pharmacist, a respiratory therapist and nurses. The roles and responsibilities of each of the MICU team members are described in Table 12.1.

While the attending physician, fellow, pharmacist and nurses worked 12-h shifts, the resident and intern worked 28-h shifts. During a 28-h shift, a resident, with support from an intern, was primarily responsible for the care delivery activities of all patients in the MICU. However, as patients often stay at the MICU for several days, patient care responsibilities were transferred among residents across multiple shifts.

MICU Workflow Terminology

At the beginning of each shift, the resident and intern in charge of patient care activities are referred to as the "on-call resident" and the "on-call intern." *During handoffs*, the on-call resident and on-call intern are referred to as the "outgoing resident" and the "outgoing intern," while the oncoming resident and intern are referred to as the on-call resident and on-call intern for the new shift. Apart from the on-call resident and intern, the oncoming team is comprised of the attending, the clinical fellow and the pharmacist. *After handoffs are completed*, the oncoming resident and oncoming intern take charge of patient care activities in the MICU. In this paper, we report on our investigation of resident handoffs in the MICU. The MICU team workflow and terminology are illustrated in Fig. 12.1.

Physician Handoffs in MICU

As there was no formal resident "sign-out" procedure at the study site, morning rounds were used for handoffs between resident teams. These transitions can be considered group handoffs, where an outgoing team (resident and/or intern) presented patient care-related information by verbalizing the written content on a handoff tool to an oncoming team (attending, fellow, resident and intern). Patient nurses, pharmacists and respiratory therapists also attended these sessions. The attending physician moderated the discussion, which often involved follow-up questions to verify the information presented by the resident and/or intern. The rest of the oncoming team played a more "passive" role, interjecting into the discussion when necessary to provide supporting information or clarification.

Theoretical Rationale

Our theoretical rationale and the supporting methods illustrate the power of utilizing a "continuity of care" based model and the results presented serve only as a "proof of concept" to emphasize the usefulness of our approach.

The clinician-centered approach to handoff evaluation utilizes a "day in the life" approach [63] and is based on identifying the contextual factors surrounding clinical workflow that have an impact on the continuity of care between clinicians during transitions.

The effectiveness (i.e., quality) and efficiency (i.e., timeliness) of information flow between clinicians is dependent on the clinicians' activities and workflow. Therefore, we argue that by adopting a clinician-centered approach (grounded in the continuity of care model) in which we shadow clinicians, we can develop a more accurate and nuanced representation of the overall handoff process with respect to the temporal sequence of the clinician's information management and transfer activities as they relate to patient care events. Capturing the nuances within such a model not only affords insights into the characteristics of a complex critical care environment [64, 65], but also provides increased clarity on the interdependencies between the various workflow components [66, 67], the challenges that arise from these interdependencies and their impact on patient care [68, 69]. Similar arguments

a

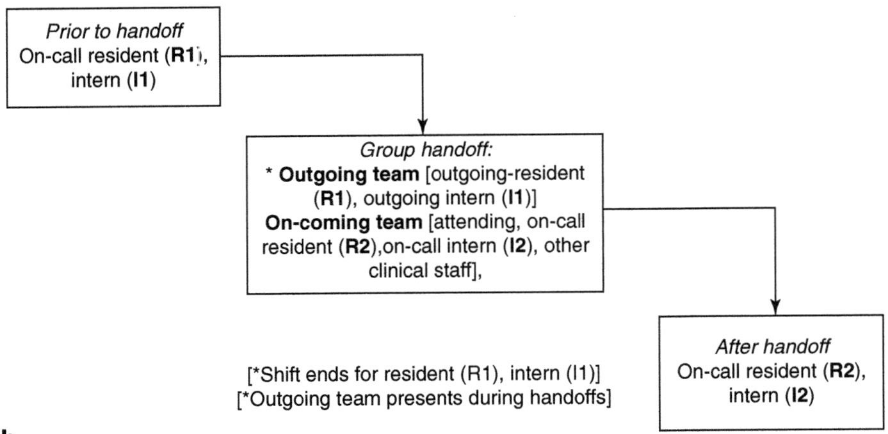

b

Preparatory Activities of the Resident Prior to Handoff

(6:00 am) on-call resident is writing her progress notes at workstation outside room1. She starts browsing the EMR of patient in room 1- reads at the values, reviews information on lab report and Xray. *(6:10 am)* **Writes down the values from the EMR onto the progress note for room 1.**
(6:14 am) She then gets interrupted by patient alarms and walks into patient room 2[...]

Handoff Communication Sequence

Outgoing resident: So MICU day 5, vent day 5. Her problems are septic shock, left thigh absyss, repiratory failure, altered mental status, acute kidney injury on CVVHD, shock liver, DICU with coliothopy and enstemy. She has a right IJ which is 5 days old, a right femaral quinten which is 5 days old, a foley, a dopp off tube, no drip, she is on ozomyl.. at 60, she's on prevacid and stds. **Medicines she is on vanc 1.25 gms, IV Q12 day 5, gent 70, IV Q day 5, merapinin 1gm IV Q 8 day 5, hydrocortizone 100 IV Q8, 100 pob IV, cena.. which actually I stopped yesterday, on latulose and (pause)**

Oncoming attending: that's good idea.

Resident Activities Immediately Following Handoffs

Attending asks the on-call resident whether they sent urine for culture for room 5. [....] The on-call resident then writes orders for comfort measures for room 1. No intubation and no CPR. Then she talks to the attending and the nurse manager about room 1. The patient is a transfer. Medicine accepted the paitnet and transferred him to ER. They transferred him here late Monday morning. We got hold of the family only today. They told him that they were okay **about DNR/DNI (Do not Reuscitate/Do not Intubate). On-call resident informs the attending that he scheduled room 6 for a protocath.**

Fig. 12.1 MICU handoff workflow and terminology (Adapted with permission from Abraham et al. [21])

were developed by Collins et al. [70], who described the importance of incorporating the handoff information elements into a continuity of care document (CCD).

Using the clinician-centered approach, we believe, we can (a) situate handoff communication events within the context of the clinician workflow; (b) highlight the complexity and interactions in handoff communication; (c) identify the points of communication breakdowns, and map them to their root contributors.

In the clinician-centered approach, we collected data of the *on-call resident during the clinician's entire shift*, i.e., from 8 am on first day to 12 pm on the following day (a total of 28 h at a time). We highlight the data collection and analysis methods that were undertaken using the clinician-centered data collection approach.

Data Collection

We employed ethnographic data collection methods including general observations, clinician shadowing, semi-structured interviews, and artifact identification and collection [71]. Similar approaches have been utilized extensively in biomedical informatics research [37, 64, 66, 67, 72].

Observation: General observations of the clinician workflow were carried out to understand the activities of the team members, and their roles in the MICU.

Clinician Shadowing: The on-call residents, primarily responsible for carrying out the patient-care tasks were closely shadowed. To support the recording of shadowing data, we meticulously documented handoff-specific data, patient-care workflow data and oncoming resident related data.

Audio Recording: Audio-recording of the communication between the outgoing and oncoming teams was collected. The audio recorder was placed in the coat pocket of the attending physician.

Semi-Structured Interviews: Interviews with the MICU attending, clinical fellows, nurses and residents were conducted. During these interviews, we asked the participants to provide their perspectives and insights on (a) handoff workflow; (b) communication content and structure (d) communication and clinical workflow challenges, and (e) recommendations and suggestions for handoff standardization.

Artifact Identification and Collection: We identified and collected the progress note that was mainly used to support verbal communication during handoffs. The progress note comprised of patient-case information structured in a SOAP (Subjective, Objective, Assessment and Plan) format. SOAP is based on the problem-oriented information organizational format that includes subjective information (e.g., patient history), objective information (e.g., vital signs), assessment information (e.g., differential diagnosis) and plan-related information (e.g., medications, orders). A SOAP-based handoff tool was used at our study setting (Fig. 12.2).

The data collection methods are detailed above in Table 12.2. Using these multiple methods, we were able to describe how the handoff process is integrated with the MICU workflow.

Data Analysis

The analysis was performed in two stages and involved a mixed *inductive-deductive* approach. *Stage 1* of data analysis was based on an inductive method of analysis using grounded theory approach [73], while *Stage 2* of data analysis was based on a

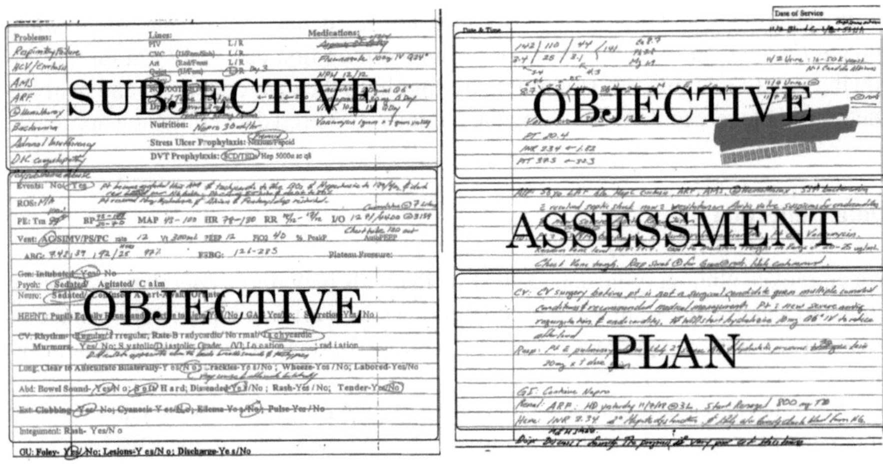

Fig. 12.2 Problem-oriented, SOAP handoff tool with subjective, objective, assessment and plan areas highlighted (Adapted with permission from Abraham et al. [21])

Table 12.2 Details of data collection in the MICU

Method	No. of participants	Participant types	Data collection time(in hours)
Observation	Varied	Healthcare-providers including: Attendings, Fellows, Residents, Nurse Manager, Nurses, Pharmacists, Nutritionists, Consults	105
Shadowing	30-40	MICU team (Attending, Fellow, Residents, Interns) during group handoffs	14
Audio-recording	80 Handoffs (5 rounds with 16 patient cases each)	Attendings, Fellows, Residents, Interns, Medical Students	15
Interviews	7	Attendings, Fellows, Residents, Nurses	2.5

structured coding template (i.e., handoff communication model) developed from Stage 1.

Stage 1 of data analysis was focused on examining the observation and shadowing data related to care provider activities using a grounded theory approach which has widely been adopted in the medical informatics domain [71]. The coding process was comprised of the following three steps – (1) *open coding* where a line-by-line analysis on the observation and shadowing data was performed in order to derive open codes related to MICU workflow and handoff communication activity. Examples of some open codes include handoff goals, roles and responsibilities, handoff activities (information presentation by sender and feedback/judgment by receiver), decisions made during handoffs (assessment and plan), interdependencies between activities, roles of participants (sender, receiver), information resources and artifacts used (progress note, computer on wheels), communication challenges (information ambiguity, loss), and strategies to overcome the challenges (information support from team). (2) *Axial coding* was performed on the open codes that were generated in order to identify repeated patterns of events and relationships between them to develop core categories relevant to handoff process. Examples of axial codes included (a) three handoff phases: pre-turnover, handoff, and post-turnover phases and their related activities such as coordination activities (one that helps manage interdependencies between individual tasks), communication events (passing of a message through a channel for a particular purpose), and patient-care delivery activities respectively, (b) team communication protocol, (c) rules of interaction, (d) decision choices (accept, reject and request information), (e) the information breakdowns during patient communication events and (f) also the decision making and collaborative problem solving cycles. *Selective coding* where the coding was iteratively performed around the core categories to develop an emerging theme related to three phases in the handoff process. For instance, by mapping the various information paths and the central decision points that lead to the final assessment and plan of care, we were able to generate a conceptual model that describes handoff communication activity in the MICU. This process was continued until we reached thematic saturation and there were no more new codes that were generated.

Second Stage: This stage of data analysis was performed on the audio-recorded communication data. Using the structured codes and the handoff communication model developed in the previous stage, we coded the audio-recorded handoff communication. Additionally, the progress note artifact that structured the communication during handoffs was analyzed. Based on the content analysis of the progress note, we identified 15 distinct communication events (CEs) that occurred during each patient handoff (details are provided in Table 12.5). For instance, the first communication event, CE1 included basic patient information – admission information & summary of some maintenance therapies.

Empirical Evaluation of Handoffs in MICU[2]

Four critical themes emerged from our analysis using the continuity of care based approach, including handoff communication model; handoff process and interdependencies; handoff breakdowns; and root contributors to handoff breakdowns. We use only a sample set of results as a "proof of concept" in this chapter.

[2] This section (including figures and tables) has been adapted with permission from Abraham et al. Bridging gaps in handoffs: A continuity of care based approach, *Journal of Biomedical Informatics*, 45(2), 240–54, and from an article in the Proceedings of the *2011 Annual Symposium American Medical Informatics Association*, Abraham et al., Falling through the cracks: information breakdowns in critical care handoff communication.

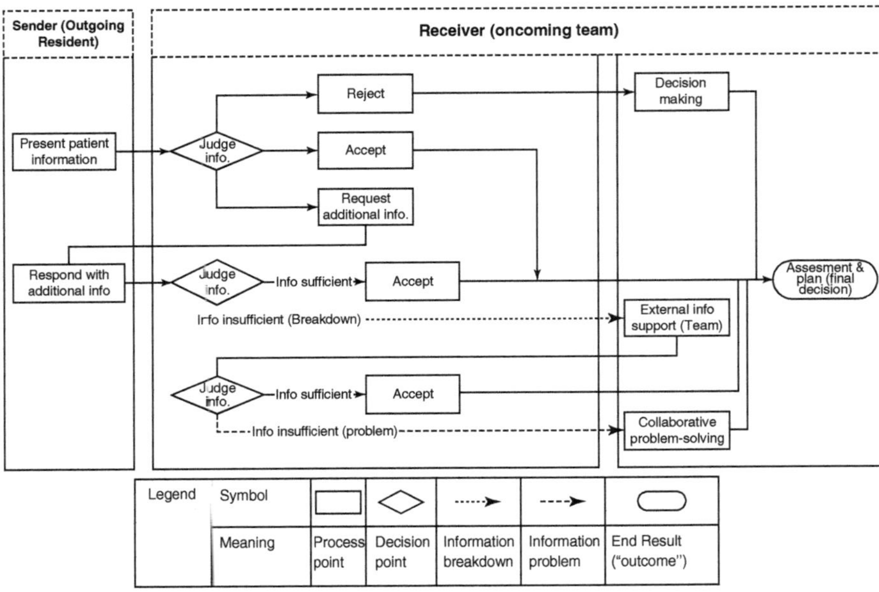

Fig. 12.3 Group Handoff Communication Model in MICU (Adapted with permission from Abraham et al. [21])

Handoff Communication Model

The model in Fig. 12.3 represents the handoff communication activity that occurred between an outgoing resident ("sender") and an oncoming MICU team ("receiver") comprised of the attending physician, fellow, resident, intern and pharmacist. The handoff was initiated by the outgoing resident presenting patient-case information (i.e., comprised of a total of 15 communication events for a single patient case), which was judged by the attending (i.e. active team member).

The attending made one of three decision choices – reject, accept and request more information. When a *reject* decision was made, a decision-making cycle was initiated. The decision-making cycle involved examining available options, establishing baseline criteria for making a decision, evaluating the available options, and finally, selecting an appropriate plan of action. The output of this cycle was incorporated into the final assessment and plan decision.

When an *accept* decision was made, the information was incorporated into the final assessment and plan of care decision. When a *request for information* decision was made, the sender tried to respond with more information, which was then evaluated for its sufficiency by the attending receiver. When the additional information was sufficient, the information was accepted by the attending. When the information was insufficient, it resulted in an information breakdown (gap in information caused by sender), which necessitated the oncoming MICU team (i.e. passive team member) to provide the additional information. If the information provided by the team was sufficient, it was accepted. Alternatively, if it was insufficient, it resulted in an information problem (gap in information caused by team), which then initiated a collaborative problem-solving cycle consisting of seeking information from sources, collectively making sense of the information, and finally, applying the understanding to solve the problem at hand. The output of this cycle was incorporated into the final assessment and plan decision. This model was repeated for the 15 communication events of each patient handoff.

Using our methodological approach, we demonstrated that the handoff phase was highly complex and interactive. The model illustrated that communication complexity arises due to several factors that influenced the effectiveness of the communication activity, such as multiple information flow paths and decision points, non-linear and recursive nature of decision-making and collaborative problem-solving activities, team interactions, and finally, the pragmatic nature of the critical care environment.

Handoff Process and Interdependencies

The handoff process consisted of three phases: pre-turnover, handoff, and post-turnover phases. While similar sub-categorization of handoffs has been previously reported [27], we extended prior research by identifying core clinician activities involved with each of these phases.

The pre-turnover phase, as the name suggests, was focused on the preparatory coordination performed by the on-call resident before the formal handoffs. These activities helped in managing interdependencies between individual tasks [74]. Table 12.3 provides five coordination activities performed by the on-call resident in the pre-turnover phase.

Following the pre-turnover phase was the handoff phase comprised of *communication events* related to specific patient cases (Table 12.4). This phase was characterized by communication events between the outgoing resident (or intern) and the oncoming MICU team related to the patient care delivery and management.

Table 12.3 Pre-turnover phase coordination activities (CA)

Coordination activity no.	Coordination activities	Description
CA1	Examine patient	Conduct physical assessment
CA2	Gather information	Seek information from different sources such as nurse, respiratory therapist, pharmacist, EMR, patient room etc.
CA3	Update information	Update patient information on patient folder
CA4	Review and analyze information	Reason-out information from different sources including EMR
CA5	Prepare progress notes	Write information on progress note form

Table 12.4 Handoff phase communication events (CE)

Communication event no.	Communication events	Description
CE1	MICU day #, vent day #, problems, lines, drips, nutrition, prophylaxis	Present basic patient information-admission information & summary of some maintenance therapies
CE2	Events ROS	Overnight patient events, review of systems
CE3	PE: Tm, BP, MAP, HR, RR, I/O	Physical exam – temp, blood pressure, heart rate, respiratory rate and ins and outs (vital signs)
CE4	Vent: rate, Vt, PEEP, FiO_2, % Peak P, AutoPeep ABG Gen: intubated – Y/N	Mechanical ventilation status & requirements and related values, arterial blood gas
CE5	Psych: sedated/agitated/calm	Psych-related issues
CE6	Neuro: sedated/confused/ alert-awake-oriented	Neurological status
CE7	HEENT: pupils equally round and reactive to light – Y/N; GAG – Yes/No, secretion –Yes/No	Head, eyes, ears, nose, and throat related information and issues; basic reflexes
CE8	CV: rhythm –regular/irregular, rate- normal/tachycardic Murmurs –Y/N, systolic, diastolic, location: …. radiaton	Cardio-vascular-related issues & examination
CE9	Lung: clear to auscultate bilaterally –Y/N; crackles –Y/N; wheeze-Yes/No, labored – Y/N	Pulmonary-related issues & examination
CE10	Abd: bowel sound- Y/N; soft/hard; distended –Y/N; rash: Yes/No; tender- Yes/No	Abdominal-related issues & examination
CE11	Ext: clubbing –Y/N; cyanosis-Y/N, edema –Y/N; Pulse- Y/N Integument: rash: Y/N	Extremities & examination
CE12	GU: foley –Y/N; lesions Y/N; discharge-Y/N	Genitourinary-related issues & examination
CE13	Labs, cultures	Lab data, culture reports
CE14	Chest X ray Other imaging	Imaging data and reports
CE15	Assessment and plan- (a) neuro, (b) endocrine, (c) resp, (d) CVS, (e) GI, (f) renal, (g) I.D., (h) heme, (i) other organs, (j) prophylaxis	Final care decision on each of the systems Analysis, decisions, and plan of care for the patient based on information above, organized by system or problem list

Adapted from Mumaw et al. [3]

A communication event is defined as the information exchange between the outgoing and oncoming teams (interaction based on give, receive and feedback of information) across a communication channel for a specific purpose [75].

Table 12.5 Post-turnover patient-care delivery activities (PA)

Patient-care activity no.	Post-turnover activities	Description
PA1	Complete pending and newly assigned tasks	Perform immediate patient care tasks pending from previous shift and newly assigned tasks for this shift
PA2	Review information	Analyze information/updates recorded on EMR in the previous shifts
PA3	Divide patient assignments	Making decision on assessment and plan of care (deciding on who should perform the patient tasks and their relative priority)

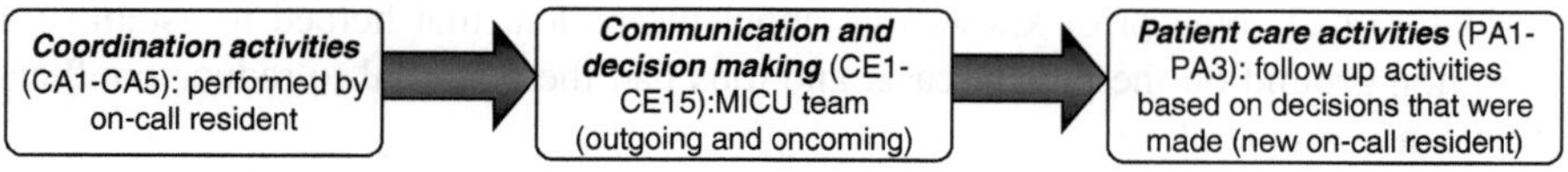

Fig. 12.4 Summary of the handoff phases and its related activities

The phase immediately following the handoff communication phases was the post-turnover phase. This phase was composed of *patient-care delivery tasks* performed by the on-call resident (i.e., the resident from the oncoming team who took charge for the current shift) after handoff (See Table 12.5).

A summary of the handoff phases and the related activities in each phase is provided in Fig. 12.4.

Handoff Breakdowns

Handoff breakdowns refer to gaps in handoff communication and were characterized as being of four possible types – Type 1 (incomplete information from sender), Type 2 (inaccurate and conflicting information), Type 3 (irrelevant information) and Type 4 (incomplete information from team). These definitions have been borrowed from [76]. Types 1, 2, and 3 were breakdowns that were immediately resolved as soon as the missing information was provided by one of the team members; Type 4 was an information breakdown that was not fixed by any of the team members, and consequently resulted in an information-related problem. Information-related problems, unlike information breakdowns, required a collective effort to be resolved. Table 12.6 (borrowed from [76]) shows examples of information breakdown counts for a sample set of ten patients.

Missing information from sender (Type 1) and incomplete/conflicting information (Type 2) were the prominent types of handoff breakdowns (shown by the column representing single day in Table 12.6). Furthermore, based on our comparison of handoff communication across consecutive days, (shown by the columns representing across 2 days in Table 12.6), we found that Type 1 continued to be the most prominent information breakdown while Type 2 was the least frequent one. This

Table 12.6 Frequency of information breakdowns on a single day and across two days

	Frequency of information breakdowns		
		Across two days	
Types of information breakdowns	On a single day	Day 1	Day 2
Type 1 (Missing by sender)	11	8	11
Type 2 (Incomplete/conflicting information)	10	7	0
Type 3 (Irrelevant information)	1	1	1
Type 4 (Missing by team)	1	1	0
Total	**23**	**17**	**12**

finding can be attributed to the fact that the team members (attending, fellow and residents) had some prior knowledge about the patient that helped to establish a common ground on the patient case, and thus had the potential to reduce conflicts between team members.

When disregarded, these information breakdowns can potentially propagate between the handoff phases and also between multiple shifts. Therefore, to address the handoff problem, our strategy was to identify the root contributors of these communication breakdowns. The following sub-section highlights the sources of the various information breakdowns.

Root Contributors to Handoff Breakdowns

Three influential factors that contributed to information breakdowns included complexity of resolving a patient case, lack of standardization format of presentation in the handoff phase, and unsuccessful completion of coordination activities in the pre-turnover phase (details are provided below). The factors that had no influence on information during group handoffs included severity of patient case, experience of sender (i.e. presenter), and frequency of follow-up questions. In this chapter, we focus on the factors that had an effect on information during handoff communication.

Complexity of Resolving a Patient Case

The first influential factor was the complexity of resolving a patient case. Complexity of resolving a patient case was defined by the difficulty in identifying the patient problem by the team (patient uncertainty/diagnosis complexity). Table 12.7 below illustrates how complexity of resolving a patient case is related to the frequency of information breakdowns in handoff communication.

The data in Table 12.7 suggests that for bed 12, as the complexity of resolving a patient case decreased (from day 1 to day 2), the frequency of information breakdowns was reduced. Similarly, for bed 17, as the complexity of resolving a patient case increased, the frequency of information breakdowns also increased.

Table 12.7 Influence of case complexity on handoff communication

	Complexity of resolving a patient case		No. of information breakdowns	
Bed no.	Day 1	Day 2	Day 1	Day 2
12	More complex	Less complex	5	0
17	Less complex	More complex	1	7

Table 12.8 Influence of standardization on handoff communication

Bed no.	Followed standardized format- Y/N?	Frequency of information breakdowns
10	N	2
2	Y	0
14	Y	3
16	Y	2

This illustrates that complexity of resolving a patient case can potentially be associated with frequency of information breakdowns.

Lack of Standardization of Handoff Presentation

The second influential factor was the lack of standardization format followed by the residents (sender) to present a patient case to the attending (receiver). Although the progress note based on the SOAP format provided a structure to follow for hand-off presentation, this information handoff format was found to be not followed by various residents. Table 12.8 below shows how standardization of handoff format influenced the frequency of information breakdowns. For instance in Table 12.8 (borrowed from [76]), a standardized handoff format was not followed for beds 10 and 15, consequently resulting in information breakdowns. Alternatively, a standardized format was followed for beds 2, 14 and 16.

Furthermore, the data suggests that a standardized format of handoff, by itself, did not always contribute to handoff communication effectiveness. While the information handoff for bed 2 did not comprise any information breakdowns, we identified the presence of information breakdowns for beds 14 and 16 despite following a standardized format of information handoff. This raised an important question as to what actually caused this inconsistency in the data, and leads us to our final influential factor.

Unsuccessful Completion of Pre-Turnover Coordination Activities

The final influential factor was unsuccessful completion of prior coordination activities in the pre-turnover phase. The five coordination activities included examining patient, gathering information, updating information, reviewing information and preparing progress notes.

Table 12.9 Status of pre-turnover coordination activities

Coordination activity no.	Coordination activity	Status of coordination activity–performed/not?
CA1	Examine patient	Performed
CA2	Gather information	Missed
CA3	Update information	Performed
CA4	Review information	Missed
CA5	Prepare progress notes	Performed

We use a detailed example of patient bed 10 (borrowed from [76]) to illustrate how coordination activities in the pre-turnover phase resulted in information breakdowns in the handoff phase. Table 12.9 below represents the status of coordination activities in the pre-turnover phase for patient bed 10. In this table, CA2 and CA4 were missed coordination activities in the pre-turnover phase (represented by shaded rows).

The 15 communication events in the handoff phase were analyzed for information breakdowns. Table 12.10 below represents the status of information breakdowns in the handoff communication phase. In this table, CE2 and CE15 comprised information breakdowns (represented by shaded rows).

We then examined the impact of the completion of coordination activities in the pre-turnover phase on the presence or absence of information breakdowns in the handoff phase by mapping the two phases and their respective activities and events. Fig. 12.5 below depicts the mapping between the phases of patient bed 10 where CA1-CA5 represent the coordination activities and CE1–CE15 represent the communication events.

Based on the mapping, we found that the information breakdowns in communication events, CE2 and CE15 in the handoff phase were caused by the missed coordination activities, CA2 and CA4 in the pre-turnover phase. This suggested that successful completion of coordination activities in the pre-turnover phase can potentially influence handoff communication. To validate this result, we revisited Table 12.8 (on the influence of standardization on handoff communication) and analyzed the status of coordination activities in the pre-turnover phase in conjunction with the standardization format data.

For bed 2, given that the standardization format was followed and the coordination activities were completed, this resulted in effective communication free of breakdowns (depicted by shaded row in Table 12.11). While, for beds 14 and 16 although the standardization format were followed, these handoffs were characterized by significant breakdowns, which was due to the unsuccessful completion of coordination activities in the pre-turnover phase. Using the information on status of coordination activities, we were able to explain the inconsistency in the data.

Therefore, based on our data, we inferred that effective handoff communication depends on standardization of handoff format and reduced complexity of patient case, and also successful completion of prior coordination activities in the pre-turnover phase.

Table 12.10 Information breakdowns in handoff communication

Communication event no.	Details of communication events	Information breakdown –Y/N?
CE1	MICU day #, vent day #, problems, lines, drips, nutrition, prophylaxis	N
CE2	Events, ROS	Y
CE3	PE: Tm, BP, MAP, HR, RR, I/O	N
CE4	Vent: rate, Vt, PEEP, FiO2, % peak P, AutoPeep	N
	ABG	
	Gen: intubated – Y/N	
CE5	Psych: sedated/agitated/calm	N
CE6	Neuro: sedated/confused/alert-awake-oriented	N
CE7	HEENT: pupils equally round and reactive to light – Y/N; GAG –Yes/No, secretion –Yes/No	N
CE8	CV: rhythm –regular/irregular, rate- normal/tachycardic	N
	Murmurs –Y/N, systolic, diastolic, location: radiation	
CE9	Lung: clear to ascultate bilaterally –Y/N; crackles –Y/N; wheeze-Yes/No, labored – Y/N	N
CE10	Abd: bowel sound- Y/N; soft/hard; distended –Y/N; rash: Yes/No; tender- Yes/No	N
CE11	Ext: clubbing –Y/N; cyanosis- Y/N, edema –Y/N; pulse- Y/N	N
	Integument: rash: Y/N	
CE12	GU: foley –Y/N; lesions Y/N; discharge-Y/N	N
CE13	Labs, cultures	N
CE14	Chest X ray	N
	Other imaging	
CE15	Assessment and plan (a) neuro, (b) endocrine, (c) resp, (d) CVS, (e) GI, (f) renal, (g) I.D., (h) heme, (i) other organs, (j) prophylaxis	Y

Discussion: Complexity and Errors in Critical Care

A process perspective to examine handoffs provided a systematic temporal and sequential analysis of the features and constraints surrounding its context including the root contributors for information breakdowns. Our methodological approach based on the continuity of care model is closely similar to other methods adopted to study long-term traces of human behavior in a variety of fields including Human Computer Interaction (see e.g., [77] on exploratory sequential data analysis), communication (see e.g.,[78]), cognitive science (see e.g., [79]) and biomedical informatics (see e.g., [80]).

Our model of handoff communication demonstrated that the communication activity is interactive and non-linear and is vulnerable to communication breakdowns. The investigation of breakdowns requires a detailed examination of the handoff problem using a handoff workflow perspective that takes into consideration

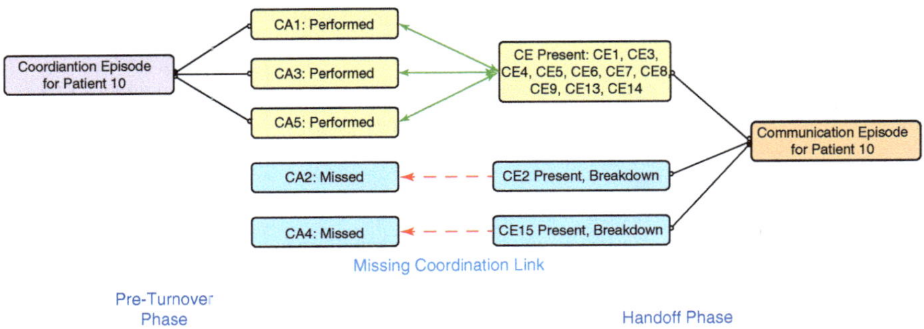

Fig. 12.5 Influence of Pre-turnover Coordination Activities on Handoff Communication (Adapted with permission from Abraham et al. [76])

Table 12.11 Influence of coordination activities on handoff communication

Bed no.	Followed standardized format – Y/N?	Frequency of information breakdowns	Coordination activity performed status – complete/incomplete
10	N	2	Incomplete
2	Y	0	Complete
14	Y	3	Incomplete
16	Y	2	Incomplete

the content and structure of communication within the overall clinical workflow context rather than solely focusing on the content of the handoff communication. We have attempted to do this by highlighting three influential factors that contribute to information breakdowns. We suggest two key strategies that can potentially ensure effectiveness and efficiency of handoff communication – (a) standardization using a handoff communication tool based on body system format and (b) streamlining pre-turnover activities using a collective information-push model. These intervention strategies have the potential to impact the MICU handoff process (pre-turnover, handoff communication, post-turnover phases) by (a) providing a structured and systematic approach to information transfer during handoff communication (b) minimizing the information breakdowns (e.gs, information loss, ambiguity) in handoff communication, and (c) ensuring the successful completion of coordination activities in the pre-turnover phase.

Our results point to two significant aspects that need to be considered for studying handoff communication is critical care settings: methodological and theoretical aspects. In terms of the methodology, we argue for a trace-based, sequential approach that captures the nuances of interactive activities during the pre-turnover, turnover and post-turnover phases. This approach relies on characterizing the workflow, thereby providing additional leverage in characterizing the handoffs within the context of work activities. In terms of the theoretical contributions, we proposed a model of handoff communication that accounts for the interactive nature of handoffs. Such models of communication are instrumental in evaluating handoff outcomes, investigating how handoffs contribute to complexity and error and also to identify the root contributors to information flow breakdowns. A detailed description of the impact of the communication model and its capabilities can be found in [21].

Discussion Questions

1. What are the some of the challenges faced in pre-turnover phase in preparation for handoffs?
2. What are the specific clinical characteristics of the information breakdowns – lost information o inaccurate information?
3. What are the effects of these information breakdowns on patient outcomes such as length of stay in the unit, re-admission rate, and infection rate?
4. Can we trace the quality of handoffs using the clinician-centered approach to clinical patient outcomes such as patient morbidity and mortality?
5. How generalizable is the handoff communication model to group handoffs at other hospitals?
6. Given that this particular setting was paper-based, what is the effect of EHR technology use on the communication model?

References

1. Patterson ES, Woods DD. Shift changes, updates, and the on-call architecture in space shuttle mission control. Comput Support Coop Work. 2001;10(3–4):317–46.
2. Helmreich RL, Foushee HC. Why crew resource management? Empirical and theoretical bases of human factors in aviation. In: Wiener EL, Kanki BG, Helmreich RL, editors. Cockpit resource management. San Diego: Academic Press; 1993. p. 3–45.
3. Mumaw RJ, Roth EM, Vicente KJ, Burns CM. There is more to monitoring a nuclear power plant than meets the eye. Hum Factors. 2000;42:36–55.
4. Roth EM, Lin L, Kerch S, Kenney SJ, Sugibayashi N. Designing a first-of-a-kind group view display for team decision making: a case study. In: Salas E, Klein G, editors. Linking expertise and naturalistic decision making. Mahwah: Lawrence Erlbaum Associates, Inc.; 2001. p. 113–35.
5. Patterson ES, Roth EM, Woods DD, Chow R, Orlando-Gomes J. Handoff strategies in settings with consequences for failure: lessons for health care operations. International J Qual Health Care. 2004;16:125–32. doi:10.1093/intqhc/mzh026.
6. Strople B, Ottani P. Can technology improve intershift report?: What the research reveals. J Prof Nurs. 2006;22(3):197–204.
7. Arora V, Johnson J, Meltzer DO, Humphrey HJ. A theoretical framework and competency-based approach to improving handoffs. Qual Saf Health Care. 2008;17(1):11–4.
8. Riesenberg L, Leitzsch J, Massucci J, Jaeger J, Rosenfeld J, Patow C, et al. Residents' and attending physicians' handoffs: a systematic review of the literature. Acad Med. 2009; 84(12):1775–87.
9. The Joint Commission on Accreditation of Healthcare Organizations (JCAHO). National patient safety goals. Critical Access Hospital and Hospital National Patient Safety Goals [Internet]. 2006. Available from: http://www.neodevices.com/resources/CR_NationalPatient SafetyGoals.pdf

10. Smith AF, Pope C, Goodwin D, Mort M. Interprofessional handover and patient safety in anaesthesia: observational study of handovers in the recovery room. Br J Anaesthesiol. 2008; 101(3):332–7.
11. Borowitz SM, Waggoner-Fountain LA, Bass EJ, Sledd RM. Adequacy of information transferred at resident sign-out (inhospital handover of care): a prospective survey. Qual Saf Health Care. 2008;17(1):6–10.
12. Powell SK. Handoffs and transitions of care: where is the lone ranger's silver bullet? Prof Case Manag. 2006;11(5):235–7.
13. Alvarado K, Lee R, Christoffersen E, Fram N, Boblin S, Poole N, et al. Transfer of accountability: transforming shift handover to enhance patient safety. Healthc Q. 2006;9:75–9.
14. Staggers N, Jennings BM. The content and context of change of shift report on medical and surgical units. J Nurs Adm. 2009;39(9):393–8.
15. Craig SS. Challenges in arranging inter-hospital transfers from a small regional hospital: an obvervational study. Emerg Med Austr. 2005;17(2):124–31.
16. Gandhi TK. Fumbled handoffs: one dropped ball after another. Ann Intern Med. 2005; 142(5):352–8.
17. Horwitz LI, Meredith T, Schuur JD, Shah NR, Kulkarni RG, Jenq GY. Dropping the baton: a qualitative analysis of failures during the transition from emergency department to inpatient care. Ann Emerg Med. 2009;53(6):701–10.
18. Donchin Y, Gopher D, Olin M, Badihi Y, Biesky M, Sprung CL, et al. A look into the nature and causes of human errors in the intensive care unit. Qual Saf Health Care. 2003;12(2): 143–7.
19. Leape LL, Bates DW, Cullen DJ, Cooper J, Demonaco HJ, Gallivan T, et al. Systems analysis of adverse drug events. JAMA. 1995;274(1):35–43.
20. Roth EM. Analysis of decision-making in nuclear power plant emergencies: an investigation of aided decision-making. in C. Zsambok and G. Klien (eds.), Naturalistic Decision Making. Mahwah: Lawrence Erlbaum Associates; 1997.
21. Abraham J, Kannampallil T, Patel VL. Bridging gaps in handoffs: a continuity of care approach. J Biomed Inform. 2012;45(2):240–54.
22. Sutcliffe K, Lewton E, Rosenthal M. Communication failures: an insidious contributor to medical mishaps. Acad Med. 2004;79(2):186–94. doi:10.1097/00001888-200402000-00019.
23. Riesenberg LA, Leitzsch J, Little BW. Systematic review of handoff mnemonics literature. Am J Med Qual. 2009;24(3):196–204.
24. Staggers N. An integrative review of research on nursing handoffs in acute care settings… transitions: unifying practice, education, and research to improve health: communicating nursing research conference and win assembly, April 13-16, 2011, rio all-suites hotel, las Vegas, nv. Commun Nurs Res. 2011;44:27–42. PubMed PMID: 2011383867. Language: English. Entry Date: 20120406. Revision Date: 20120406. Publication Type: journal article.
25. Staggers N, Jennings BM. The content and context of change of shift report on medical and surgical units. J Nurs Adm. 2009;39(9):393–8. doi:10.1097/NNA.0b013e3181b3b63a.
26. Abraham J, Kannampallil T, Patel VL. A systematic review of the literature on the evaluation of handoff tools: Implications for research and practice. J Am Med Inform Assoc amiajnl-2012-001351 Published Online First: 23 May 2013 doi:10.1136/amiajnl-2012-001351.
27. Cheung DS, Kelly JJ, Beach C, Berkeley RP, Bitterman RA, Broida RI, et al. Improving handoffs in the emergency department. Ann Emerg Med. 2009;55(2):171–80.
28. Patterson ES, Wears RL. Patient handoffs: standardized and reliable tools remain elusive. Jt Comm J Qual Patient Saf. 2010;36(2):52–61.
29. Arora V, Johnson J, Meltzer D, Humphrey H. A theoretical framework and competency-based approach to improving handoffs. Qual Saf Health Care. 2008;17:11–4. doi:10.1136/qshc.2006.018952.
30. Manias E, Street A. The handover: uncovering the hidden practices of nurses. Intensive Crit Care Nurs. 2000;16(6):373–83.
31. Crocker C. Following the patient journey to improve medicines management and reduce errors. Nurs Times. 2009;105(46):12–5.

32. Apker J, Mallak L, Gibson S. Communicating in the "gray zone": perceptions about emergency physician hospitalist handoffs and patient safety. Acad Emerg Med. 2007;14(10):884–94.
33. Arora J, Lovinger D, Humphrey HJ, Meltzer DO. Communication failures in patient sign-out and suggestions for improvement: a critical incident analysis. Qual Saf Health Care. 2005;14(6):401–7.
34. Smith AF, Pope C, Goodwin D, Mort M. Interprofessional handover and patient safety in anaesthesia: observational study of handovers in the recovery room. Br J Anaesth. 2008;101(3):332–7.
35. Philibert I. Use of strategies from high-reliability organisations to the patient hand-off by resident physicians: practical implications. Qual Saf Health Care. 2009;18(4):261–6.
36. Berkenstadt H, Haviv Y, Tuval A, Shemesh Y, Megrill A, Perry A, et al. Improving handoff communications in critical care. Chest. 2008;134(1):158–62.
37. Laxmisan A, Hakimzada F, Sayan OR, Green R, Zhang J, Patel VL. The multitasking clinician: decision-making and cognitive demand during and after team handoffs in emergency care. Int J Med Inform. 2007;76:801–11.
38. Nemeth CP, Cook RI, Kowalsky J, Brandwijk M. Understanding Sign Outs: Conversation analysis reveals ICU handoff content and form. Critical Care Medicine 2004;32(12), Supplement:A29.
39. Streitenberger K, Breen-Reid K, Harris C. Handoffs in care–can we make them safer? Pediatr Clin North Am. 2006;53(6):1185–95.
40. Clarke SP, Aiken LH. Failure to rescue: needless deaths are prime examples of the need for more nurses at the bedside. Am J Nurs. 2003;103:42–7.
41. Lofgren RP, Gottlieb D, Williams RA, Rich EC. Post-call transfer of resident responsibility: its effect on patient care. J Gen Intern Med. 1990;5:501–5.
42. Arora V, Johnson J. National patient safety goals. A model for building a standardized hand-off protocol. Jt Comm J Qual Patient Saf. 2006;32:646–55.
43. Sutker WL. The physician's role in patient safety: What's in it for me? Proc (Bayl Univ Med Cent). 2008;21(1):9–14.
44. Haig K, Sutton S, Whittington J. Sbar: a shared mental model for improving communication between clinicians. Jt Comm J Qual Patient Saf. 2006;32:167–75.
45. Nelson BA, Massey R. Implementing an electronic change-of-shift report using transforming care at the bedside processes and methods. J Nurs Adm. 2010;40(4):162–8. PubMed PMID: 20305461.
46. Ryan S, O'Riordan JM, Tierney S, Conlon KC, Ridgway PF. Impact of a new electronic handover system in surgery. Int J Surg. 2011;9(3):217–20. PubMed PMID: 21129508.
47. Wayne JD, Tyagi R, Reinhardt G, Rooney D, Makoul G, Chopra S, et al. Simple standardized patient handoff system that increases accuracy and completeness. J Surg Educ. 2008;65(6): 476–85. PubMed PMID: 19059181.
48. Beach C, Vozenilik J, Adler M, et al. Transitioning patients from the ed to the hospital: observations of handoff communication. Acad Emerg Med. 2007;14(5):205–6.
49. Campion TR, Jr., Denny JC, Weinberg ST, Lorenzi NM, Waitman LR. Analysis of a computerized sign-out tool: Identification of unanticipated uses and contradictory content. AMIA Annu Symp Proc. 2007;99–104. PubMed PMID: 18693806. Pubmed Central PMCID: 2655840.
50. Van Eaton EG, Horvath KD, Lober WB, Rossini AJ, Pellegrini CA. A randomized, controlled trial evaluating the impact of a computerized rounding and sign-out system on continuity of care and resident work hours. J Am Coll Surg. 2005;200(4):538–45. PubMed PMID: 15804467.
51. Van Eaton EG, McDonough K, Lober WB, Johnson EA, Pellegrini CA, Horvath KD. Safety of using a computerized rounding and sign-out system to reduce resident duty hours. Acad Med. 2010;85(7):1189–95. PubMed PMID: 20592514.
52. Vidyarthi AR, Arora V, Schnipper JL, Wall SD, Wachter RM. Managing discontinuity in academic medical centers: strategies for a safe and effective resident sign-out. J Hosp Med. 2006;1:257–66.
53. Landucci D, Gipe BT. The art and science of the handoff: How hospitalists share data. Hospitalist. 1999;3:4.

54. Solet DJ, Norvell JM, Rutan GH, Frankel RM. Lost in translation: challenges and opportunities in physician-to-physician communication during patient handoffs. Acad Med. 2005;80:1094–9.
55. Joint Commission (TJC) Hospital National Patient Safety Goals. 2009. Retrieved from http://www.unchealthcare.org/site/Nursing/servicelines/aircare/additionaldocuments/2009npsg (Last Accessed on September, 26, 2013).
56. Apker J, Mallak L, Applegate EB, Gibson S, Ham J, Johnson N, et al. Exploring emergency physician-hospitalist handoff interactions: development of the handoff communication assessment. Ann Emerg Med. 2009;55(2):161–70.
57. Miller A, Scheinkestel C, Limpus A, Joseph M, Karnik A, Venkatesh B. Uni- and interdisciplinary effects on round and handover content in intensive care units. Hum Factors. 2009;51(3):339–53.
58. Stevens D. Handovers and Debussy. Qual Saf Health Care. 2008;17:2–3. doi:10.1136/qshc.2007.025916.
59. Harvey C, Schuster R, Durso F, Matthews A, Surabattula D. Human factors of transition of care. In: Handbook of human factors and ergonomics in health care and patient safety. Mahwah: Lawrence Erlbaum Associates; 2007.
60. Lawrence R, Tomolo A, Garlisi A, Aron D. Conceptualizing handover strategies at change of shift in the emergency department: a grounded theory study. BMC Health Serv Res. 2008;8(1):256. doi:10.1186/1472-6963-8-256.
61. Payne B, Hardey H, Coleman P. Interactions between nurses during handovers in elderly care. J Adv Nurs. 2000;32:277–85.
62. Van Eaton E. Handoff improvement: we need to understand what we are trying to fix. Jt Comm J Qual Patient Saf. 2010;36(2):51.
63. Gillen J, Cameron CA, editors. International perspectives on early childhood research: a day in the life. Houndmills: Palgrave-Macmillan; 2010.
64. Patel VL, Kaufman DR, Magder S. The road to excellence: the acquisition of expert performance in the arts and sciences, sports and games. In: Ericsson A, editor. The acquisition of medical expertise in complex dynamic decision-making environments. Hillsdale: Erlbaum; 1996. p. 127–65.
65. Kannampallil T, Schauer GF, Cohen T, Patel VL. Considering complexity in healthcare systems. J Biomed Inform. 2011;44(6):943–7.
66. Malhotra S, Jordan MD, Shortliffe EH, Patel VL. Workflow modeling in critical care: piecing together your own puzzle. J Biomed Inform. 2007;40(2):81–92.
67. Patel VL, Zhang J, Yoskowitz NA, Green R, Sayan OR. Methodological review: translational cognition for decision support in critical care environments: a review. J Biomed Inform. 2008;41(3):413–31.
68. Unertl KM, Weinger MB, Johnson KB, Lorenzi NM. Describing and modeling workflow and information flow in chronic disease care. JAMA. 2009;16(6):826–36.
69. Randell R, Wilson S, Woodward P. The importance of the verbal shift handover report: a multi-site case study. Int J Med Inform. 2011;80(11):803–12.
70. Collins SA, Stein DM, Vawdrey DK, Stetson PD, Bakken S. Content overlap in nurse and physician handoff artifacts and the potential role of electronic health records: a systematic review. J Biomed Inform. 2011;44(4):704–12.
71. Forsythe DE, Buchanan BG, Osheroff JA, Miller RA. Expanding the concept of medical information: an observational study of physicians' information needs. Comput Biomed Res. 1992;25(2):181–200.
72. Patel VL, Cohen T, Murarka T, Olsen J, Kagita S, Myneni S, et al. Recovery at the edge of error: debunking the myth of the infallible expert. J Biomed Inform. 2011;44(3):413–24. PubMed PMID: 20869466.
73. Strauss A, Corbin J. Basics of qualitative research. Thousands Oaks: Sage Publications; 1998.
74. Malone TW, Crowston K. The interdisciplinary theory of coordination. ACM Comput Surv. 1994;26(1):87–119.

75. Woloshynowych M, Davis R, Brown R, Vincent C. Communication patterns in a uk emergency department. Ann Emerg Med. 2007;50(4):407–13.
76. Abraham J, Nguyen VC, Almoosa KF, Patel B, Patel VL. Falling through the cracks: information breakdowns in critical care handoff communication. Washington, DC: American Medical Informatics Association (AMIA); 2011.
77. Sanderson PM, Fisher C. Exploratory sequential data analysis: foundations. Hum-Comput Interact. 1994;9(3&4):251–317.
78. Frohlich D, Drew P, Monk A. Management of repair in human-computer interaction. Hum-Comput Interact. 1994;9(3–4):385–425.
79. Ritter FE, Larkin JH. Developing process models as summaries of hci action sequences. Hum-Comput Interact. 1994;9(3–4):345–83.
80. Zheng K, Guo M, Hanauer DA. Using the time and motion method to study clinical work processes and workflow: methodological inconsistencies and a call for standardized research. J Am Med Inform Assoc. 2011;18(5):704–10.

Chapter 13
Bridging Gaps in Handoff Communication: A Comparative Evaluation of Information Organization Tools

Joanna Abraham, Thomas G. Kannampallil, and Bela Patel

Introduction

Handoffs permeate the healthcare system at all levels, from the individual to the organizational level. A recent study estimated that approximately 1.6 million handoffs occur per year in a typical teaching hospital [1]. This number is likely to increase given the current ACGME (Accreditation Council on Graduate Medical Education) restrictions on resident work hours [2].

Patient Safety in Handoffs

Several reports and research studies have highlighted that handoffs, or care transition points, are high-risk areas for patient safety. Furthermore, handoffs at the different levels and within each level of the organization are highly variable and

Portions of this chapter appeared as an **open access** article in the Proceedings of the 2012 Annual Symposium American Medical Informatics Association, Abraham et al. *Ensuring patient safety in care transitions: an empirical evaluation of a handoff intervention tool.*

J. Abraham, PhD
Department of Biomedical and Health Information Sciences, College of Applied Health Sciences, University of Illinois, 1919 West Taylor Street, Chicago, IL, USA
e-mail: abrahamj@uic.edu

T.G. Kannampallil
Center for Cognitive Studies in Medicine and Public Health, New York Academy of Medicine, New York, NY 10029, USA

B. Patel, MD, DABSM, FCCP
University of Texas Health Science Center, Houston, TX USA

Division of Critical Care Medicine, Memorial Hermann Hospital, Texas Medical Center, Houston, TX 77030, USA

V.L. Patel et al. (eds.), *Cognitive Informatics in Health and Biomedicine*, Health Informatics, DOI 10.1007/978-1-4471-5490-7_13, © Springer-Verlag London 2014

potentially unreliable [3]. A number of initiatives have been launched for targeting error detection, error recovery and error prevention during care transitions, including the High 5's initiative proposed jointly by Commonwealth Fund, the WHO World Alliance for Patient Safety and the WHO Collaborating Center for patient safety [4] and the National Patient Safety Goals by the Joint Commission [5]. To support these initiatives, a number of safety solutions have been proposed that can minimize transition errors through standardization of communication. While standardization efforts have led to widespread development and implementation of handoff strategies and tools, they have had varying degrees of success in these environments [6].

Nature of Handoff Tools

Handoff tools are generally classified into two types: electronic and paper-based. Electronic tools can further be categorized into electronic medical record (EMR) integrated tools or standalone tools. The key difference between these two variants of electronic tools lies in the fact that EMR integrated tools have features that can support the automatic download and population of information fields and interface with other ancillary systems such as radiology and laboratory [7, 8]. Paper-based tools are generally in the form of a piece of paper with patient information organized into single-page [9] or tabular or checklist-based templates with basic patient information such as demographic data, reason for admission, medications, to-do lists [10], IV fluids, oxygen levels, tube feeds, and monitor settings [11, 12]. Based on a systematic review of handoff evaluation tools [13], we found that a large proportion of handoff tools are being developed for supporting physicians' handoffs [9–11, 14–27], and nursing handoffs [8, 12, 28–37], with few integrated tools to support both professions [7, 38–43].

Content and Structure of Handoff Tools

Handoff communication content in tools has been structured using one of three content models the *problem-oriented medical record* that characterizes key patient problems in a priority order (e.g., *SOAP* or *S*ubjective, *O*bjective, *A*ssessment and *P*lan) [44]; a *situation-briefing* model, that utilizes an easy-to-remember framework based on patient conditions (e.g., *SBAR* or *S*ituation, *B*ackground, *A*ssessment and *R*ecommendation) [45]; and (c) a *body-system or medical* model, where information is organized based on body-systems (e.g., cardiology, gastrointestinal, and renal systems) [46]. Our analysis from a previous systematic review has confirmed that the most common handoff content framework was the patient-problem model, followed by the situation-briefing and body-system models [13]. A detailed description of the different types of content frameworks can be found in [13].

Handoff Tool Evaluation Studies

These content models, especially the SOAP and SBAR have been adopted to structure the content for communication in a variety of clinical settings [47–50]. A majority of physician handoff tools utilize these content models as a mechanism for standardizing communication content and topics to be discussed (e.g., [18, 42]). However, their open-ended structure of topic content organization increases the potential risk for information loss and inconsistencies in communication [51]. It has been reported that SOAP-based tools decreased time needed to locate and organize information [28], improved documentation [20], reduced perceived likelihood of information omissions and missed tasks [10], and enhanced quality of information transfer [41].

Similarly, studies of SBAR-based tools have shown reliable information transfer without increasing handoff duration [8], improved patient-centered outcomes [31], and improved nurses' confidence in their communication skills [29]. Despite the support for comprehensive and systematic coverage of all body system related information, the system-based model has been used sparingly to standardize handoff communication [7].

Furthermore, the evaluation of these different content structures underlying the handoff tools have been predominantly measured using handoff-related outcomes such as information gaps [18, 20, 28], handover duration, number of patients handed off, interruptions [8], care quality, frequency of tool use [40], handoff efficiency, and length of shift-report [30].

Despite the early adoption and successes in handoff implementations [40], broader issues of handoff tool sustainability still linger. Based on our own handoff study and also other prior studies, we identified that there were two critical factors which potentially results in the ineffective use of these handoff tools in actual healthcare practice: (1) handoff tools have limited support for the completion of coordination activities such as information organization, documentation and reasoning in the preparatory phase (prior to handoff); (2) handoff tools lack a standardized structure and therefore tend to be characterized to exhibit either a very structured and rigid information organizational structure or ambiguous and flexible information structure [52]. On one hand, there is a push towards the incorporation of standardization of communication using structured methods such as templates, heuristics and communication mnemonics (e.g., SBAR). In contrast, experts have proposed guidelines for customization of communication using less-structured methods such as conveying updated patient information in summarized format. While there are tradeoffs in adopting these methods, very seldom is either one of them strictly followed in actual healthcare practice [53].

Theoretical Framings Underlying Handoff Tools

As described in Chap. 12, the seven theoretical frameworks for understanding handoff communication include information processing, stereotypical narratives, social interaction, resilience, accountability, distributed cognition, and cultural norms[54]. Most of these frameworks have been used by researchers to analyze and identify gaps in communication activity during care transitions [9, 10, 28, 30, 34, 40]. Our research analysis and that of others have confirmed [55], that information processing was the primary and most used theoretical framing [13] and the least studied theoretical perspective was resilience of tool.

Furthermore, in addition to these theoretical underpinnings that focus exclusively on the information transfer during handoffs, we identified that information organization and documentation in the preparatory phase is an important prerequisite for ensuring effective communication during handoffs [56]. There is significant evidence from other research studies by high-reliability organizations that confirms this finding [57–60]. Consequently, researchers and hospital officials have emphasized the need to develop and design tools to support clinicians in their handoff process using an evidence-based approach [61]. In other words, design of tools should focus on improving not only the standardization of the communication content but also the preparation activities such as information seeking, organization and documentation of clinical content are critical.

These factors taken together account for the limited fit of handoff tools within the social fabric of clinical workflows, consequently resulted in limited adoption and appropriation by clinicians. Towards the aim of designing a handoff intervention tool that will fit within the model of critical care practice, we designed a handoff tool and evaluated its use in a medical intensive care unit (MICU). The goals of this chapter are two-fold: first, to describe the design of the Handoff intervention tool (HAND-IT) and second, to determine the effectiveness of HAND-IT using a comparative pre-post evaluation study of handoff tools.

In this chapter, we describe the design, development and evaluation of a handoff tool to support information organization and documentation activities and its impact on the handoff workflow. We compared our body-system based handoff tool, HAND-IT (*HAND*off *I*ntervention *T*ool), with a problem-oriented, SOAP (Subject, Objective, Assessment and Plan) tool using a pre-post intervention study. The results showed the relative flexibility of HAND-IT in supporting clinical documentation and potentially preventing clinical and workflow errors.

Design of Handoff Intervention Tool

Informed by the findings from our prior study, a simple, paper-based handoff intervention tool was developed, referred to as HAND-IT. The design of the tool was based on the *spiral method* that included steps for requirement gathering, designing, building and testing of the tool.

Requirements gathering: Requirements were formulated to address the communication breakdowns and their root contributors in the overall handoff process. The two higher-level tool requirements were information organization in the pre-turnover phase and information transfer in handoff phase. The lower-level information-related requirements for our intervention tool were based on the evaluation of the information seeking and needs analysis of oncoming team.

Design: A design team for the handoff intervention tool was formed, which comprised of two senior attending physicians, a clinical fellow and the first author.

Informed by these higher- and lower-level requirements, the team collaboratively developed the basic structural format (i.e., body system-oriented and patient case-narrative) and content of HAND-IT.

Development: First, the attending physicians and the fellow individually created drafts of the tool content. The team then convened multiple times to discuss and iteratively develop a unified version of the tool including its information content and order. Through several group discussions and expert suggestions, the information elements were included/excluded based on their clinical relevance, especially to critical care.

Evaluation: The prototype was then evaluated in the MICU and based on clinician feedback through formal and informal discussions during the testing phase, the tool was modified to best fit the critical care workflow.

Theoretical Rationale for Design

The theoretical design rationale of HAND-IT was informed by our prior empirical work (described above) which found that handoff tools supporting the preparatory information organization and documentation activities prior to handoffs can result in effective communication during handoffs [56, 62]. Furthermore, handoff tools that adopt a hybrid information representation model combining features for supporting both structured and summarized information can minimize breakdowns in information and decision-making.

To address this, the design of HAND-IT was based on *content standardization* (using a body system-oriented format) and *content summarization* (using a problem-case narrative format) for standardizing information sharing during handoffs and also supporting information organization and documentation during the pre-turnover phase. Content standardization and summarization have been reported to minimize information breakdowns and support effective clinical decision-making [46, 63]. Additionally, based on the Society of Critical Care Medicine (SCCM) guidelines [64], we incorporated evidence-based concepts related to standard critical care management, which can improve patient outcomes including identification of delirium, sedation practices, prophylaxis and feeding information. Based on these functional requirements, the basic format and content of the tool were decided by the design team consisting of two ICU attending physicians (which include the MICU director and a quality officer), one MICU clinical fellow, and one researcher (first author) [See Fig. 13.1 for the final design of the HAND-IT and Table 13.1 for information categories in HAND-IT].

A *checklist-based* body system-oriented format was used to support content standardization. The patient care information within each body system was organized into fundamental categories including (a) diagnosis, (b) physical exam and labs, (c) medications, and (d) resident plan (for that particular body-system). In addition to content standardization, we incorporated a summarization feature through free-text fields to add care summaries related to (a) patient admission information, (b) problem list, (c) patient events over the last 24-h period and finally, (d) resident notes.

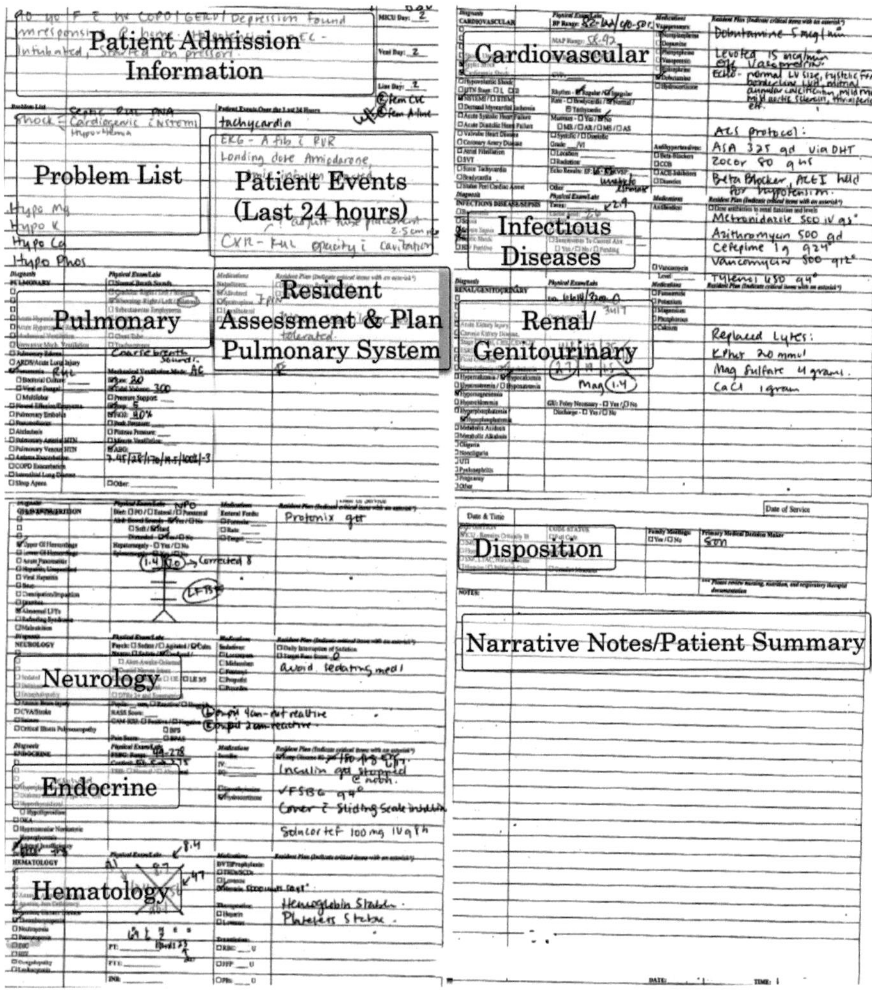

Fig. 13.1 Handoff Intervention Tool, HAND-IT (Adapted with permission from Abraham et al. [52])

Empirical Evaluation of Handoff Intervention Tool[1]

We conducted a comparative pre-post prospective intervention study to determine the effectiveness of the intervention tool for documentation. The study was based on the evaluation of two tools for supporting handoffs: SOAP note and HAND-IT,

[1]This section (including tables and figures) has been adapted from Abraham J, Kannampallil T, Patel B, Almoosa KF, Patel V L. 2012. Ensuring patient safety in care transitions: an empirical evaluation of a handoff intervention tool. Paper presented at the Proceedings of AMIA 2012, Chicago, IL.

Table 13.1 Information categories in HAND-IT

Information field	Description	Example
Date & time	The date and time stamp for the report being prepared.	10/20/11; 13:00 h
Admission information	The basic patient history and information related to patient's admissions/ transfer to the MICU.	81 year old female with HIV, CKD stage 2, HLD admitted with chest pain, shortness of breath found to be in pulmonary edema – TTE showed MR from ruptured chordae tendinae.
MICU day#, vent day#, line day#	MICU length of patient stay, Mechanical ventilation day #, day # for IVs and lines (central and peripheral).	MICU day# 3, vent day#0 and Line day#0.
Problem list	Patient problems including current and past conditions.	The patient has hypotension.
Events over the last 24 h	All noteworthy patient-related events that occurred over the last 24 h (during the last two clinician shifts).	A failed placement of a central line on a patient twice.
System diagnosis	Diagnosis information for body systems including CV, GI/GU, renal, infectious disease etc.	The data elements characterizing the CV system-oriented diagnosis include HTN stage 2, NSTEMI, valvular heart disease MR, and sinus tachycardia.
Physical exam/ labs	Information elements related to exam and labs of the patient corresponding to each organ system.	Physical exam/labs for CV system contains BP range: 90–51 and 179–75, MAP range: 61–101; HR range: 78–92; rhythm- regular, rate- normal; murmurs- Yes; MR; systolic; grade IV; echo results: EF: RVSP: 26.9>70 %.
Medications	Current, active medication orders such as name, dosage, route and interval can be entered/checked.	Medications for CV include aspirin 325, lipitor 40, plavix 75, lisinopril 10 mg, and metoprol 12.5 Q6 h.
Assessment	Plan for care and management information for each organ system.	Resident assessment and plan for the CV system for a patient case was "patient – hypotensive; NTG was weaned off; Now BP Stable; continue ACE –I, Beta blockers, aspirin, plavix for ACS protocol, continue heparin gtt, new MR – Transfer to CCU for possible MVR, TEE today to rule out endocratis."
Disposition	Disposition information for patient's continued stay in the ICU, or downgraded to an intermediate care unit (IMU) or floor service or physical transfer to an outside facility such as the skilled nursing facility (SNF) or Long-term Acute Care Hospital (LTACH) or will be under hospice/palliative care.	The patient is ready to be transferred to CCU (Cardiac Intensive Care Unit).

(continued)

Table 13.1 (continued)

Information field	Description	Example
Code status	Information on patient's code status. Three categories include full code (i.e. Full resuscitation with aggressive measures in the event of cardiac arrest), DNR/DNI (i.e., do not resuscitate or intubate) and comfort measures (eliminating sources of discomfort of a dying patient).	The patient is DNR/DNI.
Primary medical decision maker	Includes the name of relative primarily responsible for decision making for the patient.	Patient's son is the medical decision maker.
Family meetings	Includes information on whether meetings with family and care team have been held (or planned for) to explain the patient's condition and their current disposition to the family members.	
Other diagnosis and management plan	Includes any critical information that was included/not in the previous sections in a summary format in addition to a to-do and contingency list.	H and H Q12 h, Rocephin change to 1 g Q12 h, continue heparin for NSTEMI and hold diuretics.
Resident signature	Includes signature of the on-call resident primarily responsible caring for the patient and preparing the information on the tool.	
Date and time	Includes the date and time stamp of filling the information on the tool.	10/20/11; 13:30 h.

which were constructed based upon inherently different design rationales. The patient information in the SOAP note is structured upon a subjective component, an objective component, an assessment, and a plan of care. Therefore, this type of structuring follows a problem-based format, and is commonly used in a general medicine-surgery ward [65] (See Chap. 12).

In contrast to the SOAP note, the HAND-IT tool is grounded in our prior results, which show that content standardization using a body system-oriented format, and content summarization using a problem-case narrative format, would reduce the communication complexity and incidence of transition errors [56].

In the following sections, we describe the participants, design, data collection and analysis process, and evaluation measures. The setting is the same as in the previous chapter (Chap. 12), and the Institutional Review Boards (IRB) of the hospital and the university approved the study.

Participants

The study participants include the attending physician, clinical fellow, internal medicine residents, interns, respiratory therapist, pharmacist and nurses. The residents and interns were responsible for a total of 16 patients, and each were assigned up to 8 patients during a shift. The team handoffs occurred daily in the morning and took approximately 4 h to complete. At the MICU we studied, a set of three residents and three interns rotated for a period of 1 month, although their specific roles varied during different shifts (e.g., on-call, post-call or short-call). Thus there were a total of six residents and six interns during the 2-month period of the evaluation study.

Study Design

The SOAP note and HAND-IT tool were evaluated for their effectiveness as tools for supporting documentation for the handoff process. In our longitudinal pre-post prospective intervention study, two sets of residents and interns used SOAP and HAND-IT over a 2-month period (See Fig. 13.3 for the organization of the study). The effectiveness of documentation using both tools was measured during the multi-professional rounds conducted by the director of the MICU and the on-call care team (see details in the next section).

Data Collection: Multi-Professional Rounds

The multi-professional round (MPR) is a mechanism by which teams of clinical professionals perform joint evaluation. For example, such multi-professional teams often convene to evaluate quality and decision-making initiatives [66]. The director of the MICU in our study convened MPRs to evaluate the quality and completeness of the handoff note (either SOAP or HAND-IT). As they were not part of the typical MICU workflow, these MPRs (See Fig. 13.2) were conducted immediately after the morning rounds and were organized for research purposes only. Each collaborative session was attended by the MICU Director, an on-call attending physician, an on-call resident and intern, patients' nurses, a pharmacist, a respiratory therapist and the first author.

The specific patient handoff notes selected for evaluation during an MPR (in either the SOAP or HAND-IT condition) were decided upon after a brief discussion between the MICU director, the on-call attending physician and the first author of the paper. These decisions were made in a manner that ensured maximum selection variability across patient cases, patient status and patient condition complexity. Following patient cases selection, the MICU team (including each patient's nurse) convened to jointly evaluate the information documented (by the outgoing) on the tool with respect to the accuracy and completeness of patient-care information. During the MPR session, the handoff note (either SOAP or HAND-IT) was read aloud to the team. The on-call team members were then individually asked to identify any breakdowns in patient care information and patient care decisions. For instance, the patient's nurse was asked whether or not there were any identifiable omissions from a nursing standpoint for the

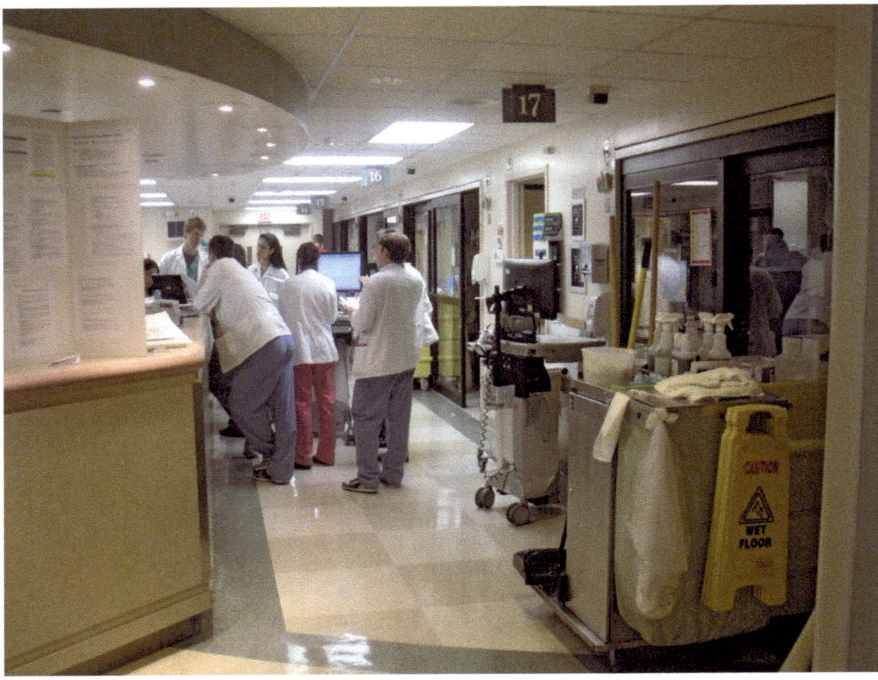

Fig. 13.2 Multi-Professional Rounds (MPR) in MICU

particular patient. Furthermore, the team members were asked if the handoff note was up-to-date and accurate. Based on their collective content analysis of the handoff note, the team characterized the breakdowns into omissions, inaccuracies, and modifications to the originally written plan of care, and missed problem lists of patients. During each MPR, the first author took meticulous notes on the analysis of the case by the team, in addition to audio-recording the sessions. Additionally, the de-identified photocopies of the evaluated SOAP and HAND-IT tools (with prior IRB approval) were collected for detailed analysis. Lastly, informal interviews with the participants (about the tool use and limitations) were conducted following each MPR.

Procedure

The experimental implementation was conducted over a 2-month period and consisted of multiple stages per month (See Fig. 13.3). During the first month, participants used the SOAP note for a period of 4 days as part of their training. This was followed by the experimental stage, during which participants used the SOAP note for 5 (High 5 s, #29) days. On the seventh, eighth, and ninth day (the last 3 days of experimental evaluation), MPRs were conducted after the morning rounds. Following

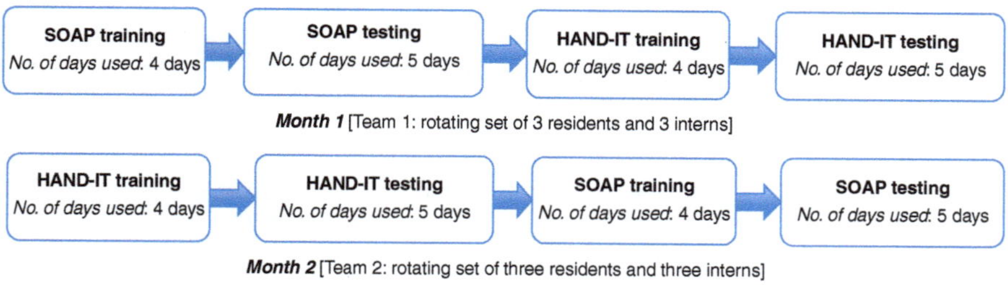

Fig. 13.3 Study Design and Procedure (Adapted with permission from Abraham et al. [52])

this period, participants were provided introductory training with the HAND-IT tool. They used HAND-IT for handoffs for the next 4 days, which helped to familiarize them with the different features with respect to content, function and format of the tool. In the last stage, we began the experimental evaluation of the use of HAND-IT for a period of 5 (High 5 s, #29) days. As with the SOAP condition, MPRs were conducted over the last 3 days of the experimental sessions. A total of five (High 5 s, #29) notes for each condition were evaluated during the MPRs: two each on days 1 and 2, and one each on day 3. The same procedure was repeated in the second month with a new MICU on-call team, but the order in which the participants used the two tools was counter-balanced with the previous month. In other words, the participants began with HAND-IT training for 4 days, followed by testing for 5 (High 5 s, #29) days. As in the previous month, a total of five (High 5 s, #29) notes from each condition were chosen for evaluation during the MPRs. As detailed in the previous section on MPRs, each handoff tool was evaluated for missed information, incorrect entries, missed problem list items and changes to plan of care.

Evaluation Measures

We employed three measures for evaluating the *effectiveness of handoff documentation* using each of the two tools: number of information breakdowns, number of decision-making breakdowns, and expertise of the clinicians. Each of these measures is described below.

Information Breakdowns: We characterized an information breakdown as a failure to appropriately gather the necessary information regarding a patient or a gap in information flow. Two variables were used in representing the information breakdowns on the handoff tool (either SOAP or HAND-IT): *number of missed information* and *number of incorrect information*.

Decision-Making Breakdowns: We characterized a decision-making breakdown as a modification (including additions/deletions) made by the attending physician to the decision-related information documented by the outgoing team (resident or intern) on the handoff tool during the MICU morning rounds. Two variables were used in representing the decision-making breakdowns: number of changes to plan of care and number of missed problem list items.

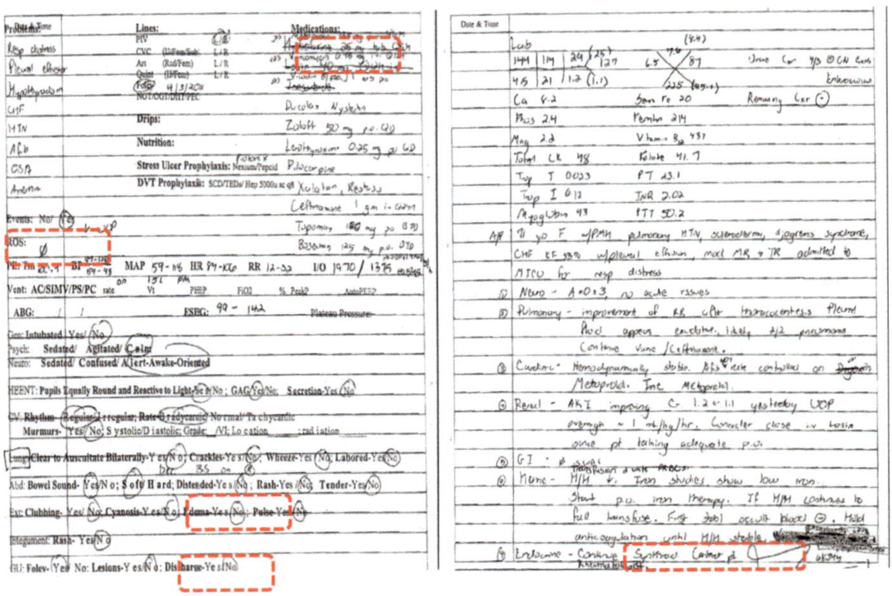

Fig. 13.4 Example of Analysis of Information and Decision Making Breakdowns using SOAP Tool

Expertise: Since patient care responsibility in the MICU was divided between an intern (a first year trainee resident) and a senior resident (third year trainee resident), we characterized the efficacy in the use of the handoff tools based on their year of residency training.

Data Analysis

For our dual-stage analysis, we used audio-recorded data, researcher notes from the MPR evaluation, and photocopies of the selected SOAP and HAND-IT tools. First, a qualitative analysis of the information on the tools was coded based on information breakdowns. Next, the frequencies of missed and incorrect information, missed problem list items, and changes to plan of care were tabulated based on the MPR recordings (See Figs. 13.4 and 13.5).

Data was organized according to *handoff tool type* (SOAP, HAND-IT) and *expertise* (resident, intern), after which a comparative analysis using student t-tests was performed. Next, the causal determinants of decision-making (i.e., number of missed problem list items and number of changes to plan of care) were evaluated while using the SOAP and HAND-IT tools. To achieve this, we developed the best-fit zero-inflated Poisson regression model with the following variables: *expertise differences* (resident, intern) and *information breakdowns* (number of missed

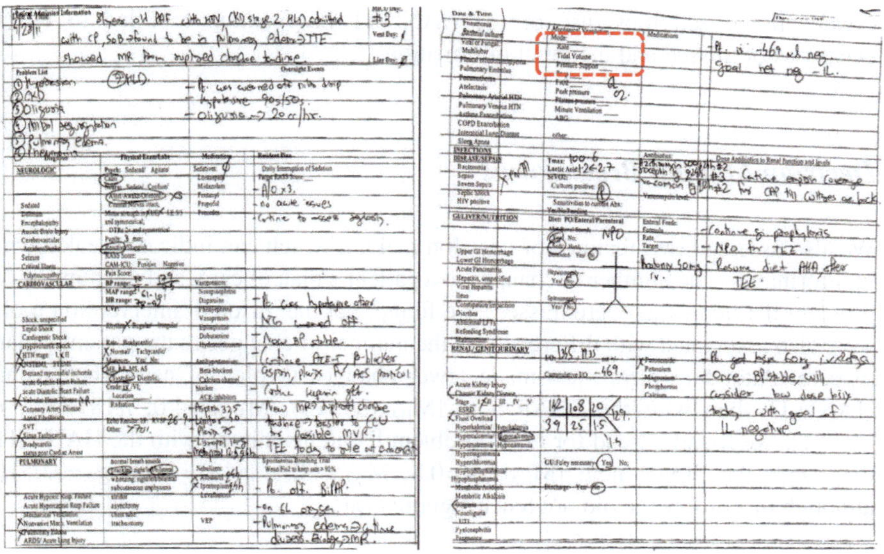

Fig. 13.5 Example of Analysis of Information and Decision Making Breakdowns using HAND-IT

information, number of incorrect information). These were the variables considered, because there was no association between expertise and information breakdowns based on Chi-square tests ($\chi^2=0.0899$, df $=1$, $p=0.76$). For the analysis of information breakdowns, an aggregate value of the number of missed information and number of incorrect information was used. For expertise differences, we used the categorized notes created by the residents and interns.

Results and Discussion[2]

Information Breakdowns

When physicians used the HAND-IT tool, they missed significantly less information than when they used the SOAP note [$M_{HAND\text{-}IT}=2.8$, $M_{SOAP}=12.5$; $t(18)=5.98$, $p<0.0001$]. In addition, when they used the HAND-IT, they recorded less incorrect information than when they used the SOAP note [$M_{HAND\text{-}IT}=0.9$, $M_{SOAP}=1.8$, $(18)=2.1$, $p<0.05$]. They differences indicate that the HAND-IT intervention tool improved the way residents and interns seek information and organize activities during the pre-turnover phase of their shifts. By changing information seeking and

[2] This section has been adapted from Abraham J, Kannampallil T, Patel B, Almoosa KF, Patel VL. 2012. Ensuring patient safety in care transitions: an empirical evaluation of a handoff intervention tool. Paper presented at the Proceedings of AMIA 2012, Chicago, IL.

organizational activities, use of the HAND-IT intervention tool led to fewer occasions of missed and incorrect information.

Decision Making Breakdowns

We also assessed two features of decision making which can indicate breakdowns in information: the number of changes to a patient's plan of care, and the number of problem list items that were missed. We found that the different intervention tools were also associated with differences in the number of changes to the patient's plan of care: Attending physicians made fewer changes to plan of care when using HAND-IT than with the SOAP note [$M_{HAND\text{-}IT}=0.8$, $M_{SOAP}=4.0$; $t(18)=3.7$, $p<0.001$]. We found a trend for fewer problem list items missed with the HAND-IT than with the SOAP note [$M_{HAND\text{-}IT}=0.8$, $M_{SOAP}=2.1$; $t(18)=1.93$, $p=0.051$], although this difference did not reach significance.

Handoff Tool Resilience

We evaluated the resilience of the handoff tools by examining the decision-making effectiveness variables (number of missed problem lists and number of changes to plan of care) in terms of both information breakdowns and expertise of the participants (residents, interns) using a Poisson regression. Based on the analysis, we found evidence that the HAND-IT was associated with fewer missed problem list items, and fewer breakdowns as a result. Specifically, when participants used the HAND-IT, an increase of 11.92 breakdowns was required before a one-unit increase in the missed problem list. In contrast, for the SOAP note, the increase in the aggregate number of breakdowns was directly proportional to the number of missed problem list items. For each unit increase in the missed problem list, we observed a unit increase in the total number of breakdowns. The number of changes in plan of care was not statistically significant in models which described the effects. This pattern of results provides evidence that the HAND-IT was more resilient in the face of breakdowns and differences in expertise than the SOAP note.

Effect of Expertise

We also evaluated effectiveness of decision-making based on the expertise of the physicians who used both tools with the regression model. Residents and interns showed different patterns of missed problem list items based on the tool they used. Residents using the SOAP note made 0.32 *fewer* missed problem list items than interns, while Residents using the HAND-IT made 2.92 *more* missed problem list items than interns. We believe this is evidence that interns, with less experience and expertise than senior residents, benefited more from the information organizational capabilities of HAND-IT than residents.

Discussion

Our results show that the HAND-IT provides effective support for the information organization activities physicians perform to prepare for handoffs, and use of HAND-IT results in fewer information breakdowns and errors. The design of HAND-IT multiple support mechanisms including a standardized checklist, organization into body systems, extensive coverage for details for the body-systems and a structured, user-friendly display for reading and writing. Our results indicate the HAND-IT use resulted in fewer changes to the plan of care created by the outgoing medical team, and fewer omitted patient diagnoses (i.e., problem lists). This was potentially afforded by the juxtaposition of body systems in a checklist and narrative cuing the physician to consider or recall information that was relevant to making diagnostic and therapeutic decisions. This also allowed physicians to draw specific inferences relevant to patient problems because the assessment and corresponding plan are formulated for each of the different body systems, and c) provided cognitive support, affording physicians' reasoning process.

Tool resiliency was also apparent as the use of HAND-IT led to fewer missed problem list items, and significantly more breakdowns were required before a missed problem list item occurred when using the HAND-IT than the SOAP note. Error resilience is one of the most frequently described characteristics of a good handoff tool, so this finding is especially relevant [54, 67]. HAND-IT was designed to summarize and systematize content in a checklist format; while resilience to breakdowns was not an explicit goal, this serendipitous outcome was likely a result of our design goals. Features of the design provided (a) transparency for the clinician's thought process via the checklist format, which could help to identify and avoid errors, and (b) support for clinicians' process of crosschecking assumptions by using the narrative to achieve a fresh perspective.

We also observed improved performance by interns using HAND-IT. Their improvement may have been due to the layered display of information, which prompted interns to attend to information relevant and appropriate for their decision-making. As a result, the significant amount of information available could be approached with a focused perspective. Additionally, HAND-IT's organization may have helped the less-experienced interns whose schemas for medical knowledge are less developed [68]. Residents, who have more developed knowledge schemas, showed a contrasting response to the HAND-IT because using a new tool forced them to re-adjust their mental models. This may have led to a higher number of breakdowns. More detailed empirical evaluation is necessary to identify the causal factors behind the differences we observed between residents and interns. A detailed discussion of the results can be found in [52].

Implications for Practice

In the current study, HAND-IT supported error detection and recovery (i.e., avoiding breakdowns in information organization and decision-making), was resilient to breakdowns, and supported education and learning, all desirable characteristics of handoff tools [54, 69, 70]. In addition, by its very design, HAND-IT supported the coordination of information flow and decision-making. This coordination inherently helps to ensuring continuity of care, and emphasizes the importance of capturing an "uninterrupted and coordinated succession" of patient events to meet their care needs. In other words, mitigating information and decision-making breakdowns improves timeliness of care delivery, reduces work duplication, minimizes patient length of stay, and most importantly, enhances patient safety and quality. Development of HAND-IT is one example of an empirically driven and theoretically grounded clinician handoff workflow tool, which takes a fundamental step toward the Joint Commission's mandate to standardize handoff communication activity. Our HAND-IT intervention tool highlights the workflow elements central to the intensive care unit model of practice.

In the modern ICU, optimal delivery of care requires consistent coordination among multiple disciplines and services, including sub-specialty consultants and supportive healthcare personnel. For example, a septic patient with multi-organ failure will require a critical care team, plus consultations from infection disease specialists to help manage the infection, and nephrology specialists to help manage acute renal failure. In addition, other services including nutrition, physical therapy, and social work frequently contribute to the general plan of care for complex patient. Our MICU observations and informal interviews with nurses and consults revealed that the HAND-IT tool improved overall continuity of care both between clinicians during transitions, and also across clinicians from different services. The tool was viewed as a "coordination artifact" that helped to manage information and task interdependencies between multiple clinicians involved in a single-patient care process.

Future Work

The next phase of our work in this area will be to evaluate handoff communication by assessing the impact of information organization on verbal communication. The *first step* in this phase is to capture the types and characteristics of communication events and breakdowns; the *second step* will be to map the handoff tool documentation to verbal communication data for a set of common patients. This process would allow us to identify the impact of information organization and documentation practices on effective communication during care transitions. Our goal in the first phase will be geared toward comparing the effectiveness of a problem-based tool (SOAP) and a body system-based tool for supporting handoff communication by analyzing the content and structure of handoff communication. Our observations and audio-recorded data of 82 resident handoffs in the MICU form the basis for our investigation in the first step of future work. While prior evaluation studies on handoff tools have primarily used survey-based and self-reported measures [7, 10, 15, 30, 50], our approach will specifically evaluate the impact that a tool's standardized content and structure has on communication effectiveness and safety.

Discussion Questions

1. What are the potential advantages and disadvantages of using a medical training model (i.e., a body system based format)? Discuss the implications of using such a model with respect to the following aspects: (a) ability to have comprehensive information regarding a patient (b) effort, time and cognitive requirements, and (c) ability to support diagnostic decision making and patient management decisions.
2. Can the medical model serve as a standardized content model for structuring handoff communication in other settings during patient transfers within a hospital and across hospitals?
3. Can the medical model be considered as a framework to train and educate multi-professional clinicians at varying levels of expertise and experience to perform better handoffs? If so, how?

References

1. Vidyarthi A. Triple handoff. Hospital Medicine, Retrieved from: http://www.webmm.ahrq.gov/case.aspx?caseID=134; Last accessed on 09/25/2013. 2006.
2. Accreditation Council for Graduate Medical Education A. Report of the work group on resident duty hours and the learning environment. 2002. Retrieved from https://www.premierinc.com/safety/safety-share/08-02_downloads/03_wkgreport_602.pdf (Last Accessed on 09/25/2013).
3. Manser TFS. Effective handover communication: an overview of research and improvement efforts. Best Pract Res Clin Anaesthesiol. 2011;25(2):181–91.
4. High 5s. High 5s project action on patient safety. 2006. Retrieved from http://www.cbo.nl/en/Patient-Safety/High5s/ (Last Accessed on 09/25/2013).
5. Joint Commission (TJC) Hospital National Patient Safety Goals. 2009. Retrieved from http://www.unchealthcare.org/site/Nursing/servicelines/aircare/additionaldocuments/2009npsg (Last Accessed on 09/25/2013).
6. Riesenberg LA, Leitzsch J, Little BW. Systematic review of handoff mnemonics literature. Am J Med Qual. 2009;24(3):196–204.
7. Palma JP, Sharek PJ, Longhurst CA. Impact of electronic medical record integration of a handoff tool on sign-out in a newborn intensive care unit. J Perinatol. 2011;31(5):311–7. PubMed PMID: 21273990.
8. Wentworth L, Diggins J, Bartel D, Johnson M, Hale J, Gaines K. Sbar: electronic handoff tool for noncomplicated procedural patients. J Nurs Care Qual. 2012;27(2):125–31. PubMed PMID: 22126852.
9. Joy BF, Elliott E, Hardy C, Sullivan C, Backer CL, Kane JM. Standardized multidisciplinary protocol improves handover of cardiac surgery patients to the intensive care unit. Pediatr Crit Care Med. 2011;12(3):304–8. PubMed PMID: 21057370.

10. Salerno SM, Arnett MV, Domanski JP. Standardized sign-out reduces intern perception of medical errors on the general internal medicine ward. Teach Learn Med. 2009;21(2):121–6. PubMed PMID: 19330690.
11. Lee LH, Levine JA, Schultz HJ. Utility of a standardized sign-out card for new medical interns. J Gen Intern Med. 1996;11(12):753–5. PubMed PMID: 9016423.
12. Wilson MJ. A template for safe and concise handovers. Medsurg Nurs. 2007;16(3):201–6. PubMed PMID: 17849931.
13. Abraham J, Kannampallil T, Patel VL. A systematic review of the literature on the evaluation of handoff tools: Implications for research and practice. Journal of American Medical Informatics Association, In Press.
14. Anderson J, Shroff D, Curtis A, Eldridge N, Cannon K, Karnani R, et al. The veterans affairs shift change physician-to-physician handoff project. Jt Comm J Qual Patient Saf. 2010;36(2):62–71. PubMed PMID: 20180438.
15. Bernstein JA, Imler DL, Sharek P, Longhurst CA. Improved physician work flow after integrating sign-out notes into the electronic medical record. Jt Comm J Qual Patient Saf. 2010;36(2):72–8. PubMed PMID: 20180439.
16. Cheah L-P, Amott DH, Pollard J, Watters D. Electronic medical handover: towards safer medical care. Med J Aust. 2005;183(7):369–72.
17. Ferran NA, Metcalfe AJ, O'Doherty D. Standardised proformas improve patient handover: audit of trauma handover practice. Patient Saf Surg. 2008;2:24.
18. Flanagan ME, Patterson ES, Frankel RM, Doebbeling BN. Evaluation of a physician informatics tool to improve patient handoffs. J Am Med Inform Assoc. 2009;16(4):509–15. PubMed PMID: 19390111. Pubmed Central PMCID: 2705254.
19. Frank G, Lawless S, Steinberg TH. Improving physician communication through an automated, integrated sign-out system. J Healthc Inf Manag. 2005;19(4):68–74.
20. Govier M, Medcalf P. Living for the weekend: electronic documentation improves patient handover. Clin Med. 2012;12(2):124–7. PubMed PMID: 22586785.
21. Ram R, Block B. Signing out patients for off-hours coverage: Comparison of manual and computer-aided methods. Proceedings of the annual symposium on Computer Applications in Medical Care. 1992;p 114–8
22. Van Eaton EG, Horvath KD, Lober WB, Rossini AJ, Pellegrini CA. A randomized, controlled trial evaluating the impact of a computerized rounding and sign-out system on continuity of care and resident work hours. J Am Coll Surg. 2005;200(4):538–45. PubMed PMID: 15804467.
23. Van Eaton EG, McDonough K, Lober WB, Johnson EA, Pellegrini CA, Horvath KD. Safety of using a computerized rounding and sign-out system to reduce resident duty hours. Acad Med. 2010;85(7):1189–95. PubMed PMID: 20592514.
24. Wayne JD, Tyagi R, Reinhardt G, Rooney D, Makoul G, Chopra S, et al. Simple standardized patient handoff system that increases accuracy and completeness. J Surg Educ. 2008;65(6): 476–85. PubMed PMID: 19059181.
25. Wohlauer MV, Rove KO, Pshak TJ, Raeburn CD, Moore EE, Chenoweth C, et al. The computerized rounding report: implementation of a model system to support transitions of care. J Surg Res. 2012;172(1):11–7. PubMed PMID: 21777923.
26. Basu A, Arora R, Fernandes N. Onsite handover of clinical care: implementing modified chaps. Clin Gov. 2011;16(3):220–30.
27. Stahl K, Palileo A, Schulman CI, Wilson K, Augenstein J, Kiffin C, et al. Enhancing patient safety in the trauma/surgical intensive care unit. J Trauma Acute Care Surg. 2009;67(3):430–5. doi:10.1097/TA.0b013e3181acbe75.
28. Chung K, Davis I, Moughrabi S, Gawlinski A. Use of an evidence-based shift report tool to improve nurses' communication. Medsurg Nurs. 2011;20(5):255–60. 68. PubMed PMID: 22165785.
29. Clark E, Squire S, Heyme A, Mickle ME, Petrie E. The pact project: improving communication at handover. Med J Aust. 2009;190(11 Suppl):S125–7. PubMed PMID: 19485860.
30. Nelson BA, Massey R. Implementing an electronic change-of-shift report using transforming care at the bedside processes and methods. J Nurs Adm. 2010;40(4):162–8. PubMed PMID: 20305461.

31. Roberts M, Putnam J, Raup GH. The interdepartmental ticket (it) factor: enhancing communication to improve quality. J Nurs Care Qual. 2012;27(3):247–52. PubMed PMID: 22437250.
32. Baldwin L, McGinnis C. A computer-generated shift report. Nurs Manag. 1994;25(9):61–4.
33. Christie P, Robinson H. Using a framework for good communication to improve quality of information at handover. Nurs Times. 2009;105:47.
34. Jukkala AM, James D, Autrey P, Azuero A, Miltner R. Developing a standardized tool to improve nurse communication during shift report. J Nurs Care Qual. 2012;27(3):240–6. doi:10.1097/NCQ.0b013e31824ebbd7.
35. Kalisch BJ, Hurley P, Hodges M, Landers D, Richter G, Stefanov S, Curley M. Pi tool patches broken communication. Nurs Manag. 2007;38(4):16. 8.
36. Raines M, Mull A. Give it to me: the development of a tool for shift change report in a level i trauma center. J Emerg Nurs. 2007;33(4):358–60.
37. Sidlow R, Katz-Sidlow RJ. Using a computerized sign-out system to improve physician-nurse communication. Jt Comm J Qual Patient Saf. 2006;32(1):32–6.
38. Barnes SL, Campbell DA, Stockman KA, Wunderlink D. From theory to practice of electronic handover. Aust Health Rev. 2011;35(3):384–91. PubMed PMID: 21871202.
39. Campion TR, Jr., Denny JC, Weinberg ST, Lorenzi NM, Waitman LR. Analysis of a computerized sign-out tool: Identification of unanticipated uses and contradictory content. Proceedings of the AMIA Annual Symposium 2007;p 99–104.
40. Rabinovitch DL, Hamill M, Zanchetta C, Bernstein M. Nurse practitioner-based sign-out system to facilitate patient communication on a neurosurgical service: a pilot study with recommendations. J Neurosci Nurs. 2009;41(6):329–35. PubMed PMID: 19998684.
41. Raptis DA, Fernandes C, Chua W, Boulos PB. Electronic software significantly improves quality of handover in a London teaching hospital. Health Informatics J. 2009;15:191–8.
42. Ryan S, O'Riordan JM, Tierney S, Conlon KC, Ridgway PF. Impact of a new electronic handover system in surgery. Int J Surg. 2011;9(3):217–20. PubMed PMID: 21129508.
43. Campion Jr TR, Weinberg ST, Lorenzi NM, Waitman LR. Evaluation of computerized free text sign-out notes: baseline understanding and recommendations. Appl Clin Inform. 2010;1(3):304–17.
44. Weed LL. Medical records that guide and teach. N Engl J Med. 1968;278(11):593–600.
45. Leonard M, Graham S, Bonacum D. The human factor: the critical importance of effective teamwork and communication in providing safe care. Quality and Safety in Health Care. 2004;13 (Suppl 1):i85–90.
46. Varon J, Acosta P. Handbook of critical and intensive care medicine. 2nd ed. New York: Springer; 2010.
47. Ardoin KB, Broussard L. Implementing handoff communication. J Nurses Staff Dev. 2011;27(3):128–35.
48. Woloshynowych M, Davis R, Brown R, Vincent C. Communication patterns in a UK Emergency Department. Ann Emerg Med. 2007;50(4):407–13.
49. White RS, Hall DM. The Bermuda triangle healthcare. An Illinois healthcare system closes the gaps in patient handoff communication. Health Manag Technol. 2008;29(7):30–1.
50. Sandlin D. Improving patient safety by implementing a standardized and consistent approach to hand-off communication. J Perianesth Nurs. 2007;22(4):289–92.
51. Braun BD. Evaluating and improving the handoff process. J Emerg Nurs. 2012;38(2): 151–5.
52. Abraham J, Kannampallil T, Patel B, Almoosa KF, Patel VL, editors. Ensuring patient safety in care transitions: An empirical evaluation of a handoff intervention tool. Proceedings of AMIA. 2012.Chicago.
53. Harvey C, Schuster R, Durso F, Matthews A, Surabattula D. Human factors of transition of care. In: Handbook of human factors and ergonomics in health care and patient safety. Mahwah, NJ: Lawrence Erlbaum Associates; 2007.
54. Cheung D, Kelly J, Beach C, Berkeley R, Bitterman R, Broida R, et al. Improving handoffs in the emergency department. Ann Emerg Med. 2009;55(2):171–80.

55. Patterson ES, Roth EM, Woods DD, Chow R, Orlando-Gomes J. Handoff strategies in settings with consequences for failure: lessons for health care operations. International J Qual Health Care. 2004;16:125–32. doi:10.1093/intqhc/mzh026.
56. Abraham J, Nguyen VC, Almoosa KF, Patel B, Patel VL. Falling through the cracks: information breakdowns in critical care handoff communication. Washington, DC: American Medical Informatics Association (AMIA); 2011.
57. Raduma-Tomàs MA, Flin R, Yule S, Williams D. Doctors' handovers in hospitals: a literature review. BMJ Qual Saf. 2011;20(2):128–33.
58. Catchpole K, De Leval M, McEwan A, Pgott N, Elliott M, McQuillan A, et al. Patient handover from surgery to intensive care: using formula 1 pit-stop and aviation models to improve safety and quality. Pediatr Anesth. 2007;17:470–8. doi:10.1111/j.1460-9592.2006.02239.x.
59. McFetridge B, Gillespie M, Goode D, Melby V. An exploration of the handover process of critically ill patients between nursing staff from the emergency department and the intensive care unit. Nurs Crit Care. 2007;12(6):261–9.
60. Jenkin A, Abelson-Mitchell N, Cooper S. Patient handover: time for a change? Accid Emerg Nurs. 2007;15:141–7. doi:10.1016/j.aaen.2007.04.004.
61. Van Eaton E. Handoff improvement: we need to understand what we are trying to fix. Jt Comm J Qual Patient Saf. 2010;36(2):51.
62. Abraham J, Patel B, Almoosa KF, Warner M, Kannampallil T, Patel VL. Minimizing communication breakdowns: an empirical evaluation of a handoff intervention tool. Crit Care Med. 2011;39(12):152.
63. Streitenberger K, Breen-Reid K, Harris C. Handoffs in care–can we make them safer? Pediatr Clin North Am. 2006;53(6):1185–95.
64. Jacobi J, Fraser GL, Coursin DB, Riker RR, Fontaine D, Wittbrodt ET, et al. Clinical practice guidelines for the sustained use of sedatives and analgesics in the critically ill adult. Crit Care Med. 2002;30(1):119–41.
65. Weed LL. Medical terminology records, medical education, and patient care. The problem-oriented record as a basic tool. Cleveland: Case Western Reserve University; 1969.
66. Gurses AP, Xiao Y. A systematic review of the literature on multidisciplinary rounds to design information technology. J Am Med Inform Assoc. 2006;13(3):267–76.
67. Cohen MD, Hilligoss PB. The published literature on handoffs in hospitals: deficiencies identified in an extensive review. Qual Saf Health Care. 2010;19(6):493–7.
68. Patel VL, Arocha JF, Kaufman DR. Diagnostic reasoning and medical expertise. Psychol Learn Motiv. 1994;31:187–252. PubMed PMID: ISI:A1994BE32M00004. English.
69. Horwitz L, Meredith T, Schuur J, Shah N, Kulkarni R, Jenq G. Dropping the baton: a qualitative analysis of failures during the transition from emergency department to inpatient care. Ann Emerg Med. 2009;53(6):701–10.
70. Lally S. An investigation into the functions of nurses' communication at the inter-shift handover. J Nurs Manag. 1999;7(1):29–36.

Chapter 14
Investigating Shared Mental Models in Critical Care

Lena Mamykina, R. Stanley Hum, and David R. Kaufman

Introduction

Clinical care is increasingly recognized as a highly collaborative practice [1]. The complexity of modern medicine, particularly of intensive care, requires deep specialization and honing of skills and expertise that can take years to acquire. As a result, clinical teams in intensive care units can include over a dozen of specialists, each contributing their unique knowledge to the overall patient care. And while speedy and successful patient recovery is an underlying objective of their combined efforts, each specialist may have their own goals and priorities, dictated by their training, experience, and focus.

The effectiveness of communication and coordination among team members has a critical impact on the quality of the patient care. Higher levels of group development, positive attitudes about teamwork, and a team approach to the management of critically ill patients were correlated with improved patient outcomes [2–5], lower risk-adjusted mortality rates [6] and reduced costs in the intensive care unit [5]. Breaks in communication among team members were shown to be significant contributors to medical errors [7]. The association between effective teamwork and medical errors is of particular importance; the recent Institute of Medicine Report on

---

A version of this chapter is under review: Mamykina L, Twohig B, Sheehan B, Hum RS, Kaufman DR, Measuring shared mental models in critical care: methodological perspective, under review. *Journal of Biomedical Informatics*, Elsevier.

L. Mamykina, PhD (✉)
Department of Biomedical Informatics, Columbia University, New York, NY 10032, USA
e-mail: lena.mamykina@dbmi.columbia.edu

R.S. Hum, MD, FRCPC
Department of Pediatrics, College of Physicians and Surgeons, Columbia University, New York, NY, USA

D.R. Kaufman, PhD
Department of Biomedical Informatics, Arizona State University, Scottsdale, AZ 85259, USA

V.L. Patel et al. (eds.), *Cognitive Informatics in Health and Biomedicine*, Health Informatics, DOI 10.1007/978-1-4471-5490-7_14,

medical errors concluded that "healthcare organizations need to promote effective team functioning" as one of five principles for improving safety of healthcare delivery [8].

One of the primary advantages of effective teamwork is that it allows for distribution of cognitive work, which is necessary given the complexity of modern medicine. However, this distribution requires that all members of a patient care team develop and maintain shared cognitive representations of the case in hand, the underlying causes of a patient's current state, the overall plan of care, and the allocation of responsibilities among clinicians on the team. Such shared representations, commonly referred to as *Shared Mental Models (SMM)*, have been shown to have positive impact on team performance in a variety of settings and domains. While research on SMM in clinical work is scarce, the few studies conducted to date suggest strong correlation between robust SMM and improved clinical performance [9]. New informatics solutions for facilitating clinical communication specifically focus on fostering and promoting shared mental models among members of clinical teams [10].

While there is a growing recognition of the importance of shared mental models and their impact on patient care, and the opportunity to facilitate them with informatics solutions, the existing research on SMM in clinical care is limited. Mental models are a construct that reference mental representations and cannot be studied directly. Researchers have identified a number of ways to study external manifestations of mental models, both individual and shared. These methods tend to fall into one of the two broad families. Many studies of mental models rely on researchers' reconstruction of an individual's internal cognitive representation based on interviews or simple tasks, which require predictions from subjects. Other studies employ a range of knowledge elicitation methods, which ask individuals to build associations between sets of concepts relevant for the domain under investigation, thus allowing individuals to directly externalize their mental models [11]. Both of these types of methods have their limitations. Qualitative methods rely on researchers' subjective interpretations, and do not allow for comparative studies. Knowledge elicitation methods require substantial time investment from the participants and have limited ecological validity; when asked to externalize their mental models, individuals may overstate their confidence in facts and relationships between them. This is compounded by the fact that laboratory testing cannot mimic the dynamically changing conditions of an ICU. As a result, we argue that there is a need for ecologically sensitive methods for studying shared mental models in clinical teams, and metrics for comparative assessment of SMM. Such metrics would be an invaluable asset for the future research in informatics interventions for facilitating development of shared mental models in clinical teams.

In this chapter, we discuss a novel approach to studying and measuring SMM of clinical teams based on clinicians' presentations of patients during handoff. The approach employs both qualitative methods that surface important aspects of clinical communication and a quantitative method that measures the degree of congruence in conversations about the same patient. Handoff—a relatively formal interview between the outgoing and the incoming clinicians during a shift change—presents a unique opportunity to study SMM. During handoff clinicians summarize each patient case to its essence and cover the most pertinent, important, and up to date information that serve as a foundation for the care provided during the new shift. We argue that the proposed approach has a higher ecological validity than more intrusive SMM research methods, yet it is more objective and less subject to interpretation than many of the observer-based methods.

In this chapter, we first present an account of teamwork and communication practices in an Intensive Care Unit of a large teaching hospital. We then discuss the new method and provide examples for how it can be used to calculate the extent of SMM of patient care teams. We then present a case-study of one of the patient cases observed over a 3 days period in our recent study of shared mental models of clinical teams in an Intensive Care Unit. Finally, we conclude with the discussion of the benefits and limitations of the proposed method and how it could be used to facilitate studies of SMM in the context of informatics interventions.

Shared Mental Models, Handoffs and Team Communication

Patient care in an ICU is a cognitively complex process with rapidly changing patient states and multiple streams of data that must be analyzed and acted upon in a short period of time [12]. This necessitates a team approach involving multiple healthcare professionals that serve to accomplish the range of clinical tasks, but also reduce cognitive complexity for decision makers. The team approach introduces an additional layer of cognitive requirements that are associated with the demands of working together effectively [13]. Clinicians that are part of an ICU team need to coordinate their activities with others who are working toward the same goal.

Handoff in critical care medicine—a research area of growing importance—is the subject of several studies in this volume. Handoff is the exchange between health professionals of information about a patient accompanying either a transfer of control over or responsibility for the patient [14]. The primary purpose of a handoff is to provide accurate information about a patient's care, treatment, current condition and any recent or anticipated changes [15]. There is a premium on ensuring accuracy in conveying information to the recipient clinician so as not to compromise patient safety. Several studies have reported that communication issues are the most common cause of sentinel events in medicine [16, 17].

In a large-scale review of the literature, Cohen and Hilligoss found that handoff was sensitive to variations in context and serves a range of communicative functions beyond the mere transmission of patient-related information [14]. It serves the goal of facilitating the integration of information into a coherent mental model of the patient. A mental model is a cognitive construct that is widely used in human computer interaction and human factors research, as well as other spheres of cognitive research. Mental models are used to describe how individuals form internal representations of systems [18]. Mental models are designed to answer questions such as "how does this work?" or "what will happen if I take the following action?"

or “why is the patient not more responsive to the medications he is currently receiving?” Running of a model corresponds to a process of mental simulation for generating possible future states of a system from an observed or hypothetical state. An individual’s mental models provide predictive and explanatory capabilities of the function of a given system [19].

As indicated, the temporal dimensions of a mental model of a patient are a defining characteristic in that they enable a clinician to project forward to a subsequent state of the patient or to reconstruct the process that precipitated the current state. It enables a clinician to anticipate how a change in course of treatment may affect a more desirable outcome or healthier future state. The intensive care unit (ICU) is designed to care for critically ill patients, who are in need of rigorous monitoring and aggressive therapy. Most ICU patients suffer from multisystem problems and the medications administered can produce severe side effects. Expert ICU clinicians or seasoned attending physicians possess robust mental models and can anticipate a causal sequence to a considerable degree of depth and when needed, adjust a therapeutic plan accordingly [12].

Shared mental models (SMMs)—an extension of the mental model concept—reflect the shared and collective knowledge of a team. SMMs provide mutual expectations, which allow teams to coordinate and make predictions about the behavior and needs of their teammates [20]. On a healthcare team, there is substantial differentiation in the roles of nurses, residents, fellows and others. As a result, some of the knowledge about a patient is shared among team members (e.g., a patient’s respiratory status); however, much of this knowledge is complementary or distributed across team members. Overlapping knowledge is essential for negotiating common task goals and objectives. Similarly, complementary knowledge enables a nurse or resident to execute their individual tasks effectively in the joint coordination of patient care.

The ICU is a high velocity environment characterized by dynamically changing conditions. A shared mental model reflects aspects of team knowledge that persist over a period of time and to a certain extent, across patients. We distinguish between teams’ shared mental models, and their *situation model*, an assessment of a patient case that develops in situ while the team is engaged in a patient care task or communication [21]. For example, an examination of the patient during bedside patient rounds may change their assessment of the patients’ current state and possibly the treatment plan. Similarly, a critical piece of information in the form of an update on the patients’ state or knowledge of the particular underlying condition introduced into a clinical communication may serve to alter the situation model as well. The important point is that the shared mental model includes knowledge elements that persist overtime whereas the situation model dynamically changes in situ.

When clinicians on a team develop a shared mental model, this contributes to an increase in their *common ground*. Common ground refers to the knowledge shared by two or more individuals engaged in a communication [22]. It is a reciprocal relationship in that shared common ground facilitates the development of more robust shared mental models. The process of checking whether individuals’ understanding is consonant with one another (i.e., validating shared knowledge) is known as grounding. Common ground is often achieved through conversational grounding— a process that involves an act of conveying a message and an indication that the message has been understood by the recipient. Two individuals who know each other, share the same role (e.g., residents in an ICU) or work in the same setting have substantial common ground prior to engaging in a communication. In handoff communication, the sender of the information will adjust her communication based on her expectation of the knowledge of the receiver. The receiver may also convey his or her understanding of the communication, although that happens less frequently in handoff communications. There are risks associated with assuming too much shared knowledge and costs (primarily time) associated with additional grounding efforts.

There are a host of factors that impact both the process and the likelihood of successful grounding during handoff. These include the clinicians' familiarity with each other and their familiarity with the patient, their workload, expectations set by more senior clinicians (i.e., attending physicians or fellows), the acuity of the patient's illness and whether the patient state or treatment protocol has changed substantially. The process of establishing common ground is essential to the formation of shared mental models. In this study, we are interested in the shared mental models that are established by different clinicians caring for the same patient and that are manifested in a handoff between pairs of clinicians with the same role on a patient care team (e.g. resident, fellow, or nurse).

A Study of Shared Mental Models in an ICU

The study was conducted during May and June of 2010 in a Cardiothoracic Intensive Care Unit (CTICU) at a large urban medical center. The CTICU is divided into the general CTICU which houses 21 patient beds and the Heart Center CTICU, which contains six beds. The unit provides post-operative care to more than 1,400 patients each year. The CTICU admits patients following heart or lung transplantation, ventricular assist device insertion (VAD), coronary artery bypass graft (CABG), valve surgery, aortic reconstructive surgery and minimally invasive surgery.

In a typical day, a medical team in the CTICU was staffed with attending physicians, fellows, second or third-year residents, and physician assistants (PAs) who were all assigned to different patients. The CTICU nursing team included staff nurses, who cared for one to two patients; many of them had over a decade of ICU experience. In the course of the study, the unit medical staff rotated once with a complete change of attending physicians, fellows and residents.

In the first part of the study, researchers rotated to observe patterns of work and communication in the CTICU for several weeks. Members of the research team alternated between shadowing individuals clinicians (n=4), for an hour at a time and observing the entire unit while positioned at the nursing station. During this time, the researchers took extensive field notes recording major events, and their impressions of the work in the unit.

The primary data collection method for the SMM analysis was audio recording of verbal handoffs of different members of patient care teams. The study used the following protocol: on the day prior to observations, the researchers, with the help of one of the attending physicians, selected a small number of patient cases (from 1 to 3) to follow in the study. We selected patients whose problems were of greater complexity (e.g. actively critical VAD patients), because mental models and communications in regards to these patients were likely to be richer and more elaborate. On the day of observations, members of the research team observed and recorded all (to the degree possible) handoffs during morning transitions of care (approximately 7:00 AM) by individual team members for the selected patients. After handoffs, researchers recorded clinical rounds, and evening handoffs (approximately 7:00 PM) for the same patients. The researchers took extensive hand-written notes throughout the study.

Finally, researchers conducted in-depth interviews with four clinicians (one nurse, one fellow, and two residents) to assess their perceptions and attitudes in regards to transitions of care. All recordings were de-identified and transcribed verbatim for analysis. The study was approved by the Institutional Review Board of New York Presbyterian Hospital/Columbia University Medical Center. We obtained informed consent from all participating clinicians.

Shared Mental Models in the ICU: Team Perceptions

In this section, we describe the results of the qualitative interviews of clinicians in the unit and our own observations of patterns of work and communication and how they impacted shared mental models of clinicians on patient care teams.

Divergent Temporal Frames and Priorities

Like in many other inpatient settings, clinicians in CTICU work in co-located teams that include an attending physician, a fellow, a resident or a PA, and a nurse, all usually physically present in the unit most of the time. In addition, many other clinicians may play different roles in patient care. For example, a patient recovering from a heart transplant will have surgeons who performed the transplant procedure, cardiologists, nutritionists, gastrointestinal (GI) specialists, physical therapists, and social workers, among others.

These clinicians have different responsibilities in regards to patient care, which often results in significant differences in their goals. While providing quality patient care is the general goal for everybody on the team, the specific priorities differ for individual team members. For example, surgeons who perform complex procedures are ultimately interested in the successful recovery from the surgical procedure. ICU physicians' primary responsibility is to stabilize the patients and transition them to less intensive and expensive step-down units. In contrast, floor clinicians are concerned with the long-term care and overall wellbeing of the patients. Sometimes these priorities come into conflict. For example, many of the aggressive medications used by ICU teams have negative side effects that may affect patients in the future. These could be of concern to their primary care providers, who need to think not only about stabilizing the patients, but also about their long-term well-being and health care needs.

These differences in focal points have an impact on the temporal frames in which different clinicians operate. For example, nurses operate in the timescale of minutes; they provide minute to minute monitoring and care, have the most direct access to the patient and the most updated patient information. Residents' time frame is somewhat wider but is often limited by temporal boundaries of one shift (12 h). Fellows, in concert with charge nurses, are responsible for managing the flow of patients and transitioning them out of the unit as soon as possible. As a result, their temporal frame includes patients' entire ICU stay; they plan their activities for speedy discharge. Surgical teams' view extends beyond ICU stay and usually covers the entire patient stay until discharge. Finally, as mentioned above, primary care providers have the widest view of the patient case that often covers the patient's lifespan.

Establishing Shared Mental Models in Rounds

Clinicians in the study perceived ward rounds as the primary formal vehicle for establishing shared mental models. Rounds allow different members of the patient care teams to come together and discuss each of their patients, including their primary issues, and plan of care. In the CTICU observed in this study, the traditional teaching rounds were led by attending physicians and included residents (or PAs who played a similar role on a team), fellows and nurses responsible for patients in the unit. Most of the fellows, residents and PAs stayed with the rounding group for the entire duration of rounds. Rounds were frequently subjected to interruptions varying in time and as a result could take up to 4 or 5 h to complete. In contrast, nurses joined rounds for the discussion of their patients only and resumed patient care responsibilities when the group moved on to the next patient.

In addition to these traditional teaching rounds, shortly prior to the study the unit introduced highly interdisciplinary rounds for patients on ventricular assist devices (VAD)—mechanical circulatory devices used to partially or completely replace the function of a failing heart. These rounds were very brief, only a few minutes per patient; however, they included extended members of patient care teams to include surgeons, cardiology consultants, nutritionists, and other consultants relevant for the different patient cases. For many junior clinicians these rounds were a rare chance to be introduced to the decision-making process of their more senior colleagues:

> So it's nice to have those rounds in the morning to figure out what's going on, and [name removed] is this like this premier VAD surgeon. So to hear what he has to say, so you hear it straight from his mouth, rather than from your attending or some other consultant is

actually the best way to figure out and learn how to take care of these patients. It actually teaches you enough stuff that I feel as if I've learned a lot from those rounds.

While both ward rounds and VAD rounds were perceived as critical to the development of shared understanding of patient cases, urgent patient care responsibilities often prevented clinicians from participating. In the teaching rounds we observed, nurses were often distracted by either patient monitoring equipment indicating changes in patients' conditions that required their attention, or by other clinicians who came to receive up-to-date account of patients' conditions. Many residents after presenting patients they were responsible for left the rounds to immediately update patients' plans of care, thus missing discussions on patients they might be responsible for in their next shifts. In regards to VAD rounds, because they happened in the early morning hours, while residents and PAs were gathering patient data in preparation for teaching rounds, very few of them were able to participate.

In addition to these formal communication events, clinicians on the patient care teams continued to informally communicate throughout their shifts, frequently synchronizing their perceptions of changes in patients' conditions, and their response to treatment. These informal information exchanges were seen as essential to maintaining continuity in shared mental models and ensuring that they stayed current and incorporated new information as it became available throughout the day. However, this frequent informal communication can result in fragmented communication and less-focused team discussions.

Transitions of Care Disrupt Continuity in Shared Mental Models

Like all hospital units, ICU follows a rotation schedule to provide 24 h of continuous care. Because clinicians within the same role and discipline are not usually present at the same time but rotate, most of the within-role communication happens during transitions of care, when new teams take over patient care. Such transitions happen twice a day, with two 12 h shifts. Teams responsible for patient care during daytime hours are considered primary, and nighttime teams are considered coverage teams. Primary teams usually carry the bulk of patient care responsibilities; most of the complex procedures are performed during the day. Nighttime teams' primary focus is maintaining the care plan agreed upon during the day shift and handling emerging crises. There are usually fewer clinicians on the night shift; as a result, the ratio of patients to clinicians increases considerably.

At the end of each shift, clinicians hand off their patients to their counterparts in a relatively formal handoff. Handoffs are usually done verbally, either at patients' bedside, or in a conference room. While there are general similarities in the purpose of handoff among team members, they vary considerably in styles and in content. For example, because each attending physician and fellow covers many patients in the unit, fellow-to-attending handoffs are very brief and focus only on the most critical aspects of patient care. However, these handoffs often go beyond transfer of information; many decisions regarding patient care are made during these handoffs.

Fellow-to-fellow handoffs are also brief in their discussion of individual patients; decisions made during these handoffs are primarily concerned with identifying patients who are ready to be moved to step-down units. Resident-to-Resident handoffs are more focused on transferring relevant information and providing context for patient care.

Generally, clinicians in the unit were concerned about the lack of continuity in patient care. Because the nighttime coverage teams don't participate in the rounds, they have to rely on handoff to ensure that the important patient information gets discussed during team meetings:

> I feel like the problem is when I leave post call, I don't -- I'm not a part of those rounds during the day so I don't know how much of that gets moved or that gets actually conveyed. You're the one who's seen that, I didn't see that, I never see that. So I don't even know after I left that day like what happened during rounds that the people discussed, what happened overnight, like what happened. Which is bad because actually you learn -- that's the way that you learn, you learn from what happened and how you maybe should have done it differently.

In summary, our observations and interviews with clinicians in the unit painted a complex picture of communication patterns in the unit. While interdisciplinary communication had both formal and informal channels, within-discipline communication was more commonly done in a formal way through handoffs. Rounds and, in particular, VAD rounds were perceived as major contributors to the development of a deeper shared understanding of patients' cases and care; however, due to their busy schedules not all clinicians on the teams were able to participate in either teaching or VAD rounds. As a result, clinicians often had to compensate with increased informal communication, further contributing to the amount of interruptions in the unit. Although informal communication is an essential part of ICU work, it is unscheduled—depending on the availability of either party and it will be variably complete depending on the two clinicians having sufficient time to establish common ground (e.g., shared perceptions of whether the patient is responding well to changes in treatment).

In the next section of this chapter, we discuss a case study of a patient we observed for 3 consecutive days and discuss how clinicians on this team developed shared mental model of the case. We then present our calculations of the SMM index and compare the changes in the index over 3 days with the qualitative changes in clinicians' understanding inferred from discussions in rounds.

Shared Mental Models: A Case Study

To illustrate how our approach can help to explicate the degree of shared mental models among members of a patient care team, we will use a case study of one of the patients we followed in the unit. The patient was a male in his 60s with a complex history of heart disease. Like most other patients in the CTICU, he was a post-surgical patient who was placed on a biventricular assist device, used to partially

Table 14.1 Changes in team composition throughout the study

Role	Day 1 AM	Day 1 PM	Day 2 AM	Day 2 PM	Day 3 AM	Day 3 PM
Attending physician	1	1	1	1	1	1
Fellow	1	2	1	2	1	2
Resident/PA	1	2	1	3	4	5
Nurse	1	2	1	2	1	2
Charge nurse	1	2	1	2	1	2

replace the function of a failing heart. He was transferred from surgery into CTICU several days prior to our observations. We will call this patient Mr. Smith (the name is changed to protect the patient's privacy). During the 3 days of observations, the team experienced 6 transitions of care, with the following changes in personnel (Table 14.1):

Developing Shared Mental Models in Rounds

We begin the discussion of the team's shared mental model of Mr. Smith's conditions and care by illustrating how the team developed SMM of the patient in rounds.

Day 1

On the first day of our observations, the patient care team had undergone significant changes, as a new attending physician and fellows joined the team. The analysis of patient discussion during rounds immediately revealed major disagreements among team members in regards to the patient state and the complexity of care, as exemplified by the following excerpt:

Attending: So he's falling apart.
Resident: He seems to be pretty good.
Attending: He's falling apart! He's got a heart rate of 120 with a blood pressure…what's the blood pressure now?
Nurse: I think it's like 70…
Attending: 70!

It is reasonable to assume that all of the participants understood that a BIVAD patient was acutely ill. However, the expert above shows that they diverged significantly in their basic understanding of how well the patient was doing and the urgency of care relative to their expectations. This lack of coherence extended to the care the patient was receiving. The attending physician, who assumed care for the patient on the morning of the observations, raised multiple concerns in regards to the choice of medication plan established as part of post-surgical treatment. In his assessment, the particular combination of medications was overburdening the patients' already weakened pulmonary system, thus further complicating his conditions and slowing recovery.

Attending: All we're doing in there? We're flogging the right heart to make the pulmonary systems basically fall apart while sedating him with stuff that makes the pulmonary fall apart which, um, he's now in increasing renal insufficiency which will make the pulmonary fall apart and he's basically got a carrying capacity which is incredibly low because he's got no…what's his CVP?
Nurse: CVP, 18 to 19. 18 to 19.
Attending: 18 to 19…Can you believe it?

When questioned by their attending physicians about reasons for the various medications the patient was on, more junior team members could not provide a reason or justification:

Attending: Why is he on Ketamine in the first place? What was the reasoning behind it?
Physician Assistant: One of your colleagues put him on it!

As the team continued discussing the case, clinicians became aware of these discrepancies and their impact on the care they were providing. The PA, an experienced clinician who has worked with the attending for many years raises the question as to the difference in treatment strategies pursued by prior attendings.

Physician Assistant: I'm wondering with all your colleagues here who have gone over him every day. Why is this the first time we're hearing about all these untoward effects of all the agents that your colleagues put him on? And I'm just trying to figure it out.

Finally, as a result, the team began developing an immediate plan of treatment that was to be pursued during the upcoming shift and made plans for developing a more comprehensive long-term plan. The attending articulated a set of goals and a general plan, but left the specifics up to the fellow and the PA. He was able to do so because of the realignment in understanding and a basic trust in the clinicians' judgment.

Attending: Do you understand what's going…what I just said here? Do you? Do you think you and [physician assistant] can get together and kinda piece this out to a functional plan of care? He has to be around for this, okay? Because now it's up to us to get one plan of care and just go with it, okay?

Day 3

Once the clinicians established the basic shared mental model during their first rounds together, their efforts during the first two days focused on slowly changing the patient's medication plan, and enacting their new approach. On day three, the patient discussion during the ward rounds was quite different from the one discussed above: it no longer focused on immediate issues, but rather tackled deeper underlying causes that contributed to the severity of the patients' illness. Specifically, the VAD device supporting the patients' heart is approved to be used a temporary solution, a "bridge", leading to a more permanent one, such as a heart transplant. However, because organs available for transplants are scarce, oftentimes, short-term solutions become long-term, and in a way "bridges to nowhere".

Attending: Okay? You'll know. The whole thing… The way we've set this up is… we've have only a couple…we've got lots of devices, lots of devices. We only have a couple of devices that are, um, long-term devices and usually, well, our initial plan of doing these devices was we were going to put them in and we were gonna actually use them as sort of transitions…to set up a bridge…a bridge to, you know, to transplantation. Um, organs have become scarcer and scarcer especially in the Eastern… well in the US and in the New York State they become less and less available. So what happens is that we have developed or have started to develop a bridge to nowhere. Okay?
Resident: Like an Alaska…
Attending: Alaska, yeah, a bridge, an absolute bridge to nowhere.

While searching for a more permanent solution, the team discussed mechanical and hydrodynamic functioning of different internal systems and forces influencing them. The attending used the analogy to pipes to help other members of the team to develop a robust mental model of pressure-flow and pressure-volume relations of the heart and blood.

Attending: What happens to the resistance in the pipe at the end of the pipe?
PA: It goes up if it stays the same. If it doesn't change…
Attending: It's not gonna change. It's fixed.
Fellow: The pressure changes.
Attending: The pressure…right.
PA: The pressure goes up if the resistance remains fixed. Right.

Once the team came to a shared understanding of what the sources of patient's problems were, they developed a plan that became a guiding principle for their coordinated actions in the next shift. Here the attending physician once again uses the reference to hemodynamics and explains how elimination of excessive fluids will cause pressures to drop and reduce cardiac output (the volume of blood being pumped out by the heart) to a more desirable level. And because of the shared understanding of the system and its internal functions, team members can independently arrive at the appropriate conclusions.

Attending: Now there are a number…there are a number of different ways to go but the most important thing for us is to pick a plan and that's what we're doing here. Pick a plan and stick to it. Okay?
Attending: What is the one thing we're supposed to do in the next 8 hours?
PA: Diurese.
Attending: Diurese, diurese, diurese. If you diurese effectively you will get to where you wanna go cause what will happen will be the cardiac output will drop because the end diastolic volume will go away… Okay? That's the method to the madness.

Summary

In summary, the transcripts of rounds captured for the patient show that the team was actively constructing a shared mental model of what was happening with the patient, and what treatment was the most appropriate. We found that the team came to the table with highly divergent perspectives on both how well the patient was doing, and the relative success of the treatment. In most of the discussion in the first day, the team came together focused on creating the required alignment between team members. The attending physician, who clearly had a very particular vision of the case, was not only communicating what was to be done, but also was working with more junior members of the team on developing a deeper underlying understanding of the dynamics of the case, patient physiology, impact of different treatment types, and the selection of the best treatment. While discussions on day one focused on creating basic alignment and making immediate modifications to the care, discussions on day three focused on understanding of the underlying reasons for the situation, and developing a long-term plan more consistent with this causal understanding.

The discussions we presented above are examples of some of the most comprehensive efforts focused on the developing of the shared mental model. However, in the course of our studies we observed widely different approaches to rounds, often dictated by temporal pressures and the specifics of patient cases. Many of the attending physicians we observed were more direct in their specification of the course of treatment (e.g., identifying particular medications) and devoted less time to fostering an understanding of the clinical state.

Measuring Shared Mental Models in Handoff

In the previous section, we used recordings of patient conversations during rounds to trace the development of shared mental models in regards to patient cases. The analysis presented above is consistent with many previous studies of shared mental modes, in which experienced observers infer SMM based on participants' discourse. In this section, we present the results of a new approach to elucidating shared mental models in patient care, based on recording of verbal handoffs of different clinicians caring for the same patient. Our expectation for such handoffs is that while each patient report will be specific to the goals and priorities of the reporting clinician, clinicians who share a robust mental model of their patient will have a substantial overlap in their presentations. Our hypothesis is that the convergence of themes and clinical concepts are meaningful indices of shared mental models.

In this analysis our main goal was to develop an approach that would allow us to assess clinicians SMM based on their handoffs, and to assign it a numeric value that would represent the extent of overlap between team members. To achieve that, we adopted the Pyramid Method a method used for automated document summarization to determine convergence of meaning in different stretches of text [23]. The full description of our method is available elsewhere (ref); below we present a summary of this approach that will be used in the rest of this chapter.

The main goal of our analysis was to compare handoffs by different clinicians on the team and generate a numeric measure of the degree of overlap in their descriptions of the patient. We also wanted to distinguish between statements based on how many team members included them in their handoffs.

Transcripts of verbal handoffs were segmented into smallest utterances with a coherent meaning [24]. We then compared all coded records for each individual patient and identified statements that appeared in multiple (at least two) transcripts. We also noted statements where team members provided contradictory information and noted them as discrepancies. Once all overlaps and discrepancies were identified, we calculated the Shared Mental Model index (SMMi) as a weighted proportion of overlapped statements (number of overlapped statements weighted by the number of team members who included them in their handoffs), adjusted by the number of discrepancies to the overall number of statements in all the handoffs given by team members for the given patient. The resulting SMMi is a numeric value between 0 and 1 that shows the relative frequency of overlapping statements to the overall statements made by the members of the team [24].

Shared Mental Models Analysis

Day 1 AM

On the first day of the observations, we recorded two morning signouts: resident-to-resident, and charge nurse-to-charge nurse. The overlap analysis showed that of all the statements made during the two captured signouts (N = 49), only four overlapped in content. Table 14.2 below shows statements that overlapped between the nurse and the resident and the codes associated with them:

As one can see from this table, the main points of the agreement between these two clinicians, beyond patients' name, included: patient's main reason for being in the unit (the heartmate, and bivad implant), and their main issue of the previous shift: weaning of nitric oxide.

In addition to these overlapping statements, there was one point of divergence between these clinicians, specifically in regards to how well the patient tolerated weaning of nitric oxide. Whereas the resident reported that the patient tolerated the weaning well ("he seems to have tolerated that pretty well"), charge nurse had a different perception ("So they don't know whether he can tolerate or not").

Table 14.2 Overlap table for handoffs captured on day 1, during morning handoff (AM)

Resident	Nurse
(1) So Smith	(1) Mr. Smith
Heartmate II	The heartmate
BIVAD implant [on May 26,]	Bivalve insertion
We gently weaned his nitric off overnight,	Main issue we tried to wean off the nitrate

The nurse provided the following explanation to her assessment of how well the patient tolerated weaning:

> Main issue we tried to wean off the nitrate. We started from 0.9 and then at 5:15 we dropped it to 0.5. CVP went up to like 18 to 20, which was previously like in the 15, and then the PA systolic went up to like 60s, so now we went back up to like 1.

The only statement the resident made about this issue was:

> He seems to have tolerated that pretty well

The analysis of the statements that did not overlap in content showed that most of them [7] were descriptions on ongoing treatments (examples), followed by clinical impressions (examples), description of what was done during the previous shift (%, examples), and previous history of the patient (%, examples).

We calculated the overlap index for this transition of care in the following way:

$$O = \frac{\sum_{i=1}^{n} o(i) \times |Ti| - D}{S} = \frac{4 * \frac{2}{5} - 1}{49} = \frac{0.6}{\frac{45}{2}} = \frac{0.6}{22.5} = 0.03$$

Comparison with Rounds

We compared the two captured handoffs with discussion of the patient case during rounds, which produced the following overlap table (Table 14.3):

Table 14.3 Overlap table for morning handoffs captured on day one (AM) and rounds

Resident	Nurse	Rounds
(1) So Smith	(1) Mr. Smith	Smith
Doing well as you sign him out to me.		He seems to be pretty good
Heartmate II	The heartmate	
BIVAD implant [on May 26,]	Bivalve insertion	
with chronic renal insufficiency,		increasing renal insufficiency
moderately diffuse RV dysfunction,		The RV's really bad.
We gently weaned his nitric off overnight,	Main issue we tried to wean off the nitrate	Tried to come off nitrous oxide, every time…
so but the mixed venous is 86		(What's his mixed venous?) 86…this morning…
only thing is that his crit is 23.4.		(I'm sorry, what's his hematocrit?) 23.4.
	CBP went up to like 18–20,	CVP, 18–19. 1–19.
	with the ketamine of 2,	(What are you on (Ketamine)?) 2.
	Lasix	He's on Lasix

Comparison with rounds highlights two interesting points. First, we can see that even though each of the observed clinicians (nurse and resident) have a relatively weak overlap with each other, or individually with rounds, when put together, they possess a more substantial amount of information about the patient and a higher degree of overlap with rounds. For example, as one can see from this table, an additional issue that overlapped between residents and rounds included right ventricular (RV) function that was listed among patient's acute issues by the resident, and was also mentioned during rounds. However, functioning of the RV was not mentioned by the Charge Nurse at all.

Moreover, the comparison with rounds also showed another point of discrepancy between team members, related to the general assessment of the patient's state. As we showed before, this discrepancy was fully revealed and elaborated on during rounds (i.e., "doing well" versus "falling apart") and led to team's reshaping of its shared mental model.

Day 1 PM

During the next transition of care that happened at 7 PM on the same day, we again captured handoffs by a resident in charge of the patient, a nurse and a charge nurse. The overlap analysis produced the following results (Table 14.4):

As one can see from this table, the level of realignment and agreement achieved during rounds on day 1 was carried through to the end-of-shift handoffs that revealed a higher level of content overlap among members of the team. Specifically, all three recorded signouts mentioned the main issue identified during rounds, namely poor function of right ventricle. In addition, all three signouts mentioned the main items on the patient's immediate treatment plan: discontinuing ketamine and epinephrine (epi), the two medications identified as problematic during rounds. In addition to a larger number of statements that overlapped, there were also no discrepancies evident among team members. Of course, the fact that two of the signoffs were conducted by nurses may have increased the degree of overlap. However, it should also be noted that bedside and charge nurses have very different roles and priorities.

This increase in SMM was reflected in the increase in the overlap index; however, the increase was relatively small because even though the number of overlapped statements increased somewhat, the total number of statements increased dramatically because of the inclusion of the very detailed nursing handoff:

$$\mathrm{O} = \frac{\sum_{i=1}^{n} \mathrm{O}(i) \times |Ti| - \mathrm{D}}{S} = \frac{4 * \frac{3}{5} + 10 * \frac{2}{5}}{275} = \frac{2.4 + 4}{275/5} = \frac{6.4}{55} = 0.12$$

Day 2 AM

On the following morning, we included the following team members in the analysis: Fellow-to-Attending; Fellow-to-Fellow; Nurse-to-Nurse; Nurse-to-Charge

Table 14.4 Overlap table for handoffs captured on day one, during evening handoffs (PM)

Resident	Nurse	Charge nurse
[patient] in Bed 9	Mr. [patient].	This is Mr. [patient].
He is 58 years old as you see,	He is a 58-year-old man,	
sleep apnea,	He has obstructive sleep apnea.	
	(cont.) aortic valve closure on 26th by Dr. [removed].	They had to close up his aortic valve and put…after they took the century-mag out. And, then he had to open his chest again to redo it.
I guess the issue with him is RV dysfunction,	RV function was really decreased	He's on…his RV is still not working that well.
I discontinued ketamine	So I stopped the ketamine 12	That [Ketamine] was D/C'd today.
and I decreased the epi.	epi, he was, I started at 3 mcg and they decreased 2 mcg at 3 p.m.	The epi was weaned down.
nonischemic dilated cardiomyopathy,	So he has a story of severe idiopathic dilated cardiomyopathy,	
a tricuspid repair,		He had a tricuspid ring repair.
	Milrinone was 0.25,	milrinone 0.25,
	Lasix was at 7.5 mg, he was on 10 mg,	Lasix 10
	He is on Seroquel too. Seroquel 12.5 mg for agitation.	They started him on Seroquel because he's been agitated…dex 1, fentanyl 100.
	Neuro wise, he is sedated, he is on Precedex 1 mcg and fentanyl 100 mcg and no more ketamine, still he is arousable, he moves is extremities, -1, he is opening his eyes,	…dex 1, fentanyl 100.
He still is hyponatremic.		He's hyponatremic.

Nurse. The overlap table for this transition of care is included. Calculating overlap index in the same way as described above, produced the following:

$$O = \frac{\sum_{i=1}^{n} O(i) \times |Ti| - D}{S} = \frac{2*\frac{5}{5} + 3*\frac{4}{5} + 8*\frac{3}{5} + 8*\frac{2}{5}}{\frac{275}{5}}$$

$$= \frac{2 + 2.4 + 4.8 + 3.2}{275/5} = \frac{12.4}{55} = 0.23$$

Table 14.5 Team Handoffs' overlap table for handoffs captured on day 2, AM (excerpt)

Fellow-attending	Fellow-fellow	Nurse-charge nurse	Charge nurse update	Charge nurse-charge nurse	Nurse-nurse
Smith	Mr. Smith				Mr. Smith…
He is on nitric of 1	Mr. Smith is on nitric of 1	Overnight we were able to wean nitric from 5 to 1 ppm	So updates, I weaned the nitric from 5 to 1		
But he is positive 1.5.	He is like 1.5 l positive.	he was positive 1.5	he is positive 1.5 l.		Positive 1.5 l.
I gave him Diuril yesterday, I gave him one dose last night.	I gave him Diuril		We gave him 500 of Diuril like 11:30 last night		and I gave him Diuril 500 … I gave it to him like 11:45
	Why, his PA pressure is actually beautiful.	His PA pressures and CVP remained stable	with PA pressures like 40s over teens		PA pressures all night, was like high 40s, highest 51/18 to like 23,
	He is on Lasix drip of 10	he was given Lasix	and Lasix is at 10	Negative he is on Lasix it is 10 mg an hour	so we increased the Lasix drip to 10 at 8 o'clock
Extubate him.		I think the plan is that they want to try to get him extubated			He is extubated
Unfortunately his right heart does not work		His right side is still really bad			He has a bad RV.

The breakdown of the statements in the pyramid is displayed in Table 14.5.

From this table, it is clear that the team has a relatively robust SMM of the patient case and the immediate plan of care. Because most of these clinicians participated in rounds on the previous day, where they had a chance to discuss their different perspective on the case and develop a shared understanding, there was more congruency in their descriptions of the patient. Most of the clinicians on the team mentioned RV as one of the main problems, the main development of the previous shift (weaning nitric from 5 to 1), the troubling fact that the patient continues to retain fluids (positive at 1.5 l), despite the fact that the patient is receiving medication to control fluids (diuril), the fact that the patients' PA pressure is at a good level (a major improvement on the one of the most critical problems of the previous day)

Table 14.6 Overlap table for handoffs captured on day 3, AM

Resident	Nurse
Okay, so Mr. [patient].	Okay. Do you know him at all, Mr. [patient]?
and an aortic valve closure (on 26th).	and aortic valve closure (on 26th).
(and an aortic valve closure) on 26th.	(and aortic valve closure) on 26th.
They also took out a centrum BIVAD.	and they explanted the BIVAD
He had a CentriMag temporary device.	Initially he was CentriMag BIVAD from 05/15. So it doesn't initially, so CentriMag BIVAD and then they moved him over to the heart center
He was extubated yesterday and he was extubated to nasal nitric …	I think yesterday they just decided that when I left in the morning, I weaned the nitric to one. He was extubated around like 11:30 (and when he was extubated, he was put on the inhaled nitric oxide).
(He was extubated yesterday and he was extubated to nasal nitric) and he was on 5 part per million of that.	I think yesterday they just decided that when I left in the morning, I weaned the nitric to one. He was extubated around like 11:30 (and when he was extubated, he was put on the inhaled nitric oxide).
[They have also had him on sildenafil] and iloprost.	and he gets iloprost q.4 h. 2.5 he gets.
They have also had him on sildenafil [Viagra]	He also gets Viagra.
3.2 at midnight.	The other night it was like as low as 3.2 but it starts at 4.
epi at 2	Is it 2 of epi
He is on milrinone at 2.5,	and 0.5 of milrinone.
and amio.	and amio was 0.5.
He must have had atrial fibrillation.	Oh yeah, he was in rapid atrial fibrillation.
and continue diuretics.	and they have been diuresing him.

and the immediate plan for extubating the patient (removing the tube that supplies oxygen through the patient's throat).

Day 3 AM

On the third day of observations, we recorded verbal handoffs of the resident and the nurse on the team. The overlap analysis of their statements produced the following results (Table 14.6).

We calculated the overlap index as follows:

$$\mathrm{O} = \frac{\sum_{i=1}^{n} \mathrm{O}(i) \times |Ti| - \mathrm{D}}{S} = \frac{15 * \frac{2}{5}}{\frac{181}{5}} = \frac{6}{36.2} = 0.17$$

As one can see from these calculations, the clinicians captured here continued to maintain a relatively robust shared mental model of the patient case. Compared with the overlap index of 0.03 calculated for day one, the corresponding index on day 3

Table 14.7 Shared mental model index across 3 days and four transitions of care

Day/time	SMM index
Day 1 AM	0.03
Day 1 PM	0.12
Day 2 AM	0.23
Day 3 AM	0.17

is considerably higher. Here, clinicians have a substantial agreement on the treatment the patient received while in the hospital (aortic valve closure, CentriMag BIVAD), the main events from the previous shift (extubated to nasal nitric), and also on the patients' current indicators pertinent to their care.

Summary

Over the 3 days of observations, we observed four transitions of care when clinicians caring for Mr. Smith transferred the information about the patient and the responsibility for his care. During these transition, the research team recorded different samples of the team members, from 2 (a resident and a nurse or a charge nurse), to 6 (including most of the team members). The overlap analysis of the patient presentations during these signouts showed drastically different levels of convergence among clinicians. These varied from only 0.03 to 0.23 (see Table 14.7 below).

As one can see from this table, the numeric results we arrived at are generally aligned with our subjective perceptions in regards to the degree of coherence among clinicians on the team exhibited during ward rounds. For example, on the first day of the study, when new members joined the team, the level of overlap was very small (0.03). However, it increased considerably for evening signouts, after clinicians discussed the specifics of the case in rounds. The next morning, when most of the team handoffs were captured by the researchers, the overlap index reached its peak (0.23). Finally, on day 3, when new clinicians joined the team, the overlap index went down somewhat to 0.17.

Discussion

Communication in critical care has come under considerable scrutiny in recent years. Communication errors are a leading cause of sentinel events. Handoff or signout has been the subject of numerous studies in recent years. The intensive care unit is typical of a high velocity and high stress workplace with competing simultaneous pressures and numerous constraints (e.g., time, resources and a lack of predictability). Furthermore, the team is comprised of clinicians who vary considerable in their backgrounds and experience. Although patient care is a common objective, there are substantial differences in the work they do and in the perspectives they develop. Formal communication is designed to update and realign the shared understanding of the patient state and how it relates to future goals (e.g, changes in the treatment plan). In this chapter, we present a novel quantitative and qualitative approach to the characterization of shared mental models.

Convergence and Divergence in Shared Mental Models

The study described in this chapter illustrated that a shared mental model is a dynamic construct that undergoes a series of transformations as the members of the team continuously negotiate their shared understanding of their patients. Our analysis of rounds and interviews with clinicians in the unit showed that interdisciplinary rounds play a critical role in shaping of SMM. During rounds, clinicians discuss relevant aspects of the case, clarify their perceptions, and resolve disagreements until they converge on a shared set of patient's problems and goals that will guide future patient care.

After rounds, however, as new patient information becomes available, clinicians form their own interpretations of these new data, and their own conclusions of how to incorporate it into their decision-making. Because formal channels of communication for the entire team are no longer available, clinicians have to rely on informal communication to maintain continuity in their shared mental models. Inevitably, with time, they experience some divergence in their understanding of the case. This divergence may be reflected in their presentations of the patients during end-of-shift handoffs. As a result, the incoming team may begin their shift with already divergent perspectives on the patient cases. This is particularly problematic for night-time coverage teams: because there are no rounds during night shifts, these clinicians lack formal methods for aligning their perspectives on the case and have to rely on informal communication only. Moreover, because the ratio of patients to clinicians is considerably higher during night shifts, time pressures may prevent clinicians from achieving the necessary alignment. In fact, clinicians have reported to us that this gap in communication does happen and its impact on patient care is a source of concern.

Quantifying SMM

The method for analyzing shared mental models we discussed in this chapter can help to capture these fluctuations in shared understanding among members of patient care teams. In the case-study of the patient we observed for 3 days and through six transitions of care, the shared mental model index changed from the almost negligible 0.03, to the considerable 0.23 and then to the somewhat moderate 0.17. These fluctuations were consistent with our subjective impressions of the level of the team's agreement during rounds: when the team had highly divergent opinions, as they did on day 1, their SMM index was at its lowest. After aligning their perceptions during rounds, their SMM index increased considerably. This suggests that the method has high face validity and deserves further exploration.

This method has a number of advantages compared to the existing ways of assessing shared mental models. Because it is based on observations of clinicians in-situ, it has a higher ecological validity than the more direct knowledge-elicitation methods. It also presents fewer demands on clinicians' time and as such has fewer barriers and is easier to deploy. Because it can be deployed frequently, it allows us to see transformations in clinicians' shared mental models and the flow of information between clinicians through their shifts. In addition, it can highlight what types of information are commonly shared among clinicians and the types that tend to be omitted in shared mental models.

At the same time, this method has a number of limitations. Most importantly, it does not allow us to easily account for common ground, or information that already became shared property of the team. In many cases in the study we found that handoffs between clinicians who previously cared for the patient were structurally different from those where clinicians were new to the case. Clinicians already familiar with the patient case tended to omit much of the patient's history and past treatments, focusing instead on the events of the previous shift, and plan of care. In contrast, when new clinicians joined the team, they received signouts with a full account of patients' facts that allowed them to build a solid foundational understanding of the patients' conditions, and provided context for the new information. These differences are only indirectly captured by our method.

We understand that there will be substantial variation in communication overlap. This is due to differences in clinicians' roles as well as other factors such as case complexity, workload and familiarity of the parties involved in the discourse. It is not possible to suggest that a particular overlap index score is optimal under all circumstances. We therefore treat it in relative terms as basis of comparison. It is reasonable to assert that a very low level of overlap may be indicative of problems in communication and presents a potential threat to patient safety.

In addition, it does not support any assessment of the accuracy of shared mental models. In their studies of SMM of combat teams, Lim and Klein (2006) found that both consistency and accuracy of shared mental models were important predictors of teams' performance [25]. We are currently investigating ways to incorporate comparison with gold standards developed by experts into our analysis.

Limitations

This study has a number of limitations. It was conducted in one ICU of a large teaching hospital with a limited number of participants and patient cases. As a result, its generalizability to other settings and participants is limited. However, data triangulation and member checks were used to increase the generalizability of findings within CTICU and correctness and appropriateness of interpretations. In addition, mental models are constructs that refer to internal representations and can only be studied indirectly. While our methods were consistent with those used in other studies of shared mental models, they provide only an approximate view of the real mental models and shared understanding. Additional research is needed to develop more accurate and reliable ways to assess clinicians' mental models of their patients. Our study did not focus on patient outcomes and we can't fully gauge the impact of the observed gaps in communication on patient care. Finally, while the observational study and interviews with clinicians suggested that the design of the EHR system and documentation practices contributed to misalignment among team members, further research is required to better understand the mediating role of documentation on communication.

Conclusions

In this chapter we discussed an approach to studying shared mental models of critical care teams and developing a quantitative index that represents the level of congruence between members of the teams. Comparison with our subjective impressions of teams' coherence showed that our method has a high face validity: when the team exhibited a low level of agreement during rounds, their SMM index was at its lowest. After aligning their respective understanding during rounds, the team received a higher SMM index.

Qualitative observations of work patterns and interviews with clinicians participating in the study highlighted the dynamic nature of shared mental models that change overtime, and fluctuate depending on teams' ability to stay aligned as new information becomes available. Rounds serve a vital role in helping teams achieve such alignment. In contrast, transitions of care present both a major threat to the teams' shared mental models, and an opportunity to maintain continuity in teams' understanding.

We believe the proposed methods can have a number of important benefits. Most importantly, it can allow for comparative studies of factors influencing shared mental models. It can also enable effectiveness studies of informatics interventions designed to facilitate teamwork.

Discussion Questions

1. Describe the concept of shared mental models and how it represents an extension of the mental model construct.
2. What is the significance of a handoff event and why is it prone to miscommunication in a clinical setting like an ICU?
3. How is common ground achieved during handoff events? Consider the nature of this process in the following set of circumstances: (1) when the two parties either

know each other well or not all; (2) the patient is rather unstable; and (3) the protocol for treatment is unclear.

4. Characterize the assumptions used in developing an SMM Index.
5. Why are discrepancies in communication so significant?

References

1. Vazirani S, Hays RD, Shapiro MF, Cowan M. Effect of a multidisciplinary intervention on communication and collaboration among physicians and nurses. Am J Crit Care. 2005;14(1):71–7.
2. Knaus WA, Draper EA, Wagner DP, Zimmerman JE. An evaluation of outcome from intensive care in major medical centers. Ann Intern Med. 1986;104:410–8.
3. Baggs JG, Ryan SA, Phelps CE, Richeson JF, Johnson JE. The association between interdisciplinary collaboration and patient outcomes in a medical intensive care unit. Heart Lung. 1992;21(1):18–24.
4. Shortell SM, Zimmerman JE, Rousseau DM, Gillies RR, Wagner DP, Draper EA, et al. The performance of intensive care units: does good management make a difference? Med Care. 1994;32(5):508–25.
5. Jain M, Miller L, Belt D, King D, Berwick DM. Decline in ICU adverse events, nosocomial infections and cost through a quality improvement initiative focusing on teamwork and culture change. Qual Saf Health Care. 2006;15(4):235–9.
6. Wheelan SA, Burchill CN, Tilin F. The link between teamwork and patients' outcomes in intensive care units. Am J Crit Care. 2003;12(6):527–34. PubMed PMID: 14619358. Epub 2003/11/19. eng.
7. Coiera E. When conversation is better than computation. J Am Med Inform Assoc. 2000; 7(3):277–86.
8. Kohn LT, Corrigan JM, Donaldson MS. To err is human: building a safer health system. Washington, DC: National Academy Press; 2000.
9. Custer JW, White E, Fackler JC, Xiao Y, Tien A, Lehmann H, et al. A qualitative study of expert and team cognition on complex patients in the pediatric intensive care unit. Pediatr Crit Care Med. 2012;13(3):278–84.
10. Wu L, Cirimele J, Card S, Klemmer S, Chu L, Harrison K. Maintaining shared mental models in anesthesia crisis care with nurse tablet input and large-screen displays. Proceedings of the 24th annual ACM symposium on User Interface Systems and Technologies, UIST'11. California, USA: Santa Barbara; 2011. p. 71–2.
11. Cooke N, Salas E, Cannon-Bowers JA, Stout R. Measuring team knowledge. Hum Factors. 2000;42:151–73.
12. Patel VL, Kaufman DR, Magder SA. The acquisition of medical expertise in complex dynamic environments. In: Ericsson A, editor. The road to excellence: the acquisition of expert performance in the arts and sciences, sports and games. Hillsdale: Lawrence Erlbaum Publishers; 1996. p. 127–65.
13. Cooke NJ, Gorman JC, Rowe LJ. An ecological perspective on team cognition. In: Salas E, Goodwin J, Burke CS, editors. Team effectiveness in complex organizations: cross-disciplinary perspectives and approaches, SIOP organizational frontiers series. New York: Taylor & Francis; 2009. p. 157–82.
14. Cohen MD, Hilligoss PB. The published literature on handoffs in hospitals: deficiencies identified in an extensive review. Qual Saf Health Care. 2010;19(6):493–7.
15. Revere A, Eldridge N. Joint Commission on Accreditation of Healthcare Organizations (JCAHO) national patient safety goals for 2008. Topics Patient Saf. 2008;12(1):1–2.

16. Coiera EW, Jayasuriya RA, Hardy J, Banna A, Thorpe ME. Communication loads on clinical staff in the emergency department. Med J Aust. 2002;176(9):415–8.
17. Eldridge N, Revere A. Joint Commission on Accreditation of Healthcare Organizations (JCAHO) national patient safety goals for 2005. Topics Patient Saf. 2005;5(1):1–2.
18. Williams MD, Hollan JD, Stevens AL. Human reasoning about a simple physical system. In: Genter D, Stevens AL, editors. Mental models. Hillsdale: Lawrence Earlbaum Publishers; 1983.
19. Patel VL, Kaufman DR. Cognitive science and biomedical informatics. In: Shortliffe EH, Cimino JJ, editors. Biomedical informatics: computer applications in health care and biomedicine. 3rd ed. New York: Springer-Verlag; 2006. p. 133–85.
20. Cannon-Bowers JA, Salas E, Converse SA. Shared mental models in expert decision-making. In: Castellan Jr NJ, editor. Individual and group decision making. Hillsdale: Lawrence Erlbaum Publishers; 1993. p. 221–46.
21. Orasanu J. Shared mental models and crew performance. 34th annual meeting of the Human Factors Society, Orlando; 1990.
22. Clark HH, Brennan SE. Grounding in communication. In: Resnick LB, Levine JM, Teasley SD, editors. Percpectives in socially shared cognition. Washington, DC: American Psychological Association; 1991. p. 127–50.
23. Nenkova A, Passonneau R, McKeown K. The pyramid method: incorporating human content selection variation in summarization evaluation. ACM Transactions on Speech and Language Processing. 2007;4(2).
24. Mamykina LM, Hum RS, Sheehan B, Twohig B, Kaufman DR. Measuring shared mental models of critical care teams: a methodological perspective. J Biomed Inform. In press.
25. Lim B-C, Klein KJ. Team mental models and team performance: a field study of the effects of team mental model similarity and accuracy. J Organ Behav. 2006;27:403–18.

Chapter 15
Clinical Artifacts as a Treasure Map to Navigate Handoff Complexity

Sarah A. Collins, Lena Mamykina, Desmond A. Jordan, and David R. Kaufman

Introduction

Why is handoff communication such an important and difficult issue to tackle in healthcare? First, let's look at why it is important. Poor teamwork and communication are associated with patient safety errors, inefficient use of resources, and excessive lengths of stay [16, 26, 29, 42, 53]. These are all critical foci of any quality and safety initiatives and are increasingly important in the context of Accountable Care Organizations and payment reform. Transitions of care are a time of heightened vulnerability to errors and delays in care [10, 39, 40].

Transitions of care occur across clinical settings and some are primarily driven by a change in the patient's physical care setting, such as: discharging a patient from the hospital to a skilled nursing facility, a primary care provider referring a patient to a specialist, or transferring a patient from the emergency department to a hospital unit. Transitions of care also occur when a patient's physical care setting does not change

Portions of this chapter appeared in Collins et al., In search of common ground in handoff documentation in an intensive care unit. *Journal of Biomedical Informatics.* 45(2):307–315, with permissions from Elsevier.

S.A. Collins, RN, PhD (✉)
Harvard Medical School and Brigham and Women's Hospital, Boston, MA 02115, USA

Partners Healthcare Systems, Boston, MA 02115, USA
e-mail: sacollins@partners.org

L. Mamykina, PhD
Department of Biomedical Informatics, Columbia University, New York, NY 10032, USA

D.A. Jordan, MD
Columbia University College of Physicians and Surgeons, New York, NY 10032, USA

D.R. Kaufman, PhD
Department of Biomedical Informatics, Arizona State University, Scottsdale, AZ 85259, USA

V.L. Patel et al. (eds.), *Cognitive Informatics in Health and Biomedicine*, Health Informatics, DOI 10.1007/978-1-4471-5490-7_15, © Springer-Verlag London 2014

but the providers caring for the patient change, such in the hospital setting. Within the intensive care unit (ICU), due to the continuous demand for monitoring and care, a transition of care typically occurs every 12-h when each patient is "handed-off" from the outgoing provider to the incoming provider and this process occurs for each discipline (e.g., nursing, medicine, respiratory therapy). Handoff is a formal structure used for clinical communication during transitions of care and is one of the most routine and frequent clinical activities in an inpatient setting [15]. In 2010, Patterson et al., defined handoff as: "The process of transferring primary authority and responsibility for providing clinical care to a patient from one departing caregiver to one oncoming caregiver" [37]. One of the central purposes of the handoff event is to establish common ground between clinicians who are transferring primary authority and responsibility and this process occurs explicitly through conversations and implicitly through shared handoff documentation tools [18].

You may ask, if handoffs occur so frequently, why is it such a complex process? An ICU transition of care does not involve a change in the physical care setting but it does involve two specific variables that significantly increase its complexity: (1) the need to establish common ground of high-volume critical care data and (2) the need to coordinate care among a multidisciplinary team. Common ground is a measure of the knowledge shared between two individuals [5]. ICU patients have high acuity and demand continuous and intense monitoring, which translates to a high-volume of clinical data. High-volume clinical data requires a significant amount of clinician time, attention, resources *and* critical thinking to analyze, filter and interpret for clinical significance. During each instance of a handoff a clinician must prioritize and convey layers of data, information, and knowledge within a temporal story-line to establish common ground with the other clinician. This typically occurs under extreme time pressures. The nature of critical care requires significant knowledge and expertise; this shared knowledge and expertise among critical care clinicians eases the complexity of discussions because it is a form of common ground established prior to the handoff encounter [7]. However, there remains a need to establish common ground for the high-volume of data and information generated during a 12 h shift for an individual patient.

Coordination of care among a multidisciplinary team complicates the effort and complexity of establishing common ground. Handoffs require communication of care plans and decisions between providers and across multiple disciplines (i.e., health professionals) that are responsible for patient care tasks [7, 10, 12, 31, 32, 39]. In reality, these are multiple parallel *and* consecutive conversations that lack formal methods for integration. We know that the increased frequency of handoff is associated with increased patient complications and longer hospital stays [23]. The potential for information loss and miscommunication is apparent at each subsequent parallel and consecutive interaction. The often cited, and highly accurate, analogy is the game of "telephone". Understanding the information flow that results from these interactions is critical to develop effective computer-based tools that support the communication and coordination of patient care in a multi-disciplinary and highly specialized critical care setting. First, to set the stage for understanding handoff interactions and information flow, we will present an overview of prior handoff and communication research. Next, as the focus of this chapter, we will walk the reader through our analysis of the structure, functionality, and content of nurses' and physicians' handoff artifacts. Our analysis will include a discussion of how handoff artifacts can be used to inform the development of an EHR handoff tool that supports the communication and coordination of patient care in a multi-disciplinary and highly specialized critical care setting and implications for future informatics work.

Overview of Prior Handoff and Communication Research

Clinicians within the ICU share a great deal of common ground pertaining to specialized knowledge, yet the care for each patient demands a robust and immediate knowledge of critical and highly complex data. The specific information conveyed during a handoff is often dynamic, patient-specific and conversational, such as information about a patient's plan of care, medication reconciliation, family issues, transport logistics, test results, follow-up care, and advanced care directives [15]. The nature of this dynamic, narrative information poses challenges for the development of structured handoff documentation tools, particularly tools shared among multiple disciplines. However, the types of content discussed should be amendable to categorizations and structured organization in automated tools. The Clinical Communication Space Theoretical Framework is useful to understand why it is challenging to develop tools that structure information and facilitate understanding and communication in the clinical setting. Dr. Enrico Coiera first described the Clinical Communication Space as a continuum along two axes – the amount of shared understanding (i.e., common ground) and the type of interaction (i.e., communication or information task). In this context, Dr. Coiera defined pre-emptive grounding and just-in-time grounding as methods to reach common ground. During Pre-emptive grounding "agents can share knowledge prior to a specific conversational task, assuming that it will be needed in the future. They elect to bear the grounding cost ahead of time and risk the effort being wasted if it is never used. This is a good strategy when task time is limited" [7] During Just-in-time grounding, "agents can choose to share only specific task knowledge at the time they have a discussion. This is a good strategy when there are no other reasons to talk to an agent. For example, if the task or encounter is rare, it probably does not make sense to expend resources in the anticipation of an unlikely event. Conversely, it is a bad strategy when there is limited task time for grounding at the time of the conversation" [7]. The optimal balance between standardized pre-emptive grounding and dynamic just-in-time grounding in the clinical setting remains unknown and is likely multifactorial.

Standardization is recognized by the Joint Commission as a solution to ensure high quality care and maintain patient safety during handoffs and intra- and interdisciplinary communication [1]. Standardization of nursing handoffs has been associated with increased communication of crucial information during handoffs, such as events from the previous shift and treatment goals for the next shift [3].

The Joint Commission and others recognize that safety is a property of systems as opposed to the individual components of care [1, 15]. Distributed Cognition, a theoretical model that posits that knowledge is distributed through the individuals (e.g, clinicians) and artifacts (e.g., computer and paper-based tools) within an activity system (e.g., ICU), supports that well-designed handoff documents and EHR tools reduce the need for clinicians to remember large amounts of information, grounds the coordination of clinical work, and, therefore, reduces information loss [21]. Paper-based documentation suffers from illegible handwriting and barriers to accessibility by multiple clinicians and from remote locations, all potential sources of error in clinical work. Computer-based documentation may reduce the need for clinicians to interrupt each other when attempting to access information [7]; yet, inaccurate data often persists, is difficult to correct, and may have broad and far-reaching consequences if not detected [44]. To support collaborative work, well-designed EHR tools embed the functionalities and infrastructure of the paper they were intended to replace [51]. With the proliferation of EHRs, methodologies from the field of computer-supported cooperative work (CSCW) are increasingly used to understand healthcare work [51]. Successful strategies include the analysis of personally developed artifacts and their use to inform the development of EHR modules that support existing workflow [7]. Insights gained through such qualitative analysis include knowledge of the functions that paper-based tools perform beyond simply conveying information. This knowledge guides the design of collaborative tools and guards against many unintended consequences that surface when paper-based systems are replaced with computer-based systems [51].

Several institutions have developed electronic handoff tools to support patient handoff communication [18, 47, 49], although few have evaluated tools for their impact on clinical processes and patient outcomes. One of the few quantitative evaluations of handoff suggests that computer-based handoff tools can reduce errors [38]. Recent systematic reviews of the handoff literature have shown a lack of consensus and poor definition of the purpose and concept of handoff [6, 37]. Patient safety literature calls for the standardization of handoffs, but the meaning of handoff standardization remains unclear, specifically in the context of the simultaneous multiple purposes that the handoff process serves in the clinical setting [6]. Unfortunately, handoff literature is saturated with anecdotally suggested strategies and mnemonics, increasing the need for high quality handoff research studies that link standardization strategies to patient outcomes to direct evidence-based care [6, 41].

Most handoff literature only focuses on the intra-disciplinary activities of handoff [38, 41, 48, 49]. Health care reform and its focus on coordinated and accountable care will necessitate expanding this myopic focus that is pervasive in the clinical literature. Without doubt, in-depth examination of the handoff process for each clinical discipline (e.g., physicians, nurses) is a significant activity that will contribute to understanding and improving handoffs. From a system perspective (and, let us not forget, the perspective of the patient), handoff is a 'parallel play' process. Nurses, physicians, and other health professionals perform handoff adjacent to each other with minimal interaction or influence between the healthcare disciplines. As these siloed conversations occur, handoff information follows a complex and winding path that is not dominated or coordinated by one particular professional group. Of course this is true! Handoff information consists of data for the *same patient*, but that patient is being cared for by different providers with different workflows and different responsibilities. These unique, complex, and winding paths alter depending on the type of handoff and the clinicians involved. The flow of patient information is often coordinated by two or more influential providers from nursing, medicine, or pharmacy [2]. As key information flows between these influential providers and parallel handoffs occur, examining information gaps and overlaps is a significant activity that will contribute to a broad and systemic understanding and improvement of handoff. With this notion, EHR tools that support handoff of multiple disciplines while enabling the sharing and reuse of pertinent patient data between disciplines may be useful to increase the efficiency of handoffs, decrease information loss, and ensure patient safety [13]. To examine and compare the gaps and overlaps in information discussed and documented between parallel handoffs and overtime for an individual patient, we first need to be able to define what information we intend to compare. In other words, how does a researcher evaluate if the same clinical information that was discussed during the nurses' morning handoff was discussed during the physicians' handoff the night before? It starts with defining types of clinical information. In this chapter we look at how we can define types of information to compare the purpose, structure, and utility of handoff documents. A subsequent chapter uses similar methods to compare the information discussed in parallel handoffs per patient across disciplines.

To define types of handoff information, we use the Interdisciplinary Handoff Information Coding (IHIC) framework. This framework is an empirically based coding framework that provides lists of handoff content that overlaps between nurses and physicians and handoff content that is specific to each discipline [13]. Recently, the applicability of this framework has been extended to analyze information discussed during rounds in an ICU setting, in addition to handoffs [11, 25]. Use of this coding framework helps delineate types of handoff information that are important to nurses and physicians and type of information that are critical to a specialized setting, such as the ICU.

The Cardiac Intensive Care Unit: World-Class Cardiac Care Peppered with Frequent, Complex, and Parallel Handoffs

The study of cognitive complexity and patient safety does not take place in a vacuum. It is intensely integrated within the setting being studied. In this book you will read about many studies and many intensive care units. The Cardio-Thoracic Intensive Care Unit (CTICU) discussed in this chapter exhibits all dimensions of a highly complex system while managing to deliver high quality care. The specific unit we studied and will refer to is a 21 bed CTICU at a large urban medical center. This unit is recognized for the highly specialized and complex cardiac surgical care that it delivers to the sickest patients from all over the world whom have undergone cardiac or thoracic surgery. The study that we will discuss was conducted during the spring 2010 and Institutional Review Board approval was obtained prior to data collection. The range of patients cared for in the CTICU are: (a) post-operative coronary artery bypass graft (CABG) surgery patients that typically require protocol driven, short-term intensive therapy and have a length of stay of a few days with an uncomplicated recovery, to (b) heart failure and transplant patients that may require a longer ICU stay and multiple intensive therapies such as an Intra-aortic Balloon Pump (IABP) or a Ventricular Assist Device (VAD) to support the body's cardiac function. These patients on multiple intensive therapies also have less predictable trajectories.

Research Methods to Analyze Handoffs

At each change of shift on the CTICU, patient responsibility is handed-off: (1) between two nurses and (2) between two resident physicians and/or physician's assistants (PAs). These two sets of highly frequent handoff offer a peak into commonly occurring complexities in the CTICU. We spent a considerable amount of time observing and collecting artifacts (i.e., documentation) from these two types of handoff. During our time on the unit, we observed that each nurse was responsible for two patients (one patient if the patient was critically unstable) and worked from 7 am until 7 pm or from 7 pm until 7 am, with equal patient care responsibilities for the daytime nurses as the nighttime nurses. Nursing handoff occurred twice a day at the 7 o'clock hour and lasted between 15 and 30 min for each patient. The residents and PAs functioned in the same role as each other with the same patient care responsibilities and coordinated patients, schedules, and handoffs mirroring that of the nurses. The residents and PAs worked daytime shifts as well as rotating evening and overnight 'on-call' shifts every few days. Handoffs also occurred twice a day for the residents/PAs at about 6:30 in the morning and anytime between 5:30 and 8:00 in the evening. During the day, each resident/PAs was responsible for 4–6 patients at a time. Overnight, fewer residents/PAs were on duty and each was responsible for as many as 11 patients. During our observations, the clinicians used a commercially developed electronic health record (EHR) for clinical documentation, however, not for handoff documentation. Nurses used two paper-based handoff tools and residents/PAs used a locally developed computer-based application that was not integrated with the EHR. We will present and analyze all of these handoff tools in detail later on in this chapter.

Observations are an important method to obtain insight into the culture of a clinical unit, and specific processes or behaviors of that clinical unit, under natural conditions. Over the course of 5 days, we observed how nurses, residents, and PAs used artifacts (i.e., documentation) during the handoff process and collected the handoff artifacts used by the clinicians. Purposive sampling was used to maximize the variability of handoff processes by CTICU patient type in the context of the patient's clinical status and expected prognosis trajectory. In other words, we sought to observe the handoff for patients that were on the CTICU for a wide-variety of reasons and were experiencing a wide range of health and sickness states and steps towards recovery. For example, we observed patients undergoing routine cardiac surgery and patients that needed emergent cardiac surgery; stable patients with a short expected length of stay and unstable patients with a variable/unknown expected length of stay; and patients undergoing long-term cardiac surgical care, such as cardiac transplant patients. Each morning we asked the charge nurse for a list of patients whose handoffs we should target based on the types of patients we still needed to observe. We observed a total of 9 changes of shifts in the morning and in the evening; during each change of shift we observed between 1–2 nursing handoffs and 1–2 resident/PAs handoffs. We did not target nurses, residents, or PAs based on their expertise or experience. Due to the highly specialized nature of the CTICU, we found that most of the nurses and PAs had at least 3–5 years of clinical and critical care experience, often on that particular unit. None of the nurses or PAs observed had less than 6 months experience. Unlike nurses and PAs, the residents rotate throughout different clinical settings as part of their training. Residents have some acute care (and sometimes critical care) clinical experience before entering the CTICU, but overall, due to the structure of resident training programs have less experience in the CTICU than nurses and PAs.

When permissible by the clinician, we collected the original paper-based artifacts (or made photo-copies of the artifacts when necessary) that the clinicians used during handoff and throughout their shift. These documents were typically filled with handwritten notes taken while receiving handoff at the beginning of their shift, throughout their shift, and for giving handoff at the end of their shift to the oncoming clinician. Therefore, the artifacts collected reflect data entry that lasted throughout the shift. In the case of the resident/PA computer-based handoff tool we collected the paper-document that each of them printed out before each shift. All of the handoffs were also audio-recorded, but the focus of this paper is on analysis of the documentation.

Handoff Artifact Analysis

Artifacts are useful for distributing information through a system [34]. It is precisely that information, and more specifically the flow and distribution of it at given points in time, which we want to understand. Observations of a handoff tend to miss information of clinical inferences, processes, and implied tasks that are a known – or assumed – between experienced clinicians and may not be stated out-loud. Asking clinicians about their handoffs is subject to recall bias. The addition of artifact analysis adds a third dimension (i.e., triangulation) to balance out the weaknesses of observations and recall and contributes to a comprehensive view and understanding of the handoff process. Artifact analysis has been successfully used to study user-designed information tools that support communication and care coordination for the purpose of developing user requirements and exploiting the functionality of the artifact in the environment [20, 51]. The distributed cognition framework characterizes divisions of labor, gaps and overlaps in domain knowledge, the representation of information within artifacts, and patterns of interactions within a system [52]. Specifically, artifacts represent a component of a system's distributed cognition and the analysis of artifacts is informative along two dimensions to understand the nature of clinical care cognitive work: (1) clinicians' creation and use of artifacts to inform clinical work, and (2) information representation with artifacts that describe the nature of the complex clinical work [34]. To understand these two dimensions of clinical care cognitive work, we combined artifact analysis with semantic coding based on a developed framework for a novel two-step data analysis approach. The first step used observational and artifact analysis techniques to analyze the structure and functionality of the artifacts. Our artifact analysis was also informed from our observations of many handoffs where we observed recurrent (largely invariant) patterns. For the second step, we analyzed the content and discipline-specific properties of the artifacts by coding each using the IHIC coding framework.

The specific methods employed for artifact analysis were based on Nemeth's cognitive artifact analysis methodology to understand distributed cognition within an operating room [24, 33]. Distributed cognition consists of four analyses: user, task, functional, and representational [24]. We identified the user as the clinicians involved in each handoff and the task as the handoff process. Nemeth's methods for artifact analysis are consistent with the functional and representational analysis from distributed cognition. We employed our observations of handoff to identify the functions that the artifact served, such as how the artifact was created and used during handoff. Consistent with representational analysis, Nemeth cites that the artifact's structure and content is a highly encoded representation that describes the complex domain work. Therefore our iterative analysis of the structure and content of each artifact, and triangulation of those findings across artifacts, were essential processes of our artifact analysis [33].

The content analysis was performed using the IHIC coding framework. The IHIC framework was developed based on analysis of handoff content from 36 nursing and physician handoff studies and includes a total of 95 handoff information elements. Forty-six percent (44/95) of the information elements are interdisciplinary content (i.e., elements were part of both nurse and physician handoffs). Thirty-six percent (34/95) of the handoff elements in the coding framework are specific to nursing handoff and 18 % (17/95) of the elements in the coding framework are specific to the physician handoff [13].

An iterative process was used to develop consensus on the artifact analysis and the application of the IHIC coding framework. Based on this iterative process, data collection and analysis was performed until data saturation was reached. Consensus for coding was reached during small group sessions which included a nurse informatician experienced in critical care nursing (SC), two informaticians with cognitive science and human factors expertise (DK, LM), a CTICU attending physician (DJ), a research assistant (AS), and a medical student [12]. During these sessions individuals presented their coding of a subset of handoff artifacts and the group agreed on interpretations of the coding framework. After the consensus for coding was established, the nurse informatician (SC) performed coding for all handoff artifacts. A physician informatician (3) performed inter-coder reliability on 32 % of the artifacts [12].

What Are These Artifacts and How Are They Part of a Complex, Sophisticated and Paper-Based System?

We analyzed a total of 22 artifacts from the CTICU. There were three types of semi-structured artifacts used during handoff: two types of nursing artifacts and one resident/PA artifact. The two nursing artifacts, a nurse admission 'Kardex' and nurse personal handoff sheet, provided different functionalities. Both of the nurses' artifacts were paper-based with pre-printed semi-structured templates for hand-written notes. The resident/PA handoff artifact was a computer-based tool that was not integrated with the EHR that the residents/PAs printed out and carried with them for reference and to take hand-written notes throughout their shift. We analyzed a total of a 6 nurse admission Kardex, 8 nurse personal handoff sheets, and 8 resident/PA handoff print-outs. The results are presented to reflect the two step analysis: (1) the analysis of the structure and functionality of the artifacts and (2) the analysis of the content of these artifacts using the IHIC coding framework.

How Do Clinicians Use and Organize Artifacts to Coordinate and Communicate Their Work?

The handoff process in the CTICU is largely similar for nurses and residents/PAs. The process consisted of a conversation between the clinician from the previous shift (i.e., outgoing clinician) and the clinician from the next shift (i.e., oncoming clinician) and was supported primarily by paper-based artifacts (including print-outs of the resident/PA computer-based handoff tool) and occasionally by reference to the EHR or other patient care monitors or devices when needed. Our observations confirmed that the artifacts analyzed in this study were the main cognitive adjuncts that the clinicians used and carried with them to record and reference patient data. The nursing handoff usually took place within sight of the patient's room and involved visual references to the patient and therapies provided. The resident/PA handoff usually occurred at the central nurses' station, not in sight of the patient, and rarely involved visual reference to the patient or the therapies provided.

In the following paragraphs we analyze the three artifacts, first discussing the structure and then the content of each artifact. The nurse admission Kardex was a highly structured and information dense sheet that reflected a consistently used process for the documentation of admission information by the nurse and discussion during handoff (see Fig. 15.1). A large portion of the Kardex included structured areas to document events that occurred during surgery such as time spent on bypass, medications and blood products given, complications and necessary interventions.

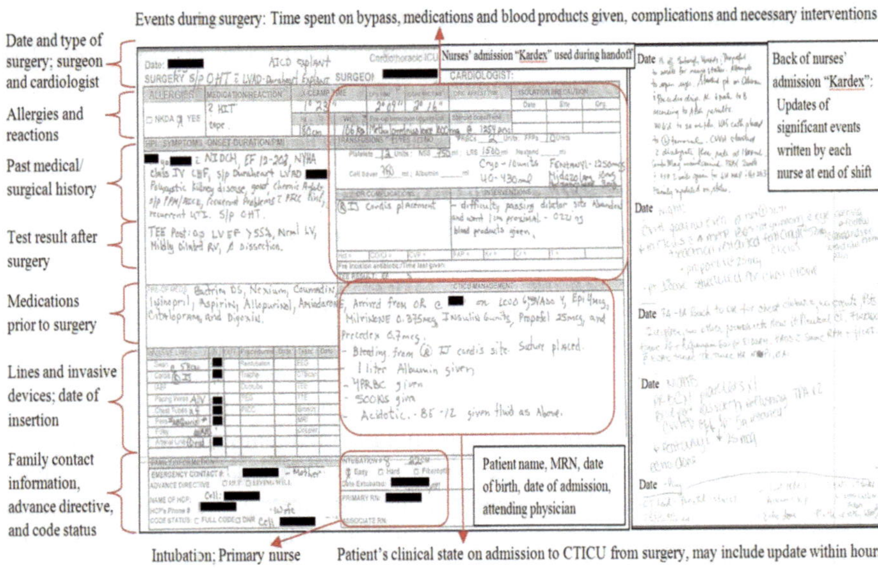

Fig. 15.1 Nurse admission Kardex annotated with descriptions and codes

There was a place to document the patient's medication list prior to surgery and the patient's current CTICU management. The CTICU nurses also wrote on the back of the Kardex, and used additional plain paper as needed, to communicate significant events that occurred during each shift (far right in Fig. 15.1).

During handoff, the outgoing nurse typically began the discussion of the patient by referring to the nursing admission Kardex. The term Kardex is derived from a traditional nursing card indexing system and refers to a paper-based semi-structured nursing tool that provides a synopsis of a patient and is written in pencil so that it could be updated easily for the purpose of communication between nursing shifts [45]. On the CTICU, the nurses' admission Kardex was filled-out once, in pen, for each patient by the nurse that admitted the patient to the CTICU – this nurse was typically designated as the patient's primary nurse who was responsible for coordinating the patient's care. At each subsequent nursing handoff, the nurses' admission Kardex was used as an information source to describe relevant background information about the patient, the surgical procedure, and the patient's clinical state upon admission to the CTICU immediately following surgery. The admission Kardex was kept in a binder at the patient's bedside or immediately outside the patient's room, was not considered a part of the patient's legal record, and was discarded after the patient was discharged. The significant events documented on the back of the Kardex were also discussed during handoff between nurses to communicate important events that occurred to date during the patient's stay in the CTICU. The nursing handoff varied in length depending on the complexity of the patient and the oncoming nurse's familiarity with the patient. For example, if the oncoming nurse cared for the patient the day before, or was the patient's primary nurse, the information on the Kardex was not discussed at all.

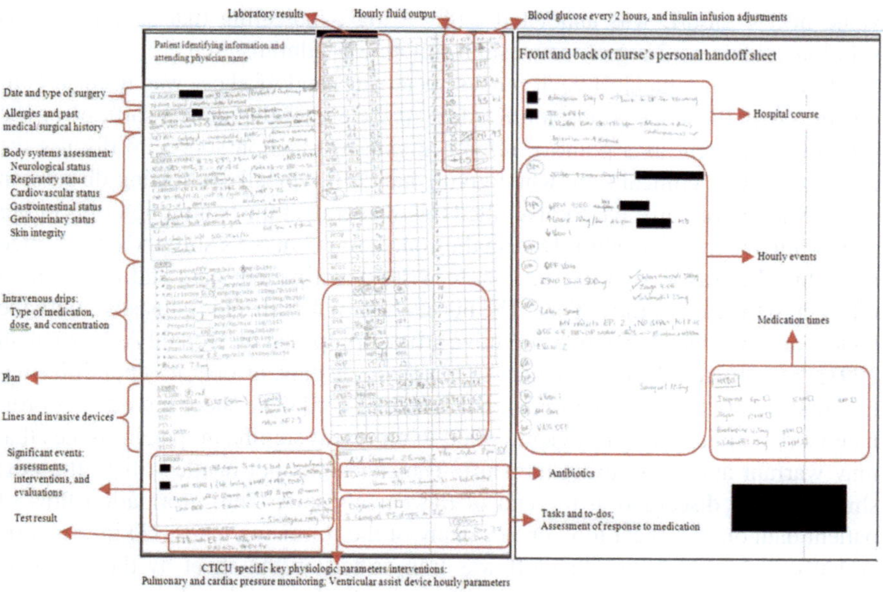

Fig. 15.2 Nurse personal handoff sheet annotated with descriptions and codes

The nurse personal handoff sheet was also paper-based and highly structured (see Fig. 15.2). The assessment of the patient corresponded to the body systems (e.g., neurological, cardiovascular, respiratory) structure. Common intravenous infusions were included in the template with dosage units and concentrations; this structure allowed the nurse to simply enter the dose in the space provided. The bottom of the sheet provided an area for the nurse to document issues and medications. Nurses used this area for a number of purposes such as: significant events, assessments, interventions, medication changes and times, tasks and to-do's, test results, and hourly parameters for interventions such as Continuous Veno-Venous Hemodialysis (CVVHD). As noted in the annotations in Fig. 15.2, the nurses' personal hand-off sheet also contained boxes for specific laboratory values measured up to seven times, boxes for hourly parameters for CTICU interventions, and boxes for measuring hourly urine output, chest-tube output and blood glucose. Nurses also used the back of the sheet to document information such as the hospital course, medication times and significant events on an hourly basis throughout his or her shift. In at least one instance on every sheet, medication information was written next to a laboratory value. For example, in Fig. 15.2, the blood glucose values in the top right corner of the front of the sheet have arrows and numbers to the right of them that indicate the change in the intravenous infusion dose of insulin in response to the blood glucose. These types of annotations were also seen to indicate the administration of potassium or magnesium in response to low potassium or magnesium laboratory values. For example, the potassium laboratory value of 3.8 mEq/L was circled and next to it "20" was written, indicating that an intravenous solution containing 20 mEq of potassium chloride was administered. On the same sheet a magnesium laboratory value of 1.9 mEq/L was annotated with "2 mg", indicating that an intravenous solution containing 2 mg of magnesium sulfate was administered.

During nursing handoff each nurses' personal handoff sheet was used in conjunction with the nurse admission Kardex. At the end of the nurse's shift, he or she used the document as a point of reference and information source to discuss the patient's current clinical state while giving handoff, typically following discussion of the Kardex. Initially, each nurse filled this sheet out at the beginning of his or her shift while receiving handoff. During the course of the nurse's shift, he or she often used this sheet as a cognitive artifact to write down patient data and information relevant to the care of the patient. The nurses' use of this sheet is consistent with the widely accepted definition of a cognitive artifact proposed by Donald A. Norman in 1991: "an artificial device designed to maintain, display, or operate upon information in order to serve a representational function" [35]. The sheet served to coordinate work activities and as a memory aid to represent significant patient issues that may warrant attention during the shift. The sheet was not handed-off to the next shift, but was discarded at the end of the nurse's shift. The information flow of patient data on this sheet took one or many of the following paths: (1) information verbally discussed during handoff was transcribed on the sheet by the receiving nurse, (2) information was transcribed from the EHR onto this sheet, (3) information was written on this sheet and later transcribed by the nurse into the EHR, (4) information was never transcribed into the EHR, (5) information was used as a reference at the end of the shift for verbal handoff to the following shift. Despite the double documentation that occurs between these paper-based handoff sheets and information contained in the EHR, these are highly structured and distinct paper-based nursing handoff artifacts, with consistent data patterns.

The resident/PA computer-based handoff artifact, which was not integrated with the EHR, consisted of four unlabeled free-text boxes that provided minimal structure; yet, social norms influenced the types of information included in each box (see Fig. 15.3). The first box on the far left included the past medical and surgical history, information about the hospital course and the patient's surgery, and test results pertinent to the surgery. The second box typically started with a date and list of the patient's intravenous infusions and may or may not include a dose (never specifying the dosing units). The intravenous infusions were followed by a list of invasive lines and devices which include the date of insertion. Next, there was often a list of the patient's antibiotics, which rarely included the dose, followed by the results of bacterial cultures. The top of the third box often was filled with a problem list, followed by recent events that were delineated by date and often carried over into the fourth box. Often, the recent events were a mix of events, tasks and to-dos and plans. Typically, the last information included was a list of tasks and to-dos which were noted as tasks by the use of an open bracket, close bracket before each task, a common physician practice (e.g., "[ ]f/u TEE result", which means follow-up on the Transesophageal Echocardiogram result) [46]. A list of all active medications was never included on the resident/PA handoff artifact. The hand-written notes on the print-out predominately included tasks and to-do's as well as significant events, plans, and updates about intravenous infusions or test results. They served an instrumental role in coordinating work, but not communication.

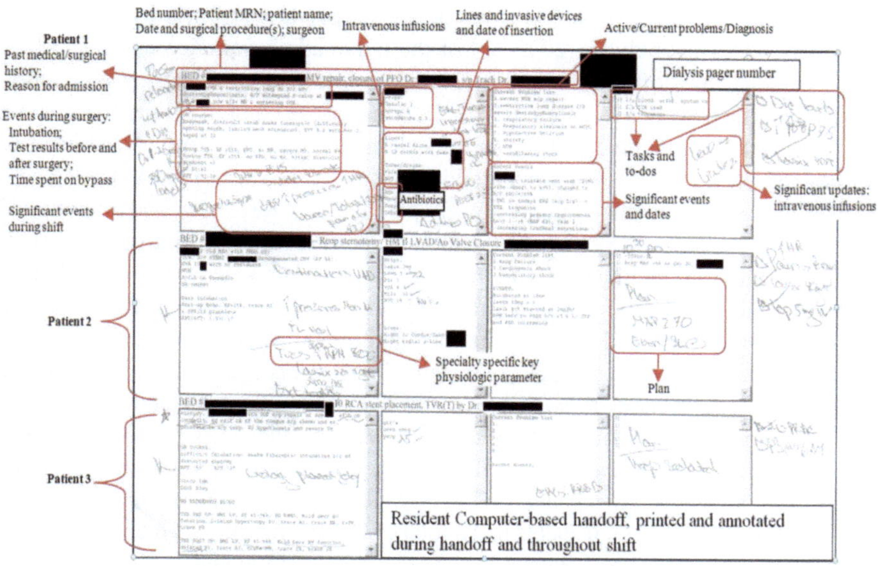

Fig. 15.3 Resident computer-based handoff print-out annotated with descriptions and codes (After this research was completed the CTICU residents began using an EHR integrated handoff application)

The computer-based application was a collaborative documentation tool used by residents and PAs – many individuals contribute to the documentation of a patient over the course of time with no historical record of the previous updates. When information was entered the resident/PA typically included a date; however, there was no record of who entered, deleted, or changed information. The system printed out a document with handoff information for three patients, organized in a landscape format. Figure 15.3 shows a print-out with 3 patients (labeled in the left hand margin of the figure) and the information for patient 1, and some of patient 2, is described and annotated. The computer-based tool was printed out by each resident/PA at the beginning of each shift as a reference and as paper for note taking while receiving handoff and during his or her shift. Additionally, each resident/PA updated the information in the computer-based tool at the end of his or her shift and used that as a reference while handing-off the patient to the oncoming resident/PA.

What Information Is Contained in These Artifacts and How Does it Compare Between Artifacts?

A total of 827 elements were coded on the 22 handoff artifacts. An element was defined as the minimum amount of content that conveyed an independent piece of clinical information, action, or goal. For example, a written reminder to decrease a medication dose was coded as one element because the notation to "decrease" is clinically insignificant without information about the medication dose. Inter-coder reliability was performed on 7 (32 %) of the 22 handoff artifacts by a physician informatician. This included 2 (25 %) of the nurse admission Kardexes, 2 (33 %) nurse personal handoff sheets, and 3 (37 %) resident/PA computer-based handoff print-outs. The percent agreement for IHIC coding of the handoff artifacts was 83 %.

There were 52 unique codes for the 827 elements on all the artifacts. Thirty-two of these 52 codes (62 %) were included in the nurses' Kardex, 42 out of 52 (81 %) of these codes were included in the nurses' personal handoff sheet, and 27 out of 52 (52 %) of these codes were included in the resident/PA handoff print-out. The IHIC coding framework includes lists of nursing handoff elements, physician handoff elements and interdisciplinary handoff elements. Our instantiation of the IHIC coding framework confirmed this mapping of handoff information elements to discipline specific lists for the artifacts analyzed. No elements from the physician list in the IHIC coding framework were present in the nursing artifacts and no elements from the nursing list in the IHIC framework were present in the physicians' artifacts. Of the 827 handoff elements, 757 (92 %) were interdisciplinary handoff elements. The nurse Kardexes had a total of 309 elements (301 interdisciplinary and 8 nursing), the nurse personal sheets had a total of 261 elements (204 interdisciplinary and 57 nursing) and the resident/PA tool had a total of 257 elements (252 interdisciplinary and 5 physician).

There was a high degree of overlap in the specific interdisciplinary codes present in the nurses' and physicians' artifacts. Table 15.1 presents the codes that were present in at least half of the nurses' handoff artifacts and half of the physicians' handoff artifacts. CTICU specific key physiologic parameters and interventions were present in greater than 50 % of the nursing and physician artifacts. Other information that is critical to the care of ICU patients such as intravenous infusions, lines and invasive devices, and antibiotics were included in both nurses' and physicians' handoff artifacts the majority of the time.

Implications for e-Artifacts

Our analysis of CTICU nurses' and physicians' *paper-based* handoff artifacts demonstrated a non-technical, yet sophisticated, system with a high degree of structure for the organization and communication of patient data that functions to coordinate the work of multiple disciplines in a highly specialized unit of patient care. Therefore, computer-based tools, or "e-artifacts", developed to support handoff must further facilitate the communication of patient data and coordination of work above and beyond the existing paper-based system. Specifically, further research should investigate if mobile and touch-pad devices can support the cognitive functions that paper-based handoff artifacts currently provide to clinicians and determine the sustained need for print-outs from computer-based tools. The artifact analysis also highlighted the limitations of a system that is not integrated with the EHR, including a high degree of transcription and siloed information, that have been linked to ineffective communication and potential sources of error in patient care [8]. Our findings of CTICU social norms, semi-structured handoff templates,

Table 15.1 Presence of codes in >50 % handoff artifacts by type of artifact

Presence in BOTH physician and nurse handoff >50 % of time	
Interdisciplinary[a]	
1. Antibiotics	9. Patient sex
2. Clinicians involved in case	10. Patient's hospital MRN
3. Hospital course/summary/current history	11. Plan
4. Intravenous infusions	12. Reason for admission/transfer
5. Lines and invasive devices	13. Significant events during last shift/overnight
6. Past medical/surgical history	14. Specialty specific key physiologic parameters/ interventions
7. Patient age	15. Tasks/To-dos
8. Patient name	16. Test/procedure results
Presence in ONLY nurse handoff[b] *>50 % of time*	
Interdisciplinary[a]	
1. Active medication list	5. Intake and output/hydration status
2. Admission information and date/hospital day	6. Laboratory Data
3. Allergies	7. Patient date of birth
4. Family contact information	8. Patient weight
Nurse[a]	
1. Blood glucose	6. Neurological status
2. Cardiovascular status	7. Patient height
3. Gastrointestinal status	8. Respiratory status
4. Genitourinary status	9. Skin integrity
5. Medication times	
Presence in ONLY physician handoff >50 % of time	
Interdisciplinary[a]	
1. Active/Current problems/Diagnosis	
2. Patient floor/bed number	
Physician[a]	
1. Cultures	

[a]Discipline mapping from Interdisciplinary Handoff Information Coding (IHIC) framework
[b]Presence in either nurse report >50 % of time or nurse Kardex >50 % of time

and the high degree of common ground and specialty-specific handoff content on nurses' and physicians' handoff artifacts makes the case for the development of handoff tools with interdisciplinary views and reuse of data that are tailored to specialty areas. The concept of tailoring handoff content to settings has been cited elsewhere in handoff literature [1, 36].

Artifacts Coordinate Work and Serve as Communication Tools

Handoff tools function to communicate accounts of historical events deemed significant by the clinicians present at the time of the event. Our analysis demonstrated that these tools coordinated work activities and served as a memory aid.

The observational nature of our study cannot conclude if the highly structured handoff artifacts impacted the largely invariant patterns of the handoff process that we observed. We can conclude from our observations of artifact use during handoff that the structure of the handoff discussion was consistent with the structure of the handoff artifacts. Physicians use team checklists in physician handoff notes to organize, manage, and hand off critical patient-based tasks, and that these tasks are often delineated by a preceding use of open and closed brackets in computer-based systems [46]. The communication function of these handoff artifacts was also evident by the nurses' and physicians' practice of documenting significant events on a shift to shift basis and verbally reviewing those events during handoff. Traditionally, a nursing Kardex and paper-based nursing flowsheets display patient information at a glance [4, 19] and narrative notes tell the story of the patient [9]. Yet, summarization is a difficult problem to solve within an EHR [50]. One of the challenges of summarization is capturing the temporal nuances of patient data. For example, the free-text discussion of significant events on the handoff artifacts included information about the precipitating factors of an event, the event, subsequent interventions, evaluation of the patient response to interventions, changes to the plan of care, and anticipatory guidance for next time the event occurs. Capturing such a rich, and clinically important, story is not possible using all structured data. Our analysis and previous work highlight the need for structured narrative handoff tools, a design that blends coded data elements for selection by the clinicians with options for free-text data entry [27].

Another challenge for the summarization and structuring of handoff data is supporting the individual needs of clinicians. For example, we found that nurses who cared for a patient the previous day did not reference the information on the Kardex during handoff, demonstrating that they did not require the same information than clinicians who were unfamiliar with the patient. This finding indicates that flexibility and tailored displays may be useful for computer-based handoff solutions in specialty units.

The annotation of structured data with free-text to convey temporal information is a well established nursing practice [19] and has been demonstrated as an effective practice in aviation to facilitate critical thinking and maintain the safety of air traffic. This link between free-text annotations and critical thinking has been cited as a rationale for why paper artifacts persisted in aviation after the implementation of computer-based systems [30]. These practices may persist in clinical care because they increase situational awareness and serve an important role in maintaining patient safety. For example, we found that nurses circled potassium values and indicated the amount of potassium that was administered in response to that value; potassium and magnesium are important electrolytes to monitor and replace intravenously in cardiac ICU patients, but an overdose can be lethal. This simple annotation conveys (1) acknowledgment of the critical value, (2) and an unambiguous statement that potassium was administered for that particular critical value, possibly preventing confusion that could lead to a potassium over-dose error. The potential for potassium over-dosing errors, propagated by a series of ambiguous and fragmented displays in an EHR, is well documented in the informatics literature [22]. A paper-based handoff sheet is not the solution to medication errors for many reasons, including the inability to share information among multiple providers; however, rigorous analysis of the clinicians' strategic use of handoff artifacts to support communication, coordination and maintain patient safety must play a significant role in the development of specifications for EHR handoff tools.

The inclusion of medication information on handoff artifacts took many forms and differed between nurses and physicians. Nurses included many details about the hourly titration of intravenous infusions and the times that medications were due for administration; the residents/PAs specified the type of intravenous infusions and rarely included medication times, only dates. The Kardex provided an area for the documentation of the patient's medication list prior to surgery, but there was no documentation of an active medication list after the CTICU admission in any of handoff artifacts. Medication data within the handoff artifacts did not provide medication reconciliation functionality, but rather a means to highlight certain types of medications, the addition of a medication, and as a cognitive artifact to support medication tasks. This is in contrast to the assumed importance of medication reconciliation as a critical part of patient handoff [14].

Content Overlap as a Marker of Common-Ground for Patient Safety

Our coding using the IHIC framework demonstrated that the content of the nurse and physician handoff artifacts highly overlapped. Most of the handoff items, according to the IHIC framework, were interdisciplinary and many were specific to the specialized CTICU. The high interdisciplinary nature of these items may indicate that these are the items *perceived* by collaborating clinicians as clinically significant to establish common ground for the purpose of maintaining safe, effective, and collaborative care in the CTICU. Our study was not designed to detect information loss associated with compromised patient safety. Our study was designed to detect overlapping clinical content as evidence of common ground between nurse and physician handoff artifacts. Based on prior work described on this chapter, we posit that evidence of common ground in handoff artifacts is associated with safe, effective, and collaborative care.

This is a first attempt to code artifacts using this coding framework to inform the development of a computer-based handoff tool in a specialty setting. Based on our systematic review of nurse and physician handoff that informed the development of the IHIC framework, the structure of the handoff artifacts analyzed for this study are consistent with the general structure of handoff tools in the literature [13]. Consistent with our findings, a few handoff studies also discuss the use of specialty specific data; Van Eaton et al. demonstrated that a handoff tool that supported specialty areas improved workflow efficiency and patient care [49]. Distributed cognition posits that the way in which information is represented is a critical element of artifacts and the functions and tasks that artifacts support [24]. Consistent with the artifact analysis literature, we found that the structure, organization, and physical location of data elements are critical to understanding handoff artifacts [43]. For example, the physical location of data elements within the document influenced the IHIC coding category because in a given document the same clinical concept (e.g., blood pressure) may be discussed as part of a patient's past medical history, cardiovascular status, vital signs, or a significant event from last night.

The IHIC coding supports the development of interdisciplinary handoff tools that offer tailored views and reuse of data and we suggest its future use for the analysis of nursing and physician handoff content. Nurses tended to include data at a finer level of granularity; therefore, their handoff artifacts contained more data elements than the physicians. Disciplines may need the same type of content but the structure of data input and output may fit the workspace differently for nurses and physicians. Needs may also differ based on clinicians' variable levels of clinical experience. Our findings confirmed that clinicians use siloed discipline-specific handoff documentation. We know that ineffective communication is a patient safety problem within critical care settings [40] and future research should investigate the role of siloed information sources among disciplines as a potential source of error.

A greater commonality of information may exist between disciplines on a specialized unit. Furthermore, a specialized unit may have needs for a greater degree of customization of handoff tools; our application of the IHIC coding framework to the highly specialized CTICU setting supports that notion. The frequent use of specialty specific content in the handoff artifacts, including the consistent use of structured detailed information of events and interventions during surgery, indicated a need to tailor handoff tools to specialty settings. Forcing clinicians to use a less specialized handoff tool that hinders the documentation of critical specialty specific information may, at best, proliferate clinically irrelevant information and, at worst, facilitate information loss.

Treating handoff as a discipline specific process may narrow our view of information flow within a clinical setting. Our findings, while limited by a small sample size, demonstrate the potential value of approaching handoff investigations from a patient-centered view to evaluate the flow of information among all disciplines. The analysis of handoff artifacts from multiple disciplines aids in the understanding of distributed cognition within a setting. We analyzed artifacts that were saved for the duration of a patient's time on the CTICU and used as a communication tool from shift to shift and artifacts that were discarded at the end of each shift. Further research should evaluate the intra-disciplinary content discussed during handoff and the patient-centered information flow of this content between disciplines. Computer-based tools should leverage the type of information that clinicians perceive as clinically significant and, therefore, communicate through paper-based handoff systems. Additionally, the handoff literature should analyze the use of individual clinician's artifacts that are discarded at the end of a shift. Our findings demonstrated that these artifacts support cognitive processes and may maintain patient safety. The successful development of computer-based systems is dependent on a robust knowledge of the distributed cognition of a system, including the integration of the functionalities performed by paper-based artifacts. Artifact analysis facilitates a multi-dimensional understanding of clinical processes and cognitive work [33, 34]. We found that the analysis was greatly informed by our observations of the use of the artifacts by clinicians during handoff. Additionally, we recommended a triangulated analysis of structure, function, and content of the artifact as a methodology to increase confidence of findings and interpretation of results.

In summary, there is a high degree of overlapping handoff content between nurses and physicians. We recommend the design of patient-centered interdisciplinary computer-based handoff tools tailored to specialty settings to facilitate the establishment of common ground. The IHIC coding indicated that physician, nursing, and interdisciplinary handoff element lists may be employed to organize and manage handoff content. The artifacts analyzed were semi-structured which supported the development of computer-based handoff tools that utilize a structured-narrative design [27]. For example, the documentation of medications on a handoff tool may be amendable to structured data entry and the documentation of 'family contact information' may be best amenable to narrative, free-text data entry. The structured narrative design allows a computer-based handoff tool to fuse unstructured text and coded handoff data elements into a single document, similar to the semi-structured organization on the paper-based artifacts analyzed in this study [27]. The scope of data content desired by clinicians for handoff is also significant to the design of handoff tools. Our findings indicated that clinicians included content that is comprehensive of the patient's CTICU length of stay (e.g., admission information through short and long-term care plans) on their handoff artifacts. Other studies cite that clinicians only want content that is pertinent to the next shift [37]; therefore, future analysis should look at the scope of data content for the patient's stay to include in handoff tools.

Looking Toward Other Settings

The data presented in this chapter were from an analysis of one CTICU. There are some differences and some similarities among ICUs. We believe the methods used to collect and analyze the data lend confidence to the discussed themes and conclusions drawn from this study. For example, purposive sampling, data saturation (i.e., no new content and structure themes were identified), and triangulation of data for the artifact analysis increase the generalizability of the findings within the CTICU. Analyzing the types of information included on handoff artifacts across ICU settings and clinician types will help us to understand and define the core type of ICU handoff information that should comprise a patient-centered handoff tool and the information that is appropriate for tailored handoffs in specialty care settings.

A Treasure Map of Complexity, Common Ground, and Implications to Informatics

Effective handoff communication requires clinicians to maintain continuity of care by conveying and documenting intermediate (daily) goals and tasks that are aligned with the intra- and interdisciplinary plan of care [28]. Nurses' and physicians' handoff artifacts in the CTICU were highly structured and allowed for annotations and note taking during handoff and patient care activities. Our artifact analysis indicated that the clinicians used these documentation tools to support individual cognitive process as well as communication and collaboration within a discipline. These types of functionalities help trace how individual cognitive processes are related to the flow of information within a system – they serve as a treasure map to piece together and navigate the complexities and common ground that exists within the ICU. Handoff tools remained siloed between disciplines, yet, there was a high degree of overlap in content between the information contained in the nurses' and physicians' handoff artifacts which is evident of established common ground. Yet, consistent with the Interdisciplinary Handoff Information Coding framework, the level of granularity used to capture clinical concepts differed between nurses and physicians for some types of data. The handoff artifacts were semi-structured and contained consistent types of specialty specific information. Due to the observational nature of the study, we could not conclude if the artifact structure was optimal for handoff. However, our compilation of CTICU handoff data elements based on our artifact analysis indicates that the future development and evaluation of semi-structured patient-centered handoff tools with discipline specific views customized for specialty settings may support handoff communication and patient safety. Future work to design computer-based handoff tools integrated with the EHR in a highly specialized critical care setting needs to include an in-depth analysis of the use of paper and computer-based artifacts among different disciplines and clinicians with variable clinical experience. Computer-based handoff tools that are customized to the clinical setting and enable the sharing of interdisciplinary data may support the cognitive work of individuals and the communication of critical patient-centered data.

Discussion Questions

1. How can the concept of content overlap be used to design handoff tools that support best clinical practices?
2. How can we investigate the ideal balance of content that overlaps between disciplines and content that is discipline-specific in handoff tools?
3. How can content overlap be used to increase our understanding of the level of complexity in patient handoffs?

4. How could artifact analysis and content overlap be used to measure common ground between clinicians during patient handoff?
5. Could the concepts of content overlap and common ground be used to develop a standardized measure of complexity in patient handoffs? If so, how?

Acknowledgment We acknowledge Dr. Dan Stein for his contribution to the inter-coder reliability, Alisabeth Shine, Paul Reyfman, and all the clinicians who participated in the study described in this chapter.

References

1. Arora V, Johnson J. A model for building a standardized hand-off protocol. Jt Comm J Qual Patient Saf. 2006;32(11):646–55.
2. Benham-Hutchins MM, Effken JA. Multi-professional patterns and methods of communication during patient handoffs. Int J Med Inform. 2010;79(4):252–67. doi:10.1016/j.ijmedinf.2009.12.005.
3. Berkenstadt H, Haviv Y, Tuval A, Shemesh Y, Megrill A, Perry A, Rubin O, et al. Improving handoff communications in critical care: utilizing simulation-based training toward process improvement in managing patient risk. Chest. 2008;134(1):158–62. doi:10.1378/chest.08-0914.
4. Brown P, Borowitz SM, Novicoff W. Information exchange in the NICU: what sources of patient data do physicians prefer to use? Int J Med Inform. 2004;73(4):349–55. doi:10.1016/j.ijmedinf.2004.03.001.
5. Clarke H, Brennan S. Grounding in communication. In: Resnick L, Levine J, Behreno S, editors. Perspectives on Socially Shared Cognition. Washington, D.C.: American Psychological Association; 1991.
6. Cohen MD, Hilligoss PB. The published literature on handoffs in hospitals: deficiencies identified in an extensive review. Qual Saf Health Care. 2010;19(6):493–7. doi:10.1136/qshc.2009.033480.
7. Coiera E. When conversation is better than computation. J Am Med Inform Assoc. 2000;7(3):277–86.
8. Collins S, Bakken S, Vawdrey DK, Coiera E, Currie L. Model development for EHR interdisciplinary information exchange of ICU common goals. Int J Med Inform. 2011;80(8):e141–9. doi:10.1016/j.ijmedinf.2010.09.009.
9. Collins S, Bakken S, Vawdrey DK, Coiera E, Currie LM. Discuss now, document later: CIS/CPOE perceived to be a " shift behind " in the ICU. Stud Health Technol Inform. 2010;160(1):178–82. doi:10.3233/978-1-60750-588-4-178.
10. Collins S, Bakken S, Vawdrey DK, Coiera E, Currie LM. Agreement between common goals discussed and documented in the ICU. J Am Med Inform Assoc. 2011;18(1):45–50. doi:10.1136/jamia.2010.006437.
11. Collins S, Hurley A, Chang F, Benoit A, Illa A, Laperle S. DP. Content and functional specifications for a standards-based multidisciplinary rounding tool to maintain continuity across acute and critical care. J Am Med Inform Assoc. 2013; [in press].
12. Collins S, Mamykina L, Jordan D, Stein D, Shin A, Reyfman P, Kaufman D. In search of common ground in handoff documentation in an intensive care unit. J Biomed Inform. 2012;45(2):307–15. doi:10.1016/j.jbi.2011.11.007.
13. Collins S, Stein DM, Vawdrey DK, Stetson PD, Bakken S. Content overlap in nurse and physician handoff artifacts and the potential role of electronic health records: a systematic review. J Biomed Inform. 2011. doi:10.1016/j.jbi.2011.01.013.

14. Daniel DM, Casey DE, Levine JL, Kaye ST, Dardik RB, Varkey P, Pierce-boggs K. Taking a unified approach to teaching and implementing quality improvements across multiple residency programs: the Atlantic Health experience. Acad Med. 2009;84(12):1788–95.
15. Dayton E, Henriksen K. Communication failure: basic components, contributing factors, and the call for structure. Jt Comm J Qual Patient Saf. 2007;33(1):34–47.
16. Fagin CM. Collaboration between nurses and physicians: no longer a choice. Acad Med. 1992;67(5):295–303.
17. Flanagan ME, Patterson ES, Frankel RM, Doebbeling BN. Evaluation of a physician informatics tool to improve patient handoffs. J Am Med Inform Assoc. 2009;16(4):509–15. doi:10.1197/jamia.M2892.
18. Groah L. Patient safety first. AORN Journal. 2006;83(1):227–30.
19. Gurman G, Steiner Z, Kriemerman S. A new intensive care worksheet. Int J Clin Monit Comput. 1988;5(1):27–30.
20. Gurses AP, Xiao Y, Hu P. User-designed information tools to support communication and care coordination in a trauma hospital. J Biomed Inform. 2009;42(4):667–77. doi:10.1016/j.jbi.2009.03.007.
21. Hazlehurst B, Gorman PN, McMullen CK. Distributed cognition: an alternative model of cognition for medical informatics. Int J Med Inform. 2008;77(4):226–34. doi:10.1016/j.ijmedinf.2007.04.008.
22. Horsky J, Kuperman GJ, Patel VL. Comprehensive analysis of a medication dosing error related to CPOE. J Am Med Inform Assoc. 2005;12(4):377–82. doi:10.1197/jamia.M1740.
23. Horwitz LI, Moin T, Krumholz HM, Wang L, Bradley EH. What are covering doctors told about their patients? Analysis of sign-out among internal medicine house staff. Qual Saf Health Care. 2009;18(4):248–55. doi:10.1136/qshc.2008.028654.
24. Hutchins E. Cognition in the wild. Cambridge: The MIT Press; 1995.
25. Illa A, Dykes P, Hurley A, Chang F, Benoit A, Collins S. Mapping HL7 vMR to CCD and hospital handoff codes. AMIA Annu Symp Proc. 2012 Oct 23: 1786.
26. Jain M, Miller L, Belt D, King D, Berwick DM. Decline in ICU adverse events, nosocomial infections and cost through a quality improvement initiative focusing on teamwork and culture change. Qual Saf Health Care. 2006;15(4):235–9. doi:10.1136/qshc.2005.016576.
27. Johnson S, Bakken S, Dine D, Hyun S, Mendonça E, Morrison F, Bright T, et al. An electronic health record based on structured narrative. J Am Med Inform Assoc. 2008;15(1):54–64. doi:10.1197/jamia.M2131.
28. Keenan G, Yakel E. Promoting safe nursing care by bringing visibility to the disciplinary aspects of interdisciplinary care. AMIA Annu Symp Proc. 2005:385–9.
29. Larson E. The impact of physician-nurse interaction on patient care. Holist Nurs Pract. 1999;13(2):38–46.
30. MacKay W. Is paper safer? The role of paper flight strips in air traffic control. ACM Trans Comput Hum Interact. 1999;6(4):311–40. doi:10.1145/331490.331491.
31. Mador RL, Shaw NT. The impact of a Critical Care Information System (CCIS) on time spent charting and in direct patient care by staff in the ICU: a review of the literature. Int J Med Inform. 2009;78(7):435–45. doi:10.1016/j.ijmedinf.2009.01.002.
32. Miller A, Scheinkestel C, Hospital A, Limpus A, Nursing Q. Uni- and interdisciplinary effects on round and handover content in intensive care units. Hum Factors. 2009;51(3):339–53. doi:10.1177/0018720809338188.
33. Nemeth C, Cook R, O'Connor M, Klock P. Using cognitive artifacts to understand distributed cognition. IEEE Trans Syst Man Cybern. 2004;34(6):726–35. doi:10.1109/TSMCA.2004.836798.
34. Nemeth C, O'Connor M, Klock P, Cook R. Cognitive artifacts' implications for health care information technology: revealing How practitioners create and share their understanding of daily work. In: Henriksen K, Battles J, Marks E, Lewin D, editors. Advances in patient safety: from research to implementation, vol. 2. Rockville: Agency for Healthcare Research and Quality (US); 2005. p. 279–92.
35. Norman DA. Cognitive artifacts. In: Carroll JM, editor. Designing interaction psychology at the human-computer interface. Cambridge: Cambridge University Press; 1991. p. 17–38.

36. Patterson ES, Roth EM, Woods DD, Chow R, Gomes JO. Handoff strategies in settings with high consequences for failure: lessons for health care operations. Int J Qual Health Care. 2004;16(2):125–32. doi:10.1093/intqhc/mzh026.
37. Patterson ES, Wears RL. Patient handoffs: standardized and reliable measurement tools remain elusive. Jt Comm J Qual Patient Saf. 2010;36(2):52–61.
38. Petersen LA, Orav EJ, Teich JM, O'Neil AC, Brennan TA. Using a computerized sign-out program to improve continuity of inpatient care and prevent adverse events. Jt Comm J Qual Improv. 1998;24(2):77–87.
39. Pronovost P, Berenholtz S, Dorman T, Lipsett P, Simmonds T, Haraden C. Improving communication in the ICU using daily goals. J Crit Care. 2003;18(2):71–5. doi:10.1053/jcrc.2003.50008.
40. Pronovost P, Wu A, Sexton J. Acute decompensation after removing a central line: practical approaches to increasing safety in the intensive care unit. Ann Intern Med. 2004;140(12):1025–33.
41. Riesenberg L, Leitzsch J, Massucci J, Jaeger J, Rosenfeld J, Patow C, Padmore J, et al. Residents' and attending physicians' handoffs: a systematic review of the literature. Acad Med. 2009;84(12):1775–87.
42. Sexton JB, Thomas EJ, Helmreich RL. Error, stress, and teamwork in medicine and aviation: cross sectional surveys. BMJ. 2000;320(7237):745–9.
43. Sharma N, Furnas G. Artifact usefulness and usage in sensemaking handoffs. ProcAm Soc Inf Sci Tech. 2009;46(1):1–19. doi:10.1002/meet.2009.1450460219.
44. Staroselsky M, Volk LA, Tsurikova R, Newmark LP, Lippincott M, Litvak I, Kittler A, et al. An effort to improve electronic health record medication list accuracy between visits: patients' and physicians' response. Int J Med Inform. 2008;77(3):153–60. doi:10.1016/j.ijmedinf.2007.03.001.
45. Steffen L. Ode to the Kardex. Creat Nurs. 2009;15(1):53–4.
46. Stein DM, Vawdrey DK, Stetson PD, Bakken S. An analysis of team checklists in physician signout notes. AMIA Annu Symp Proc. 2010;13:767–71.
47. Stein DM, Wrenn JO, Johnson SB, Stetson PD. Signout: a collaborative document with implications for the future of clinical information systems. AMIA Annu Symp Proc. 2007 11:696–700.
48. Strople B, Ottani P. Can technology improve intershift report? What the research reveals. J Prof Nurs. 2006;22(3):197–204. doi:10.1016/j.profnurs.2006.03.007.
49. Van Eaton EG, Horvath KD, Lober WB, Rossini AJ, Pellegrini CA. A randomized, controlled trial evaluating the impact of a computerized rounding and sign-out system on continuity of care and resident work hours. J Am Coll Surg. 2005;200(4):538–45. doi:10.1016/j.jamcollsurg.2004.11.009.
50. Van Vleck T, Elhadad N. Corpus-based problem selection for EHR note summarization. AMIA Annu Symp Proc. 2010;2010:817–21.
51. Xiao Y. Artifacts and collaborative work in healthcare: methodological, theoretical, and technological implications of the tangible. J Biomed Inform. 2005;38(1):26–33. doi:10.1016/j.jbi.2004.11.004.
52. Zhang J, Patel V, Johnson K, Smith J, Malin J. Designing human-centered distributed information systems. IEEE Intell Syst. 2002;17:42–7.
53. Zwarenstein M, Reeves S. Working together but apart: barriers and routes to nurse–physician collaboration. Jt Comm J Qual Improv. 2002;28(5):242–7, 209.

Part III
Clinical Workflow

Chapter 16
Re-thinking Complexity in the Critical Care Environment

Thomas G. Kannampallil, Trevor Cohen, David R. Kaufman, and Vimla L. Patel

Introduction

The term "complexity" is used to define tasks or systems ranging from complicated to intractable, and to generally mean "not simple." As noted by a Nobel laureate Murray Gell-Mann, "a variety of different measures would be required to capture all our intuitive ideas about what is meant by complexity and by its opposite, simplicity" [1]. But, it is generally acknowledged that complexity is context-dependent [2], and subjective [1]. While the implications for complexity has been discussed within the context of several settings [3–8], some of these discussions have been met with skepticism (e.g., [9, 10]), provoking responses that the key ideas of complexity theory used in healthcare are often distorted ideas, "trotted out in the guise of complexity" [9], and are merely the "emperor's new toolkit" [10].

Portions of this chapter (including figures) have been adapted from Kannampallil et al., Considering complexity in healthcare systems. *Journal of Biomedical Informatics*. 44(6): 443–447, with permissions from Elsevier.

T.G. Kannampallil (✉)
Center for Cognitive Studies in Medicine and Public Health,
New York Academy of Medicine, New York, NY 10029, USA
e-mail: tkannampallil@nyam.org

T. Cohen, MB ChB, PhD
School of Biomedical Informatics, University of Texas Health Science Center, Houston, TX 77054, USA

D.R. Kaufman, PhD
Department of Biomedical Informatics, Arizona State University, Scottsdale, AZ 85259, USA

V.L. Patel, PhD, DSc, FRSC
Center for Cognitive Studies in Medicine and Public Health,
New York Academy of Medicine, New York, NY 10029, USA

Department of Biomedical Informatics, Arizona State University, Scottsdale, AZ 85259, USA

Department of Biomedical Informatics, Columbia University, New York, NY 10032, USA

V.L. Patel et al. (eds.), *Cognitive Informatics in Health and Biomedicine*, Health Informatics, DOI 10.1007/978-1-4471-5490-7_16,

Complexity theory has been used for studying healthcare management [5], continuity of care [11], nursing [12], and decision-making [13]. While Bar-Yam [3] describes the complexity of the overall healthcare system, Innes and colleagues [14] considered the individual patient consultation as their unit of analysis, and highlighted features of complex adaptive systems, such as non-linearity (leading to uncertainty) and adaptation to the influence of outside agencies [15]. Most of the prior work on healthcare complexity is descriptive, with limited analysis, and thus provides limited insights for researchers and practitioners on how to study and understand complex systems.

Defining Complexity and its Properties

Characterizations of complexity have been adapted from statistical mechanics, physics (e.g., chaos theory, network complexity), computer science (e.g., computational complexity, cellular automata) [16, 17], economics, biology, and philosophy (e.g., time-space dimensions of complexity) [1]. Other related characterizations have used the nature of the task (or problem): "wicked" [18] or "ill-structured" [19] problems have described as "complex problems." While there is considerable overlap among the many definitions [1], significant unresolved issues about the notion of complexity and the nature of complexity science remains [15].

In general complex systems are said to possess the following properties: nonlinearity, open interaction with the environment, self-organization (and co-evolution) and emergence [15]. Several researchers have nominally used these properties to explain the complexity of healthcare systems with examples. *Nonlinearity* is a property by which the responses of a system are not proportional to the applied stimulus, potentially leading to sudden and often, stochastic changes within the system. For example, an increase in the number of patients in the waiting room of an emergency room (ER) above a threshold can cause significant effects on the efficiency of the functioning of the ER – potentially leading to exponential increases in wait times for patients, or shortage of resources and personnel.

Openness refers to the continuous interaction with the external environment, with changes in the environment affecting the outcomes within the complex system. For example, policy decisions such as the health care law have significant impact on the healthcare system. *Self-organization* is a property of a complex system by which higher order coordination is achieved through the interaction of lower order entities. A key aspect of self-organization is that there is no overseeing controller (internal or external) and is triggered through recursive feedback loops. *Emergence* is a coalescence of multiple entities (or agents) to operate together with properties that are significantly different from any one (or more) of the individual entities. From a systems perspective, Kurtz and Snowden [20] explain complexity using cause and effects – the "known" (where cause and effects are known and easily replicable), the "knowable" (where cause and effect are separated by time), "chaos" (where cause and effect relationships are not perceivable) and finally, "complexity" (where cause and effect are not replicable).

The earlier views on complexity (e.g.,[21]) used a functional decomposition perspective – i.e., decomposing a complex system that consists of multiple interacting components into its constituent components. This conflict between the reductionist approach and complex systems approach is well acknowledged [22]. Heng (2008) cites examples of failed efforts of reductionist approaches in medicine – increasing the glucose levels through intensive glucose therapy led to increased morbidity [23]. Other examples include the lack of improvement for survival patients through aggressive chemotherapy sessions [24]. While a reductionist approach is currently considered to be unproductive with current thinking on healthcare complexity, much of the reported research in biomedical informatics still uses such an approach (or a variant of it) to address the challenges of arising out of complexity in clinical settings.

Sources of Complexity in Critical Care Settings

Critical care settings (e.g., intensive care units, ER) represent a prototypical complex system. Complexity arises due to a number of factors – the volume and variety of patients that are attended to, the number of clinical professionals involved in the care process (e.g., physicians, residents, medical students, nurses and other auxiliary clinical support personnel), and the depth and breadth of clinical (and technical knowledge) that is required.

Recent reports suggest that there are about 90,000 ICU and 330,000 ER patient admissions per day in the United States. These patients vary significantly in terms of presenting complaints, demographics and clinical conditions requiring significantly different, individualized approaches with several associated tasks (and actions). Donchin et al. [25] found that on average of 178 actions are performed per patient, per day in a critical care setting. Additionally, the clinical knowledge and skills needed to complete these tasks is ever expanding with increasing disease classifications, newer protocols, methods and strategies for improving practice.

These aspects of complexity arise from what Durso and Drews [26] describe as the complexity of "natural systems" (i.e., the patient). Clinical activities are also significantly mediated by health information technology (HIT) – including medical devices, electronic health records (EHR), barcode medication administration systems (BCMA), computerized order entry systems (CPOE), clinical decision support systems and communication devices that help coordinate and manage activities among clinicians. Though the role of HIT in clinical settings is seen a positive light, the evolution and utilization of HIT is fraught with challenges including its effective use. While the uncertainties and complexities of HIT can be considered as "engineered complexity" (Durso and Drews [26]), the interplay between the users, the clinical needs and their use of technology contributes towards the overall complexity of the healthcare system. Such interplay, often described within a socio-technical framework, is a key characteristic of the critical care environment.

An Approach for Studying Complex Critical Care Settings

We propose an approach for studying complexity that draws on both the complex systems and the reductionist paradigms by understanding the operation of a system (e.g., critical care) at various levels of granularity (e.g., at the level of a physician or at the level of a task). This involves characterizing the interactions between components and the failures that arise during system functioning. This requires a detailed understanding of the system functioning and also new methodologies that help in developing such an understanding.

Our definition of complexity uses a commonly accepted paradigm based on *the interrelatedness of components of a system* [19, 21, 27]. Here, interrelatedness refers to relative influence and impact among the system components increasing with the number of components and the number of interconnected components. In other words, the number of components of a system may make it "complicated," it is the degree and number of relationships between the components, both manifest and latent, that make it inherently complex. This interrelatedness among components of complex systems manifests as properties, or features, of the system, such as non-decomposability and emergence, nonlinear behavior, and in some cases self-organization.

Several researchers (e.g., [18, 19, 21, 27]) have described these properties as identifying characteristics of complex systems. These properties, however, can also be understood as *consequences* of the interrelatedness of system components. *Non-decomposability* is often a consequence of the interrelationships between system components. In other words, such systems cannot be understood studying their individual components. It is important to consider, however, that some interrelations are usually more substantial than others, such that non-decomposability is not absolute. Non-decomposability does not mean that complex systems cannot be studied; rather, it implies that the focus or granularity in studying such systems needs to accommodate the constraints that are introduced as a result of the interrelationships.

An important behavioral outcome of interrelations, a sort of "non-decomposability of actions," is that of *emergence* [28–30]. Interactions between components of complex systems, due to their interrelations, often lead to unexpected behavioral properties of such systems. These properties typically cannot be predicted from the behavioral characteristics of individual system components. A particular form of emergence, self-organizing system behavior, may also occur.

Interrelations between system components tend to complicate responses of complex systems to external influence. That is, as systems become more complex, they tend toward increasingly *nonlinear behavior*. Linearity is characterized as predictability and proportionality of behaviors in response to external influences; increasingly complex systems tend to behave less predictably and proportionately [5].

Summary

In the rest of this chapter, we further explicate our approach to studying complexity. Drawing from a range of studies in critical care including studies on errors, communication during care transitions, and decision-making, we describe how our described approach provides a foundational and realistic platform for studying complex critical care settings. The current focus is to use the complexity perspective to identify, investigate and potentially solve current problems in the healthcare domain. For this purpose, we consider the various senses of the term "complexity" and how they relate to modern healthcare practice, with the aim of facilitating better-informed research approaches to studying complex healthcare settings. The rest of this chapter provides a detailed description of complexity, effects and our approach to complexity, adapted from Kannampallil et al. [31].

Effects of Complexity

One of the critical effects of system complexity is on its "computability.[1] " In other words, there is a cost involved—in terms of cognitive, temporal, or physical resources required or expended—when working within or on such systems. This is the case for individuals working within these systems and external observers who study (or try to understand) these systems. *Understanding, describing, predicting,* and *managing* are fundamental goals for individuals who work within complex systems, as well as for those who study them.

How the number of components and (unique) interrelations between components instantiates system complexity, can be characterized by considering different combinations of these. While it is possible to consider a plethora of conditions, here, we consider four specific combinations. Below we describe the four conditions along with an example for each (Fig. 16.1).

1. *Few components, low interrelatedness*. These are *simple* systems, with low computational costs, making them relatively easy to understand, describe, predict, and manage. These are also readily decomposable with near-linear behavior

[1] Computability is not related to computational complexity.

Fig. 16.1 The range of complexity depending on number of and degree of interrelatedness between components

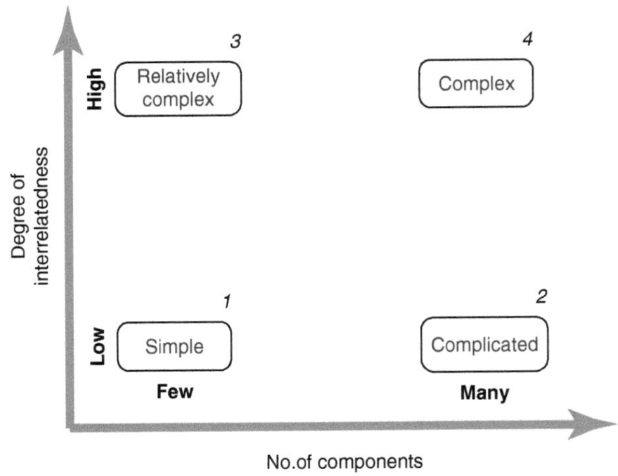

under most circumstances. An example of few components (physician, note, and computer interface) and relations (inputs and computer responses) would be a physician simply copying patient medical information from their hand-written note into an electronic medical record (EMR) interface.

2. *Many components, low interrelatedness.* These systems are *complicated* with a large number of components but with few relations between those components. Computational costs increase with the number of components. These systems can be described, predicted, and managed, albeit at a linearly higher computational cost in comparison to simple systems. For example, consider an EMR system used by multiple personnel (physicians, nurses, pharmacists, and billing administrators), each interacting with the system in a limited manner for their specific role-based tasks.
3. *Few components, high interrelatedness.* These systems are *relatively complex* and require significant computational costs. Fewer components makes them amenable to description but significantly difficult to predict or manage. The interrelatedness also affects its decomposability. Such systems are best studied as a "whole" (due to their relatively small number of components). For example, consider the interactions between team members in a critical care unit during a trauma situation (e.g., a "code blue"). The team responding to a code may include only a few members, but the interaction between team members can be extremely divergent, depending on the situation. Shetty et al. [32], for example, found considerable divergence in the performance (deviation from protocol, errors) between two similar teams for identical resuscitation simulation scenarios, showing the significantly varied behavior of highly interdependent small critical care teams. Similar work on deviations showed variations between clinicians of varying expertise [33].
4. *Many components, high interrelatedness.* These systems are *complex* and have high computational costs. Due to the significant interrelatedness between their large numbers of components, such systems are challenging to describe and even more challenging to predict or manage. For example, multiple critical teams

attending to traumas from a mass casualty event have to deal with multiple patients with different conditions with a significantly changed work environment (e.g., trauma protocols). Such a scenario would be a compounded case of the example presented in case 3 above, resulting in significant number of components (i.e., a significantly greater number of patients and patient care teams) and high interrelatedness (within and across team members) to manage the workflow in the critical care setting.

In order to study the behavior of systems, one has to understand the nature of organization of the components [34]—that is, identify components and interrelationships between components. In conditions (1) and (2), where the degree of interrelatedness is low, it is possible to describe, predict and manage the behavior of the system. In conditions (3) and (4), the significant number of interrelationships between components can cause highly erratic and unpredictable system behavior.

Studying Complex Systems

As researchers in the healthcare domain, we cannot effectively characterize complex systems from a global perspective alone. Given the significant size of the healthcare system with all its components (e.g., patient care, organizational management, insurance, billing, policy, etc.) a more nuanced approach is potentially necessary. As presciently observed by Herbert Simon, decades before the emergence of complexity science as a unified field, one cannot study the complexity of a system without "specifying the content of complexity" [27]. Simon made a case for complex systems to be *decomposed, wherever possible, into smaller functional components* and the relations between them in order to better study and understand these systems. The functional decomposition involves the organization of a system into subsystems, or components, and specifying the relations between these subsystems.

The challenge, then, is to identify the appropriate components and their existing interrelationships. In other words, "one must focus on the right level of description" [35] to cut the system at its seams. This requires significant study of behaviors of components, component interrelationships, and most importantly, whether the isolated subset of the system is representative and appropriate for studying the problem at hand. In other words, a key concern is to focus on the *granularity and seams of functional components* that can be further studied. This is often context-specific and must account for the nature of the problem being solved, and the purpose of studying the complex system (i.e., describe, understand, predict, or manage) [35].

In order to decompose a complex system into its constituent components, one has to first *identify components* (at an appropriate level of granularity). Next, the degree (or strength), uniqueness, and number of relationships between the various components must be determined. For example, while tight coupling between two components signifies linked behavior, a weak relationship indicates lesser dependence. Relationships could also be as probabilistic, correlational, or directional. Slicing, or disregarding, strong or unique interrelationships may have significantly greater effects than disregarding weak or redundant relationships in overall system behavior. For example, for studying physician handoff practices within emergency care settings, it is likely that issues related to the transfer of patient-related information are more important to consider than those related to resource availability or bed management. In other words, the functional slices have to be context-dependent accounting for the important parameters under consideration.

The nature of the problem being solved and the purpose of studying the complex system are often driven by the research objectives and the context within which the problem is studied. In the example presented above regarding physician handoff practices in critical care settings, the creation of a functional slice was driven by the research question (i.e., studying handoff practices). Accordingly, researchers and clinicians should make appropriate, conscious decisions regarding which relationships to ignore and which to preserve, rather than implicitly making such decisions. Toward that aim, the possibility of "latent" interrelationships between components should also be considered. System behavior often varies under different conditions that may or many not expose the nature of relationships between the various components within the system. Some relationships remain latent under most conditions and appear only under certain specific conditions. Such "perturbation" states are important for understanding the behavior under varying conditions. For example, an ED functioning during the time of a sudden influx of patients from a mass casualty event. During this time, workflow, clinician activities, group behavior, and handoff processes tend to be significantly different from normal working conditions. Several aspects of the ED workflow changes, including that off-service personnel are brought in for clinical support, trauma protocols are adopted, and teaching (i.e., in teaching hospitals) are suspended [36]. In such situations, apparently new dependencies arise or weak ones may be strengthened (such as the activation of trauma protocols or suspending teaching, in the example). Depending on the complex problem being studied, it is important to consider varied system conditions and relationships that such conditions can expose.

Another metaphorical representation that can be used to describe our approach is the foreground-background metaphor. For example, one can shine a bright light on the foreground highlighting the considered phenomena. The background from that image will have lesser illumination but would still be relevant in interpreting the context of the foreground. Similar ideas were utilized in the development of graphical representations using the "Focus+Context" [37] views large datasets can be visualized with certain parts in focus with related parts in a contextual background.

Studying Complex Critical Care Environments: Some Examples

One of the purposes of this chapter is to develop an approach for the study of complex systems. As previously mentioned, our perspective is based on the principle of *functional decomposition* of a complex system: the problem to be solved has to be specified, followed by delineating the components of the system and the relationships among them, and, finally, isolating appropriate components of the system for study. While there is no set of general heuristics that can be applied for functional decomposition of every system, the above-mentioned stages can be used as a high-level road map.

Errors Recovery and Correction

Our research on errors (reported in Chaps. 2, 3, 4, 5 and 6) provides a classic example of how our approach for studying complexity was used in practice. The overall research program on errors and error recovery was based on a multitude of studies that first characterized the nature of errors in critical care [38], followed by detailed evaluation studies that helped in isolating the potential causes for these errors [39]. These were followed by a series of studies by Patel and her colleagues that progressively investigated the nature of errors in a variety of treatment conditions thereby identifying the potential contributors, causes and the underlying cognitive mechanisms of error generation, detection and recovery [40] in laboratory-based (also in Chap. 3) and semi-naturalistic settings (Chap. 4). Some of the key factors that were identified that influenced error detection and recovery include the nature of expertise, case complexity, task complexity, and team interactions.

The authors extended these studies to the naturalistic clinical environment (In vivo), where the constraints in the natural environments on error generation, detection and recovery are different (Chap. 5). Finally, Cohen and colleagues began to address the issues of training for error detection and correction in virtual environments [37]. The successful identification of the error correction and detection mechanisms was instrumental in re-creating the evaluation studies on error in virtual environments (Chap. 6).

Communication During Care Transitions

One of the key aspects of clinical work is communication between the care providers. Effective communication between care providers affects the quality of patient care, reduces the potential for errors and improves patient safety. Communication takes an even more central role in the case of care transitions (or handoffs) (Chap. 12 and 13) where care responsibility is transferred from an outgoing clinician to an incoming clinician. Prior research had often focused on characterizing and understanding these transitions as a discrete communication activity, independent of other surrounding activities that are relevant for handoffs. This would be representative of a typical reductionist approach to studying the complex process of handoffs.

Studies conducted over a 3-year period that included observations, clinician shadowing and interviews contextualized the latent relationships that existed during handoffs. In other words, while handoff in itself was an isolated care-related activity, it must be considered within the context of the workflow within the critical care setting. Based on this understanding, our approach to studying handoff was situated on evaluating the communication of handoff workflow rather than the communication alone. This led to the development of a handoff intervention tool [41] that was designed to support the overall handoff workflow as opposed to the communication aspect alone.

Handoff is also part of a series of formal communication events that serve to realign the shared mental models (SMM) that enable the coordination of care (Chap. 14). A clinical ICU team is constituted by a wide range of providers with different levels of expertise, background and roles. However, care coordination is predicated on whether clinicians can converge on common understanding regarding the current state of the patient, the change of the state over time and common objectives regarding treatment. Handoffs serve to locally realign SMM between two individuals from a common discipline (e.g., residents, nurses) and rounds may provide an opportunity for a broader realignment. Mamykina and colleagues developed a measure or index for characterizing SMM by quantifying the overlap in discourse. The overlap analysis of hand showed highly variable levels of convergence among clinicians. Interestingly, Collins et al. (Chap. 15) studied the structure of clinical documents and found that there is a high degree of overlapping handoff content between nurses and physicians. This manifested itself in the kinds of content, rather than in the specific detail. Although there are a host of factors that contribute to misalignment and fragmentation, it is our contention that improvements in EHRs can play an important mediating role in bolstering SMM.

Methodological Approaches

One of the insightful aspects of our multi-year study on the complexity and error in critical care is the significant developments that we made in terms of the methodological improvements to capture the variance and changes in a critical care unit. For example, one of the aspects we have been successful in obtaining in terms of a systems complexity perspective is the analysis of the activities of clinicians in critical care settings using Radio-frequency identification (RFID) tags [42, 43]. Using RFID sensors we were able to unobtrusively characterize the activities of clinicians thereby able to reliably predict their tasks, interaction with other clinicians, movement patterns in the ER, and patterns of collaboration and predicting the work practices.

Another example of the methodological approach that we used to account for the complexity is to adopt a temporally oriented evaluation approach. In other words, as opposed to collecting data on discrete events, we captured events (and activities) that unfolded over the course of hours (and sometimes, days). Such an approach was used in several studies including those studying shared mental models in communications (Chap. 14), handoffs (Chap. 12) and deviations from protocols (Chap. 8).

To analyze communication, one needs to be able to segment time to both characterize discrete events and continuity over multiple events stretching over longer periods of time. A shared mental model approach is predicated on understanding how clinicians individually and jointly understand the prior state or states of a patient that have resulted or contributed to the current patient state and they need to project forward to a future state. Handoffs are communication events that focus most intently on the prior 12 h that correspond with a typical shift by a clinician completing a shift and they project forward to the subsequent 12 h for the clinician beginning their shift (See Chap. 14). In many critical settings, multiple handoffs occur in parallel and the degree of convergence is highly variable. This can lead to gaps in communication and can compromise patient safety.

In related research on handoffs we utilized a clinician-centered approach to capture the handoff process. Such an approach helped in identifying the intricate dependencies that existed between the handoffs and the clinical workflow activities that would otherwise have been impossible to identify. A similar trace-based approach was used to identify the nature and evolution of deviations from trauma protocols [33]. This research continues to evolve using technological innovations afforded by sensors, and algorithmic techniques to capture the work activities in a challenging clinical environment.

Conclusion

The specific nature of modern healthcare work renders it particularly amenable to functional decomposition, as work is distributed between actors (physicians, nurses, residents, and other clinical support staff) and artifacts (information technology, machines, paper notes) (e.g., see [44–46]). There is often a *structure* in the relationships that exist between care providers, artifacts, and patients. While some relationships are apparent, others manifest only under certain conditions. As such, it is possible to characterize it as a network of actors, where (at a high level of decomposition) the nodes are actors (or artifacts) and the edges are their relationships. For example, the ED can be considered as a complex network of clinicians (attending physicians, residents, nurses), patients, and information technologies that are used to manage patient care. To study handoff activities in the ED, one has to consider the clinicians involved (actors), artifacts used (paper and electronic records) and information being transferred. Handoff activities can be considered as a sub-network within the larger ED network. In short, the distributed and fairly structured organization of health care settings makes the functional decomposition approach viable.

As with any research approach, there are potential disadvantages to functional decomposition. First, the process of selectively including some components or interrelations and disregarding others may lead to oversimplification of the problem. Second, creating progressively smaller slices of a complex system imposes greater demands toward understanding components and their intricate web of interrelationships to other components. Moreover, using a microstructure level of explanation maybe difficult for people outside the field to conceptualize. In spite of these limitations, we believe that our approach is a useful and systematic mechanism for understanding complexity in healthcare settings.

References

1. Gell-Mann M. What is complexity. Complexity. 1995;1(1):16–9.
2. Mainzer K. Thinking in complexity. New York: Springer; 1997.
3. Bar-Yam Y. Improving the effectiveness of health care and public health: a multiscale complex systems analysis. Am J Public Health. 2006;96:459–66.
4. Leape LL, Berwick DM. Five years after to err is human what have we learned? J Am Med Assoc. 2005;293(19):2384–90.
5. Plsek PE, Greenhalgh T. Complexity science: the challenge of complexity in health care. BMJ. 2001;323(7313):625–8.
6. Wilson T, Holt T, Greenhalgh T. Complexity science: complexity and clinical care. BMJ. 2001;323(7314):685–8.
7. Patel VL, Cohen T. New perspectives on error in critical care. Curr Opin Crit Care. 2008;14(4):456–9.
8. Smith M, Feied C. The emergency department as a complex system: New England Complex Systems Institute; 2006. Cited 30 July 2010. Available from: http://www.necsi.edu/projects/yaneer/emergencydeptcx.pdf.
9. Paley J. Complex adaptive systems and nursing. Nurs Inq. 2007;14(3):233–42.
10. Reid I. Let them eat complexity: the emperor's new toolkit. BMJ. 2002;324(7330):171.
11. Strumberg JP. Continuity of care: a systems based approach. Asia Pac Fam Med. 2003;2:136–42.
12. MacDonald MA. From miasma to fractals: the epidemiology revoluation and public health nursing. Public Health Nurs. 2004;21:380–91.
13. Clancy TR, Delaney CW. Complex nursing systems. J Nurs Manag. 2005;13:192–201.
14. Innes AD, Campion PD, Griffiths FE. Complex consultations and the 'edge of chaos'. Br J Gen Pract. 2005;55(510):47.
15. Phelan SE. What is complexity science, really? Emergence. 2001;3(1):120–6.
16. Hartmanis J, Stearns R. On the computational complexity of algorithms. Trans Am Math Soc. 1965;117:285–306.
17. Turing A. On computable numbers, with an application to the Etscheidungs problem. Proceedings of the London Mathematical Society; 1936;2(42):230–65.
18. Rittel H, Webber M. Dilemmas in a general theory of planning. Policy Sci. 1973;4:155–69.
19. Simon HA. Structure of ill-structured problems. Artif Intell. 1973;4(3–4):181–201.
20. Kurtz CF, Snowden DJ. The dynamics of strategy: sense-making in a complex and complicated world. IBM Syst J. 2003;42(3):462–83.
21. Simon HA. The architecture of complexity. Proceedings of the American Philosophical Society; 1962. p. 467–82.
22. Heng HQ. The conflict between complex systems and reductionism. JAMA. 2008;300(13):1580–1.
23. Gerstein HC, Miller ME, Byington RP, et al. Effects of intensive glucose lowering in type 2 diabetes. N Engl J Med. 2008;358(24):2545–59.
24. Savage L. High-intensity chemotherapy does not improve survival in small cell lung cancer. J Natl Canc Inst. 2008;100:519.

25. Donchin Y, Gopher D, Olin M, Badihi Y, Biesky M, Sprung CL, et al. A look into the nature and causes of human errors in the intensive care unit. Crit Care Med. 1995;23(2):294–300.
26. Durso FT, Drews F. Health care, aviation, and ecosystems: a socio-natural systems perspective. Curr Dir Psychol Sci. 2010;19:71–5.
27. Simon HA. The sciences of the artificial. Cambridge: MIT Press; 1996.
28. Coveney P, Highfield R. Frontiers of complexity: the search for order in a chaotic world. New York: Ballantine Publishing Group; 1995.
29. Gallagher R, Appenzeller T. Beyond reductionism. Science. 1999;248:79.
30. Johnson S. Emergence: the connected lives of ants, brain, cities, and software. New York: Simon and Shuster; 2001.
31. Kannampallil TG, Schauer GF, Cohen T, Patel VL. Considering complexity in healthcare systems. J Biomed Inform. 2011;44(6):443–7.
32. Shetty P, Cohen T, Patel B, Patel VL. The cognitive basis of effective team performance: features of failure and success in simulated cardiac resuscitation. Proceedings of the 2009 AMIA Annu Symp. 2009. p. 599–603.
33. Kahol K, Vankipuram M, Patel VL, Smith ML. Deviations from protocol in a complex trauma environment: errors or innovations? J Biomed Inform. 2011;44(3):425–31.
34. Weaver W. Science and complexity. Am Sci. 1948;36(4):536.
35. Goldenfeld N, Kadanoff LP. Simple lessons from complexity. Science. 1999;284(5411):87–9.
36. Reddy M, Paul S, Abraham J, McNeese M, DeFlitch C, Yen J. Challenges to effective crisis management: using information and communication technologies to coordinate emergency medical services and emergency department teams. Int J Med Inform. 2009;78:259–69.
37. Razzouk E, Cohen T, Almoosa KF, Patel VL, editors. Approaching the limits of knowledge: the influence of priming on error detection in simulated clinical rounds. Proceedings of the annual American Medical Informatics Association (AMIA) symposium, Washington DC, 2011.
38. Zhang J, Patel VL, Johnson TR, Shortliffe EH. A cognitive taxonomy of medical errors. J Biomed Inform. 2004;37(3):193–204.
39. Kubose TT, Patel VL, Jordan D. Dynamic adaptation to critical care medical environment: error recovery as cognitive activity. Proceedings of the 2002 Cognitive Science Society; 2002. p. 43.
40. Patel VL, Cohen T, Murarka T, Olsen J, Kagita S, Myneni S, et al. Recovery at the edge of error: debunking the myth of the infallible expert. J Biomed Inform. 2010;44(3):413–24. PubMed PMID: 20869466.
41. Abraham J, Kannampallil T, Patel VL. Bridging gaps in handoffs: a continuity of care approach. J Biomed Inform. 2012;45(2):240–54.
42. Kannampallil TG, Li Z, Zhang M, Cohen T, Robinson DJ, Franklin A, et al. Making sense: sensor-based investigation of clinician activities in complex critical care environments. J Biomed Inform. 2011;44(3):441–54. Epub 2011/02/25. eng.
43. Vankipuram M, Kahol K, Cohen T, Patel VL. Toward automated workflow analysis and visualization in clinical environments. J Biomed Inform. 2011;44(3):432–40.
44. Bardram JE. Activity-based computing for medical work in hospitals. ACM Trans Comput Hum Interact. 2009;16(2):1–36.
45. Berg M. Accumulating and coordinating: occasions for information technologies in medical work. J Comput Support Coop Work. 1999;8(4):373–401.
46. Cohen T, Blatter B, Almeida C, Shortliffe E, Patel VL. Distributed cognition in the psychiatric emergency department: a cognitive blueprint of a collaboration in context. Artif Intell Med. 2006;37:73–83.

Chapter 17
Automated Workflow Analysis and Tracking Using Radio Frequency Identification Technology

Mithra Vankipuram, Thomas G. Kannampallil, Zhe (Eric) Li, and Kanav Kahol

Introduction

The health care industry faces a number of challenges and arguably one of the most important ones lies in maintaining high levels of patient safety. A much-cited report released by the Institute of Medicine [1] estimates that as many as 98,000 people die each year due to medical errors [1]. The causal determinants of these errors can be traced to a variety of medical, cognitive and social challenges in the clinical workplace. These challenges are exacerbated in critical care environments that are characterized by distributed, interdependent, episodic and non-linear work activities. The dynamic nature of the care process in critical care environment affects the nature and timing of work activities of clinicians, and often increases the possibility

---

Portions of this chapter has appeared in (a) Vankipuram et al., Toward automated workflow analysis and visualization in clinical environments. *Journal of Biomedical Informatics*. 44(3): 432–440, with permissions from Elsevier; (b) Kannampallil et al., Making sense: sensor-based investigation of clinician activities in complex critical care environments, *Journal of Biomedical Informatics*. 44(3), 441–454, with permissions from Elsevier and (c) an article in the Proceedings of the 2009 Annual Symposium American Medical Informatics Association, Vankipuram et al., *Visualization and analysis of activities in critical care environments*.

M. Vankipuram, MS, PhD (✉)
Analytics Lab, Hewlett-Packard (HP) Labs, Palo Alto, CA 94304, USA
e-mail: vankipuram.mithra@gmail.com

T.G. Kannampallil
Center for Cognitive Studies in Medicine and Public Health, New York Academy of Medicine, New York, NY 10029, USA

Z. (Eric) Li, MS
Drchrono Inc., Mountain View, CA 94043, USA

K. Kahol, PhD
Affordable Health Technologies Division, Public Health Foundation of India, New Delhi, India

Health Informatics, DOI 10.1007/978-1-4471-5490-7_17,

of errors. Studying the work activities of clinicians in such environments can help in understanding the care delivery process, workflow, and interruptions that affect clinical work.

Exploratory investigations of clinician activities are often performed using observational methods. While these methods provide a descriptive depth that cannot be matched by automated methods, use of participant observation methods [2, 3] in a critical care setting is often challenging, as capturing the work activities of multiple clinicians requires several observers who must be closely synchronized during their data capture sessions. The tools currently used for workflow analysis in clinical environments include methods such as ethnographic observation, shadowing of individual clinicians, surveys and questionnaires [4]. The data collected by these methods can be used to model work activities centered on a particular individual (or a group) and their activities [5]. Such approaches sometimes are inadequate to develop a holistic and complete picture of work activities. For example, observations are gathered from an individual's point of view and may not be adequate to capture multiple activities occurring within a clinical environment. Though it is plausible to capture additional activities by increasing the number of observers, such an approach is highly likely to disrupt clinical activities. Given these constraints in complex critical care environments, there is a need for an unobtrusive alternative that can augment existing methods of data collection and enable piecing together a more complete workflow, understanding the nuances of underlying activities, interactions and dependencies.

Tools that can be used to monitor continuous activities in clinical environments can provide significant insights into the work activities in clinical environments. Radio-frequency Identification (RFID) technology offers a seamless, cheap and effective mechanism for monitoring and tracking events within clinical environments. In this chapter, we describe the potential and use of RFID-based sensors for reliably capturing the activities, mobility and interactions of clinicians. This chapter is based on aggregated results from our previously published work that on the use of RFID technology in critical care settings [6–8].

Background

Complexity and Critical Care Workflow

The study of complex systems draws together emerging approaches from several diverse fields including economics, physics, biology, mathematics and computer science on the common ground of complexity. This interdisciplinary effort seeks to formulate unifying principles of complexity. Several authors have proposed that the healthcare system or elements thereof can be characterized as a complex system [9–13]. For example, Smith and Feied [13] argue that an emergency department is a *paradigmatic complex system*. This argument rests on the unpredictability of both patients' clinical conditions and clinicians' work patterns, the vast decision space and incomplete evidence that complicate clinical decision-making and the inherent unpredictability of the system as a whole.

Several concepts drawn from the complex systems literature are pertinent to the study of a critical care unit as a complex cognitive system. A cogent and readable account of the ways in which concepts from the complexity literature might be applied to social systems has been developed by the Complexity in Social Science [14] project [14]. Complex systems are by their nature non-deterministic and dynamically structured. That is to say, it is not possible to predict the behavior of a complex system by studying the function of its components in isolation, and furthermore the study of the behavior of any such component reveals little about the system as a whole. Likewise, the process of clinical care emerges from a series of dynamic and flexible interactions between patients, health-care providers and outside influences [15]. While this argument applies readily to workflow, it also relates to the cognitive processes that underlie critical care decision making, as the cognitive processes in critical care settings are distributed across the minds of the clinical team and a range of physical media [16]. Given the complex nature of system behavior, it is not possible to predict the knowledge, expertise and information that will be available at the point in time at which clinical decisions are made. Similarly, for transfer of information, it has been observed that within complex social systems the flow of information is determined somewhat serendipitously by the geographical location of team members [17], which is influenced in turn by the complex dynamics of the system as a whole.

These aspects of the critical care workplace present challenges for the human-intensive ethnographic methods that have been previously employed. However, complex systems theory suggests that only limited insight into system behavior can be obtained through the study of component parts. Consequently, there is a role for automated sensors to complement the human-intensive data collection methods that have been employed previously. While not able to capture the depth and richness of representation that are possible through ethnographic methods, these sensors offer certain advantages in that it is possible to collect data concerning a geographically mobile clinical team over an entire shift. This is desirable, as even an exceptionally well-funded research program that may be able to employ multiple well-trained human observers is likely to experience problems integrating a team of observers into a busy clinical environment without obstructing patient care.

RFID Sensor Technology

Recent times have seen a prolific increase in the use of radio frequency identification (RFID) devices in clinical settings. This is driven by early research results that have shown that RFID technology can improve better tracking of patients, more effective and safer drug administration and lower monitoring costs. Potential advantages not withstanding, the widespread adoption has been tempered by the lack of consistent results regarding the viability of real time location systems (RTLS) in clinical settings. RFID tools have been used in a variety of applications including locating healthcare professionals, tracking patient flows, equipment and medication, and improving hospital-wide throughput, bed management, and workflow [18–21].

Sensors typically used for entity activity recognition include passive infrared sensors, radio identification tags and pressure sensors. For example, Fry and Lenert [22] developed a system for location tracking of patients, staff and equipment called MASCAL. RFID sensors were used to track clinicians and equipment during mass casualty events. Sensor tracking data was combined with personnel and clinical information to centralize the management of resources. In a related study, Chen et al. [23] describe the use of RFID sensors to identify patients, and notify clinicians on patient related information that decreased the waiting time for patients in intensive care units.

Sensor technology used for the studies described in this chapter was an active RFID system. The system is composed of *tags* and *base stations* that are used to capture the movement and interactions between the clinicians in critical care settings. Tags are mobile devices that help in the tracking of moving objects. Base stations are stationary devices that provide radio coverage and tracking of the tags. The tags and base stations communicate using a vendor-customized *IP-Lite* radio connection protocol. During data collection sessions, clinicians carried the RFID tags (i.e., the sensors) in the pockets of their coats. Base stations were placed at key locations to capture their movements and the transitions between spaces such as patient rooms. As a clinician carrying a tag comes in close physical proximity with a base station, a ping event is registered with that base station. This is referred to as a *tag-base* ping. The strength of ping event is measured in terms of received signal strength index (RSSI). Additionally, when two clinicians come in close proximity to each other, a *tag-tag* ping is registered. As with the tag-base pings, the relative physical distance between the clinicians is reflected in the signal strength of the tag-tag pings. The tags and base stations send pings at approximately 3-s intervals. In other words, for every 3 s, each tag registered with a corresponding base station in its vicinity.

Figure 17.1 shows the configuration of tags and base stations and how ping events are registered between them. In Fig. 17.1, interactions between three tags and one base station are shown. The tags register pings with each other (tag-tag pings, represented as n1, n2 and n3) and, concurrently register pings to the common base station (m1, m2 and m3 pings). The tag-tag and the tag-base pings are used for the identification of the location of a clinician (or multiple clinicians) and their collaborators at any particular point in time. The tag-tag interactions provide an additional dimension (of co-location of clinicians) through which to interpret the actions of the clinicians.

We use an illustrative example of how some activities in the clinical environments can be captured by appropriate placement of tags and base stations. Consider the scenario representing patient arrival is depicted in Fig. 17.2. First, key members

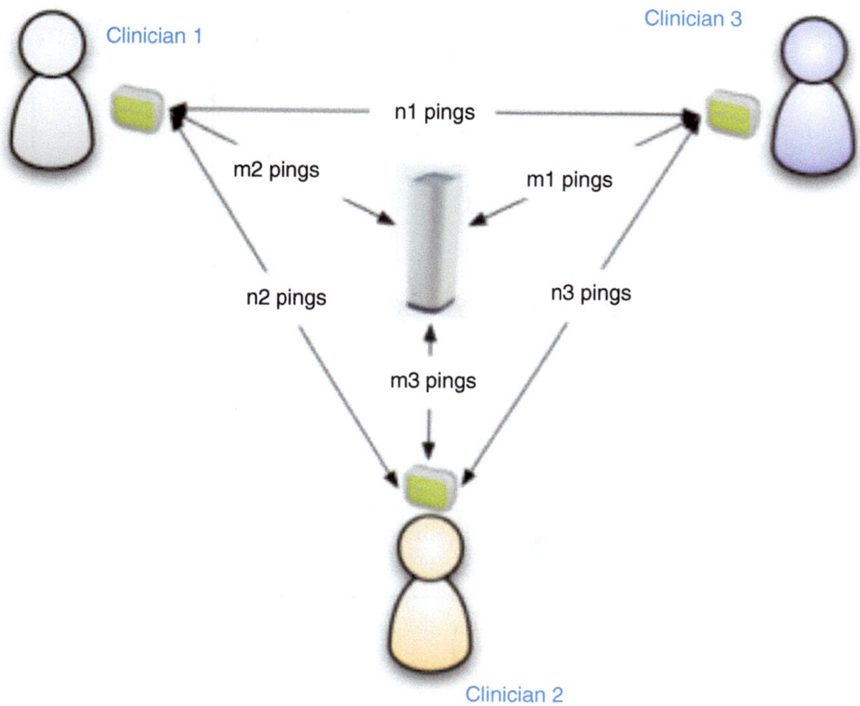

Fig. 17.1 Tag-Tag and Tag-Base configuration. Three tags and one base station is shown in the figure with interactions between them represented by pings (tag-tag and tag-base).

of the patient care team (resident, nurse and so on) gather by the bed of the patient. Following this, examination of the patient takes place. A resident may move to the telephone to consult or the nurse may move to the nurse's station to document details of the encounter. All these activities are linked to entities performing some type of movement in the environment.

Formally we can express this sequence of activities in terms of time as

(i) At time t_1: Patient arrives at the trauma unit and is sent to the trauma bay
(ii) At time t_2: The nurse and a resident check in on the patient
(iii) At time t_3: The resident seeks a phone consult while the nurse heads over to the station to continue with documentation.

In the figure, 'P' refers to the patient; 'N' refers to the nurse and 'R' to the resident on call. The black solid dots denote location of base stations (B_{1-6}). Base stations were placed at various key locations; one at each trauma bay, one near the phone and the other near the computer. For these given sequence of events, the following are the trends we see in the data derived from the tags.

(i) At time t_2: Tags R and N get close to B_1.
(ii) At time t_3: Tag N is very close to B_5 and Tag R is very close to B_6.

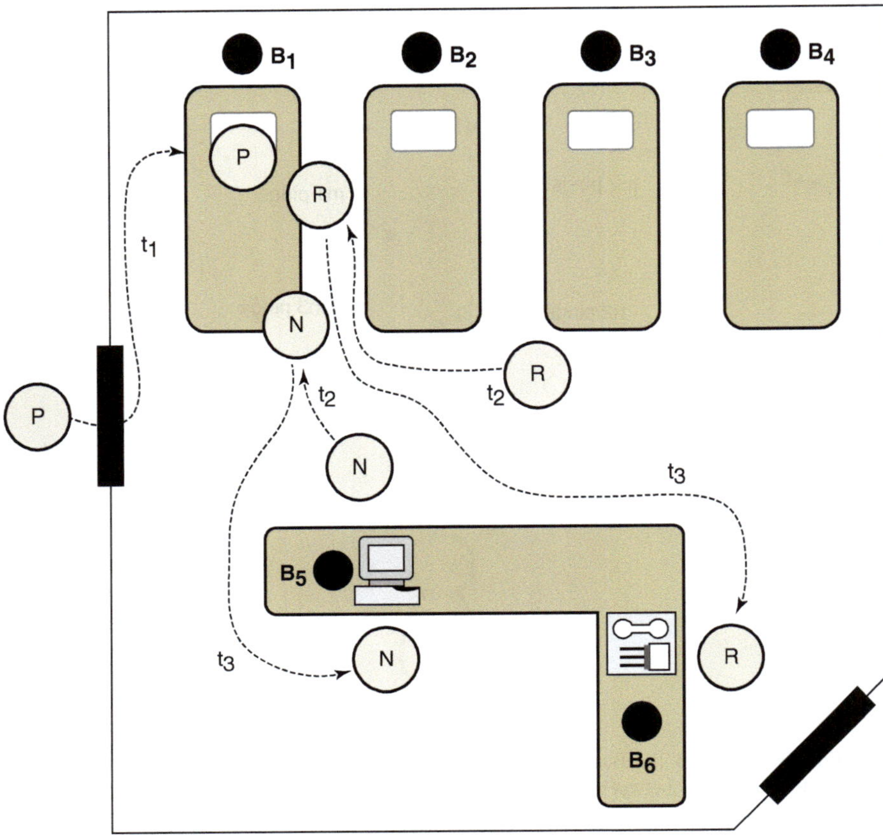

Fig. 17.2 Example scenario: patient arrival at a trauma unit

With the initial setup phase we know that B_1 is trauma bay 1, we can assume that the patient is being managed by the nurse and resident at time t_2 and that the patient arrived at the unit sometime before t_2. Therefore, at time t_3, the system can probabilistically estimate that the nurse was documenting the patient report, and the resident was seeking a phone consult. While the scenario presented is a simplification of the total process, it provides a conceptual view of how we can track activities through tags. In reality, activity models generated can be more complex. The models would be required to handle variations in activities performed while classifying them accurately.

Capturing Clinical Work Activities: Two Evaluation Studies

In the rest of this chapter, we describe two evaluation studies that describe the use of RFID technology. In the first study, sensor data is used to predict a set of clinician activities in a simulated trauma scenario. In the second, sensors are used to characterize the nature of clinician interactions and collaboration in an emergency care setting. Using both these studies we describe the potential scope of using RFID technology in the clinical work environment. We also discuss potential applications of its use in training, monitoring and administration in critical care settings.

Predicting Clinical Workflow from Through Automated Analysis

Many processes produce outputs that may be characterized as observable signals. In the case of RFID tags carried by clinicians, these signals are the discrete received signal strength values captured by the base stations. Hidden Markov modeling is a well-known method for characterizing real-world signals in terms of signal models [23]. The models can provide a theoretical description of the underlying system from which deviations from the norm can be identified.

Activity Modeling Using Hidden Markov Models

Hidden Markov Modeling (HMM) is a probabilistic modeling tool that is usually employed for temporal sequence analysis and has been effectively used in movement analysis, gesture and speech recognition applications. An HMM models a temporal sequence of events (called an observation sequence) in terms of a state machine, in which the current state of the model is probabilistically dependent on the previous states. A well-trained HMM activity model can detect the temporal activities that the HMM has been trained for.

As with any method, HMM based activity recognition has certain advantages and disadvantages. The key disadvantage of HMMs lies in the fact that the amount of data that is required to train an HMM is very large. Another issue with HMMs is that they require positive data to train with, i.e. in order to effectively train an HMM to recognize a class of activities, we require a carefully constructed training set that best describes the activity. However, these disadvantages are outweighed by a trained HMM's capability to handle variations in the final style of execution of an activity. Activities may be performed in a different manner in critical care environments and it is important that the model of activities accounts for these variations. By training the HMM system in a robust manner, it is possible to recognize the motion and some communication activities regardless of the deviations for our application. In addition, HMMs scale well as they can be trained to learn activities incrementally. New activities can be trained for without affecting models of previously learned activities. For these reasons, we chose HMMs for the development of activity models and activity recognition.

Activity recognition using HMMs is a two-step process. It involves (i) *training* HMMs for specific activity models and (ii) *testing* the HMMs for their recognition accuracy with annotated test samples. In order to develop robust activity HMMs, we first require data that describes the activity. This data is obtained from the RFID tags. More specifically, the data utilized is the RSSI value of each tag-base encounter gathered during data collection. We collect this data for the activities of interest in multiple samples. We utilize half of the samples for training the HMMs and retain the rest for testing the developed models. A database of samples for each activity facilitates training the HMMs for each activity, thereby creating a library of HMM activity models for each activity. The training of HMM activity models is achieved using the Baum-Welch algorithm.

Once a library of HMMs is built with one HMM for each activity, the developed models can be tested. The testing of an activity sample proceeds by firstly, estimating the probability that the sample movement belongs to the library. This is achieved using the Forward-Backward procedure for each of the HMM's in the library. The HMM that yields the highest probability for the test sequence is determined to be the type of activity that the movement sequence belongs to. The accuracy of recognition is measured as the ratio of the number of correctly identified test sequences to the total number of test sequences. In this manner, activity models are developed and tested for activity recognition.

Data Collection

We collected two sets of data: (a) Qualitative data from observers, and, (b) Quantitative data gathered from the RID tags.

Both the qualitative data and quantitative data are obtained from standardized sources. While time-stamped quantitative data is retrieved from the RFID tags, observations were generated by observers using an activity tracking software tool. The tool contains a list of commonly occurring activities for the Nurse and Physician. The activities chosen were based on an ontology developed by Zhang and colleagues based on their prior work on analyzing the workflow in emergency departments [24]. Observers may select an appropriate activity from the list provided and add detailed comments a description text box. The observations are then automatically dated and timed and stored in the output observation file. In this way time-stamped data is obtained for both qualitative and quantitative data sources. This makes synchronization of the two data streams possible.

Quantitative data is obtained using *active* RFID tags to gather data. The tags record encounters with other tags (tag-tag encounter) and base stations (tag-base encounter). For each encounter or interaction, the tags record (a) identification number of the tag or base station detected, (b) time and date of encounter, and (c) the received signal strength indication (RSSI) value.

In order to test the HMM based activity recognition system, we simulated 15 Trauma activities (listed in Table 17.1) in a lab setting, (depicted in Fig. 17.3) with

Table 17.1 Activity list and corresponding clinical descriptions

Activity	Movement	Clinical description
A1	1-to-2	Paged physician/nurse tends to patient on bed 1
A2	2-to-3	Physician/nurse moves to treat patient on bed 2
A3	3-to-4	Physician/nurse leaves trauma through entry/exit 1 after visiting patient on bed 2
A4	4-to-5	Physician/nurse enters trauma through entry/exit 1 and attends to the phone
A5	5-to-6	Physician/nurse after attending to a phone call move to use the computer at the nurse station
A6	6-to-1	Physician/nurse leaves Trauma through entry/exit 2
A7	1-to-4	Physician/nurse enter and leave trauma
A8	4-to-6	Physician/nurse enter trauma through entry/exit 1 and move to use the computer at the nurse station
A9	6-to-2	After using the computer physician/nurse move to treat patient on bed 1
A10	2-to-4	After visiting patient on bed 1, physician/nurse leaves trauma through entry/exit 1
A11	5-to-1	After attending a phone call, physician/nurse leaves trauma through entry/exit 2
A12	1-to-3	Paged physician/nurse attends to patient on bed 2
A13	3-to-5	After visiting patient on bed 2 physician seeks a phone consult
A14	5-to-2	After completing a phone call physician/nurse moves to treat patient on bed 1
A15	3-to-6	After treating patient on bed 2 physician/nurse move to use the computer at the nurse station

ten tags and six base stations. These activities were simulations of clinical activities. In order to simulate potential activities in a lab setting we observed commonly occurring movement tasks in the Trauma unit, an example being "physician moving to phone for a consult" (Activity A13). Figure 17.3 depicts the lab setup for testing.

The setup for the testing involved the creation of a 20 ft by 20 ft grid in a lab setting. Six base stations (depicted by black solid circles) we placed in predefined locations (Base 1 and 4 at Entry/Exit points 2 and 1 respectively; Bases 2 and 3 at Beds 1 and 2; Base 5 at the phone on nurse station; Base 6 at the computer on the nurse station). This is congruous with base station setup in the real-world scenario. We gathered movement data for the 15 sample activities listed in Table 17.1. For each RFID tag-base pair or tag-tag pair an encounter is recorded every 3–4.5 s. This data is captured in a time-modulated manner, i.e., encounter information is communicated by detecting differences in the time of the encounter rather than the frequency. This results in a sparse matrix when considering the entire tag-base station configuration. Figure 17.4 depicts a sample of the matrix generated. The encounter of a tag X with base stations A, B and C (gray filled boxes) are shown in a 60 s long timeline. We use linear interpolation to fill missing data in this sparse matrix. While this methodology provides an RSSI value for all base stations at all instances, it adds some noise to our system that may affect the overall activity recognition accuracy.

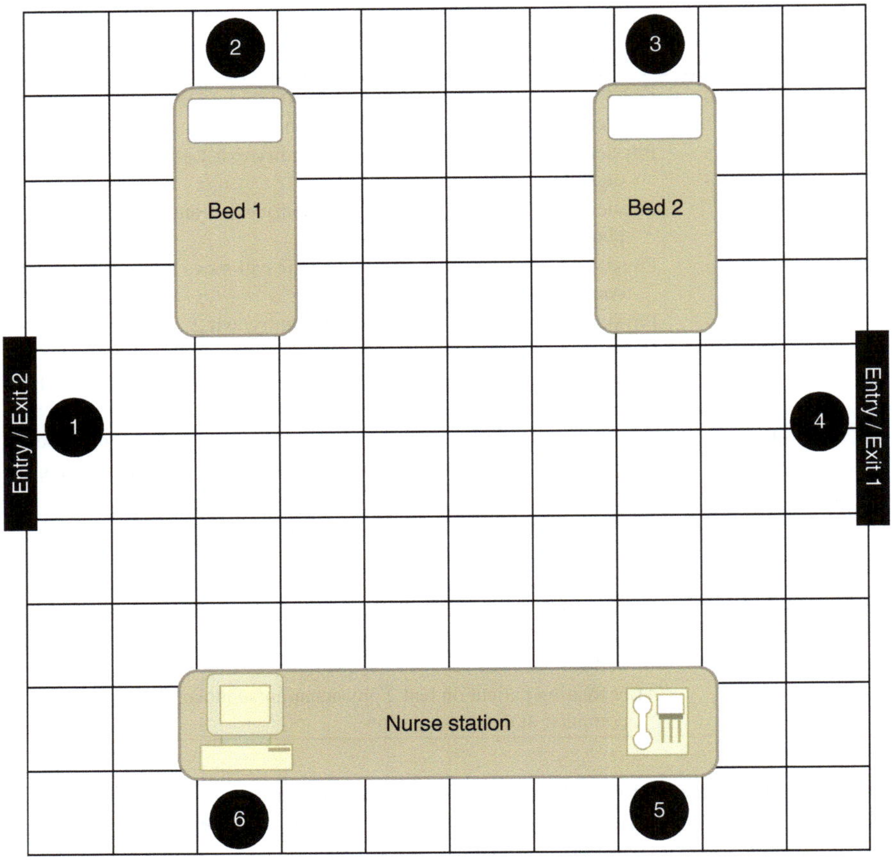

Fig. 17.3 Test setup for simulated clinical activities

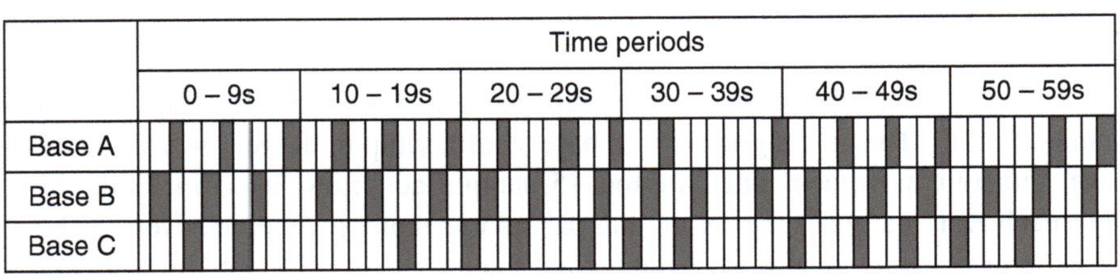

Fig. 17.4 Sparse matrix of tag-base encounters (*gray* fill indicating an encounter record with some tag)

For each of these activities, we gathered ten samples of data. Each sample involved a tagged entity (researcher) following the movement pattern prescribed for the activity. Each sample performed with ten different tags, totaling 100 samples for each activity. This ensured sufficient randomization of activity movements, accounting for inter-tag variability as well. A total of 1,500 samples (15 activities × 10 samples × 10 tags) were gathered for testing. Out of the 100 samples

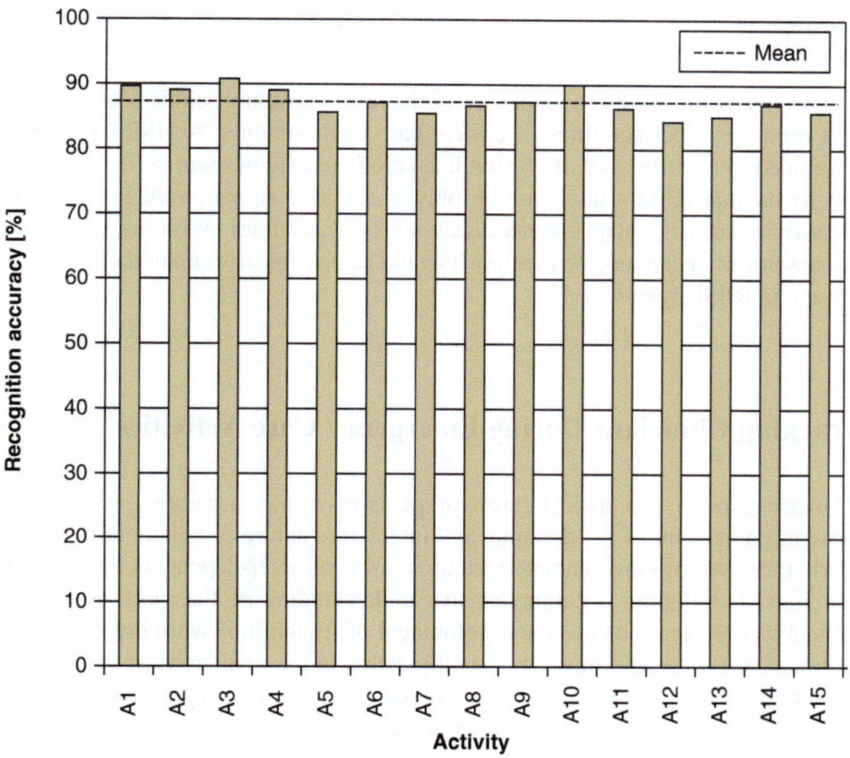

Fig. 17.5 Hidden Markov Model (HMM) based activity recognition results

gathered for each activity, 50 samples were used to train the HMM for activity recognition, and the other 50 were used as a testing set to evaluate the algorithms' accuracy.

Results of HMM-Based Evaluation

Figure 17.5 summarizes the recognition accuracy for the 15 motion patterns (A1–A15). Recognition accuracy is the ratio of the number of activities correctly identified to the total number of activities used for testing. A mean recognition accuracy of 87.5 % was obtained, with a maximum of 90.5 % and minimum of 84.5 %. The analysis of the incorrectly classified test samples revealed that misclassifications were a result of variations in the training set. As discussed previously, HMMs require to be trained on a controlled sample that best represent the activity. Obtaining training data from real-world scenarios are likely to have variations that may compromise the quality of models generated. This is a limitation of utilizing HMM models with RSSI values alone for activity recognition. Additional sensors such as accelerometers could be utilized in conjunction with RFID tags to improve the activity recognition rates.

Summary

RFID sensors were used to record of motion and location of clinical teams, which was used to model activities in critical care environments. A HMM model was developed to identify a set of 15 simulated clinical activities with 87.5 % accuracy. We found that RSSI values, as the only observable signal, were insufficient in identifying activities with the necessary levels of accuracy. With the use of additional sensors such as accelerometers it would be possible to counter the noise levels present in RSSI signals.

Tracking Clinicians During Emergency Care Activities

In many respects, the critical care workplace resembles a paradigmatic complex system: on account of the dynamic and interactive nature of collaborative clinical work, these settings are characterized by non-linear, inter-dependent and emergent activities. Developing a comprehensive understanding of the work activities in critical care settings enables the development of streamlined work practices, better clinician workflow and most importantly, helps in the avoidance of and recovery from potential errors. We used sensor-based technology to capture the movement and interactions of clinicians in the Trauma Center of an Emergency Department (ED). Remarkable consistency was found between sensor data and human observations in terms of clinician locations and interactions. With this validation and greater precision with sensors, ED environment was characterized in terms of (a) the movement patterns of clinicians, (b) interactions with other clinicians and finally, (c) patterns of collaborative organization with team aggregation and dispersion.

Study Setting

The study was conducted in a certified Level 1 Trauma Center in the Emergency Department of a large teaching hospital located in the United States. The hospital provides 24/7 emergency and trauma care to approximately 52,000 patients a year. The ED is separated into distinct units caring for pediatric patients, general medicine patients and those requiring trauma care. The physical set-up of the trauma side of the ED includes eight trauma patient beds and five urgent care beds. In times of high patient volume, additional chairs and beds are placed in the open spaces as needed. The care team for trauma ED typically includes one attending physician, two resident physicians and two trauma nurses, an urgent care nurse, a charge nurse, one technician, and a respiratory therapist shared by the entire ED. The trauma center is also supported by a dedicated trauma team, consulting physicians and the staff from other units of the ED (including off-service providers) as needed.

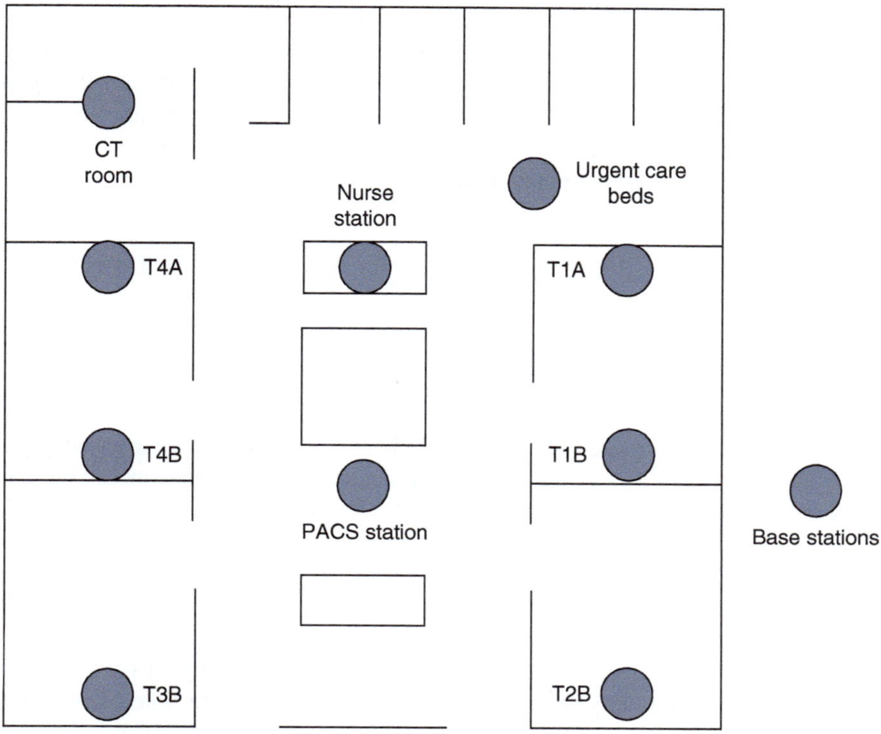

Fig. 17.6 Spatial orientation of the base stations in the ED. Each circle represents a base station at that location. The locations were CT room (*CT*), Nurse station (*NS*), Image browsing station (PACS), Trauma bed 1A (*T1A*), Trauma bed 1B (*T1B*), Trauma bed 2B (*T2B*), Trauma bed 3B (*T3B*), Trauma bed 4A (*T4A*), Urgent care beds

Participants

Observation and tagging occurred on four separate shifts over a 2-month period at the trauma center. During each observation session, the attending physician, two resident physicians, and two trauma room nurses, were solicited for participation. Informed consent was obtained from all participants before the start of each data collection session. Participants were instructed to go about their usual activities.

Sensor Setup

A total of ten (10) base stations were placed across the trauma rooms, physician station, nurse station, CT room and urgent care rooms. The tags were distributed among the attending physician (1), residents (2) and nurses (2). The sensor data included the tag-tag and tag-base pings along with their corresponding signal strength and time-stamp. Sensor data on the tags and base stations was then formatted and uploaded to a MySQL database server. The spatial orientation of the base stations is shown in Fig. 17.6.

One of the critical factors in effectively using the sensor technology is the calibration of the sensors to filter "good" signals from noise. Prior research has used a variety of mechanisms to filter the sensor signals. In general, *threshold signal strength* is often established as a baseline measure. In our experiments, we used a RSSI signal strength value of −70 dB (decibel) as our cut off signal strength. This value was based on the manufacturer's specification and our calibration tests verified this threshold.

Shadowing

In order to validate and complement the information provided by the sensor data, human observers shadowed the "tagged" clinicians. The purpose of shadowing the clinicians was twofold: first, to confirm the accuracy of the location estimations made by the tags and second, to get additional information on the activities of clinicians. The attending physician was shadowed for two sessions, while in the other sessions, a resident and nurse was followed.

To assist observers with their shadowing tasks, we used the UObserve suite of data logging tool [25]. UObserve is a mobile platform that provides researchers with the ability to conduct field observations using standard templates to ease data collection, and importantly the capacity to precisely record the time of recorded events. The UObserve tool is based on the work domain ontology of the ED environment. The use of UObserve allowed for precision and ease in capturing events (e.g. time, place, participants, activities) and synchronization with the tagging data. For this study, observers were provided with a version of UObserve, which had a list of ED-specific locations (based on the base-station locations) and collaborating clinicians at that location. At every instance when the tagged subject changed location, the observer noted the location on the UObserve tool. Additionally, other clinicians who came in direct contact with the shadowed-clinician were also noted.

For each location selection, a time-stamp was automatically added by the system. This time-stamp was synchronized with the time-stamps on the sensors. The data from UObserve was uploaded from the mobile device to an encrypted server. A companion application was developed to export the data in customizable data formats. A sample screen shot from one template in the UObserve interface is shown in Fig. 17.7.

Data Collection

Four data observations of the core trauma care team (1 attending, 2 residents, 2 trauma nurses) occurred over a 2-month period. One clinician was shadowed per session by an observer. Prior to collecting the data in the ED, the tags and

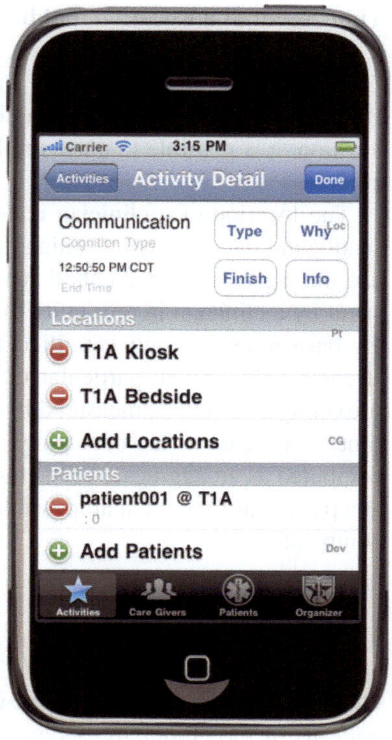

Fig. 17.7 UObserve iPhone interface with the location details and activity template is shown

base stations were extensively tested in the laboratory and in the ED (in pilot experiments) to ascertain their accuracy and effectiveness. During each of these sessions, both sensor and shadowing data were captured. On average, each of the data collection sessions lasted about 3 h (mean = 3.2 h, s.d. = 0.14 h) and was conducted from the start of attending shifts during both afternoon and night periods. While all five team members wore RFID tags, only selected team members were shadowed. Clinicians varied across the sessions.

Data Analysis

In this section, a detailed explanation of the various measures that were used to analyze the sensor and observation data is provided. Particular attention is given to the manner in which the data from the sensors are extracted, processed and analyzed. We specifically investigate two characteristics of clinician activities: *movement of clinicians* and their *interactions* with each other. Based on these two specific characteristics, we investigate the following: time spent at a location, time spent with other clinicians, transition between various locations and collaborative work activities.

Time Spent at a Location and in Proximity to Other Clinicians

Collaborative work is often done within the specific context of location and people. By ascertaining the location of a clinician and subsequently the time spent at that location, it is possible to make preliminary judgments on the work activities of the clinicians.

The location of a clinician is determined based on the tag-base pings and the shadowing data. For determining the time spent by the clinicians at a location, we use the tag-base ping events that were retrieved from the base stations. The time spent by a clinician in proximity to a base station is determined by aggregating the tag-base pings at each identified base station with the highest threshold signal strength value at that particular time. Like time spent in a location, time spent in proximity to others is measured by pings over the threshold response level. Unlike time at a location (tag-base pings), time spent in proximity to other clinicians is computed as an aggregate of the tag-tag pings. If there were multiple tag-tag pings at a particular time, then all possible pairs of tag-tag pings were aggregated for this computation.

Transitions Between Locations

One of the ways to investigate the workflow of clinicians is to trace the movement patterns of the clinicians. As explained earlier, work activities are often context (and location) dependent. In other words, locations can be used as a general proxy for certain types of activities. For example, the presence of an attending or resident at a trauma bedside can be considered as a "patient care" activity. Similarly, a physician at a physician workstation can be construed as the physician performing a documentation task. On account of the hands-on nature of clinical work in this setting, transitions between locations provide a preliminary account of the workflow in a collaborative setting. For example, the movement of the attending physician across various locations within the ED over the period of a shift can be used to gauge their work pattern. If the attending physician was at their workstation for most of a shift, then we can make predictions about the low degree of activity during that shift. In contrast, if there is significant amount of movement by the attending physician across various trauma rooms, then we can make predictions about the high degree of activity during a shift. While these examples are extreme scenarios, it is important to note that transitions between different locations can be used as a basis for determining the nature of activities in the ED. In short, the transition between locations provides a trace-based illustration of the workflow.

In order to develop the transitions between locations in the ED, we identified ten locations in the ED where the base-stations captured significant signal strength. These locations were: CT Room (CT), Nurse Station (NS), Image Browsing Station (PACS), Trauma Bed 1A (T1A), Trauma Bed 1B (T1B), Trauma Bed 2B (T2B), Trauma Bed 3B (T3B), Trauma Bed 4A (T4A), Urgent Care Beds. Based on the tag-base pings at these locations, we first developed a transition probability matrix of location transitions for each clinician.

A location-based transition probability matrix represents the transitions between a set of selected locations. Each cell in the matrix represents the total count of the transitions between the two locations. For example, if the cell value between the CT room and the Nurse's Station for the attending physician was 25, it means that the physician moved from the CT room and the Nurse's Station a total of 25 times during the shift. The transition probability matrix is also often referred to as an *antecedent-consequent* matrix, since it provides the counts of the number of transitions between the antecedent and consequent events. We developed a 10×10 matrix for the location-based transitions (for the ten locations described earlier in this section) for each of the clinicians, per session.

In order to develop the transition probability matrix, we first filtered the tag-base pings that were above the threshold value. Using a sliding window with an interval of 15 s, we temporally collected the locations of all clinicians within this time-window. The location with the highest RSSI strength per clinician was then separated out. This process was applied to the entire data set till all locations of all clinicians were obtained over their entire shifts. The temporal sequence of locations was then converted into a matrix of location-based transitions for further analysis.

Collaboration: Aggregation and Dispersion

Highly complex environments are often characterized by collaborative interactions to maintain the continuity of work activities. The collaborative interactions can be characterized in terms of three key concepts: the *size* of the collaborating team of clinicians, the *length* of their collaboration and the *location* at which the interactions of the team occurs. The knowledge of these three concepts is useful in developing a "blueprint" of the collaborative activities within the ED. We use the tag-tag pings between clinicians to estimate the collaborative interactions between them. Using physical proximity as an indicator for interaction, we identify the following: first, the pair-wise interactions between all the clinicians and the locations at which these interactions take place were identified (based on tag-base pings). Then, the location and size of the largest group of clinicians are detected using matrix-based algorithm.

While, we use the term "interaction" in a general sense, meaning physical proximity between clinicians, it can be argued that close proximity at a particular location in an emergency care setting (e.g., at a specific trauma bed) would indicate that the clinicians are together for a common purpose or goal (e.g., care for a patient at a location). Thus, even though the clinicians may not be verbally communicating with each other, a common goal of being at the same location can be considered as a measure of a shared collaborative activity. We use this concept to measure the degree of team aggregation and dispersion in the ED.

As explained earlier, we first identify the pair-wise interactions between all pairs of clinicians. For the sensor data, we focus primarily on the pair-wise interactions of the attending physician, as they are central to controlling the workflow in the ED. For ascertaining the pair-wise interactions, the sensor data was first "chunked" into intervals of 30 s, after testing with intervals ranging from 30 to 180 s. To be considered as a "valid tag-tag ping" at a particular location several conditions were first evaluated. We describe these conditions with an example. Consider two tags, tag1 and tag2 at a location B1 (base station location). A valid tag-tag ping between these two tags would involve the following interactions: tag1-tag2 ping, tag2-tag1 ping, tag1-B1 ping and tag2-B1 ping. Additionally, all these pings have to occur within the selected 30-s interval.

After obtaining the pair-wise interactions (and their locations), we evaluated the formation (aggregation) and dissipation (dispersion) of larger clinician groups. The identification of large groups was progressively more complex than the pair-wise comparisons. Since groups (size > 2) take longer time to form (and disperse), we considered time intervals of 100 s for this analysis. The time period of 100 s was arrived after testing with various "time-chunks", discussions with ED attending physicians and our own observation data. Based on our observation data and discussion with ED clinicians, we evaluated the average group formation (for groups of different sizes) time across each shift. A 100-s interval was found to be an appropriate time-span for capturing the formation (and dispersion) of groups of sizes varying from two to four. The groups were ascertained in the following manner: first, the presence of a group within the considered time interval was determined. Second, it was verified whether the interactions were occurring within the same location. We explain the aggregation algorithm with an example.

For every 100-s interval that we considered, we developed a two-dimensional matrix similar to the one shown in Fig. 17.4. There are two types of information that is encoded in the matrix: the tag-tag interactions (represented as a binary operator between tags T1–T5 in the left half of the matrix) and the tag-base interaction (represented as a binary operator between base stations B1–B10). From the example matrix (see Fig. 17.4), we generate all possible tag-tag interactions. In this case, the only tag-tag interactions are with tag 1 (T1) with (T2 and T3). The interactions of all other tags (T2, T3 and T4) are with only with T1. Thus, the direct interactions in this period of time are {T1, T2, T3}. Next, we investigate the reverse tag pings (i.e., from T2 to T1, T3 to T1, etc.). For this, we evaluate the column values for T1: {T2, T3, T4}. The intersection set between direct and reverse set of tag-tag pings gives us the set of tags that were interacting in this time period. In our case, we get the set of tags as {T1, T2, T3}. This means that the clinicians carrying the tags T1, T2 and T3 were in close physical proximity to each other.

The last step in the algorithm is to establish the location where the clinicians were together. For this, we use the identified set of tags and compare it with the common set of locations at which these tags were present. In other words, we explore the columns for the base stations (B1–B10) that have non-zero values in the cells for the set of identified interacting tags. In the case of the example provided, the only location where the base station has non-zero value is for the column

	Tags					Base stations									
	T1	T2	T3	T4	T5	B1	B2	B3	B4	B5	B6	B7	B8	B9	B10
T1	0	1	1	0	0	1	1	1	1	0	0	0	0	1	1
T2	1	0	0	0	0	0	1	0	0	1	0	0	1	1	0
T3	1	0	0	0	0	0	1	1	0	1	0	1	0	0	1
T4	1	0	0	0	0	0	0	0	1	0	0	0	0	0	0
T5	0	0	0	0	0	0	0	1	0	0	0	0	0	0	0

Fig. 17.8 Mechanism for identifying group aggregation and dispersion. The matrix has two components: the tag-tag interactions (between tags T1–T5) and between tags and base stations (B1–B10). The presence of a tag-tag or tag-base interaction between tags/base stations is denoted by 1 in the corresponding cell

pertaining to B2 (see Fig. 17.8). Consequently, a group will only be considered as such if all members ping one another, as well as the location base station during the same 100-s time period. Thus, we can identify the largest group during this time period as {T1, T2, T3} at location {B1}. The highest signal threshold values were taken into consideration if there were multiple possible locations for the identified group. There was less than 5 % incidence of multiple locations for a group across all sessions. We computed the size of the largest group for every 100-s interval for the all the four sessions.

Results

In this section, we report on the results from the sensor and observation data. First, we validate the correlation between sensor and observed data. Based on this validation (i.e., the plausibility of using tags as a data collection mechanism), we investigated the relative entropy of the ED system. Then we report on the workflow of the ED clinicians based on their location transitions and interactions with other clinicians. Finally, we describe the formation and dispersion of teams as a measure of collaboration in the ED.

Validating Sensor and Shadowing Data

In order to evaluate the degree of association between the sensor and shadowing data, we computed the correlation between these data sets for both mobility and interactions among clinicians. A high correlation between the sensor and observed data validates the accuracy of the sensor data in capturing the location and interactions among the clinicians. We computed the Pearson moment-correlation between the location determined by the sensor data and location determined by human observers. We obtained a statistically significant correlation between the observed and sensor-based location data ($p < 0.01$, $R = 0.96$) (See Fig. 17.9a).

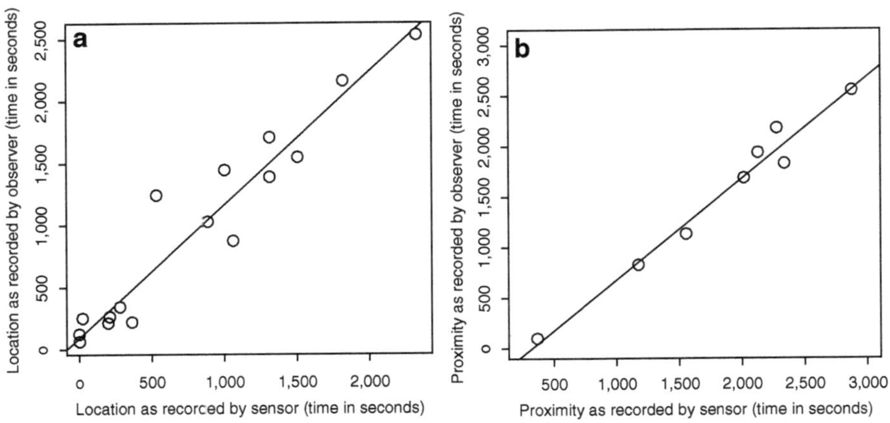

Fig. 17.9 (**a**) Correlation between location as determined by the sensor and location as determined by the shadowing observer over time and (**b**) correlation between interactions between physicians as determined by the sensor and as determined by the shadowing observer over time (across all four data collection sessions)

Similarly, we also computed the correlation of proximity between the clinicians as determined by the sensors and shadowing observer. Based on Pearson product-moment correlation, we found significant correlation between co-location of the physicians as determined by the sensors and by the observers ($R = 0.98$, $p < 0.001$) (See Fig. 17.9b). In other words, physicians (attending and the two residents) were more likely to be co-located than the nurses. The inherent lack of co-location of nurses can be attributed to the significant percentage of nurse activities are often performed in isolation from other physicians (e.g., documentation, care coordination). Hendrich et al. [26] reported similar results where they found that that nurses spend significant amount of their time at nurse stations performing documentation and care coordination activities. The mobility and interaction correlations were computed from data across all sessions.

The significant correlation between the sensor and observed data provides an initial validation for the accuracy of the sensor data in capturing the location and interactions of clinicians in the ED. A comprehensive knowledge about the location and interactions is instrumental in real-time monitoring of emergency environments. Such monitoring can provide useful insights into the activities around specific events such as arrival of a patient with severe acuity or a mass emergency event (e.g., a train accident) and for the study of errors. These concepts are further explored in the discussion section.

Time Spent at Locations and in Proximity with Other Clinicians

Based on the tag-base pings, we computed the time spent by the clinicians in various ED locations. As described earlier, the time spent was computed based on

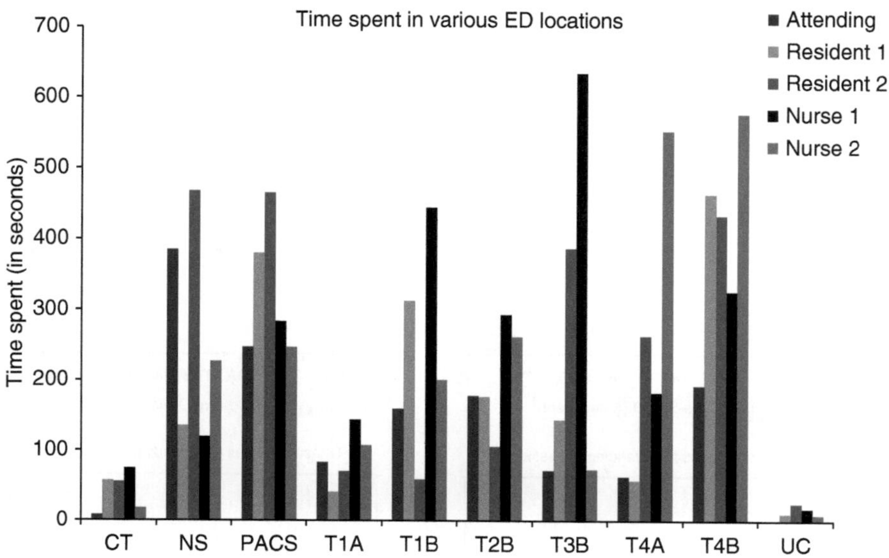

Fig. 17.10 Time spent by all clinicians at various ED locations across all sessions. The locations are *CT* CT room, *NS* Nurse station, *PACS* Image browsing station (and physician station), *T1A* Trauma bed 1A, *T1B* Trauma bed 1B, *T2B* Trauma bed 2B, *T3B* Trauma bed 3B, *T4A* Trauma bed 4A, *UC* Urgent care beds

the aggregation of tag-base pings at each location over time. Figure 17.10 shows the time spent by the clinicians at the various locations in the ED. The x-axis shows the different ED locations (same as those marked up in Fig. 17.2) and y-axis is the time spent at each location in seconds. From Fig. 17.10, we found that: clinicians spent most of their time in the trauma rooms (at the various trauma beds 1A, 1B, 2B, 3B, 4A and 4B); the residents and nurses spent significantly more time in the trauma rooms (i.e., beside the patients) than the attending physician. This is primarily a function of the care process in large teaching hospitals where residents (along with the support of nurses) manage the care process under the supervision of the attending physician.

In a similar manner, we also computed the time spent by the attending physician with other clinicians based on the tag-tag pings. We found that the attending physician spent considerably more time with other physicians (residents) compared to time spent with nurses ($p < 0.01$). This was expected considering as the study was conducted at a teaching hospital.

Transition Between Locations

In order to investigate the clinician workflow we traced the transitions between various locations by the clinicians. The transitions were determined based on the transition probability matrices. Figure 17.11 shows the counts of transitions between

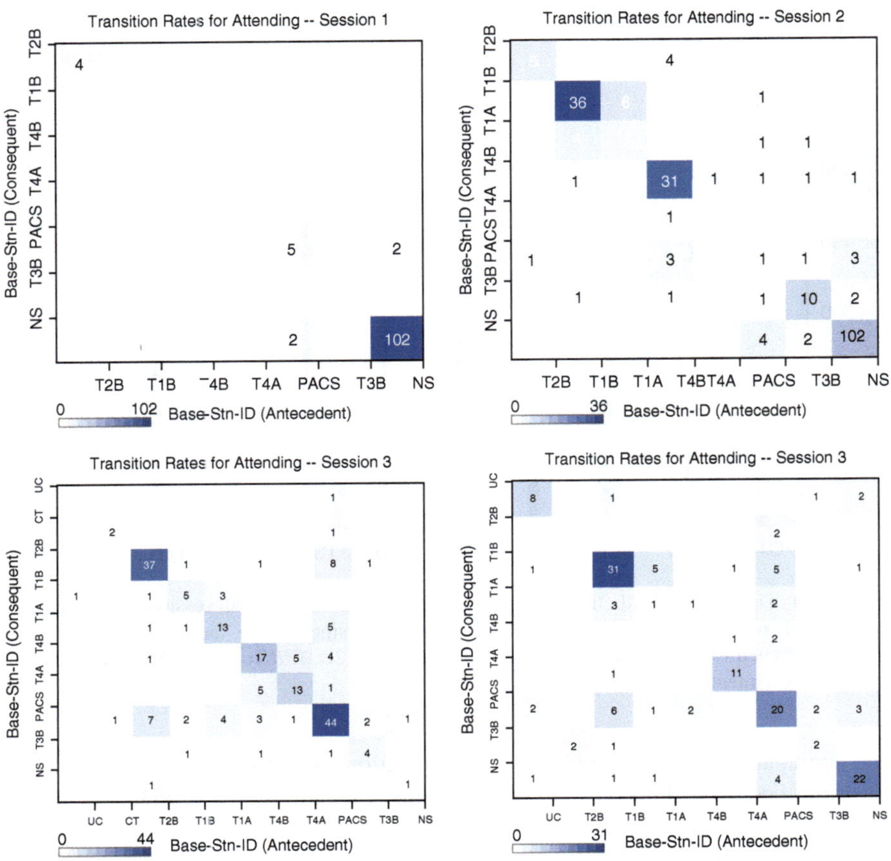

Fig. 17.11 Location transition matrix for the attending physician from the four sessions. The x-axis shows the originating location and the y-axis shows the terminating location during the transition. The counts in the diagonal matrix shows the instances where the attending physician did not move in consecutive time intervals

various locations by the attending physician in the four sessions. The x-axis represents the originating location and y-axis represents the terminating location for each transition. The diagonal of the matrix represents instances where the attending physician was in the same location for consecutive time intervals. Significant differences in the transition patterns can be gleaned from the analysis of the four graphs. In session 1, the attending physician was fairly sedentary at the nurse station (NS). This was probably due to a relatively slow shift.[1] In sessions 2–4, we can see that the attending physician moved across the various trauma rooms and had a “foot print” across all the locations in the ED. It can also be observed that a significant

[1] In fact, our observation data shows that during this session, the attending physician spent a considerable portion of this slow shift teaching the residents at the Nurse’s station.

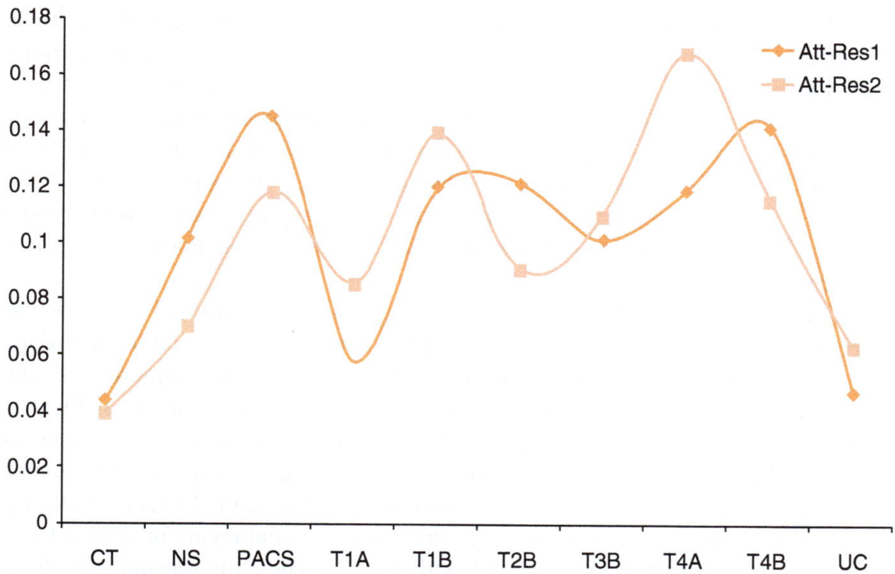

Fig. 17.12 Pair-wise co-location probability between the attending and the residents

time was spent in the trauma rooms (darker squares in the cells representing the trauma rooms).

We also developed similar location matrices for other clinicians. In the case of residents, we found that the transition pattern of one resident was complementary to the other. In other words, we found that, one resident was invariably present at a set of trauma rooms (and absent from the rest of the trauma rooms), while the second resident was present at the remaining trauma rooms. This is consistent with the demands of their shared workload and division of patient care duties. This is further investigated in the next section on collaborative patterns. We found no consistent patterns in the location transitions among the nurses.

Collaboration: Aggregation and Dispersion

We computed all pair-wise co-occurrences between the attending physician and other clinicians. As expected, we found consistent co-location of the attending and the residents in the trauma rooms. This was further confirmatory evidence for the likely complementary role that each of the residents took for the patient care activities. In other words, we found that one resident had a prominent "role" with respect to the treatment of a specific patient. This can be seen in terms of the pair-wise co-location probability (see Fig. 17.12) where one resident is more likely to be present along with the attending physician in a trauma room. The high co-location probability of one resident was highly correlated with a low co-location probability of the other resident being in the same trauma room. We did not find any consistent patterns with respect to the co-location between nurses and the attending physician.

While the interaction between pairs of clinicians is interesting, complex settings are characterized by a significant amount of collaborative activity. Consequently, we were interested in the behavior of the team as a unit, in addition to that of individual clinicians or clinician pairs. We investigated the formation and dispersion of larger groups (>3) in the ED. Based on our algorithm described earlier we computed the team size dispersion over the data collection sessions. On average we found that there was a high percentage of two and three-clinician groups across all sessions. We found several interesting patterns with respect to the aggregation and dispersion of teams across the ED.

First, the incidence of larger clinician groups (4 and above) was very low. On average, there were less than 15 such group occurrences. These clinician groups always included the physician, both residents and one of the nurses. The low occurrence of the larger groups was probably due to a combination of factors: first, such large groups would entail the majority of the care team. From observations, we know that these large groups typically come together during a major trauma and quickly disperse to care for the other patients in the ED center. During occasion of lower patient volume, large groups might congregate in central locations with team members entering and exiting freely. These circumstances of high demand and low volume are relatively infrequent. Second, our algorithm that determined the presence of teams was extremely stringent in terms of the requirements that ascertained the presence of a group (multiple tag-tag and tag-base pings within a short interval). While, this may ignore extremely slow forming groups, we believe that the ED is an extremely fast-paced environment where the formation and dispersion of groups are in response to rapidly emerging situations.

Second, larger clinician groups (size greater than or equal to four) always congregated in one of the trauma rooms. This is highly likely in ED settings where the arrival of a patient with high acuity levels triggers significant activity around that patient. While, we cannot directly verify the acuity of the patient at the times where the larger groups congregated, in our future work we plan to retrospectively investigate the arrival acuity levels of patients for the sessions in which we collected sensor data. Third, team size of three almost always (90 % of the cases) involved at least one resident and a nurse. The third participant in such three-person groups was either the resident or the attending physician. About 60 % of such three-person groups were formed in the trauma rooms, while the rest were primarily split between the nurse station (NS) and physician station (PACS). Two clinician pairs were very common and we found significant variability among these pairs. But, about 50 % of the two-clinician groups identified consisted of the physician and one of the residents. This is typical considering the dual role of the attending physician in patient care and medical education.

An example of how the overall size of the largest ED team changes over a data collection session is shown in Fig. 17.13. The x-axis shows the time while the y-axis represents the size of the largest group at that point in time. As can be seen from the figure, the size of the group varies between 2 and 3 and for a short time a group of size 4 congregates together.

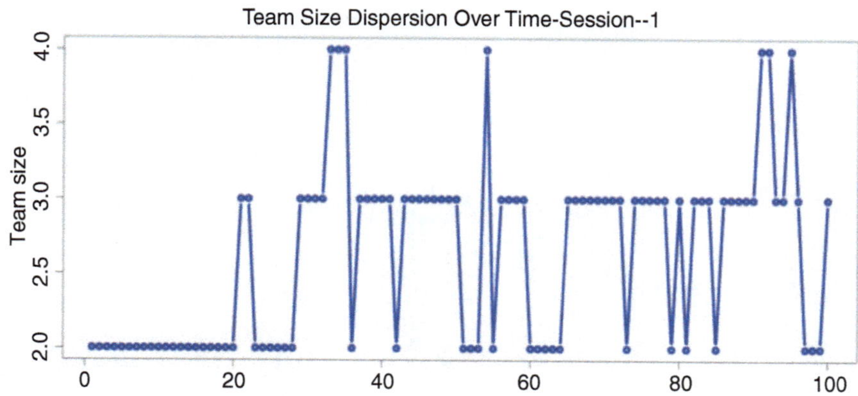

Fig. 17.13 Team size dispersion across a data collection session (session 2). The x-axis shows the time distribution (i.e., the time over a data collection session). The y-axis shows the size of the team

Discussion

We used RFID sensors to simulate and predict workflow and to capture the work activities of clinicians in critical care settings. The results from two studies reported in this chapter show the *appropriateness of using sensors to study work activities in complex critical care environment.* While, we used limited data collection sessions, our results provide significant support for more extensive use of sensors for studying complex activities. Though human observers are definitely required to collect highly nuanced information about the activities in complex environments, sensors are a reasonably reliable complementary data collection mechanism. Combining sensor data with other readily available clinical information (such as patient arrival information, condition, acuity, etc.) can help in developing flexible mechanisms for monitoring and managing the resources of complex environments. We further describe potential applications and uses of sensor technology including its role in visualization and training, management of resources and tracking of errors in critical care environments.

Visualization of Workflows

Visualizing workflow in 3D enables researchers and clinicians alike to easily grasp the activities that make up the workflow. In addition to enabling researchers review workflow in a novel way, the configurable virtual reality (VR) visualizations can also be employed for educational purposes. For example, a resident would be able to go experience a trauma from the perspective of the attending or nurse. This kind of configurability would enable the cross-training of clinical teams.

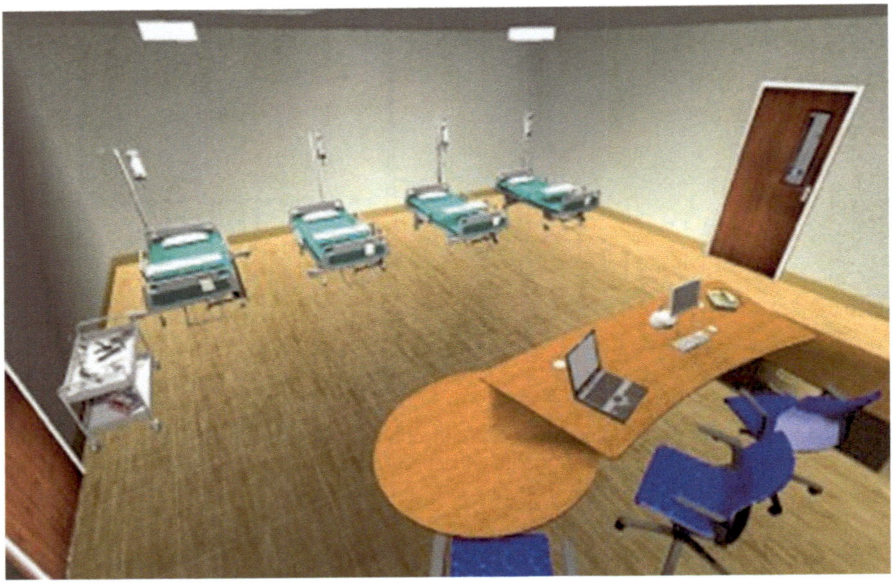

Fig. 17.14 Virtual trauma unit for workflow visualization

The visualizations can also be used to educate clinicians by illustrating cases of optimal workflow in relation to error-prone workflow.

In the domain of healthcare, virtual reality has been used to develop simulations for training of cognitive and psychomotor surgical skills and clinical decision making skills [27–29]. However, there is a lack of VR-based solutions for visualization of workflows and error scenarios even though such systems may have a major role to play in error prevention and mitigation. We can employ online VR environments such as Second Life® (http://secondlife.com/) and Active Worlds® (http://www.activeworlds.com/) for such visualizations. In this stage of the work, we have developed a standalone system that could be employed for such visualizations employing an open source gaming engine called Irrlicht (www.irrlicht.net).

A sample virtual trauma unit (see Fig. 17.14) was developed to mimic the trauma unit at Banner Good Samaritan Medical Center, which is the site of development for the project. The virtual trauma room consists of four trauma pods or beds. The nurses' station faces the trauma pods. A computer and phone are key components that are included in the design of the nurses' station. Two exit doors are present in either side of the trauma room. These details are synchronous with the test and real world set up. The current simulation contains three basic characters – the patient, resident and the nurse. The number and type of models to be utilized depend on the entities studied in the real-world. Models of the characters are built using modeling software (Maya and 3dMax; http://usa.autodesk.com/). Once the models are developed they can be controlled in the simulated world programmatically.

In order to obtain VR simulations of the workflow, the system generates a list of activities making up the workflow. These activities are then manually fed into the visualization engine to create the simulations. Currently, this stage of visualization process is completed offline. VR simulations created in this manner present a simulated view of real-world events. This is valuable to clinicians and researchers in highlighting the main events in the workflow within the context of the clinical environment.

Recent research [7] has reported on the potential of online 3-D virtual environments for medical education and learning. Online virtual environments provides an informal environment in which the learners can understand the norms, practices and challenges of working in a complex environment and integrate such information through repetition and group interactions.

Real-Time Monitoring of Activities and Resources in the ED

Sensor technology has been significantly useful in the remote and real-time monitoring of activities in various environments such as nursing activities, elderly care and telemedicine. Monitoring and management of resources in a highly dynamic and complex setting requires significant amount of data with respect to the activities and happenings within that setting. Data from the sensors (both mobility and interaction) provide information regarding the clinician (in terms of their location and co-location with other clinicians) with great precision and detail. Additionally, this information is time-sequenced. As a result, a real-time feed from the sensor data can be used to develop a trace of events in the ED. For example, the rapid formation and dispersion of large teams at different trauma beds may indicate the possible arrival of several patients with high acuity. Hospital administrators can use the data from the sensors to ascertain the "status of the ED". This information is critical in deploying additional resources, both in terms of personnel and equipment, to the ED. Additionally sensor data can have potential applications when changes are introduced in a critical care environment. For example, the introduction of new health information technology (HIT) creates significant changes in work activities.

Framework for Studying Errors

The study of errors in emergency care settings has received significant attention in recent times. While sensor technology has been minimally used in the investigation of origin and propagation of errors in the ED, it is a viable mechanism for this purpose. From our sensor data, we developed normative and predictive models of clinician activities in the ED. These activities can be retrospectively used to investigate the temporal events and activities that surround reported error incidents.

What is missing from most prior studies on the tracing of errors in critical care environments is the detailed information regarding clinician activities around the time at which the error occurred. The continuous monitoring using sensors provides a large database of clinician location, movement and interaction events. Using the methods described earlier (e.g., transition patterns, group formation and interactions), it is possible to re-create the distribution of attention and resources in the ED around the time at which the error was reported. Such a "replay" of events can help in tracing potential activities that could have been avoided and may have contributed to the error. We will use an example to describe this.

Consider that an attending physician self-reports an error regarding the delayed administration of a drug to a patient in trauma-bed 4 at 530 ET on June 1, 2010. The error report also includes the arrival condition of the patient, history and other patient-relevant information. There are two sets of information that can be used to develop a trace of the events that happened prior and after the error occurred. The sensor data can be used to identify the patterns of interactions, movement and collaboration among the clinicians around the time at which the error happened (say, from 5 to 6 PM on June 1, 2010). The clinical information on the patient along with observation (audio or field notes) can be used as complementary evidence to develop a much richer perspective of the activities surrounding the reported error event. Thus, a detailed sequence of events can be used to track the possible contributory activities that possibly led to the error event. This framework, which combines sensor data and clinical data, for studying errors is shown in Fig. 17.15.

This framework for investigating the origin and propagation of errors has several advantages. First, the data collected from using the sensors can be retroactively combined with the clinical data. Self-reported errors in an emergency setting are usually very low. As such, it is important to be able to trace the events that happened around the time the error incident was reported. Sensors provide a viable mechanism by which data can be collected for extended periods of time and then be retrospectively used for evaluation and analysis. Second, sensors can be used as a passive data collection mechanism with minimal interference with the clinician's work activities. Third, the relatively long battery life of most sensors makes it feasible for running long data collection sessions (e.g., 20–30 days) without any breaks in data capture. Such an arrangement with human observers is extremely costly and labor-intensive. Our future research work involves the use of the framework to investigate the activities of clinicians in the ED around self-reported errors.

Challenges and Lessons Learned

In summary, there are several potential research and applied opportunities for the use of sensor technology in complex critical care environments. In spite of the significant challenges for designing, calibrating, collecting and analyzing sensor data, we believe that sensor technology has exciting prospects for developing

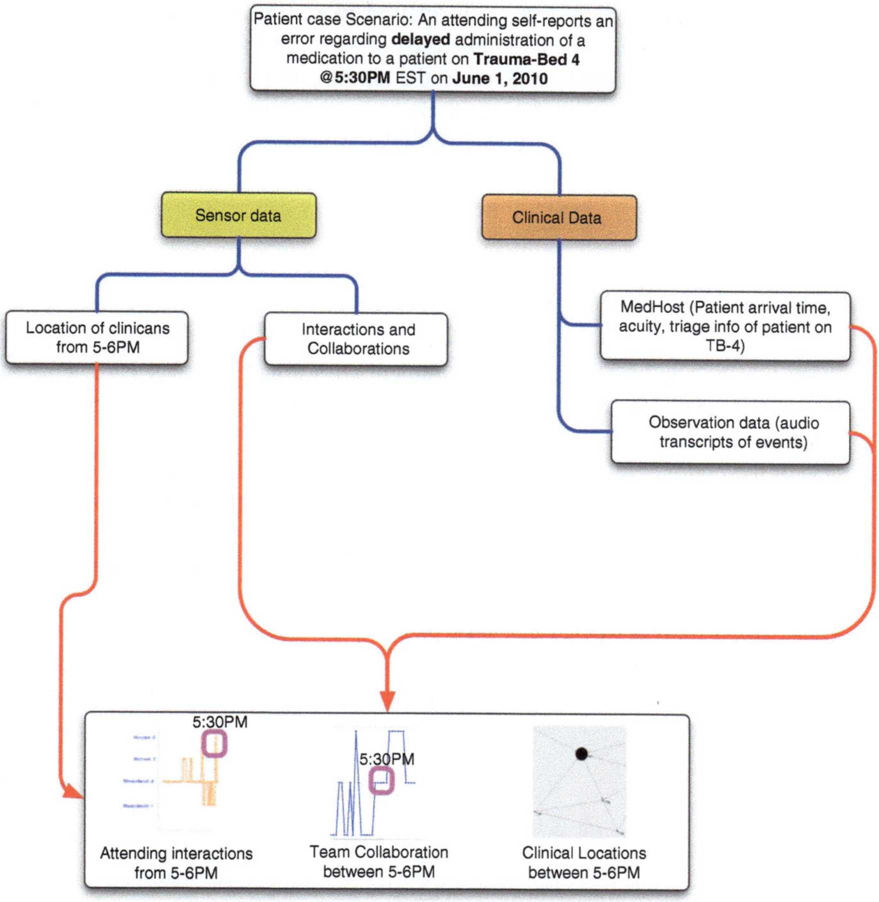

Fig. 17.15 Framework for studying errors

insights of the work of complex critical care environments, which would otherwise be impossible due to significant time and cost burden of using human observers. The calibrating and setting up of the sensors often requires extensive pilot testing to ascertain the exact positioning of the base stations to get maximum coverage. We also had to ensure that our technology did not cause adverse effects on medical equipment and devices. Per our manufacturer's description, our sensor technology operates in the same frequency range as the WiFi (Wireless), which is ubiquitous in hospital settings. While, we did not extensively test for adverse effects of sensors, we believe that our technology does not cause adverse effects on medical devices as argued by van der Togt et al. [30]. Some clinicians were concerned about their privacy issues due to the use of sensors during their shifts. We collected no physician or patient-identifying information and all IRB-regulated protocols were followed for assuring data protection and privacy. For example, all data was saved on an encrypted drive and all identifying information (e.g., time) was removed prior to data analysis. Another significant challenge that we faced was the cost involved in managing the sensor technology. Due to the significant amount of data generated from the sensors, we developed algorithms for compressing and storing the data. This volume of data also required us to develop computationally efficient algorithms for analysis.

Discussion Questions

1. What are the challenges of tracking clinical workflow in critical care settings? What are some of the potential solutions for collecting high-fidelity data in such settings?
2. One of the major challenges with capturing micro-level data (e.g., using sensors) is the significant volume of data. What are some of the approaches to streamline data collection using sensors?
3. How can we minimize the "noise" in sensor data? What are some of the algorithmic approaches for doing so?
4. There are several activities that take place in a hospital setting that may be of interest from the patient safety point of view. Hand washing is one example. Can you provide other activities related to patient safety that would be interesting to track and quantify?

References

1. Institute of Medicine (IOM), U.S. Committee on Quality of Health Care in America. In: Kohn LT, Corrigan JM, Donaldson MS, editors. To err is human: building a safer health system. Washington, D.C: The National Academies Press; 2000.
2. Abraham J, Kannampallil T, Patel VL. Bridging gaps in handoffs: a continuity of care approach. J Biomed Inform. 2012;45(2):240–54.
3. Laxmisan A, Hakimzada F, Sayan OR, Green RA, Zhang J, Patel VL. The multitasking clinician: decision-making and cognitive demand during and after team handoffs in emergency care. Int J Med Inform. 2007;76:801–11.
4. Horsky J, Gutnik L, Patel VL, editors. Technology for emergency care: cognitive and workflow considerations. AMIA Annu Symp Proc. 2006; 334–8.
5. Malhotra S, Jordan D, Shortliffe E, Patel VL. Workflow modeling in critical care: piecing together your own puzzle. J Biomed Inform. 2007;40:81–92.
6. Kannampallil TG, Li Z, Zhang M, Cohen T, Robinson DJ, Franklin A, et al. Making sense: sensor-based investigation of clinician activities in complex critical care environments. J Biomed Inform. 2011;44(3):441–54. Epub 2011/02/25. eng.
7. Vankipuram M, Kahol K, Cohen T, Patel VL. Visualization and analysis of activities in critical care environments. AMIA Annu Symp Proc. 2009;2009:662–6.
8. Vankipuram M, Kahol K, Cohen T, Patel VL. Toward automated workflow analysis and visualization in clinical environments. J Biomed Inform. 2011;44(3):432–40.

9. Bar-Yam Y. Improving the effectiveness of health care and public health: a multiscale complex systems analysis. Am J Public Health. 2006;96:459–66.
10. Patel VL, Cohen T. New perspectives on error in critical care. Curr Opin Crit Care. 2008;14(4): 456–9.
11. Plsek PE, Greenhalgh T. Complexity science: the challenge of complexity in health care. BMJ. 2001;323(7313):625–8.
12. Plsek PE, Wilson T. Complexity, leadership, and management in healthcare organisations. BMJ. 2001;323(7315):746–9.
13. Smith M, Feied C. The emergency department as a complex system: New England Complex Systems Institute; 2006. Cited 30 July 2010. Available from: http://www.necsi.edu/projects/yaneer/emergencydeptcx.pdf.
14. COSI. COSI http://www.irit.fr/COSI/. Cited 20 June 2010. Available from: http://www.irit.fr/COSI/.
15. Berg M. Patient care information systems and health care work: a sociotechnical approach. Int J Med Inform. 1999;55:87–101.
16. Cohen T, Blatter B, Almeida C, Shortliffe E, Patel VL. A cognitive blueprint of collaboration in context: distributed cognition in the psychiatric emergency department. Artif Intell Med. 2006;37:73–83.
17. Celler BG, Earnshaw W, Ilsar ED, Betbeder-Matibet L, Harris ME, Clark R, et al. Remote monitoring of health status of the elderly at home. A multidisciplinary project on aging at the University of New South Wales. Int J Biomed Comput. 1995;40:147–55.
18. Alwan M, Dalal S, Mack D, Kell SW, Turner B, Leachtenauer J, et al. Impact of monitoring technology in assisted living: outcome pilot. IEEE Trans Inf Technol Biomed. 2006;10(1): 192–8.
19. Østbye T, Lobach DF, Cheesborough D, Lee AMM, Krause KM, Hasselblad V, et al. Evaluation of an infrared/radiofrequency equipment-tracking system in a tertiary care hospital. J Med Syst. 2003;27(4):367–80.
20. Schrooyen F, Baert I, Truijen S, Pieters L, Denis T, Williame K, et al. Real time location system over WiFi in a healthcare environment. J Inf Technol Healthcare. 2006;4(6):401–16.
21. Stanford V. Using pervasive computing to deliver elder care. IEEE Pervasive Comput. 2002;1(1):10–13.
22. Fry EA, Lenert LA. MASCAL: RFID tracking of patients, staff and equipment to enhance hospital response to mass casualty events. AMIA Annu Symp Proc. 2005:261–5.
23. Chen C, Liu C, Li Y, Chao C, Liu C, Chen C, et al. Pervasive observation medicine: the application of RFID to improve patient safety in observation unit of hospital emergency department. Stud Health Technol Inform. 2005;116:311–5. IOS Press.
24. Brixey JJ, Robinson DJ, Turley JP, Zhang J. The roles of MDs and RNs as initiators and recipients of interruptions in workflow. Int J Med Inform. 2010;79:e109–15.
25. Li Z, Robinson DJ, Zhang J. UObserve: a mobile app for the study of emergency department workflow. Ann Emerg Med. 2010;56(3):S121. American College of Emergency Physicians Research Forum.
26. Hendrich A, Chow M, Skierczynski BA, Lu Z. A 36-hospital time and motion study: How do medical surgical nurses spend their time? Perm J. 2008;12(3):25–34.
27. Seymour NE, Gallagher AG, Roman SA, O'Brien MK, Bansal VK, Andersen DK, et al. Virtual reality training improves operating room performance – results of a randomized. Double-blinded study. Ann Surg. 2002;236(4):458–64.
28. Kahol K, Vankipuram M, Smith ML. Cognitive simulators for medical education and training. J Biomed Inform. 2009;42(4):593–604.
29. Ahlberg G, Heikkinen T, Iselius L, Leijonmarck CE, Rutqvist J, Arvidsson D. Does training in a virtual reality simulator improve surgical performance? Surg Endosc. 2002;16(1):126–9.
30. van der Togt R, van Lieshout E, Hensbroek R, Beinat E, Binnekade JM, Bakker PJM. Electromagnetic interference from radio frequency identification inducing potentially hazardous incidents in critical care medical equipment. JAMA. 2008;299(24):2884–990.

Chapter 18
Sub-optimal Patterns of Information Use: A Rational Analysis of Information Seeking Behavior in Critical Care

Thomas G. Kannampallil, Amy Franklin, Trevor Cohen, and Timothy G. Buchman

Introduction

Human information seeking is driven by their need to satisfy their various needs [1] related to specific tasks and activities. The effectiveness of information seeking is critical in achieving high throughput and efficiency. Nevertheless, given the plethora of available data it is impossible to effectively focus on specific data – cognitive barriers such as information load, memory capacity and strategies significantly affect the effectiveness of information seeking and gathering. While much is known about the information needs and sources of information that are typically used by

---

Portions of this chapter, including sections 2, 3 & 4 (along with tables and figures) appeared in Kannampallil et al. Understanding the nature of information seeking behavior in critical care: implications for the design of health information technology. *Artificial Intelligence in Medicine*. 57(1):21–9.

T.G. Kannampallil (✉)
Center for Cognitive Studies in Medicine and Public Health, New York Academy of Medicine, New York, NY 10029, USA
e-mail: tkannampallil@nyam.org

A. Franklin, PhD
School of Biomedical Informatics, University of Texas Health Science Center, Houston, TX 77030, USA

National Center for Cognitive Informatics and Decision Making in Healthcare (NCCD), Houston, TX 77030, USA
e-mail: amy.franklin@uth.tmc.edu

T. Cohen, MB ChB, PhD
School of Biomedical Informatics, University of Texas Health Science Center, Houston, TX 77054, USA
e-mail: trevor.cohen@uth.tmc.edu

T.G. Buchman, PhD, MD, FACS, FCCP, MCCM
Emory Center for Critical Care, Emory University School of Medicine, Woodruff Health Sciences Center, Emory University, Atlanta, GA 30322, USA
e-mail: tbuchma@emory.edu

V.L. Patel et al. (eds.), *Cognitive Informatics in Health and Biomedicine*, Health Informatics, DOI 10.1007/978-1-4471-5490-7_18, © Springer-Verlag London 2014

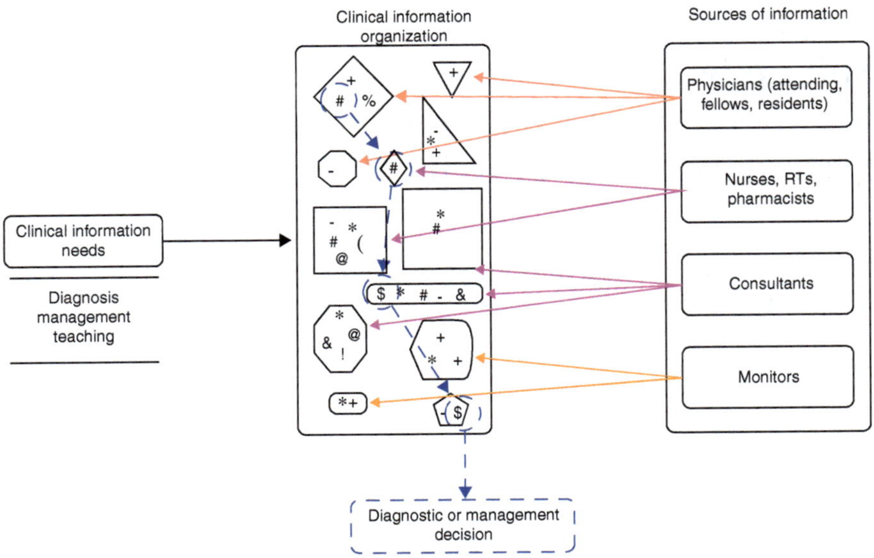

Fig. 18.1 Information sources and their organization in critical care environments: the distributed nature of clinical information organization is shown in the *central box* and the *dotted lines* show the trace of the relevant information that is abstracted for a diagnostic decision

clinicians (both physicians, nurses and other healthcare professionals) [2–6] very little is known about the processes and mechanisms that underlie the clinicians' use of the information sources. Additionally, most of the prior work on information needs and use has been conducted in primary care settings.

The process of information seeking is likely to be significantly different in the highly information-intensive and collaborative environment of critical care, where clinicians are face the arduous task of finding the right information to complete their tasks in a timely manner. Additional challenges arise due to the significantly collaborative nature of critical care work that requires significant interaction between the clinicians to manage a smooth and efficient patient care process. For example, patient information is often added to a central patient record repository by different clinicians – attending physicians, residents, nurses and other support personnel. As a result, when a physician has to develop a concrete understanding of the patient's Fig. 18.1 shows how different clinicians incorporate information into a patient's chart and how they have to locate the relevant information for making diagnostic and management decisions (dotted lines show the trace of the relevant information that is abstracted for diagnosis decisions). As highlighted in Fig. 18.1, the distributed nature of information organization in critical care settings has significant effect on the process of information seeking including: (a) *increased patient diagnosis time* resulting from longer time for filtering and organizing information. This leads to inefficiencies in diagnosis and decision-making. (b) Additionally, it also increases the potential for the *loss of information* when the necessary information cannot be found in a timely manner, consequently, increasing the potential for errors, and (c) the presence of multiple sources of similar information results in *redundancy of available information* and also increases the need for the physician to constantly switch among these resources to find appropriate information for their needs. In this chapter, we investigate how such challenges manifest during clinical information seeking tasks for making patient diagnosis decisions in critical care.

We specifically focus on the following: (a) develop an overall perspective on the nature of information seeking in critical care contexts, (b) time utilization across various resources during the information seeking process, (c) relative usefulness (or utility) of the information gathered from various sources during clinical decision-making, and (d) nature and structure of medical knowledge that is gleaned from the various sources.

Method

This section describes the setting, participants, data collection, and data analysis that were used for this study. A detailed description can be found in [7].

Setting and Participants

The study was conducted at a large academic hospital in the Gulf Coast area that had over 33,000 admissions in 2010. Our study focuses on a 16-bed "closed" [8] MICU (medical intensive care unit) managed by intensivists. In the unit, both paper and electronic charts were simultaneously maintained and used for patient care documentation (See Table 18.1 for a description).

Eight (n=8) MICU physicians participated in the study (6 attending physicians, 1 third-year resident, 1 clinical fellow). Given their training status, the data from the third-year resident was not used for our analysis. The Institutional Review Board (IRB) approved the study.

Procedure

Participants were asked to walk through the steps needed to create a clinical summary reviewing the details from a single patient case using information from charts (electronic and paper), and interactions with other clinicians. Clinicians verbalized ("thought-aloud") the relevant information related to their actions [9]. For example, the participants demographics and history were described (e.g., "this is a 34-year old African American male with a history smoking related issues"). The participants also nominally mentioned the sources from which they gleaned the information (e.g., "on resident notes") and their rationale as to why the considered information was important. Verbal think aloud techniques are commonly used in biomedical informatics research (e.g., [10, 11]) and are powerful mechanisms for developing

Table 18.1 Information sources and their related sub-sources of information along with the specific types of information that is present in these sources

Information source	Information sub-source	Information category (content)
Paper chart	Resident notes	History, physical exam, lab and xray results, list of diagnoses and problems, analysis and plan of care
	Attending notes	Same as residents notes, attending notes, problem list and expanded plan
	Consult notes	Data (history, physical exam, relevant labs and x-rays and other tests related to the consultant's specialty), problem list, assessment and plan
	Orders/labs	Some labs, usually of same day or day prior
	Imaging	Summary of the report or analysis by the tech
	Medications	List of relevant medication (usually an incomplete list)
	Nursing notes & physiology data	Flow sheets
Electronic record	Resident notes	Same as above, in greater detail
	Attending notes	Same as above, in greater detail (with analysis and plan)
	Consult notes	Initial notes, has full details as above, as relevant to the consultant's specialty
	Orders/labs	All labs and results – official record, from admission and prior admissions as well.
	Imaging	Pictures of images as well as reports – official records
	Medications	List of current and past medications, including dosages, routes, types
	Nursing notes & physiology data	Nursing notes, or data directly downloaded from bedside, such as vital signs (BP, pulse, oxygenation, respiratory rate), with trends over time (24 h). Also, some other test results such as glucose that are done at the bedside by the nurse.

insights on human cognition and decision-making. At the end of their information seeking process, participants provided a clinical summary of the patient where they described the patient case followed by their assessment and plan for that patient. Each verbal report was audio recorded and then transcribed for further analysis.

Data Collection

All data collection sessions were conducted after morning rounds (late morning or early afternoon) between October and December of 2010. Study participants were not present during morning rounds and were unfamiliar with the cases that were assigned to them. The data collection sessions were run on 3 separate days using two medical cases: day 1 (three participants, *sepsis*), day 2 (two participants, *renal failure*), and day 3 (three participants, *sepsis*). While there were marginal differences between the sepsis and renal failure cases, our clinical research collaborators ensured that the patient mix was similar across the 3 days.

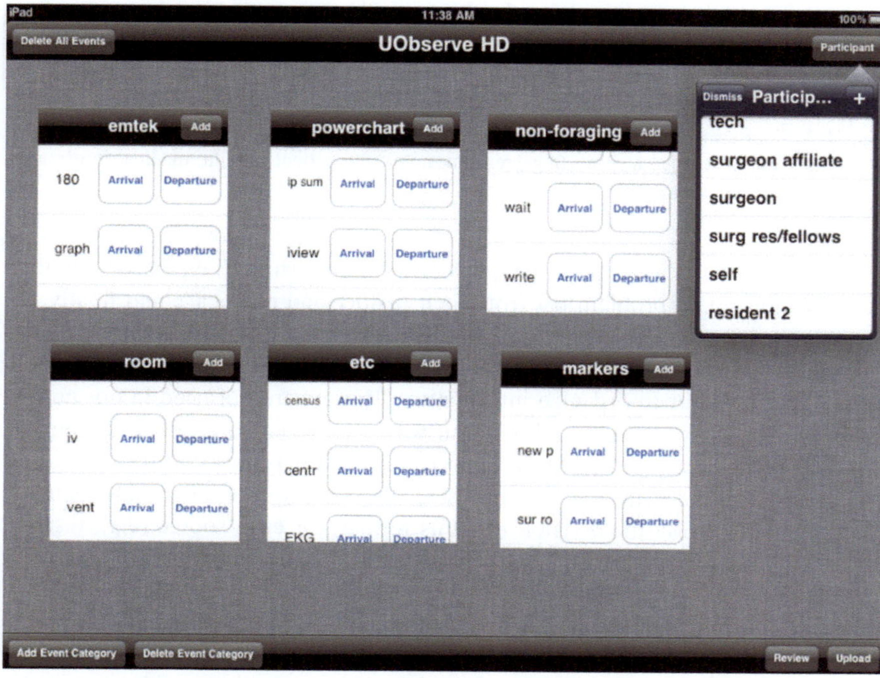

Fig. 18.2 iPad application used for data collection

For each session, one researcher wrote down detailed notes regarding the physician actions, sources used, and clinical personnel they interacted with and all other task related activities. Simultaneously, the second researcher captured the duration of each action (or task) using an iPad application [12]. The application provided a simple touch-based mechanism to capture the duration of access of each source (e.g., resident note, see Fig. 18.2) using a pre-created template of sources and sub-sources. The time captured from the iPad-recording was verified by comparing it with the time on the audio recording. Verbalized transitions (e.g., "now I am going to look at the resident notes from today's rounds") assisted partially with the reconciliation across sources.

Data Analysis

Audio recordings and field notes were transcribed and then verified by a physician collaborator for accuracy and completeness. Data from these recordings were organized into a structured format shown in Fig. 18.3. The columns represent the type of information source (paper or electronic), information sub-source (e.g., resident note), time at which the source was accessed, the information category (e.g., history and physicals from resident note, based on categories provided in Table 18.1),

Information source	Information sub-source	Start time	Information category	Information sub-category	Information unit
Paper	Resident note	3.3	Resident H & P	Age	Heart disease
				Problem list	Renal failure
					ESRD

Fig. 18.3 Transcribed format: the columns show the source, time at which the source was first used, the specific source category (e.g., resident note), the patient-specific medical information (in the "detail" column)

the information sub-category the physicians were using (i.e., based on their verbalization) (e.g., problem list from their history and physical), and finally, the patient-specific medical information that was referred to as an "information unit." The category and sub-category of information were based on suggestions by our clinical collaborator to organize information. These were not used in our current analysis. The "information unit" column was used to capture clinically relevant information and was used extensively in our current analysis.

In analyzing the data, we first separated the sources into paper and electronic categories. Following the division into this format, for each source (e.g., resident note or attending note), we identified the content including number of unique mentions of information that was verbalized from that source. For example, in Fig. 18.3, from the resident's note the physician noted the following patient-condition related information: heart disease, renal failure and ESRD (provided in the "information unit" column). Further description of the identification and use of "unique mentions" of information is provided in the data analysis section.

Rate of Information Gain: Time Utilization for Information Seeking

In addition to evaluating the *time spent on documentation* and *utilization of medical knowledge categories*, we computed the *information gain* and *utility* of the retrieved information. *Overall rate of information gain* is a measure of the total information gathered from the various sources over a period of time. Based on the number of information units gained from each sub-source and the time spent, we computed the overall rate of information gain, G_o

$$G_o = \frac{Total\ no. information\ units\ in\ sub\text{-}source}{Time\ spent\ on\ sub\text{-}source}$$

Here, the sub-source would include categories mentioned in Table 18.1 and an information unit was the clinically relevant information provided in the "information unit" column in Fig. 18.3. G_o provides a measure of the overall rate of information gained from a source.

An important aspect of information rich environments is that repeated occurrence of information reduces the potential value of that information. That is, when the same information is encountered multiple times within the same document, its relative value for the reader decreases. This is the basis of Charnov's marginal value

Table 18.2 Calculation of the rate of information gain and relative rate of information gain

Sub-source	Info. units (IU)	No. of new IU	Repeat (within-source)	Repeat (across-source)	Total info. gain	Time spent (s)	Rel. info gain [17]
Resident note	27	24	3	0	[24 * 1 + 3 * 0.5] = **25.5**	158	[25.5/27]/158 = 0.005

theorem [13–15]. Detailed analysis of the use of marginal value theorem and its use in information use in a variety of decision making settings can be found in Pirolli and Card [1] or in Pirolli [16, 17]. Information gain has implications for the choice of sources that are used for information gathering. While a source may contain a large quantity of information, if the overall information gain is low, then the utility of that source is likely to be lower.

We utilized the marginal value theorem to compute the *relative rate of information gain* [18] across the various sub-sources. For this, we identified the repeated information within and across sub-sources and assigned different weights to the repeated and unique information. The assignment of weights was done in the following manner: patient-condition related information that was never repeated across the whole transcript was given a score of 1 (high utility information: *Unique*); patient-condition related information that was not repeated within the same sub-source but in a different sub-source was given a score of 0.75 (medium utility information). For example, if the heart disease was first mentioned in a resident note, and then repeated in the attending note (i.e., a different source), the second time it was used, it was given the lower score. Patient-condition related information that was repeated within the same source (e.g., heart disease repeated within same resident note again) was given a score of 0.5 (low utility information). The scoring mechanism was based on a modified version of Charnoff's marginal value theorem. *Relative rate of information gain* [18] was computed by dividing the information gain per sub-source, by the time spent on utilizing that source. An example of how the information gain was computed is shown in Table 18.2.

In our scoring mechanism, while we did weight the uniqueness of information we did not consider the relative importance of a piece of information. For example, information regarding a patient's age is perhaps less important than their past history of MI for a patient presenting with chest pain (age may also be a factor is the patient is older). While, considering the relative importance of each patient-condition related information would greatly improve our information-theoretic analysis, information importance or relevance is highly variable (by both condition and across participants). As such, we did not consider it in our current analysis.

Structure of Medical Knowledge

The patient-related detail (see "Information Unit" column in Fig. 18.3) was categorized using the medical knowledge framework [19, 20]. It provides an epistemological framework for characterizing the knowledge used for clinical comprehension and problem solving, and represents a formalization of medical knowledge. The framework differentiates the levels at which a physician organizes the available knowledge and provides insights into the clinical practitioners' medical knowledge. We have utilized similar approaches to describe physician-patient interactions [21], diagnostic reasoning [22, 23], nature of clinical expertise [23] and clinical comprehension [24]. We utilize the framework to categorize and understand the nature of information that is retrieved by physicians during their information seeking process. This also aids in developing an understanding of the clinical reasoning processes that underlie the information seeking process.

The hierarchical framework consists of five levels of medical knowledge, with empirium at the lowest level, followed by observations, findings, facets and diagnoses at higher levels. Empirium corresponds to basic description of sensory information and often contains no medical interpretation (e.g., skin color). Observations are perceptual categories and require medical knowledge for interpretation. For example, a patient reporting dry skin or chest pain during a physician encounter. Findings are groups of observations that are interpreted in terms of their clinical significance. For example, shortness of breath is interpreted within the context of a myocardial infarction. Facets refer to cluster of findings indicating a medical condition or a cluster of conditions (e.g., embolic phenomena are interpreted from a cluster of chest pain, DVT in calf muscles and V/Q). The clustering of findings together helps in exploring a particular condition (i.e., embolic phenomena) while ignoring others. These represent general pathological conditions and help the clinician to partition the diagnosis problem space. The diagnosis level is the highest level with known therapeutic or explanatory models. The diagnosis category subsumes all the previous categories. As reported elsewhere (e.g., [25]), this hierarchy of medical knowledge is useful for narrowing down the diagnosis search space. In other words, as the physician collects data regarding a patient, the diagnosis search space is narrowed till the final diagnosis and management decisions are made.

Consider the following example: a physician notes that a patient presented to the emergency department with chest pain, shortness of breath, leg swelling, excessive sweating and a weak pulse. As described earlier, chest pain, leg swelling and excessive sweating would be considered as observations in the framework. The presence of a deep vein thrombosis (DVT) through a Doppler scan is a finding that is developed from a preliminary observation of leg swelling. These deductions (along with other evidence) can lead the physician to reach an intermediary conclusion regarding the presence of embolic phenomena in the patient. The final stage is the diagnosis of pulmonary embolism (where one or more arteries are blocked) in the patient. A summary of the categories and a brief explanation is provided in Table 18.3.

All transcripts were coded using the knowledge categories provided in Table 18.3. By having these knowledge categories, we were able to organize the structure of medical knowledge gathered from paper and electronic records.

Two researchers coded the data into the categories described above (one a practicing Internal Medicine physician and the other a graduate student with a

Table 18.3 Summary of medical knowledge categories and examples

Category	Explanation	Example
Empirium	Lowest level of information	Age
Observations	Units of information that are recognized as potentially relevant in the problem-solving context	Chest pain
Findings	Groups of observations that have potential clinical significance	V/Q (Ventillation-Perfusion) mismatch, DVT in calf muscles (Deep Vein Thrombosis on Doppler scan)
Facets	Clusters of findings that indicate an underlying problem or class of problems, often reflecting pathological descriptions ("interim hypothesis or constructs")	Embolic phenomenon
Diagnosis	Subsumes all previous levels	Pulmonary embolism

medical degree). There was a high degree of agreement between the coders, and any discrepancies in the coding were resolved through collaborative discussion and agreement between the coders. Given the small sample size and exploratory nature of the experimental design, comparisons between electronic and paper records between the various variables (time spent, relative rate of information gain, medical knowledge categories) were analyzed using paired t-tests.

Results

Qualitative Evaluation: Information Seeking Process

First, we provide a brief overview of the information seeking process in the MICU. Similar to what was reported in prior studies (e.g., [26–28]), we found that information was distributed among various sources: paper and electronic records, monitors, and people (nurses, pharmacists, respiratory therapists, and residents). During their information seeking process, physicians gathered information from paper charts, electronic records, through patient evaluation, and indirectly, from other clinicians involved in the care process. Based on our field notes and observations, we found that paper charts were used as the information source that contained notes by residents at patient admission, attending notes and summary, orders, tests, and other administrative material. While paper records were information-rich and mostly current, they provided the physician only a snapshot view of a patient. Most of our participants also described that the updates to the paper records were manual and, hence slow. As one of our participants noted, "*I usually cannot depend on the paper charts for the most updated information…these are usually slow in getting up-to-date*".

In contrast, electronic charts contained updated information about test results, information from bed-side monitors and vitals. Electronic records were often used in conjunction with the paper charts to "fill-in" information that is often unavailable or missing in the paper charts. Several participants mentioned that they had to go back and forth between both sources to find the most up-to-date information, "*you just learn to figure out where to find the most updated information. It may be idiosyncratic but you develop habits and preferences*." For example, we observed that the physicians sometimes switched back and forth between paper and electronic charts to find some pertinent information regarding a patient condition (or status). Most often, this was to determine whether there were updates regarding a lab test or X-ray. In addition to serving as an electronic data storage, electronic records also afforded flexible mechanisms for visual representation (e.g., zooming of x-ray images), alternate mechanisms for information representation (e.g., using graphs to visualize trends or comparisons) and structured organization of information content (e.g., orders, lab results are organized in separate tabs). As one of our participants observed, "*I have to use the electronic charts for certain things..such as graphs and charts as it is gives the flexibility to manipulate and view from different perspectives*." Physicians also interacted with clinical support staff including fellows, residents, nurses, and respiratory therapists to update their knowledge about the patient's current condition.

The distributed nature of information led to a fragmented process of information seeking, aggregation and organization. Physicians differed in the order in which they utilized the various information sources. While, most physicians started their diagnosis process with the paper chart others depended heavily on the electronic charts for patient related information. While the use of electronic records and patient interaction were an integral part of all physicians information seeking process, the use of paper charts and interactions with other clinicians depended on several factors including complexity of the patient case, familiarity with the patient case, physician's personal preferences, and the patient LOS in the MICU. Based on our analysis, we found that the information seeking process to be *exploratory*, *cumulative*, and *iterative* (this is further discussed in the section "Discussion"). The information sources and a preliminary framework of physician information seeking during clinical decision-making tasks is shown in Fig. 18.4. The figure shows three separate sources (and modalities) of information that differ in the nature, type and structure of available information. The arrows between the sources shows the iterative nature of the utilization of information for clinical decision making process.

Quantitative Evaluation: Structure of Information Seeking

In this section, we describe the time spent on information sources, information gain from various sources, and the nature of knowledge utilization from these sources.

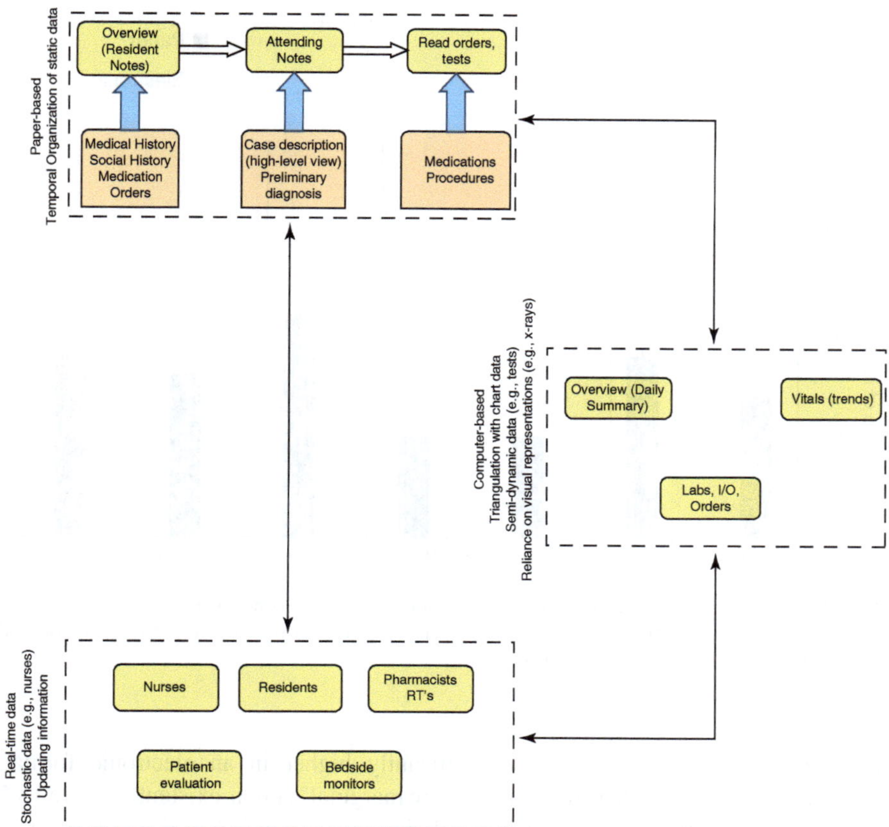

Fig. 18.4 Sources and utilization of information resources

Time Spent on Information Sources

There was no significant difference in the overall time spent on paper when compared to electronic charts ($M_{\text{electronic}} = 661.3$ s, $M_{\text{paper}} = 528.3$ s, $p = 0.296$). As expected, more time was spent on evaluating the physician notes (both attending and resident notes) on the paper record than on the electronic record ($t(6) = 2.38$, $p = 0.05$). Meanwhile, significantly more time was spent on electronic records for retrieving information regarding orders, medications and laboratory results.

Rate of Information Gain from Various Sources

The overall rate of information gain, G_o, was greater for paper records when compared to electronic records ($t(6) = 3.262$, $p < 0.005$). The *relative rate of information gain*, R_g, was marginally greater when using electronic records ($t(6) = 1.89$, $p = 0.1$). More specifically, the relative rate of information gain for attending notes,

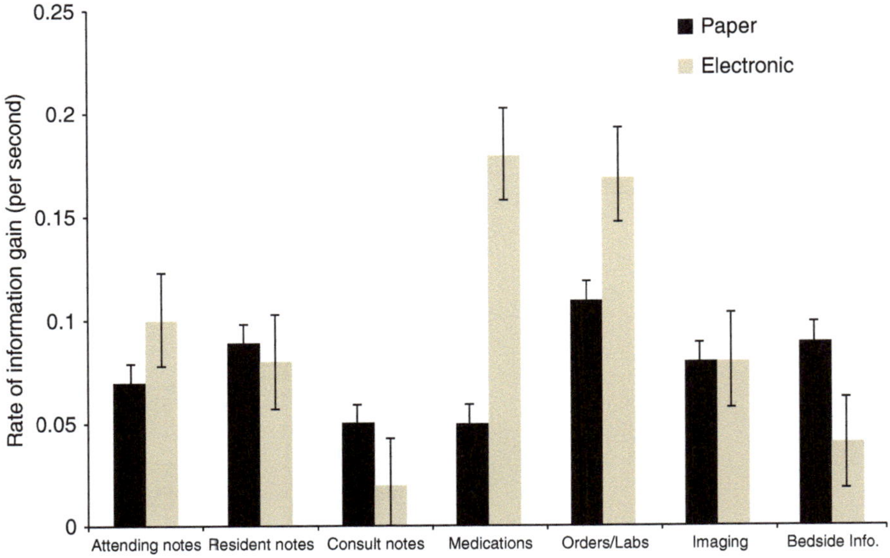

Fig. 18.5 Relative rate of information gain (i.e., information gain/time spent) of the various information sources in the MICU. The x-axis represents the various sub-sources of information and y-axis represents the information gained

medications and orders/labs was significantly higher in an electronic format. The differences in the other sub-sources were marginal (or non-existent). Figure 18.5 shows the differences between paper and electronic records based on the relative rate of information gain (rate was measured per second).

This effect was more prominent in the case of medications and orders/labs from the electronic records and was due to the highly structured representation that was afforded by the electronic interfaces. This was not particularly surprising as prior research has shown the positive effect of structured representation on human cognition [29]. For example, tables and graphs aid in easier interpretation and comprehension of information.

Optimal Rate of Information Gain

From our data, we computed the optimal time spent on a resource that resulted in the highest rate of information gain. This was computed by aggregating the rate of gain of information for each source per document plotting against time (see Fig. 18.6) on a log-log scale.

In the figure, the light-shaded line (marked "data line") shows the rate of gain of information. The dark-shaded line (marked "trend line") shows the best-fit trend line based on the available data. The slope of the trend line gives the optimal time spent within a data source with maximum information gain. The *x*-axis and *y*-axis

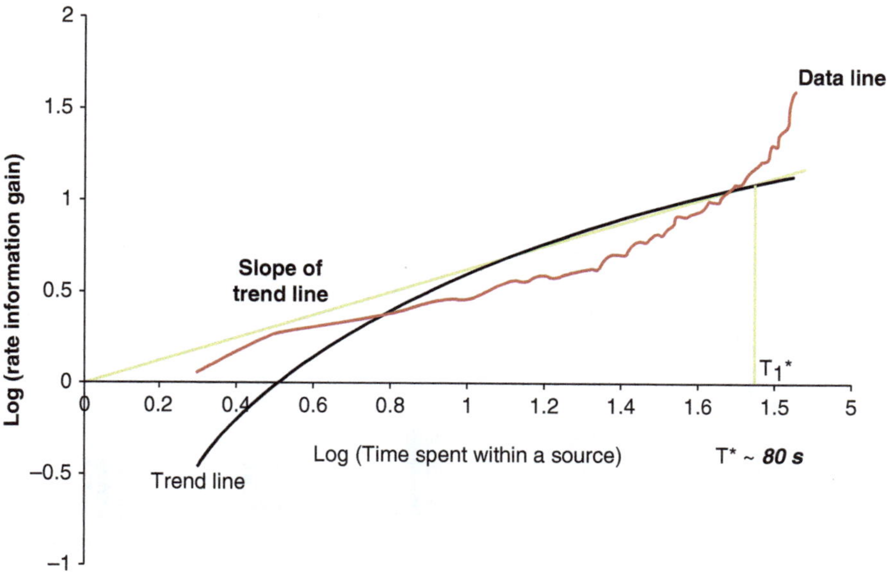

Fig. 18.6 Log-log plot of rate of information gain versus time spent within the resource. The graph shows the "data line", the rate of gain of information across sources (with increasing time), the "trend line", which represents the best fit of the data, and the "slope of the trend line"

represent the time spent on a resource and rate of information gain respectively on a log-scale. From our data, this optimal time spent (t^*) to be around 80 s.

We found that physicians spent around 80 s predominantly on orders/labs (electronic), pre-ICU notes (paper), and bedside information/flow sheets (paper). In other words, the optimal time spent for highest information gain, was achieved for those sources that had high rate of information gain (see Fig. 18.5 for sources that had the highest rate of information gain). The optimal time spent (t*) was based on a small data set for specific disease conditions and using the format at our study site. We also found that physicians spend significantly more time on resident notes (mean =240 s) and attending notes with lesser rate of information gain (see Fig. 18.6).

Knowledge Utilization from Various Sources

There were no differences in the overall utilization of the medical knowledge categories across paper and electronic records ($t(6)=-0.22$, $p=0.83$). The distribution of medical knowledge categories across paper and electronic records is shown in Fig. 18.7. Nevertheless, there were nuanced differences in the individual knowledge categories. We found that there was *significantly more* retrieval of medical knowledge categories related to observations ($t(6)=4.2285$, $p<0.001$) and findings ($t(6)=2.2163$, $p=0.05$) from electronic charts. In contrast, more empirium type of

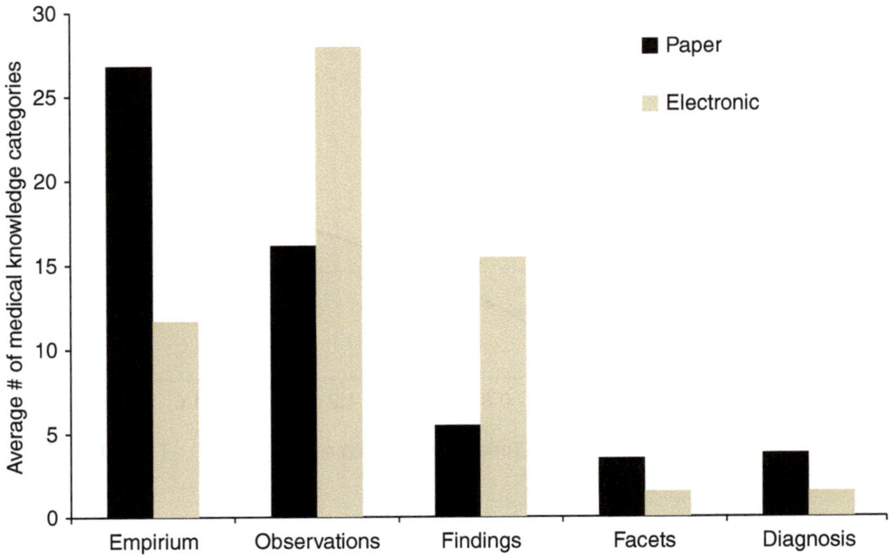

Fig. 18.7 Average number of medical knowledge categories in paper and electronic records

information was retrieved from paper charts ($t(6)=2.5342$, $p<0.05$). No significant differences were observed for facets or diagnosis. The difference in the nature of medical knowledge retrieved is also likely related to the functional organization of information.

Additionally, we wanted to explore if the medical knowledge categories of a certain type were retrieved from specific information sub-sources. We found a high degree of correlation between the information category (e.g., specific information within an information sub-source) in the electronic records and the medical knowledge categories: observations and medications ($r=0.56$, $p<0.05$); observations and orders/labs ($r=0.57$, $p<0.05$), findings and medications ($r=0.66$, $p<0.05$) and findings and orders/labs ($r=0.61$, $p<0.05$). Other comparisons in the electronic charts were not significant. In particular, the correlations show that structured organization of information in electronic charts prompts quicker retrieval of higher order medical information. For example, medication lists and laboratory results are organized in a structured template in electronic charts that aids in quicker reasoning and abstraction of information within the context of the clinical problem. While we cannot show causal association, this points to the fact that the organization of information potentially drives the reasoning process. We discuss this further in the next section.

Discussion

We investigated information seeking behavior of physicians during clinical decision-making, focusing on the *time spent* on various sources from which the information was retrieved, the *relative information gained* and the *structure of medical knowledge* retrieved from the various sources. We found that physicians spent relatively equal amount of time on electronic and paper records for retrieving information during their decision making process. Overall, more information was retrieved from paper records, but the information retrieved from electronic records was significantly more unique and consequently, led to a higher information gain. Additionally, we also found that there were inherent differences in the epistemology of the medical knowledge that was retrieved: physicians retrieved significantly more higher-level medical knowledge (observations and findings) from electronic charts, while more basic information (empirium) was retrieved from paper charts.

An interesting deduction that can be made from our findings is the principle of *local optimization* during the information seeking process. Physicians optimized their information seeking process by accessing resources that they believed maximized their information gain and aided in their medical reasoning and decision-making process. In other words, the information seeking process was driven by the socio-technical organization within the environment. This led physicians to depend on certain resources for certain types of information (e.g., orders and labs on electronic charts as they were highly structured). Information sub-sources that had higher information gain were utilized for retrieving certain information. For example, we found that patient medications and orders for laboratory tests and labs were retrieved from electronic records. These information sub-sources (medications and orders) were highly structured and allowed for easy access and retrieval. In the same vein, paper charts were used for retrieving basic information regarding patients (of type empirium, e.g., age). Additionally, higher-level medical knowledge (e.g., findings) was more easily retrieved from structured sources leading them closer to clinical diagnosis.

Such a process of contextually-centered information seeking has several disadvantages: first, it requires significant switching between resources leading to loss in time and effort; Second, considerable amount of expertise and experience is necessary before a physician settles on a successful search process and strategy; and third, there is no uniformity within this process across physicians and hence requires a physician to constantly develop new strategies with systemic and organizational changes. It is often acknowledged that a considerable part of the information seeking process (in any environment) involves an organic adaptation to the environment that leads to learning appropriate and potentially efficient mechanisms for information seeking. While physicians showed marginal difference in the relative rate of information gain across paper and electronic charts, the significant nuances within individual information sub-sources (e.g., paper for lower level information and electronic charts for structured information) showed the propensity of physicians to adapt their information seeking strategies to synchronize with the choices available in the environment. In other words, an *adaptable* and *local* information seeking strategy is utilized.

While global optimization strategies are potentially unachievable in complex critical care settings, integrated systems that simultaneously support the cognitive and reasoning processes of physicians are likely to be highly beneficial. We discuss design implications that can potentially mitigate the inefficiencies of the local optimization during information seeking.

Enriching the External Representation

One of the important drivers for physicians depending on certain sources for certain types of information is the ease of retrieving information from these sources. For example, we found that *significantly more unique information was gained from electronic records than paper records*. As previously described, this effect was likely due to the structured representations in electronic records (for example, tables and charts). In contrast, during our observation sessions we found that physicians relied on the paper charts for reading through the notes (and briefly looked over the typed electronic notes). As one of our participants observed, "*I like to get an overall view of this patient from the paper chart and then I can look at the tests*." This was likely due to the fact that electronic charts did not offer any specific advantages for reading the physician notes (for example, highlighting key events or information in the notes) while the paper notes afforded easy perusal through annotation and markups. Augmenting some of the electronic notes by increasing its affordability for quick reading and evaluation is likely to increase the efficacy of using electronic notes.

The concept of enrichment of a source is derived from information foraging theory [17, 30] where the rate of gain of information from a resource can be improved by providing better mechanisms for information identification and retrieval. For example, organizing laboratory test results in a tabular form (with graphical plotting) helps in quicker retrieval of information than a listing of values. Providing mechanisms for structured enrichment, such as highlighting key results or important aspects of the past medical history, can potentially improve the rate of information retrieval and correspondingly lead to quicker and more accurate decisions. Similar results have also been reported by Sharda et al. [31] who found that enrichment of psychiatric narratives through structured presentations (e.g., through highlighting key concepts) led to expert-like clinical comprehension among novice clinicians. As we move towards complete electronic adoption by 2014, the importance of enriching aspects of Electronic Health Record (EHR) use is very important.

Supporting Clinical Decision Making and Reasoning

Based on our observations, we found that the information seeking process was exploratory, cumulative, and iterative. During information seeking process physicians had to constantly find and re-find information from multiple sources to confirm or invalidate their various hypotheses. In particular, physicians depended on certain sources for certain types of information resulting in them returning to previously encountered information for confirmation. For example, most physicians viewed imaging on the electronic charts and often returned to the paper charts to verify and confirm their deductions from the imaging results. Such a process led to the iterative back-and-forth switching between multiple sources (a process driven by the contextual organization of information). Such switching increases the cognitive load on physicians to effectively filter the information for diagnostic reasoning and decision-making [10, 20].

In addition to the switching, the nature of the information across sources that was utilized by physicians was inherently different: we found that physicians retrieved a significant amount of lower level medical information from paper records. This points to a *data-driven* approach to reasoning about the clinical case (e.g., [21]). In contrast, the presence of significantly more high-level medical information of type "findings" suggests a *hypothesis-driven* reasoning strategy while using the electronic records. While expert clinicians can effectively manage such switching for routine cases, it can pose significant challenges for a novice (e.g., medical student) or intermediate (junior medical resident) level physicians [32].

In short, the local optimization within the information seeking process by physicians can affect the logical flow of their reasoning process (e.g., switching between data-driven and hypothesis-driven strategies). While we did not explicitly measure the effectiveness of the reasoning strategies, it is evident that the reasoning strategies were a combination of both data- and hypothesis-driven strategies. For effective development of systems and tools that support clinical reasoning and decision-making within the complex critical care domain, designers need to consider the clinical workflow and the socio-technical aspects within the design process [33].

Based on our evaluation and analysis, we found that the information seeking process is *exploratory*, *cumulative*, and *iterative*. During information seeking process physicians had to constantly *find* and *re-find* information from multiple sources to confirm or invalidate a hypothesis. In particular, they depended on certain sources for certain types of information and this resulted in physicians requiring to return to previously encountered information to confirm the information that was previously gathered. For example, most physicians viewed imaging on the electronic charts and often returned to the paper charts to verify and confirm their deductions from the imaging results. Such a process led to the constant iterative back-and-forth switching between multiple sources.

As described elsewhere [10, 34, 35], information filtering occurs during diagnostic reasoning and requires significant cognitive effort from the physician. The distributed nature of information in critical care created extra information load: both in terms of finding the appropriate information and in using the appropriate resource to find the right information. Hence, even with the availability of structured electronic records, most physicians preferred to switch between the resources to find information necessary for making their decisions. Such switching added extra time and steps to their tasks, consequently, decreasing the efficiency of their work.

Limitations: There are some limitations that we hope to address in the future iterations of this study. We did not assign different weights for information or their sources. In other words, all information was considered as equal. While, we realize this may not be the ideal, such an approach provided a baseline for establishing the viability of the information-theoretic approach for studying information seeking behavior. We have started a secondary analysis of data by re-classifying it based on its relative clinical importance. We also did not control the order in which the clinicians sought and retrieved information. It is possible that the information gain and medical knowledge structure are affected by the order in which the different sources (paper, electronic) are accessed.

Additionally, we did not have access to the complete patient record to investigate whether the information retrieved was indeed complete. It must also be noted that this study was conducted in a single MICU and further evaluation studies must be conducted to explore the generalizability of the results across settings. Nevertheless, we believe that our study is a first of its kind that investigates the information seeking process from an information-centric perspective providing insights into the rationale behind the strategies adopted during the information seeking process.

Directions for Future Work

In this chapter, we discussed an information-theoretic approach to evaluating information seeking practices among clinicians. As previously discussed, the process of information seeking in clinical environments is not well understood – an understanding that can potentially have significant effect on clinical and management outcomes. For example, differences that exist in the information seeking practices of experts (e.g., attending physicians) and novices (e.g., interns or medical students) can have significant consequences for a number of things including the design of health information technology that supports clinicians' activities, cognitive load during work activities, and the management of clinical workflow.

In an ongoing exploratory study, we investigated the differences in processes and strategies of information seeking between residents and affiliate providers (nurse practitioners [NPs] and physician assistants [PAs]). Initial results from the study showed fundamental differences in the information seeking strategies of residents and affiliates: residents predominantly utilized a *patient-based* approach of aggregating all relevant information for one patient at a time. In contrast, the affiliates used a *source-based* approach in which similar (or equivalent) information was aggregated for multiple patients at a time (e.g., x-rays for all patients).

Similar studies that explore the information seeking strategies of clinicians during various critical clinical activities (e.g., handoffs) can provide significant insights are multiple levels: understand the information needs, characterize the challenges faced during information seeking, the tools (or technology) that can potentially support these activities, potential for errors or missed information and other socio-technical issues.

Discussion Questions

1. What are some of challenges that clinicians face for information gathering in critical care environments? How can we mitigate the effects of such challenges?

2. What role does health information technology play in mitigating the information overload challenges? What technological support can aid the streamlining of the information seeking in clinical workflows?
3. The use of electronic health records (EHR) has been shown to affect clinical reasoning relative to paper charts. How does the use of EHR as a primary data gathering (information seeking) tool affect the reasoning process? Are there any detrimental effects?

References

1. Pirolli P, Card S. Information foraging. Psychol Rev. 1999;106:643–75.
2. Covell DG, Uman GC, Manning PR. Information needs in office practice. Ann Intern Med. 1985;103(4):596–9.
3. Gorman PN, Helfand M. Information seeking in primary care: how physicians choose which clinical questions to pursue and which to leave unanswered. Med Decis Making. 1995;15(2): 113–9.
4. Cogdill KW, Friedman CP, Jenkins CG, Mays BE, Sharp MC. Information needs and information seeking in community medical education. Acad Med. 2000;75:484–6.
5. Davies K, Harrison J. The information-seeking behaviour of doctors: a review of the evidence. Health Info Libr J. 2007;24(2):78–94.
6. Green ML, Ciampi MA, Ellis PJ. Residents' medical information needs in clinic: are they being met? Am J Med. 2000;109:218–23.
7. Kannampallil T.G, Franklin A, Mishra R, Cohen T, Almoosa KF, Patel VL. Understanding the Nature of Information Seeking Behavior in Critical Care: Implications for the Design of Health Information Technology. Artif Intell Med. 2013;57(1):21–29.
8. Safar P, Grenvik A. Organization and physician education in critical care medicine. Anesthesiology. 1977;47(2):82–95.
9. Ericsson KA, Simon HA. Verbal protocol analysis: verbal reports as data. Cambridge: MIT Press; 1993.
10. Patel VL, Yoskowitz NA, Arocha JF, Shortliffe EH. Cognitive and learning sciences in biomedical and health instructional design: a review with lessons for biomedical informatics education. J Biomed Inform. 2009;42(1):176–97.
11. Patel VL, Zhang J, Yoskowitz NA, Green R, Sayan OR. Translational cognition for decision support in critical care environments: a review. J Biomed Inform. 2008;41(3):413–31. PubMed PMID: 18343731. Pubmed Central PMCID: 2459228. Epub 2008/03/18. eng.
12. Li Z, Robinson DJ, Zhang J. UObserve: a mobile app for the study of emergency department workflow. Annals of Emergency Medicine 2010;56(3): S121.
13. Charnov EL. Optimal foraging: the marginal value theorem. Theor Popul Biol. 1976;9:129–36.
14. Stephens DW, Charnov EL. Optimal foraging: some simple stochastic models. Behav Ecol Sociobiol. 1982;10:251–63.
15. Stephens DW, Krebs JR. Foraging theory. Princeton: Princeton University Press; 1986.
16. Pirolli P. Rational analyses of information foraging on the web. Cognit Sci. 2005;29(3):343–73.
17. Pirolli P. Information foraging: a theory of adaptive interaction with information. New York: Oxford University Press; 2007.
18. Ely JW, Osheroff JA, Ebell MH, Bergus GR, Levy BT, Chambliss ML, et al. Analysis of questions asked by family doctors regarding patient care. BMJ. 1999;319(7206):358–61.
19. Evans DA, Gadd CS. Managing coherence and context in medical problem-solving discourse. In: Evans DA, Patel VL, editors. Cognitive science in medicine: biomedical modeling. Cambridge: MIT Press; 1989. p. 211–55.

20. Patel VL, Kaufman DR. Medical informatics and the science of cognition. J Am Med Inform Assoc. 1998;5(6):493–502. PubMed PMID: 9824797. Pubmed Central PMCID: 61330. Epub 1998/11/24. eng.
21. Patel VL, Arocha JF, Kaufman DR. Diagnostic reasoning and medical expertise. In: Medin D, editor. Psychology of learning and motivation – advances in research and theory. San Diego: Academic; 1994. p. 187–252.
22. Patel VL, Kaufman DR, Arocha JF. Emerging paradigms of cognition in medical decision-making. J Biomed Inform. 2002;35(1):52–75. PubMed PMID: 12415726. Epub 2002/11/06. eng.
23. Patel VL, Groen GJ, Scott HS. Biomedical knowledge in explanations of clinical problems by medical students. Med Educ. 1988;22(5):398–406.
24. Patel VL, Kushniruk AW, Yang S, Yale JF. Impact of a computerized patient record system on medical data collection, organization and reasoning. J Am Med Inform Assoc. 2000;7(6): 569–85.
25. Arocha JF, Wang D, Patel VL. Identifying reasoning strategies in medical decision making: a methodological guide. J Biomed Inform. 2005;38(2):154–71.
26. Laxmisan A, Hakimzada F, Sayan OR, Green RA, Zhang J, Patel VL. The multitasking clinician: decision-making and cognitive demand during and after team handoffs in emergency care. Int J Med Inform. 2007;76(11–12):801–11. PubMed PMID: 17059892. Epub 2006/10/25. eng.
27. Malhotra S, Jordan D, Shortliffe E, Patel VL. Workflow modeling in critical care: piecing together your own puzzle. J Biomed Inform. 2007;40:81–92.
28. Patel VL, Cohen T. New perspectives on error in critical care. Curr Opin Crit Care. 2008; 14(4):456–9.
29. Zhang J, Norman DA. Representations in distributed cognitive tasks. Cognit Sci. 1994; 18(1):87–122.
30. Sandstrom PE. Scholarly communication as a socioecological system. Scientometrics. 2001; 51(3):573–605.
31. Sharda P, Das AK, Cohen T, Patel VL. Customizing clinical narratives for the electronic medical record interface using cognitive methods. Int J Med Inform. 2006;75(5):346–68.
32. Patel VL, Groen GJ. Real versus artificial expertise: the development of cognitive models of clinical reasoning. In: Stefanelli M, Hasman A, Fieschi M, Talmon J, editors. Proceedings of the third conference on AI in medicine, Lecture notes in medical informatics (44). Maastricht: Springer; 1991. p. 25–37.
33. Patel VL, Shortliffe EH, Stefanelli M, Szolovits P, Berthold MR, Bellazzi R, et al. The coming of age of artificial intelligence in medicine. Artif Intell Med. 2009;46:5–17.
34. Patel VL, Arocha JF, Kaufman DR. Diagnostic reasoning and expertise. In: Medin D, editor. The psychology of learning and motivation: advances in research and theory, vol. 31. San Diego: Academic; 1994. p. 137–252.
35. Evans D, Gadd C. Managing coherence and context in medical problem-solving discourse. In: Cognitive science in medicine: biomedical modeling. Cambridge: MIT Press; 1989. p. 45.

Chapter 19
The Effects of Structuring Clinical Rounds on Communication and Efficiency

Laura K. Jones, Amy Franklin, Thomas G. Kannampallil, and Timothy G. Buchman

Introduction

Clinical rounds are a critical time for determining a patient's daily and long-term goals, for communicating these goals to a patients' healthcare team and to family, and for teaching medical students and other clinicians. However, these discussions are highly variable ranging from highly structured monologues at some sites to free form dialogues in other units [1–7]. Best practices and standards for round discussions are still emerging. As discussed in Lane et al.'s [8] review of the literature, known barriers to round quality include interruptions, long rounding times, and poor information retrieval. Given rounds' importance for team communication [9–11] and patient care, significant effort is being put forth to improve round quality. For example, tools such as scripts and checklists are proven to hasten the rounds process and increase the rounding teams' satisfaction [1, 3, 5, 7, 12–14].

L.K. Jones, PhD (✉)
Department of Surgery, Emory University School of Medicine, Atlanta, GA 30322, USA
e-mail: lkjones@emory.edu

A. Franklin, PhD
School of Biomedical Informatics, University of Texas Health Science Center, Houston, TX 77054, USA

National Center for Cognitive Informatics and Decision Making in Healthcare (NCCD), Houston, TX 77030, USA
e-mail: amy.franklin@uth.tmc.edu

T.G. Kannampallil
Center for Cognitive Studies in Medicine and Public Health, New York Academy of Medicine, New York, NY 10029, USA
e-mail: tkannampallil@nyam.org

T.G. Buchman, PhD, MD, FACS, FCCP, MCCM
Emory University School of Medicine, Atlanta, GA 30322, USA

Emory Center for Critical Care, Woodruff Health Sciences Center, Emory University, Atlanta, GA 30322, USA
e-mail: tbuchma@emory.edu

V.L. Patel et al. (eds.), *Cognitive Informatics in Health and Biomedicine*, Health Informatics, DOI 10.1007/978-1-4471-5490-7_19,

Our team studied a much larger tool for improving round quality—the use of a team theater. This theater is a room that sequesters the rounding team from the rest of the unit. Many hospital sites have implemented conference rooms [15–17] for rounding purposes, however, these rooms are often separate from the patients and the hospital unit itself. Our team theater, on the other hand, is situated within the unit and allows line of sight to patients and staff through its glass walls. It is intended to mitigate interruptions from passersby and reduce fatigue, as the rounding team sits instead of stands. Based on studies from the field of aviation, where decisions are made from sterile cockpits [18, 19], we investigated if the rounding in the team theater would be effective in helping to reduce barriers to round quality introduced by the clinical environment [20, 21]. We hypothesize that sequestering the rounding team could be the key to establishing and maintaining structure during rounds by reducing the variation in length of discussion and content.

Method

Setting

Our study was conducted in a cardiothoracic intensive care unit (CT-ICU) in a large, urban, academic hospital. During the course of observation, a new CT-ICU was built and staffed by our clinical team. In this natural experiment, we were able to capture rounds of the same CT-ICU team in two configurations, one with, and one without a team theater. For ease of discussion, we will refer to the initial configuration, of the unit as Unit A and the new configuration will be referred to as Unit B (team theater). Following the same participants through a physical change of space, we observe the impact of sequestering a team during round discussions.

The team theater (depicted below in Fig. 19.1) is centrally located in Unit B. Its glass walls allow occupants to remain aware of hallway activity while blocking minor interruptions. The rounding team is able to sit for the duration of rounds at desks that can be arranged into a circular formation.

Rounding Procedure

For both units, rounds would commence when the intensivist arrived and the affiliate providers (i.e., nurse practitioners and/or physician assistants), and/or residents concurred that they were ready to begin. Prior to the move to the team theater, rounds in Unit A occurred in the hallway outside of the patients' rooms and peripheral to the large, centralized nursing station. Rounds in Unit B utilized the theater space.

Following a semi-structured format, the teams would gather and one affiliate would commandeer a computer, load the patients' medical record and deliver their

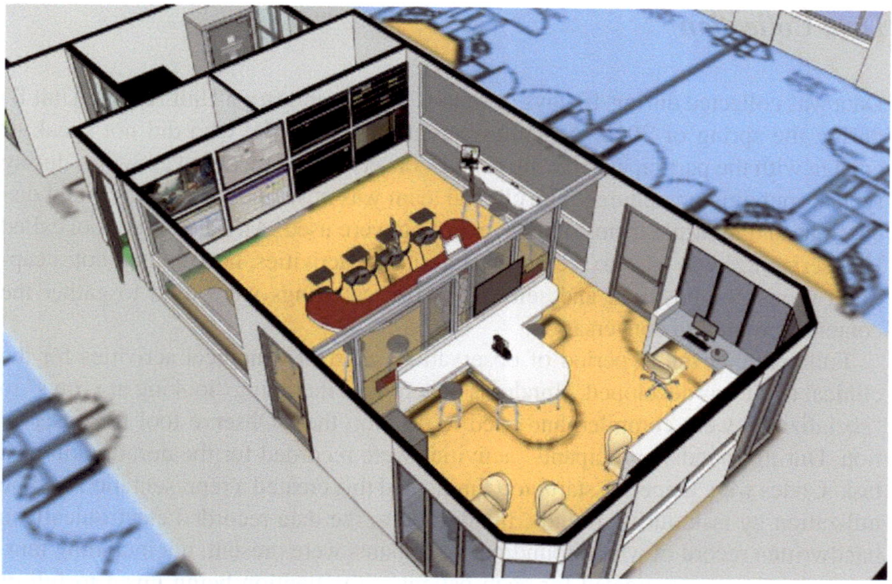

Fig. 19.1 The team theater, depicted above, has changed rounding behaviors

updates on each patient. Periodically, the patient's nurse would interject to add additional information on the patient. The composition of the team during discussion varied, ranging from 2 to 6 participants. The intensivist and affiliates were sometimes joined by the patient's nurse, a pharmacist, respiratory therapist, fellow or medical student and the occasional dietician. Family members were also were included in Unit A discussions. After reviewing each patient's current status, the affiliate would state his or her daily and long-term plans. Finally, the intensivist would share his/her thoughts and then open the case for discussion with the rest of the team.

Participants

Five affiliate providers and 5 intensivists form the core of the rounding team. Additional clinical team members such as pharmacists, nurses and therapists were included when present. Families and alert patients were taken aside to make sure they understood the purpose of the research and its risks.[1] Verbal consent was obtained from all participants in this institutional review board approved study.

[1] All participants were made aware that they could withdraw their participation at any time. No participants chose to withdraw, and the little concern from potential participants (save the ten intensivists) that did arise about the research was allayed.

Data Collection

Data was collected during 10 days of rounds in each unit (n = 5 Unit A, n = 5 Unit B) during the spring of 2012. An anthropologist with a PhD, who did not speak or engage with the participants during rounds, observed and recorded activities during typical rounding procedures. The clinical team was observed throughout round discussions and multiple forms of data recording were used. An iPad based tool called UObserve [22] was used to record the duration of activities, handwritten notes captured group composition, and selected audio recordings were used to gather the content of rounding conversation.

Following an initial period of observation, a list of canonical activities for the clinical team was developed. Hundreds of activities including "looking at x-rays" to "socializing" were compiled and used to develop the UObserve tool for observation. During rounds, participants' activities were recorded for the duration of each task. Codes were tapped to start/stop timing and this created a representation of time utilization by task during rounds. In addition to the data recorded electronically, a handwritten record of which rounding participants were present, not including family and patient, was created for each patient with attention being given to full or part-time participation in the discussion. Group composition and contributions were pulled from this data.

In addition to the observations made by the researcher, audio recordings were captured for the group by placing microphones on the intensivist and as well as the other clinical team members presenting patients (i.e. affiliates, medical students). As the data collection agreement only allowed for encrypted recordings that were destroyed after 24 h, data transcription was limited to the longest and the shortest patient presentations. The names of people and pharmaceuticals were anonymized in the transcriptions.

Data were analyzed considering the unit in which the discussion occurred, the composition of the group at the time, and the proportion of time spent during the rounds on each patient. Additionally, we considered the nature of communication during each discussion.

Time Spent During Rounds

While rounds accomplish many goals from coordinating patient care, providing opportunities for interaction between clinical team members, and educating trainees, rounds consume a significant amount of clinical time (on average 105 min) [23]. Concerns for the maintenance of attention and consistency across patients have given rise to studies exploring the amount of time spent during high and low patient loads [24] as well as the amount of time attributed to each patient [25–27]. Here we consider the amount of time spent discussing each patient, including their position in that discussion in both units observed.

The time spent on each patient was organized according to the order in which the patients were discussed. The patients were sequentially ordered and the total time spent per patient was computed for both ICU configurations. Next, for each session, the time spent per patient was normalized as a proportion of the total time spent during that session. For example, if the total time for a session was 2,400 s (i.e., 40 min), and the time spent for the first patient was 600 s, then the proportion of time spent for the first patient was 600/2,400 = 0.25. Similarly, the order of patients was also normalized as a proportion of the total number of patients seen during that session. Kendall's τ correlations were calculated for each session to evaluate whether there was a significant negative correlation between the order of patients seen and the proportion of time spent on each patient.

In addition to this, we also identified the number of clinical staff that was present during the rounds. Full-time members of the rounding team generally included the attending physician and the affiliate who presented the case under discussion. Part-time members of the rounding team generally included a second affiliate and a pharmacist. If they were present, fellows, medical students, other affiliates, nurses, consults, and others were generally present part-time. Changes in the composition of the group could potentially alter the length of rounds.

Content of Rounds: Qualitative Analysis

Changes to the content of rounds often include the use of tools such as checklists or standardized content [1, 7, 12–14]. The aim of these processes is to eliminate information loss and communication gaps by ensuring discussion of all relevant details. These lists often cover information at the level of capturing each body system or process (e.g. discussion of current breathing function and input/outputs overnight.) Other rich descriptions of ICU effort or round discussions such as Sung et al.'s [27] compare times spent discussing new patients, established patients, data review and staff communication. Here, we add an additional layer of description. Given our two settings of sequestered and open rounds along with the two sets of shortest and longest patient discussions, we explore what distinguishes these conversations. That is, what beyond duration changes?

We focus at the pragmatic level to consider what is the intent of each utterance is and how many of such turns are used to organize the discussion in addition to sharing patient data.

The longest and shortest patient discussion for each observed round was transcribed within 24 h of collection. Identifying information such as patient name was not included in the transcript. The written transcription of the discussion was separated into turns by speaker and further broken down by utterance. Each utterance roughly captures a thought, and multiple utterances may be contained in a single turn of conversation. 5,431 utterances were transcribed (average 400 utterances in long discussion and 143 utterances on average in short patient discussions).

Twenty patient cases are presented and each case represents a different individual with unique history and needs. While we did confirm that each patient's discussion includes some mention of all major body systems (e.g. discussion of cardiac function, state of extremities, labs, medications, renal function etc.), it is beyond the

Table 19.1 Categories of utterances spoken during rounds

Category	Description	Example
Describing	Follows the designated format and describes the patient's case	Mr. X is a 62 year-old patient
Seeking	Requests information	What is his white count?
Coordinating	Aligns members of the rounding team	We will diurese her tomorrow
Clarifying	Clears ambiguity	You said we were getting another x-ray?
Other	Covers all other communicative acts include rhetoric and social communication	Thank you; continue

scope of the current paper to determine if the length and coverage of each discussion is appropriately thorough. Here, we are not exploring if duration of conversation is influenced by the complexity, relevance of information given, or amount of training provided by case. Instead, we explore whether or not different communicative processes such as information seeking and coordinating across the group differ based on environment of conversation and length of discussion.

We used grounded theory to discover the communication themes occurring during rounds. Our dataset was coded by the lead investigator into 1 of 5 categories of speech acts. These categories include describing, seeking, coordinating, clarifying and other forms communicative practices (see Table 19.1 below). As we are focused entirely on rounds, describing as a category encompasses all forms of reporting or summarization of patient state, history or other declarative knowledge of the patient. This description is provided in a semi-structured format (e.g. regular structure and order to the presentation such as giving name, gender, patient age, recent procedures, and other details in order). Utterances were coded as information seeking if there was an explicit request for information and typically given as a question. Similarly, clarifying questions requested confirmation, clarification, or other negotiation. Coordinating statements included utterances that establish roles, plans and agreement regarding the alignment of shared activities and goals. Finally, a remaining category of other was used to capture social communication, rhetoric and non-patient related content.

Results

Time Spent on Rounds

In the team theater, i.e. ICU Unit B, there was no effect on the time spent per patient based on the order of patients seen or the number of full-time staff that were present during the rounds. But, there was significant effect on the presence of part-time staff members, with the proportion of time spent per patient increasing at a rate of 0.019

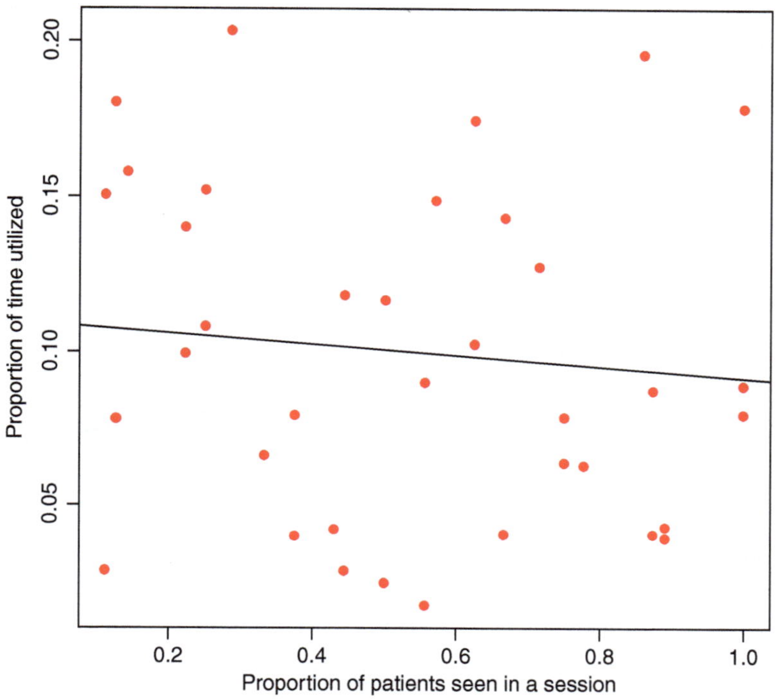

Fig. 19.2 Proportion of patient seen as a function of the proportion of time spent per patient in the team theater (Unit B). There was no significant decrease in the time spent on each additional patient

(*p* <0.001) with each additional patient that was discussed during the rounds. It seems that in a controlled environment, the part-time presence of staff increases the discussion time, potentially giving the patients they see a greater allotment of time. While sequestering the rounding team may reduce the effect of interruptions and other events that might lead to spending a disproportionate amount of time with each patient, the introduction of new variables, such as more staff members, may increase discrepancies.

In contrast, in Unit A, there was a marginal effect of the order of the patients seen on the proportion of time spent per patient. In other words, the proportion of time spent per patient increased at a rate of 0.04 (p=0.072) with each new patient that was discussed during the rounds. The number of full-time or part-time staff that was present did not affect this increase the per-patient rounding time. Figures 19.2 and 19.3 shows the relation between the proportion of time spent and patients seen across all sessions for the team theater and traditional rounding sessions. Additionally, the Kendall's τ correlations were not significant for any of the sessions in either unit (sequestered or not), providing further overall evidence of no significant negative correlations between the order of patients seen and the time spent for discussing each patient.

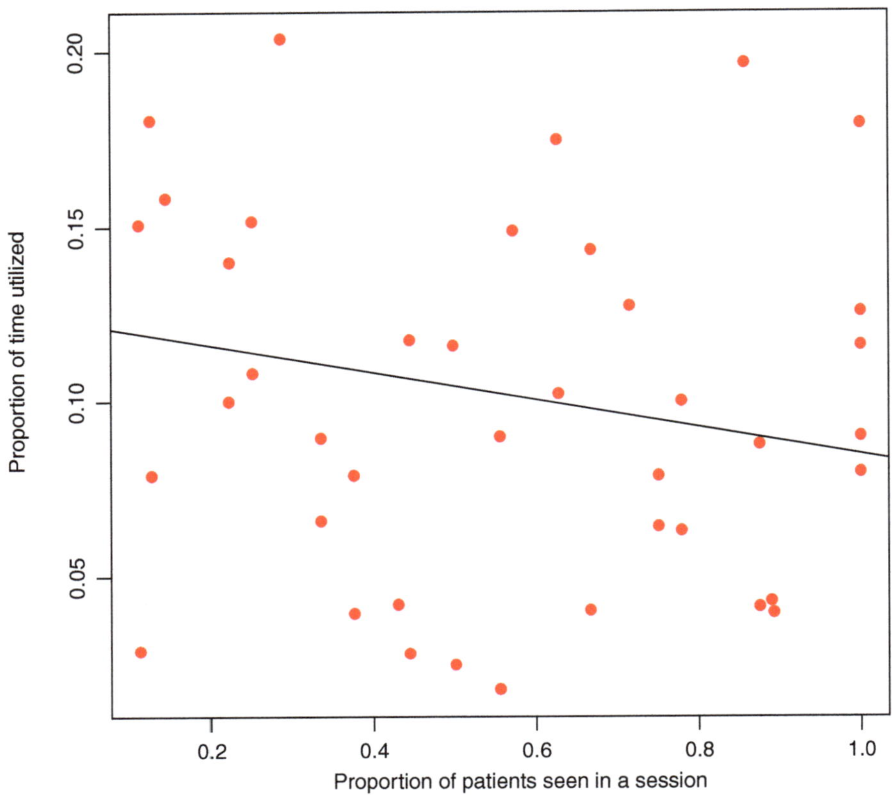

Fig. 19.3 Proportion of patients seen as a function of the proportion of time spent per patient in Unit A. There was a slight increase ($p < 0.1$) in the time spent on each additional patient

Our results are in contrast to previous findings that suggested a decrement in time spent per patient based on position in rounding discussion. We found an increase in time spent per patient in our traditional unit as well as an increase with group size in the sequestered unit. Differences in our findings and the previous may reflect variability created by contextual factors such as day of the week, acuity of patients, and group dynamics.

Comparing by Duration: Longest Versus Shortest Patient Discussions

While the above analyses considered the duration of all presentations, we continue our analysis by exploring differences between the longest and shortest discussions within a rounding session to determine if there are any meaningful differences.

One potential impact of interdisciplinary rounds may be simply more people equals more being said. Sequestering the teams is intended to prevent group attrition and limit interruptions. Our analysis indicates, however, when the longest discussions were considered there were no differences between the two ICUs in terms of the number of utterances ($M_{21\text{-}ICU}$=6.8 ($S.D._{21\text{-}ICU}$=1.09), $M_{11\text{-}ICU}$=6.0 ($S.D._{11\text{-}ICU}$=1.87), $t(4)=0.827$, $p=0.45$), speakers ($M_{21\text{-}ICU}$=443.0 ($S.D._{21\text{-}ICU}$=64.94), $M_{11\text{-}ICU}$=387 ($S.D._{11\text{-}ICU}$=113.09), $t(4)=1.081$, $p=0.34$), or turns ($M_{21\text{-}ICU}$=173.4 ($S.D._{21\text{-}ICU}$=48.74), $M_{11\text{-}ICU}$=154.6 ($S.D._{11\text{-}ICU}$=63.38), $t(4)=0.496$, $p=0.64$). However, when we consider the shortest discussions for each session in both units, there was a significant difference in the number of utterances in the shorter sessions with the non-sequestered ICU having fewer utterances ($M_{21\text{-}ICU}$=128.4 ($S.D._{21\text{-}ICU}$= 33.34), $M_{11\text{-}ICU}$=169.2 ($S.D._{11\text{-}ICU}$=53.76), $t(4)=-3.327$, $p<0.05$).

There were no differences in the number of speakers ($M_{21\text{-}ICU}$=3.8 ($S.D._{21\text{-}ICU}$= 1.92), $M_{11\text{-}ICU}$=4.6 ($S.D._{11\text{-}ICU}$=1.67), $t(4)=-0.82$, $p=0.45$) or the number of turns ($M_{21\text{-}ICU}$=43 ($S.D._{21\text{-}ICU}$=22.21), $M_{11\text{-}ICU}$=53.8 ($S.D._{11\text{-}ICU}$=24.12), $t(4)=-1.92$, $p=0.12$). We then consider if the variation seen is duration only or in fact there are differences in the content of discussions.

Content of the Rounds

As you would expect given the updating and planning goal of rounds, 63.49 % of round discussions are spent in description. 4.7 % of utterances seek information while 4.4 % in general are used for clarification. A sizeable portion (21.36 %) is found to cover rhetorical statements, social conversation and other types of communication not directly functioning to support the patient case. In both configurations A and B, we observed interruptions from both outside and inside the group, relevant and irrelevant to the patient under discussion, that would often cause deviation from this semi-structured format.

With our goal of exploring length and location, we first compare the longest and shortest discussion within each unit to determine if the differences in duration are due to quantity of discussion or content conveyed. Only the coordinating category ($t(4)$ =2.95, $p<0.05$) varied between the long and short rounds and only for the sequestered unit.

While the intent of sequestering to reduce interruptions and fatigue, there seems to be an impact on group attrition. The larger groups found in the sequestered units may require additional coordination which is seen in the above result as well as contributes to the lengthier duration of discussion. It is a limitation of our analysis that we did not consider the paralinguistic features of the utterances of coordination. It is ambiguous as to whether or not we have captured greater agreement in coordination (e.g. Yes, we will do X today) or request for coordination (e.g. We will do X, right?) as such differences may be conveyed only using tone of voice. Future work is needed to tease apart the kinds of coordination in different implementations.

When we consider other differences across units (looking again at location while comparing short to short and long to long), it is generally only in the shorter rounds[2] that differences are found across the configurations. Activities of describing

[2] Seeking($t(4)=4.18$, $p<0.05$) between units for long.

($t(4) = -6.92, p < 0.05$) coordinating($t(4) = -1.21, p < 0.05$), and clarifying ($t(4) = 6.34$, $p < 0.05$) differed between the sequestered and non-sequestered units. This suggests that the shorter patient discussions in the non-sequestered units are both lesser in terms of time spent, content covered, and coordinating activities.

Conclusion

As efforts are made to improve the quality of rounds, it is important to consider the influence of the environment as well as the format of the round and the use of tools such as checklists. Our results suggest the potential for sequestering clinical teams in team theaters is one way of supporting round discussions. From interest in remote presence through robot-physicians on rounds to the use of team theaters, we must continue to expand the body of research investigating the impact of design (including artifacts and physical space) on performance. From rich descriptions such as Sung et al. to comparative studies of different configurations [28], future work is needed to better understand the sources of variability during rounds and their impact on patient outcomes.

Discussion Questions

(a) If the presence of more care team members increases variability in rounds, should the care team size be capped during rounds? What are the pros and cons of having more participants in interdisciplinary rounds? Is variability always a negative?
(b) Communication is complex and especially challenging to study. How did our mixed methods, both quantitative and qualitative, substantiate each other? What other methods could be used to study communication in healthcare?
(c) Bedside rounds are becoming less common and team theater-style configurations and telemedicine more common. Are we ready for rounds be conducted completely outside of the ICU? Why or why not?

References

1. Dodek PM, Raboud J. Explicit approach to rounds in an ICU improves communication and satisfaction of providers. Intensive Care Med. 2003;29(9):1584–8. PubMed PMID: 12898001. Epub 2003/08/05.
2. Geary S, Cale DD, Quinn B, Winchell J. Daily rapid rounds: decreasing length of stay and improving professional practice. J Nurs Adm. 2009;39(6):293–8. PubMed PMID: 19509604. Epub 2009/06/11.

3. Gurses AP, Xiao Y. A systematic review of the literature on multidisciplinary rounds to design information technology. J Am Med Inform Assoc. 2006;13(3):267–76. PubMed PMID: 16501176. Pubmed Central PMCID: 1513658. Epub 2006/02/28.
4. Mansell A, Uttley J, Player P, Nolan O, Jackson S. Is the post-take ward round standardised? Clin Teach. 2012;9(5):334–7. PubMed PMID: 22994475.
5. Gonzalo J. The return of bedside rounds. J Gen Intern Med. 2010;25(8):792–8. PubMed PMID: 21061081. Pubmed Central PMCID: 3019335. Epub 2010/11/10.
6. Sen A, Xiao Y, Lee SA, Hu P, Dutton RP, Haan J, et al. Daily multidisciplinary discharge rounds in a trauma center: a little time, well spent. J Trauma. 2009;66(3):880–7. PubMed PMID: 19276768. Epub 2009/03/12.
7. Cardarelli M, Vaidya V, Conway D, Jarin J, Xiao Y. Dissecting multidisciplinary cardiac surgery rounds. Ann Thorac Surg. 2009;88(3):809–13. PubMed PMID: 19699903. Epub 2009/08/25.
8. Lane D, Ferri M, Lemaire J, McLaughlin K, Stelfox HT. A systematic review of evidence-informed practices for patient care rounds in the ICU. Crit Care Med. 2013;41(8):2015–29. PubMed PMID: 23666096.
9. Reader TW, Flin R, Cuthbertson BH. Communication skills and error in the intensive care unit. Curr Opin Crit Care. 2007;13(6):732–6. PubMed PMID: 17975399. Epub 2007/11/03.
10. Reader TW, Flin R, Mearns K, Cuthbertson BH. Team situation awareness and the anticipation of patient progress during ICU rounds. BMJ Qual Saf. 2011;20(12):1035–42. PubMed PMID: 21700727. Epub 2011/06/28.
11. Reader TW, Flin R, Mearns K, Cuthbertson BH. Developing a team performance framework for the intensive care unit. Crit Care Med. 2009;37(5):1787–93. PubMed PMID: 19325474. Epub 2009/03/28.
12. Carroll K, Iedema R, Kerridge R. Reshaping ICU ward round practices using video-reflexive ethnography. Qual Health Res. 2008;18(3):380–90. PubMed PMID: 18235161. Epub 2008/02/01.
13. Rehder KJ, Uhl TL, Meliones JN, Turner DA, Smith PB, Mistry KP. Targeted interventions improve shared agreement of daily goals in the pediatric intensive care unit. Pediatr Crit Care Med. 2012;13(1):6–10. PubMed PMID: 21478796. Pubmed Central PMCID: 3163112. Epub 2011/04/12.
14. Stahl K, Palileo A, Schulman CI, Wilson K, Augenstein J, Kiffin C, et al. Enhancing patient safety in the trauma/surgical intensive care unit. J Trauma. 2009;67(3):430–3; discussion 3–5. PubMed PMID: 1974138. Epub 2009/09/11.
15. Miller M, Johnson B, Greene HL, Baier M, Nowlin S. An observational study of attending rounds. J Gen Intern Med. 1992;7(6):646–8. PubMed PMID: 1453250.
16. Elliot DL, Hickam DH. Attending rounds on in-patient units: differences between medical and non-medical services. Med Educ. 1993;27(6):503–8. PubMed PMID: 8208158.
17. Stickrath C, Noble M, Prochazka A, Anderson M, Griffiths M, Manheim J, et al. Attending rounds in the current era: what is and is not happening. JAMA Intern Med. 2013;173(12): 1084–9. PubMed PMID: 23649040.
18. Gawande A. The checklist manifesto: how to get things right, vol. x. 1st ed. New York: Metropolitan Books; 2010. p. 209.
19. Nance JJ. Why hospitals should fly: the ultimate flight plan to patient safety and quality care, vol. ix. Bozeman: Second River Healthcare Press; 2008. p. 225.
20. Hohenhaus S, Powell S. Distractions and interruptions: development of a healthcare sterile cockpit. Infant Nurs Rev. 2008;8(2):108–10.
21. Fore AM, Sculli GL, Albee D, Neily J. Improving patient safety using the sterile cockpit principle during medication administration: a collaborative, unit-based project. J Nurs Manage. 2013;21(1):106–11. PubMed PMID: 23339500.
22. Li Z, Robinson DJ, Zhang J. UObserve: a mobile app for the study of emergency department workflow. Annals of Emergency Medicine 2010;56(3):S121.

23. Priest JR, Bereknyei S, Hooper K, Braddock 3rd CH. Relationships of the location and content of rounds to specialty, institution, patient-census, and team size. PLoS One. 2010;5(6):e11246. PubMed PMID: 20574534. Pubmed Central PMCID: 2888591. Epub 2010/06/25.
24. Pardo D, Rey M, Weinreb S, Cooney E, Gabler NB, Howell MD, et al. Intensivist rounding time allocation during times of high and low ICU capacity strain. 2013. doi:10.1164/ajrccm-conference.2013.187.1_MeetingAbstracts.A5316.
25. Kannampallil T, Jones L, Buchman T, Franklin A. Last patients finish last: end of round time compression during CT ICU clinical rounds. Crit Care Med. 2011;39(12):176.
26. Cohen MD, Ilan R, Garrett L, Lebaron C, Christianson MK. The earlier the longer: disproportionate time allocated to patients discussed early in attending physician handoff sessions. Arch Intern Med. 2012;172(22):1762–4. PubMed PMID: 23403737.
27. Sung N, Weiss CH, Rho J, DiBardino DM, Collander B, Wunderink RG. Rounding order as a predictor of individual patient rounding times. 2012. doi:10.1164/ajrccm-conference.2012.185.1_MeetingAbstracts.A6562.
28. Landry MA, Lafrenaye S, Roy MC, Cyr C. A randomized, controlled trial of bedside versus conference-room case presentation in a pediatric intensive care unit. Pediatrics. 2007;120(2):275–80. PubMed PMID: 17671052.

Part IV
Looking into the Future

Chapter 20
Clinical Implications of Cognitive Complexity in Critical Care

Khalid F. Almoosa, R. Stanley Hum, Timothy G. Buchman, Bela Patel, Vafa Ghaemmaghami, and Trevor Cohen

Introduction

The evolution of critical care medicine and the Intensive Care Unit (ICU) has been a major advance in the success of modern medicine. Critical care medicine is a subspecialty that provides intensive life-sustaining monitoring and therapies for patients with life-threatening conditions in a very specialized setting. Each year, more than five million patients are admitted to the 5,000 ICUs in the United States [1], and the cost to sustain this care exceeds $90 billion annually [2]. Critical care is very dynamic, fast-paced, and complex in content and delivery, and optimal critical care is provided round-the-clock by a highly specialized, multi-disciplinary team.

K.F. Almoosa, MD, MS, FCCP (✉)
Division of Critical Care Medicine, Memorial Hermann Hospital, University of Texas Health Science Center, Texas Medical Center, Houston, TX 77030, USA
e-mail: khalid.f.almoosa@uth.tmc.edu

R.S. Hum, MD, FRCPC
Department of Pediatrics, College of Physicians and Surgeons, Columbia University, New York, NY, USA

T.G. Buchman, PhD, MD, FACS, FCCP, MCCM
Emory Center for Critical Care, Emory University School of Medicine, Woodruff Health Sciences Center, Emory University, Atlanta, GA 30322, USA

B. Patel, MD, DABSM, FCCP
Critical Care Medicine, Memorial Hermann Hospital, University of Texas Health Science Center, Texas Medical Center, Houston, TX 77030, USA

V. Ghaemmaghami, MD, FACS
Trauma Division, Department of Surgery, Banner Good Samaritan Hospital, Phoenix, AZ 85006, USA

University of Arizona College of Medicine, Phoenix, AZ USA

T. Cohen, MB ChB, PhD
School of Biomedical Informatics, University of Texas Health Science Center, Houston, TX 77054, USA

V.L. Patel et al. (eds.), *Cognitive Informatics in Health and Biomedicine*, Health Informatics, DOI 10.1007/978-1-4471-5490-7_20, © Springer-Verlag London 2014

The provision of critical care has improved outcomes such as mortality and has prolonged and saved countless lives since its inception.

The landmark Institute of Medicine report "To Err is Human" awoke our nation to the reality of our unsafe healthcare system [3], where deaths from medical errors are the sixth leading cause of death. This error-ridden and failure-prone system continues to grow in size and complexity, in part due to the growth of medical science and technology, information systems and capabilities, public health needs, and population growth and aging. Because the ICU exemplifies the breadth and depth of a complex healthcare system, it is a high-risk environment prone to risk, errors, and failures. In this capacity, it can significantly contribute to patient harm as indicated by the IOM report and thus remains a vital focus of efforts to improve patient safety and quality of care.

Many facets of critical care expose it to the risks of injury and harm. Clearly, the plethora of illnesses and their various manifestations and complications require a broad and deep knowledge of clinical critical care medicine, and any deficiency of this can lead to delayed or erroneous diagnoses. The need to acquire and maintain procedural skills is important to avoid injury from invasive procedures. The multi-disciplinary ICU team model mandates clear, timely, and structured communication of patient information and plan of care among team members. The availability of immediate and accurate information is paramount to avoid delays or inappropriate treatments or decisions. The multitude of interventions, consultations, and care transitions provide ample opportunity to delay or hinder workflow. The implementation of protocols and policies are vital to standardizing patient care and ensuring adherence to evidence-based practices, but their application requires understanding and engagement to be effective. Most importantly, skilled clinical decision-making is foundational to developing an effective and timely plan of care that directly affects patient outcomes in particular and healthcare delivery in general. This chapter explores some of these facets of critical care practice from the perspective of cognitive informatics and its clinical application to improve patient care delivery in the complex ICU environment.

Clinical Decision-Making

Of all the duties and challenges of today's ICU clinician, clinical decision-making perhaps the most complex and challenging; yet it is also the most important. Clearly, knowledge of clinical science coupled with the critical thinking and procedural skills required to apply that knowledge are foundational to successful clinical practice. However, since the realm of clinical medicine lies within the larger healthcare delivery system, the determinants of good clinical practice extend beyond medical knowledge and clinical reasoning to include many other concepts. This section explores some of these concepts.

Heuristics

Clinical decision-making in high velocity environments such as the ICU has many constraints, including limited time, urgency of patients' conditions and needs, multi-tasking, high stress and high-risk situations, and nuances based on patient preferences. These conditions provide ample opportunities for the use of heuristics, or mental shortcuts in decision-making. In many circumstances, these heuristics are effective decision aids. However, they inherently have limitations and can potentially lead to bias if not used properly. Decision-making involves many different approaches and types, each of which has its own advantages and limitations. Despite the prevalent use of heuristics in clinical care, the manner in which they are used in high intensity environments such as the Emergency Center or the Intensive Care Unit has not been formally studied. To characterize physicians' use of cognitive heuristics in clinical decision-making when caring for critically ill patients, Payne et al. performed a national pilot study to ascertain critical care and emergency medicine attending physicians' perception of the frequency of use of heuristics and biases during clinical reasoning using an electronic survey instrument [4]. In this study, subjects were given a semi-structured questionnaire that contained a definition and 37 clinical examples of heuristics and biases, and they were asked to rate the prevalence of their use in clinical practice. The researchers found that physicians reported the use of several types of heuristics that differed between emergency medicine and critical care physicians. The most common ones reported by critical care physicians include: confirmation bias (tendency to look for confirming evidence to support a diagnosis, and ignore evidence to the contrary), availability (when a diagnosis is triggered by similar recent cases), planning fallacy (tendency to underestimate the time to complete a task), in-group bias (tendency to have positive views of, and give preferential treatment to, patients they perceive to be members of their own group), and deformation professional (tendency to view things according to the conventions of one's own profession).

The researchers then performed a proof-of-concept study, where data were collected during morning rounds in an adult medical ICU at a large teaching hospital [4]. Clinical team interactions were recorded and "single purpose phrases" – phrases deemed to represent a single decision, thought or action – were identified and coded based on information utilized, decision quality, outcome, and the use of heuristics. Many types of heuristics, in addition to those mentioned above, were identified and were part of one of the three main steps in the critical care process: immediate need assessment, addressing problem, and patient management. In each of these steps, the authors identified potential reasoning errors that may lead to erroneous decisions which included neglecting or not considering pertinent data, considering data not associated with the correct diagnosis, inaccurate mapping of the patient's situation, not considering all possible diagnoses, not noticing a change in the patient's status, not fully investigating all diagnostic possibilities, and not recognizing a pre-existing condition that may impact the current clinical state.

This work demonstrated that heuristics are prevalent throughout the spectrum of critical care practice. The ICU environment is ideal for the use of heuristics when applied appropriately, and their use can have a powerful salutary effect on decision-making and efficiency of care. On the other hand, their misuse can result in flawed reasoning and ultimately incorrect decisions that lead to poor, delayed, or even dangerous patient care. In fact, this study's results are impressive but not surprising in the extent and scope of biases prevalent among critical care physicians, and one can only hypothesize the effect of this cognitive "habit" on diagnostic accuracy. Because of the great positive and negative potential of the use of heuristics, it is imperative that knowledge gained from this and other studies on heuristics be extended and integrated into clinical training, where it can nicely complement the reasoning and thinking patterns taught through the use of the scientific method and deductive reasoning. This incorporation of heuristics in daily clinical decision-making is particularly important not only because of growing workloads reducing thinking time, but also from the increased transitions of care (shift work), increasing complexity of patients' illnesses, and increasing sub-specialization of all branches of clinical science and care delivery. The fast pace of the ICU and the need to immediately address urgent patient care issues can easily lead to a "cookbook" approach to medicine, which may be appropriate most of the time but detrimental for the more unique cases. On the other hand, the contentious nature of clinical practice and diagnostics would benefit from a more standardized approach to decision-making. The incorporation of heuristics – and the knowledge and increased awareness of its potential biases – can facilitate physicians' reasoning and decision-making while at the same time caution them from its pitfalls. In fact, Croskerry et al. suggested that cognitive de-biasing strategies, where clinicians are educated about biases and how to avoid them, can reduce diagnostic errors, a major component of medical errors [5].

Error Management by Individuals

Risk and error are pervasive components of complex systems. In healthcare, the Institute of Medicine estimated that between 44,000 and 98,000 patients die every year from preventable medical error [3], a projection that many today believe is underestimated. Furthermore, since this report's publication in 1999, there has been little improvement in patient safety as a result of risk mitigation and error reduction, and medical errors cause more deaths in the United States than AIDS, breast cancer, or motor vehicle accidents [6]. The traditional approach to error mitigation has been to focus on the individual through blame, education, re-training, or punishment. This approach fails to incorporate the concept of systems improvement in complex settings, where the interaction of multiple factors in the system is more likely to contribute to risk and error than individual limitations or bad intentions. The scientist Hutchins pioneered work on cognition in complex systems and shifted the focus from individuals functioning in their environment to groups of individuals interacting with all the components in their real-world system [7]. Furthermore, the traditional approach has been predicated on the belief that increased knowledge and expertise reduce error and poor outcomes, a concept that is increasingly refuted and replaced by a systems improvement and human factors interaction approach. It is currently believed that error and risk are inevitable components of complex systems, and the main focus therefore should be on risk and error detection and recovery in addition to error mitigation to control adverse outcomes [8]. Prior studies have reported that both experts and non-experts commit errors in complex clinical environments, but the nature and management of these errors rather than their number differ significantly. In addition, experts detect more errors and correct them more efficiently than non-experts, particularly more complex ones [9, 10]. Cognitive complexity work has become increasingly focused on these aspects of risk and error mitigation [11, 12].

Building on prior work, Patel et al. conducted an in vitro study of error detection and recovery on 25 attending (expert) and resident (non-expert) physicians in makeshift laboratory settings at 2 sites [13]. Participants were presented with two clinical problem cases in paper form that contained a range of knowledge-based and procedural management errors embedded within them, such as inappropriate antibiotics, contraindications for procedures, and missed diagnoses. Subjects were not informed beforehand (primed) that errors were present in the cases and were asked to evaluate their management. Analysis of natural language responses were analyzed in areas such as error detection, error corrections, and justification of clinical decisions. Results demonstrated that experts were somewhat better able to detect errors, particularly the most complex types, and did so as they were working through the problem. However, error detection by experts fell short of expectations, with no participant detecting more than half of the embedded errors, regardless of expertise. Error detection by non-experts was more likely related to adverse events, and more often detected after reading through the entire case. Experts more frequently provided justifications for their detection of errors than non-experts, perhaps reflecting their teaching role and skills. Non-experts demonstrated a more cautious detection of errors and had a slower recovery time. This study implies that error detection and recovery are dependent on expertise and that although all clinicians at all levels make errors, the type, effect, and recovery from these errors differ by expertise.

In a follow-up study, Razzouk et al. studied error recovery in vivo through the use of virtual world technology to simulate the verbal presentation of cases in a clinical setting [14]. The objective was to determine whether failed error detection was due to lack of knowledge or other reasons. The experiment involved 17 physicians-in-training at various levels of their post-graduate programs (interns, residents, and fellows) who were presented with two verbal case scenarios on OpenSim (an open source project that provides a host server for virtual worlds; http://opensimulator.org) representing common ICU cases that contained embedded errors with varying degrees of complexity. Subjects observed a case presentation in the context of a virtual ICU environment, then summarized their impressions of the case. Subsequently, they answered a set of knowledge-based questions designed to test for the knowledge prerequisite to the detection of each embedded error. For the second case, they repeated this procedure after being primed to focus on error detection. Results demonstrated that priming had a significant effect on error detection. The authors concluded that while detection of embedded errors by non-expert physician learners was limited, it improved significantly with priming.

This implies that performance can be substantially improved with specific training and may ultimately have a salutary effect on patient outcomes and safety.

These studies and others focusing on error and risk detection, prevention, and recovery have direct implications on how critical care medicine is practiced. Critical care physicians will increasingly encounter complex patients, utilize complex technologies and data, interact with complex specialties and policies, and function in an accountable public and professional climate. Cognitive demands such as decision-making, team-leading, multi-tasking, information analysis, and communication require continuous attention and effort and may interfere with clinical duties needed more urgently in critically ill situations. In addition, these studies build on prior knowledge regarding teams' response to error. Error detection and recovery by teams is better compared to individuals working alone (see below), although new errors may be generated by team discussions [15]. A solid understanding of how clinicians at all levels of expertise function effectively and safely is vital to improving the quality of our patients' care and outcomes, and these studies on risk and error management provide a foundational perspective to improve our clinical practice.

Expertise in knowledge and skills is vital to good clinical practice but has a limited effect on error occurrence. As clinicians and human beings managing patients in complex and risky environments, we must acknowledge that we will always make errors – albeit different types – and that most may not even be recognized by us or others. Attention should therefore focus on improved error detection and recovery rather than error elimination, as evidenced by an increased body of literature reporting that error elimination is an impractical and unobtainable goal. Fortunately, while error management is a skill that can be acquired with expertise, it may also be learned by non-experts earlier in their careers through specific training. Clearly, experience can increase vigilance about potential specific dangers and lead to rapid intervention to prevent or control them. But as Razzouk et al. demonstrated in their study, perhaps "priming" physicians at the start of their careers during their training using interactive formats may accelerate this knowledge and incorporate it into their practice earlier. Priming may have a major effect on adverse outcome reduction in academic institutions in particular, which are often the most complex and error-prone healthcare facilities due to the presence of trainees managing the sickest patients. Furthermore, contrary to popular belief, other studies have reported that the greatest number of errors may occur at low workloads and the least at high workloads [16]. However, error detection at high workloads is decreased, leading to a higher level of adverse outcomes. In addition, with training the total number of errors remains the same, but error detection improves. Earlier error detection can have important clinical consequences in patients with high acuity illnesses such as in the ICU environment.

Error Management by Teams

From exploring error management by individuals [12], Patel et al. extended their work to decision-making within clinical teams. Using a semi-naturalistic approach, two cases with embedded errors were presented to 5 ICU teams (including a total of 32 clinician subjects) during rounds, and the teams were instructed to discuss and comment on the cases' management. Error generation, detection, and recovery were evaluated and compared between individuals and teams. Teams detected a mean of 4.8 ± 1.3 of a total of 8 errors in both cases, accounting for 60 % of all errors and performing better than individuals, none of whom identified more than half of the embedded errors in any experiment (these results are not strictly comparable, as different case scenarios were used in each experiment, but the suggestion of better performance by teams is nonetheless encouraging and intuitively appealing). Teams performed better at detecting complex and knowledge-based errors than simple and procedure-based ones. Interestingly, longer team discussions resulted in generation of new errors. However, the likelihood of recovery from errors also increased with the number of interactive dialogue episodes. At the same time, errors were being generated as the length of the dialogue increased, suggesting that at some point in time, dialogue about patient care moves away to discussion of more general issues related to developing broader understanding of the problem.

The notion that teams almost always perform better than individuals is again reaffirmed by this study. Indeed, team-based learning is rapidly replacing traditional formats as a core model for education in medical schools, where the focus is on team-centered decision-making and cognition [17]. Many factors of teamwork may contribute to improved decision-making and error management: sharing of individual knowledge, social interactions stimulating generation of ideas, correction of mistakes and slips, aligning and focusing on common objectives, lack of social or organizational hierarchy hindering discussions, safety culture, and shared responsibility and accountability. While involving several perspectives adds to the collective knowledge, a more important concept demonstrated by this study is the fact that increased discussion time increased the likelihood of error detection and recovery despite generating more errors! This underscores the power and value of distributed cognition through open discussion among professionals in high-risk, time-limited, and dynamic situations such as the ICU. It would be of interest to re-evaluate this concept during varying levels of workload, work complexity, and team interpersonal relationships. The growing complexity of patient illnesses and needs demand a more team-focused approach to clinical management to optimize safety and efficiency of the delivery of care.

Hand-offs

Communication failures in healthcare remain a leading cause of medical errors and adverse events, and almost half of them occur during the handoff process [18, 19]. A handoff in clinical care refers to the transfer of information, responsibility, and authority between two or more providers to ensure the continuity of patient care [20, 21]. The dynamic complexity and needs of round-the-clock ICU environment, coupled with changing demands on healthcare providers such as limited residents' duty hours and growing shortages of nurses and physicians, emphasize the increasing reliance on information exchange among providers and hospitals during shift changes and patient transfers. Several tools have been utilized to facilitate handoffs, including structured notes, electronic programs, and checklists [22–24]. However, handoffs remain misunderstood, error-prone [25], and underutilized [26], contributing to a lack of consistency in their use [27]. A better understanding of the handoff process is vital to improving the design of handoff tools and their effective use in clinical practice. Several recent studies have shed light on this vital communication event.

One approach to studying handoffs is to study the tools or materials used by clinicians. Collins et al. analyzed nurses', physicians', and physician assistants' (PA) handoff artifacts at change-of-shift in a specialty surgical ICU at a large urban medical center [28]. The 22 document types were typically semi-structured handwritten forms and observation of their use in practice revealed that nurses and physicians/PAs' handoff process was largely similar, consisting of a conversation between providers of the outgoing and incoming shifts supported by these artifacts and the occasional use of the electronic medical records. There was also significant overlap of the specific content of the artifacts between nurses and physicians. This may suggest that the development of an interdisciplinary handoff tool is a reasonable approach to standardizing communication among disciplines, contrary to the current segregated approach.

The study of handoff tools in isolation cannot capture the interplay between use of these tools and the state of the clinical unit, hence the need for a more holistic approach. In their pursuit to study handoffs in a dynamic ICU environment, Abraham et al. developed a clinician-centered approach where the effectiveness of handoff tools was evaluated in the context of their use and the current patient workload [29]. This approach utilized multiple methods including direct observation and shadowing, interviews, artifact evaluation, surveys, and audio recordings. Their subsequent studies discussed below were also largely based on this methodology.

To evaluate the current handoff process in a clinical environment, Abraham et al. conducted a qualitative study on group handoffs in the ICU setting in a large academic center. The main handoff in the ICU occurred during morning rounds where residents formally presented the patient cases to the oncoming team. The study researchers evaluated the handoff process through the clinician-centered approach described above, using a combination of direct observation, shadowing providers during their work, interviews of the providers, and audio-recordings of handoff communication. The handoff process was divided into three phases: pre-turnover phase, where the provider collected and prepared the information for the handoff; the handoff phase, comprised of the communication activity during the rounds; and the post-turn-over phase, comprised of the patient care activities as a result of the handoff. Outcomes of the handoffs included acceptance of the information, rejection of the information, or requests for further information. Results indicated that there were two critical sources of information breakdown. One was the inconsistent use of the available SOAP note (*S*ubjective, *O*bjective, *A*ssessment, and *P*lan) for handoff, which demonstrated the suboptimal use of a structured tool consistent with the information needs at handoff time. The other critical source of information breakdown was the lack of completion of the pre-turnover activities that are required for effective handoff. Based on these findings, the authors suggested a more structured handoff tool that can direct information exchange better: one that is based on a body-systems format, and an information-push approach to handoffs that emphasize information being sent to users without their explicit request.

Based on this information, Abraham et al. conducted a follow-up study to determine the effectiveness of a structured handoff tool compared to the commonly used SOAP handoff note in the same ICU setting [30]. The new *H*andoff *I*ntervention *T*ool (HAND-IT) is based on a body system-oriented format with two design requirements: content standardization and content summarization (problem-case narrative format). Handoffs on morning multidisciplinary rounds were evaluated by the research team and the use of the tools was evaluated for missed or incorrect information and missed problem list items (information breakdown), changes to plan of care (decision-making breakdowns), and expertise of the clinicians. The study team found that significantly more information was missed or incorrect, more changes to the plan of care were made, and more missed problem list items occurred using the SOAP tool compared to the HAND-IT tool. Furthermore, interns' performance (first year residents with less experience and expertise) was significantly improved by the better information organization in the HAND-IT tool. The authors concluded that the HAND-IT tool improved handoffs and was more resilient, requiring more breakdowns before it resulted in missed information. These findings suggest improved information transfer tools of this nature may enhance clinical efficiency and potentially patient safety.

Poor handoffs remain a threat to safety and quality of patient care [18]. Poor handoffs may result in information loss, compromised decision-making, reduced communication and teamwork, errors and adverse outcomes, and increased costs. The quality of handoffs can be affected by a plethora of factors: stress, fatigue, memory overload, multitasking, interruptions, training and education, team dynamics and relationships, levels of expertise, and professional hierarchies [31]. An effective handoff tool should therefore be structured and focused, and should integrate information technology. Standardization of handoffs is associated with improved communication and information flow [32], and Abraham et al. confirmed this concept by demonstrating that a standardized tool facilitates information flow and decision-making. Furthermore, a good handoff tool encourages discussion among clinicians that not only supports patient care but promotes shared learning and cultivates professional relationships. Finally, a structured tool reduces the risk of information loss or errors by non-experts and would be particularly helpful in academic settings or for physicians starting out their careers, mitigating the risk inherent in clinicians-in-training.

The growing need to improve this aspect of clinical care is reflected by the Joint Commission mandate to standardize communication activities between clinicians during transitions of care [23]. Since handoffs occur in all transitions of care settings, they are vital to the safety and continuity of care of any patient but particularly the critically ill or complex patient. However, the development of a structured tool to facilitate handoffs is an important yet insufficient step towards this goal. Like the use of any tool, training, monitoring, and adaptation of the use of the handoff tool is necessary, with feedback to the users and customization of the tool as needed.

Tools may need to be modified according to the setting of their use: emergency center to ward, or operating room to ICU, or inpatient to outpatient. Additional studies on the handoff process are needed to optimize this foundational aspect of communication, teamwork, decision-making, and ultimately good clinical practice.

Workflow

Workflow is a sequence of activities or operations performed in a system by variously involved agents and resources. It provides an overview of the conditions or context in which processes within a system occur and all the factors that can contribute to those processes. Workflow analysis is vital to improving any system and its outcomes; in healthcare, workflow has a direct correlation to patient outcomes, as it can influence timing of care, decision-making, and compliance with protocols and policies. However, since workflow is a multidimensional concept, it is inherently difficult to study in its entirety. Typical methods of workflow analysis include ethnographic observations, interviews and surveys. However, these approaches are limited by the inability to capture information from various perspectives simultaneously, an important perspective since workflow entails interactions among various systems, needs, and resources. Nevertheless, the need to understand it better is vital to improving healthcare delivery.

Vankipuram et al. have offered a new model to augment the traditional approaches to studying workflow in complex clinical environments [33]. In their paper, they describe the use of radio identification technology (RID) for quantitative continuous monitoring to supplement the traditional qualitative methodology, analogous to the use of the "black box" in aviation. RID-enabled tags are worn by clinicians and communicate with base units that measure distances, locations, and time at particular locations within a selected environment, providing information on the interactions of agents and artifacts in the said environment. The Hidden Markov Modeling technique (HMM) was then used to develop a prediction model of 15 simulated trauma activities in a laboratory based on observations in a trauma unit, and the model predicted 87.5 % of the clinician activities. While clinical trials are still pending, this appealing model has great potential to provide information on the efficiency and structure of workflow in a clinical environment during various levels of demand and resource needs. In addition, it can be used to generate information on teamwork coordination, real-time conditions during which errors or failures develop, and changing needs based on changing demands, personnel, and resources. This may help in improving outcomes, such as reducing waiting times in the ICU, as reported by Chen et al. [34].

To further understand the nature and impact of interruptions on clinical workflow, Mamykina et al. performed an observational study of 34 nurses and physicians in a pediatric ICU [35]. The researchers shadowed individual subjects for an hour during their shifts and recorded information on number, types, sources, timing, and resumption lag (time to return to original task) of interruptions. A total of 547 interruptions were recorded, averaging 9.85 times/h for residents and 9.52 times/h for nurses. The most common source of interruptions was by clinicians on the same team or the same unit for both professionals (more than 60 % of interruptions). Other types of interruptions included clinicians outside of the unit, phone and pagers, patients and visitors, and patient monitoring equipment. Nurses were more likely to get interrupted by patients and visitors and monitoring equipment, while physicians were more likely to get interrupted by pagers and clinicians from outside the unit. Some types of interruptions such as those from clinicians outside of the unit peaked in the morning hours, while interruptions between team members steadily increased during the day. Interruptions among team members were uncommon when the team was together performing patient rounds but increased after rounds. The root causes of interruptions were categorized as follows: coordinating work (provide directives and instructions, request for help, obtain or share information, and determine responsibilities), situation awareness (updates and current activities, events, state of resources), mutual understanding (clarifying expectations), shared decision-making, mentoring, patient/family requests, emotional affiliation (seeking or offering emotional support to colleagues), social (work unrelated), and device alarm. The most common groups were coordinating work, situation awareness, and mutual understanding, accounting for about 60 % of all interruptions. Although not common, patient/family requests and shared decision-making resulted in the longest resumption lag (average 20 min).

This study confirms what almost all clinicians will acknowledge: interruptions in daily clinical workflow are common and varied and occur throughout the shift. Interruptions not only disrupt the work routines but can affect the decision-making process that occurs almost continually in high intensity environments such as the ICU. This may have a detrimental impact on patient safety and efficiency of clinical work. While the types of interruptions are many, they overlap among specialties, such as nurses and physicians, and may characterize a particular unit or department depending on their unique characteristics. Finally, interruptions may be an indicator for potentially improved workflow, highlighting areas where increased efficiency was needed such as communication, information flow, and determination of roles and responsibilities. Better tools such as information displays or handoff processes may attenuate interruptions and facilitate improved flow and patient care. Better rules or policies such as the "sterile cockpit" – where the person performing a task is protected from interruptions due to the serious and important nature of the task – can not only reduce interruptions but improve safety and reduce the likelihood of errors. Of course, one must always consider the emotional and psychological toll interruptions have on the busy professional, contributing to stress, team dynamics, and burnout.

Information Seeking Behavior

A major determinant of effective and safe clinical decision-making is the availability of accurate, specific, and timely data at the bedside. Technology and electronic medical records form a growing facilitative role on data collection and ultimately on healthcare decisions and outcomes. Our healthcare system finds itself in the midst of a major transition from the traditional paper-based medical record and order entry to an electronic, nationally compatible information system. How clinicians utilize and access their information sources, and how hospitals and healthcare systems collect information on their clinicians' activities and needs, will significantly affect workflow, decision-making, resource use, and ultimately patient care. Two studies have investigated information seeking methods, each providing a unique perspective on clinician activities.

Kannampallil et al. combined human observation with sensor-based technology to investigate clinician activities in a complex clinical environment [36]. Sensor-based technologies have been used to study mobility and interactions of clinicians [37]. This study was conducted in the Emergency Center (EC) of a Level I Trauma center teaching hospital and utilized *tags* attached to clinicians (attending physicians, residents, nurses) and stationary *base stations* placed at key locations to capture the tracking of the tags. The information captured described the movements and interactions of the clinicians within the ED that can be used to study and even predict models of clinician activities. These data included: location and time spent at that location, transitions among locations, and aggregation with other clinicians. Human observers followed the tagged subjects and collected specific information to confirm the accuracy of the information made by the tags as well as obtain additional information. Results demonstrated good correlation between locations of the clinicians from tag (sensors) and observers' data. Residents and nurses spent more time in the trauma rooms at the bedside, while attending physicians spent more time with other physicians than with nurses. There were few consistent patterns of location, particularly among nurses.

Sensor data technology is a potentially valuable tool to improve clinical care by measuring the complexity of a clinical environment. Data collected on movement and interactions among clinicians can measure and provide valuable insight into clinician effort and activities, teamwork and collaboration, resource and time utilization, workflow patterns and efficiency measurements (see prior "Workflow" section), and retrospective review of environmental conditions when an error or bad outcome is investigated. This information can be used by clinicians and hospital leadership in several ways. First, it can help plan resource needs and allocation of specific units, time periods, and workloads that more precisely control costs, inventory, and waste and reflect real-time changing needs that characterize busy clinical settings. Second, it can monitor changes in processes or structures within a clinical environment and adjust that change accordingly. Third, sensor data technology can offer real-world education and training opportunities to identify and mitigate disruptions, risks, errors, inefficiencies, and process failures, but also to promote teamwork, efficiency, and prioritization. Finally, by complementing clinical forums such as the Morbidity and Mortality Conference or Multi-disciplinary Rounds, it can provide a valuable framework to study origin and progression of errors and unexpected patient outcomes. Information such as clinician activities, demands, and needs can be assessed around the time an adverse outcome occurred, improving our ability to learn about these situations and prevent them in the future.

From a different perspective, another report by Kannampallil et al. studied the information-seeking behaviors of physicians in a complex environment. Under direct observation of the study team, seven expert physicians reviewed the entire medical record of a single patient case in the ICU. The type of data retrieved (subdivided into categories), the time and source for data retrieval, and the *information gain* (number of information units in a sub-source divided by the time spent on that source, with greater gain for newly-encountered information than redundant information) were collected and analyzed. Results indicated that information was distributed among various sources; these sources were utilized for different types of data collection and the information gain differed among sources. Structured organization of information facilitated accelerated retrieval by the physicians. Physicians toggled between the paper and electronic records, but the total time spent on each did not differ. Information gain was greater for electronic medical records, mostly because of the uniqueness of the data. The total amount of information obtained, however, was greater for the paper records.

This study underscores several important clinical concepts. First, it highlights the efficiency of data collection by physicians. This study demonstrates the extensive time and cognitive energy spent by physicians seeking, filtering, and organizing data from a myriad of sources. This lost time and energy distract from clinical care provided by the physician. In addition, searching for information from multiple sources may disrupt the logical flow of reasoning during clinical decision-making. Second, information seeking challenges may contribute to data loss and misinterpretation. In the context of a busy clinical situation, difficulties in data acquisition may not be tolerated for a prolonged period of time, tempting the discouraged physician to obviate further data pursuit and potentially affecting the clinical decision and plan of care. Third, the distributive nature of clinical data may contribute to missing or conflicting information, requiring additional time and effort to confirm or even rectify the void or discordance. This is not only inefficient but can be directly harmful to patient safety. Finally, there is a "learning curve" inherent in navigating data sources, which may continue to escalate as sources of data change. This further burdens the physician with the need to relearn processes and needlessly expend further time and energy.

The efforts demonstrated by these studies to characterize information-seeking behaviors are vital to promoting efficient, timely, and safe clinical care. The use of sensor-data technology to study clinicians' activities can inform hospital and physician leadership about resource needs and workloads, monitor and adapt new programs or policies based on real-time data, and facilitate teamwork and collaboration. Similarly, understanding how physicians seek information can facilitate and redesign decision-making, workflow, and other value-added activities. In addition, the development of standardized data platforms may attenuate the challenges of cognitive barriers such as knowledge deficits, memory-capacity limitations, and information overload that impede decision-making.

Protocol-Based Practice

Protocols and guidelines are important tools in complex environments and have demonstrated beneficial effects on patients' safety and outcomes in the ICU [38, 39]. Protocol-based practice improves care by reducing reliance on memory, decreases variation and non-value added work by clinicians, guides care based on scientific evidence, adds structure and predictability to complex tasks, and promotes standardization of practice [40–42]. More importantly, in the clinical arena where unexpected events and patient deterioration are common, protocols cannot be followed for all patients all of the time. Deviations from protocols are often regarded as "errors," but in the complex and constantly changing arena of healthcare, some deviations may be necessary and indeed beneficial to care. How and when to apply, modify, or deviate from them is an important area for further study to improve the development and application of this important tool and to promote the development of the "shared mental model" characteristic of high reliability teams.

To understand the socio-technical factors that affect the use of a protocol in a complex clinical setting, Myneni et al. evaluated a common computerized weaning protocol (CWP) in a medical intensive care unit (MICU) [43]. The initial step was to create a FRAM-based model (Functional Resonance Accident Method) of the CWP to categorize the specific components of the protocol and to learn how they interact to produce desired or unexpected outcomes. This indicated that there were many factors in the CWP that were inadequate and unpredictable, which may ultimately affect how the protocol is used and the outcomes it produces. Most of these factors could be rectified through education, improved communication among users, and impact demonstration. The next step in this study involved the observation of 65 weaning sessions using the CWP, and each session was categorized as favorable (45, 69 %), unfavorable (4, 6 %), and near-miss (16, 25 %). Major problems identified with the CWP and potentially leading to the unfavorable or near-miss outcomes related to misinterpretation of specific steps, on-time delivery support, inadequate communication and collaboration among clinicians, and insufficient feedback of the protocol's impact on quality of care delivery. While several implications arise from this study, the most important is that it demonstrates that the introduction of a clinical practice protocol does not ensure its consistent or even accurate application.

Deviations from standardized polices or protocols are a common component of complex clinical care and occur for various reasons. Building on a prior study by Kahol et al. [44], Vankipuram et al. investigated the adaptive behavior of clinicians in following the standardized Advanced Trauma Life Support (ATLS) guideline [45] in a busy Level I Trauma center [46]. Field observations of junior (non-expert) and senior (expert) residents occurred for 30 trauma cases to identify if deviations from the management protocol occurred, their types, and reasons. Deviations were categorized into errors (violated standards), innovations (provided potentially beneficial novel perspective), proactive (potentially beneficial activity performed in anticipation of future need) and reactive (activity performed in reaction to an unanticipated event). A total of 153 deviations occurred whose types were related to the clinician's experience level. Proactive deviations were similar among groups, but innovations were greater among experts and reactive deviations and errors were greater among non-experts. More deviations occurred later in the management process. Errors occurred throughout the patient care period, but innovations occurred after the initial patient evaluation (primary patient survey) where more flexibility in the protocol is permitted.

In healthcare, more often than not, a policy or protocol is developed and implemented without any follow-up monitoring or analysis on its use or effect. The assumptions underlying this practice are that the protocol is self-explanatory;

it will demonstrate benefit based on the literature or others' experience; it will be easily integrated into the current workflow, and it does not add further time or effort on the user. A weaning protocol is a strong evidence-based and well-accepted intervention in the critical care community that has been in use at the study institution for a while. Yet the study indicated that 31 % of cases resulted in an unfavorable or near-miss outcome. This suggests that even the application of a common and well-established protocol is fraught with difficulties and variation. Clinicians and nurses in particular can attest to the myriad of instances when leadership implements a policy that is ineffective, unclear, and unmonitored and only contributes to the added workload without any clear indication of benefit such as safety or efficiency. Therefore, the application of a protocol should include regular re-evaluation to provide amendments when necessary to optimize its effectiveness. Protocols need to evolve to accommodate changing patient needs, new technology and medical science, and personnel turnover. The use of a tool like FRAM should be a routine practice at healthcare facilities to ensure that protocol-based practice is updated, efficient, and effective with minimal disruption to current workflow. In fact, routine revisions of protocols may even indicate that their utility and role have expired, prompting their retraction from the practice setting. Furthermore, optimum use of a protocol will encourage its use and support the standardization of practice.

Ineffective use of protocols can also affect deviations by increasing errors and reduce innovations and proactive interventions. Since deviations from protocols are a common and often expected component of protocol-based practice, it is vital to minimize unwanted deviations by ensuring the protocol is used optimally and appropriately. Protocol implementation should be supplemented by robust training in its use, not only to increase effectiveness and promote engagement as explained above, but to guide the user to incorporate positive deviations as needed and minimize error or reactive deviations. More effective understanding of the protocol may mitigate other reasons for non-beneficial deviations, such as individual preferences, habits, or outside influences. Of note, the rigid implementation of protocol, particularly those based on extrapolations of evidence from the study population to a broader unstudied population, may not demonstrate the intended benefit and may in fact be harmful. Tight glucose control is a classic example of how a single study resulted in a rapid development and implementation of hyperglycemia protocols nationally that required strict control parameters and resulted in increased mortality due to hypoglycemic events [47]. Again, this demonstrates that protocols are tools for to be used and adapted to the clinical situation.

Conclusion

The increasing complexity of the ICU milieu, coupled with the growing demands on critical care, the integration of multiple informational systems and sources, and the accelerating growth in medical science and technology all mandate a greater need to integrate, coordinate, and facilitate ICU workflow, handoffs, information collection and analysis, and decision-making. The studies discussed in this chapter have reported on different models used to evaluate these multidimensional aspects of critical care and have shed considerable light on how clinicians practice from a practical and applied perspective. They have also demonstrated the potential for new models and tools to improve safety, efficiency, and the effective application of evidence-based medicine. This increased understanding of cognitive systems in clinical care can lead to the development of new models to deliver care, more effective training approaches to teach aspiring clinicians, and better use of technology to facilitate safe and efficient medical care. Critical care medicine – in fact, all medical specialties – must incorporate this dimension to their practices to elevate their quality of care to the level of a highly reliable organization such as the aviation industry or the military. The twentieth century has focused on increasing and applying knowledge gained from medical science to improve diagnostics and therapeutics to treat disease and prolong lives. As our healthcare system grows in size and complexity, we must complement this exponential growth in medical science with the equal understanding and application of cognitive science to improve healthcare delivery and ultimately offer the level of care the twenty-first century will demand.

References

1. Angus DC, Kelley MA, Schmitz RJ, White A, Popovich Jr J. Caring for the critically ill patient. Current and projected workforce requirements for care of the critically ill and patients with pulmonary disease: can we meet the requirements of an aging population? JAMA. 2000;284(21):2762–70. PubMed PMID: 11105183. Epub 2000/12/06. eng.
2. Pronovost PJ, Needham DM, Waters H, Birkmeyer CM, Calinawan JR, Birkmeyer JD, et al. Intensive care unit physician staffing: financial modeling of the Leapfrog standard. Crit Care Med. 2006;34(3 Suppl):S18–24. PubMed PMID: 16477199. Epub 2006/02/16. eng.
3. I.O.M. To err is human. Institute of Medicine Washington, DC: National Academy Press; 1999.
4. Payne VP, Vimla L. Heuristics and biases in critical care decision-making. In: Patel VL, Kaufman DR, Cohen T, editors. Cognitive informatics: case studies on critical care, complexity, and errors. London: Springer; 2013.
5. Croskerry P. The importance of cognitive errors in diagnosis and strategies to minimize them. Acad Med. 2003;78(8):775–80. PubMed PMID: 12915363. Epub 2003/08/14. eng.
6. Leape LL, Berwick DM. Five years after to err is human: what have we learned? JAMA. 2005;293(19):2384–90. PubMed PMID: 15900009. Epub 2005/05/19. eng.
7. Hutchins EB. How a cockpit remembers its speeds. Cogn Sci. 1995;19:265–88.
8. Rasmussen JG. The role of error in organizing behavior. Ergonomics. 1990;33:1185–99.
9. Patel VL, Groen CJ, Patel YC. Cognitive aspects of clinical performance during patient workup: the role of medical expertise. Adv Health Sci Educ Theory Pract. 1997;2(2):95–114. PubMed PMID: 12386402. Epub 1997/01/01. Eng.
10. Patel VL, Groen GJ, Arocha JF. Medical expertise as a function of task difficulty. Mem Cognit. 1990;18(4):394–406. PubMed PMID: 2381318.Epub 1990/07/01. eng.
11. Patel VL, Cohen T. New perspectives on error in critical care. Curr Opin Crit Care. 2008;14(4):456–9. PubMed PMID: 18614912. Epub 2008/07/11. eng.
12. Cohen TP, Patel VL. A framework for understanding error and complexity. In: Patel VK, Kaufman DR, Cohen T, editors. Cognitive informatics: case studies on critical care, complexity, and errors. London: Springer; 2013.

13. Patel VL, Cohen T, Murarka T, Olsen J, Kagita S, Myneni S, et al. Recovery at the edge of error: debunking the myth of the infallible expert. J Biomed Inform. 2011;44(3):413–24. PubMed PMID: 20869466. Epub 2010/09/28. eng.
14. Razzouk E, Cohen T, Almoosa K, Patel V. Approaching the limits of knowledge: the influence of priming on error detection in simulated clinical rounds. AMIA Annu Symp Proc. 2011;2011:1155–64. PubMed PMID: 22195176. Pubmed Central PMCID: 3243217. Epub 2011/12/24. eng.
15. Kubose T, Patel V, Jordan J. Dynamic adaptation to critical care medical environment: error recovery as cognitive activity. In: Annual meeting of the cognitive science society, 2002;8–10.
16. Amalberti R, Wioland, L. In: Soekka H, editor. Human error in aviation safety: human factors, system engineering, flight operations, economics, strategies, management. Brill Academic Publishers; The Netherlands 1997.
17. Schmitt MH, Gilbert JH, Brandt BF, Weinstein RS. The coming of age for interprofessional education and practice. Am J Med. 2013;126(4):284–8. PubMed PMID: 23415053. Epub 2013/02/19. eng.
18. Horwitz LI, Meredith T, Schuur JD, Shah NR, Kulkarni RG, Jenq GY. Dropping the baton: a qualitative analysis of failures during the transition from emergency department to inpatient care. Ann Emerg Med. 2009;53(6):701–10.e4. PubMed PMID: 18555560. Epub 2008/06/17. eng.
19. Sutcliffe KM, Lewton E, Rosenthal MM. Communication failures: an insidious contributor to medical mishaps. Acad Med. 2004;79(2):186–94. PubMed PMID: 14744724. Epub 2004/01/28. eng.
20. Riesenberg LA, Leitzsch J, Massucci JL, Jaeger J, Rosenfeld JC, Patow C, et al. Residents' and attending physicians' handoffs: a systematic review of the literature. Acad Med. 2009; 84(12):1775–87. PubMed PMID: 19940588. Epub 2009/11/27. eng.
21. Arora VM, Johnson JK, Meltzer DO, Humphrey HJ. A theoretical framework and competency-based approach to improving handoffs. Qual Saf Health Care. 2008;17(1):11–4. PubMed PMID: 18245213. Epub 2008/02/05. eng.
22. Van Eaton EG, Horvath KD, Lober WB, Pellegrini CA. Organizing the transfer of patient care information: the development of a computerized resident sign-out system. Surgery. 2004; 136(1):5–13. PubMed PMID: 15232532. Epub 2004/07/03. eng.
23. Arora V, Johnson J. A model for building a standardized hand-off protocol. Jt Comm J Qual Patient Saf. 2006;32(11):646–55. PubMed PMID: 17120925. Epub 2006/11/24. eng.
24. Stein DM, Vawdrey DK, Stetson PD, Bakken S. An analysis of team checklists in physician signout notes. AMIA Annu Symp Proc. 2010;2010:767–71. PubMed PMID: 21347082. Pubmed Central PMCID: 3041400. Epub 2011/02/25. eng.
25. Mistry KP, Jaggers J, Lodge AJ, Alton M, Mericle JM, Frush KS, et al. Performance and tools. In: Henriksen K, Batties JB, Keyes MA, Grad ML. Rockville Maryland, editors. Tools and Practices Using six sigma(R) methodology to improve handoff communication in high-risk patients performance and tools. 2008. PubMed PMID: 21249919. Epub 2011/01/21. eng.
26. Harvey CM, Schuster RJ, Durso FT, Matthews AL, Surabattula D. Human factors of transition of care. In: Carayon P, editor. Handbook of human factors and ergonomics in healthcare and patient safety. Mahwah: Lawrence Erlbaum Associates; 2007.
27. Riesenberg LA, Leitzsch J, Little BW. Systematic review of handoff mnemonics literature. Am J Med Qual. 2009;24(3):196–204. PubMed PMID: 19269930. Epub 2009/03/10. eng.
28. Collins SA, Mamykina L, Jordan D, Stein DM, Shine A, Reyfman P, et al. In search of common ground in handoff documentation in an intensive care unit. J Biomed Inform. 2012;45(2):307–15. PubMed PMID: 22142947. Pubmed Central PMCID: 3306473. Epub 2011/12/07. eng.
29. Abraham J, Kannampallil TG, Patel VL. Bridging gaps in handoffs: a continuity of care based approach. J Biomed Inform. 2012;45(2):240–54. PubMed PMID: 22094355. Epub 2011/11/19. eng.

30. Abraham JA, Almoosa K. Falling through the cracks: investigation of care continuity in critical care handoffs. In: Patel VL, Kaufman DR, Cohen T, editors. Cognitive informatics: case studies on critical care, complexity, and errors. London: Springer; 2013.
31. Streitenberger K, Breen-Reid K, Harris C. Handoffs in care–can we make them safer? Pediatr Clin North Am. 2006;53(6):1185–95. PubMed PMID: 17126690. Epub 2006/11/28. eng.
32. Berkenstadt H, Haviv Y, Tuval A, Shemesh Y, Megrill A, Perry A, et al. Improving handoff communications in critical care: utilizing simulation-based training toward process improvement in managing patient risk. Chest. 2008;134(1):158–62. PubMed PMID: 18628218. Epub 2008/07/17. eng.
33. Vankipuram M, Kahol K, Cohen T, Patel VL. Toward automated workflow analysis and visualization in clinical environments. J Biomed Inform. 2011;44(3):432–40. PubMed PMID: 20685315. Epub 2010/08/06. eng.
34. Chen CI, Liu CY, Li YC, Chao CC, Liu CT, Chen CF, et al. Pervasive observation medicine: the application of RFID to improve patient safety in observation unit of hospital emergency department. Stud Health Technol Inform. 2005;116:311–5. PubMed PMID: 16160277. Epub 2005/09/15. eng.
35. Mamykina LH, Hum S, Kaufman D. Investigating shared mental models in critical care. In: Patel VK, Kaufman DR, Cohen T, editors. Cognitive informatics: case studies on critical care, complexity, and errors. London: Springer; 2013.
36. Kannampallil T, Li Z, Zhang M, Cohen T, Robinson DJ, Franklin A, et al. Making sense: sensor-based investigation of clinician activities in complex critical care environments. J Biomed Inform. 2011;44(3):441–54. PubMed PMID: 21345380. Epub 2011/02/25. eng.
37. Vankipuram M, Kahol K, Cohen T, Patel VL. Visualization and analysis of activities in critical care environments. AMIA Annu Symp Proc. 2009;2009:662–6. PubMed PMID: 20351937. Pubmed Central PMCID: 2815477. Epub 2009/01/01. eng.
38. Pronovost P, Needham D, Berenholtz S, Sinopoli D, Chu H, Cosgrove S, et al. An intervention to decrease catheter-related bloodstream infections in the ICU. N Engl J Med. 2006; 355(26):2725–32. PubMed PMID: 17192537. Epub 2006/12/29. eng.
39. Barr J, Fraser GL, Puntillo K, Ely EW, Gelinas C, Dasta JF, et al. Clinical practice guidelines for the management of pain, agitation, and delirium in adult patients in the intensive care unit. Crit Care Med. 2013;41(1):263–306. PubMed PMID: 23269131. Epub 2012/12/28. eng.
40. Wood KA, Angus DC. Reducing variation and standardizing practice in the intensive care unit. Curr Opin Crit Care. 2001;7(4):281–3. PubMed PMID: 11571427. Epub 2001/09/26. eng.
41. Holcomb BW, Wheeler AP, Ely EW. New ways to reduce unnecessary variation and improve outcomes in the intensive care unit. Curr Opin Crit Care. 2001;7(4):304–11. PubMed PMID: 11571430. Epub 2001/09/26. eng.
42. Rozich JD, Howard RJ, Justeson JM, Macken PD, Lindsay ME, Resar RK. Standardization as a mechanism to improve safety in health care. Jt Comm J Qual Saf. 2004;30(1):5–14. PubMed PMID: 14738031. Epub 2004/01/24. eng.
43. Myneni SC, Cohen T, Almoosa KF, Patel VL. Standard solutions for complex settings: the idiosyncrasies of a weaning protocol use in practice. In: Patel VK, Kaufman DR, Cohen T, editors. Cognitive informatics: case studies on critical care, complexity, and errors. London: Springer; 2013.
44. Kahol K, Vankipuram M, Patel VL, Smith ML. Deviations from protocol in a complex trauma environment: errors or innovations? J Biomed Inform. 2011;44(3):425–31. PubMed PMID: 21496496. Epub 2011/04/19. eng.
45. ACS. Advanced trauma life support for doctors. Chicago: American College of Surgeons (ACS) Committee on Trauma; 2004.
46. Vankipuram MG, Ghaemmaghami V, Patel VL. Adaptive behaviors in complex clinical environments. In: Patel VK, Kaufman DR, Cohen T, editors. Cognitive informatics: case studies in critical care, complexity, and errors. London: Springer; 2013.
47. van den Berghe G, Wouters P, Weekers F, Verwaest C, Bruyninckx F, Schetz M, et al. Intensive insulin therapy in critically ill patients. N Engl J Med. 2001;345(19):1359–67. PubMed PMID: 11794168. Epub 2002/01/17. eng.

Chapter 21
Large Scale Cognitive Error in Critical Care: The Adoption of "Best Practices" That Are Either Ineffective or Harm Patients

Timothy G. Buchman

1. The devil leads him by the nose with a false hypothesis. (For this he deserves our pity.)
2. His arguments are erroneous and sloppy. (For this he deserves a beating.)

- Albert Einstein, on two paths to incorrect cognition [1]

Introduction

Cognitive error is common in critical care medicine. One or more caregivers reaches an erroneous conclusion based on (a) failure to receive/perceive data; (b) failure to comprehend data; (c) failure to accurately project the consequences of decisions based on the data. Any of these failures will lead to loss of situation awareness [2]. This loss of situation awareness predisposes to a decision/action sequence that is a poor (or even adverse) choice for the patient. A simple example relates to a drug allergy. If a provider is unaware of a drug allergy, or fails to comprehend that a drug allergy is general to a class of drugs, or prescribes a drug in the class and fails to anticipate the allergic reaction, the probability of that reaction and adverse outcome rises.

Such cognitive errors are common. Moreover, they commonly cause harm. It is therefore appropriate and important to reduce their frequency and mitigate their effects. Common strategies include improved data presentation, automated alerting, optimizing handovers and creation of shared mental models.

Identification of an error presupposes the existence of a better and more correct alternative. What is "correct" in critical care emerges from scientific investigation, clinical trials and published reports. The purpose of this chapter is to review and abstract an increasingly common phenomenon in critical care, namely the adoption of a "best practice" that is subsequently shown to be worthless or even harmful to the patient. It is organized as critical care clinicians typically review the condition of each patient, that is by body systems. For each body system, we identify important clinical problems, discuss the evolution of a new "best practice," and then

T.G. Buchman, PhD, MD, FACS, FCCP, MCCM
Emory Center for Critical Care, Emory University School of Medicine,
Woodruff Health Sciences Center, Emory University, Atlanta, GA 30322, USA
e-mail: tbuchma@emory.edu

V.L. Patel et al. (eds.), *Cognitive Informatics in Health and Biomedicine*, 441
Health Informatics, DOI 10.1007/978-1-4471-5490-7_21, © Springer-Verlag London 2014

explore the subsequent events that led to discarding that new "best practice." We conclude the chapter with a synthesis and abstraction of the faulty reasoning and make suggestions to reduce the likelihood that the critical care community will repeat these costly and dangerous experiences.

Neurological System

Injuries to the spinal cord (spinal cord injuries, SCI) are unfortunately common and devastating. Vehicular accidents, work-related trauma and falls account for the majority of these injuries, which cause devastating paralysis that currently afflicts around 1.3 million patients in the USA alone.

Given the severity of the injuries and consequent disability, an international effort beginning in the 1980s was undertaken to identify drugs that could improve outcome. Even a minor improvement (meaning that examination showed clinical improvement such that injury appeared to be one or two vertebra caudal to the original examination) could mean independence from a ventilator, use of upper limbs and so on. This led to a series of trials, well chronicled in a recent review of pharmacological therapy for acute spinal cord injury [3]. In the USA, the initial study was called the National Acute Spinal Cord Injury Study, or NASCIS. Three such studies were undertaken. The first of these trials, reported in 1984, reported no favorable effect from the administration of the potent anti-inflammatory steroid, methyl prednisolone [4]. As that trial concluded, the investigators reviewed animal data that suggested that the human dose might have been insufficient. As a consequence, a second trial (NASCIS-II) was conducted increasing the dose and adding a third arm to the trial using an alternative drug [5]. The NACSIS-II trial of 487 patients with SCI, published in the prestigious *New England Journal of Medicine*, showed favorable effects with methylprednisolone in the higher dose, but only via post-hoc analysis and only in patients who received the drug within 8 h of the injury. Patients who received the drug more than 8 h were excluded, and thus the final conclusions of the study were based on only 66 patients versus 69 controls. Moreover, analysis of patients treated beyond the 8-h window showed the drug to have a harmful effect. Nevertheless, there was near-immediate adoption of high-dose methylprednisolone as standard care for SCI. International trials also led to mixed results. Finally a third study involving 14 centers in the USA and 2 in Canada was performed. In this NACSIS-III study, 499 patients presenting within 8 h of spinal cord injury were randomized into three arms, two that included high-dose methylprednisolone for 24 and 48 h respectively, and a third arm including an engineered "super-steroid" with enhanced antioxidant properties. A placebo arm was not included because methylprednisolone administration had become standard care.

As these and other prospective, randomized controlled trials were collected for meta-analysis, it became apparent that while no consistent benefit for methylprednisolone therapy could be demonstrated, there were clear findings of harm. Wound infections, hyperglycemia and gastrointenstinal hemorrhage were significant.

There was additional evidence for higher risk of systemic infections. Even more compelling evidence of harm was observed in a 10,000 patient randomized control trial of methylprednisolone for head injury [6].

In 2013, an international panel of neuroscientists and clinicians made a Level I recommendation: "*Administration of methylprednisolone (MP) for the treatment of acute spinal cord injury (SCI) is not recommended. Clinicians considering MP therapy should bear in mind that the drug is not Food and Drug Administration (FDA) approved for this application. There is no Class I or Class II medical evidence supporting the clinical benefit of MP in the treatment of acute SCI. Scattered reports of Class III evidence claim inconsistent effects likely related to random chance or selection bias. However, Class I, II, and III evidence exists that high-dose steroids are associated with harmful side effects including death*" [3]. The prestigious Cochrane Review on steroids for spinal cord injury which still takes the position that methylprednisolone is indicated is singly authored by the principal investigator of the NACSIS studies.

The error arose from a hope that steroids would be the "magic bullet" in mitigating spinal cord injuries. As soon as there was the slimmest evidence of benefit, investigator and the clinical community saw what they wanted to see, namely an improvement in the lives of patients devastated by neurological trauma. The search for an effective therapy continues: the current "magic bullet" for spinal cord injury under investigation is hyperbaric oxygen therapy.

Heart and Vascular System

Through 1970, sudden cardiac death was a large and rising cause of death in the USA. Prehospital care was poor, cardiopulmonary resuscitation and defibrillation were still in their infancy and interventional cardiology has not yet been conceived. Electrocardiographic data showed that patients who had gone on to cardiac death exhibited premature ventricular contractions. In 1971, Lown and Wolf proposed that, "since sudden cardiac death is due to an arrhythmia, drug prophylaxis might prove effective." Indeed, with the proliferation of ambulatory heart monitors (Holter monitors) in the 1980s, several investigators observed that sudden cardiac death was preceded by ventricular fibrillation. It was only logical that suppression of premature ventricular contractions (PVCs, sometimes seen prior to ventricular fibrillation) would reduce the risk of sudden cardiac death. For two decades, inpatients were routinely treated with infusions of lidocaine to suppress premature ventricular contractions. However it was only in the mid-1980s that oral agents were developed that could suppress the premature beats.

In June 1987 the first patients were enrolled in the Cardiac Arrhythmia Suppression Trial (CAST). This double-blind, randomized controlled study enrolled more than 1,700 patients in 27 centers. The entry criteria included a history of myocardial infarction (6 days-2 years in the past); the presence of asymptomatic premature ventricular beats documented by Holter monitor; and the suppressibility of those beats by oral medication. Patients were randomized to the medications versus placebo controls.

The findings prompted an early report in the *New England Journal of Medicine* [7]. Patients receiving the oral agents had a significantly higher risk of death. Those oral agents disappeared from the marketplace. A second trial, CAST II, was initiated with yet a different oral agent. The enrollment criteria were made more stringent—the myocardial infarction could have occurred no more than 90 days previously, the heart muscle had to be demonstrably compromised and so on. CAST II was terminated early when an excess of early (within 2 weeks) cardiac death in the treatment group.

There is no question that PVCs are associated with premature death. Modern studies continue to demonstrate that the presence of any PVC on a single electrocardiogram (much less a continuous Holter monitor) is a very strong predictor of both cardiovascular as well as all-cause mortality [8]. The difficult lessons for critical care professionals coming from the CAST trials are that (1) association is not causation; and (2) the treatment may be more dangerous than the condition intended to treat.

The more general cognitive error is that critical care professionals have focused on "correcting physiologic abnormalities" versus identifying and mitigating the underlying cause. This is perhaps the most important cognitive error made in critical care: there is repeated confusion between an abnormal finding (a symptom or sign) and the pathologic state that leads to the abnormal finding.

Another common cognitive error involves the apparent validation of a "some is good therefore more must be better" strategy. In the cardiac system, this took the form of supranormal oxygen delivery.

In the early 1990s, circulatory shock came to be redefined as a physiology consequent to sustained imbalance between oxygen supply and oxygen demand. In 1992, Shoemaker and colleagues published a provocative study of 253 high risk surgical patients where they calculated the gap between measured oxygen consumption and an estimated oxygen demand based on the patient's own preoperative data [9]. The abstract telegraphed the authors' beliefs: "The data demonstrate a strong relationship between the magnitude and duration of the oxygen uptake deficit in the intraoperative and early postoperative period and the subsequent appearance of organ failure and death. The latter may be reduced when oxygen debts were prevented or minimized by augmenting naturally occurring compensations that increased oxygen delivery."

In 1998, the authors reported their first trial supporting their belief [10]. Trials of the strategy for other forms of shock followed [11]. All seemed rosy until two issues were brought to light. First, there was a systematic error ("mathematical coupling") in the calculations of oxygen delivery and oxygen uptake. When this error was accounted for, the general salutary effect of "more delivery is better" vanished [12]. Perhaps more important, the patients who survived were not those who were merely treated to increase oxygen delivery—it was those patients who actually responded to the treatment. In other words, it was the patient's capacity to respond more than the treatment itself that marked survivors. Even then, the proponents of increasing oxygen delivery beyond the patient's ordinary physiologic levels would not let go of the concept [13]. By 2002, reports began to appear that supranormal resuscitation strategies did not in fact improve outcome [14]. The following year, it was reported that supranormal resuscitation caused significant harm [15]. The practice has been largely abandoned.

Shock is an ancient and formidable foe. What happened in this vignette was the use –some would say abuse—of the pulmonary artery catheter to measure and modify hemodynamics and oxygen delivery. So strong was the desire to overcome shock, so strong was the belief that paying off the oxygen debt could be enhanced by putting oxygen in a bank –driving high delivery to enhance greater uptake--that the early investigators saw what they wanted to see. In fact, there is no storage form of oxygen other than hemoglobin and myoglobin, a reservoir of about 5 min duration in humans. Yet it took years to dissuade adherents that their therapy was causing harms.

Pulmonary/Respiratory System

The adult respiratory distress syndrome (ARDS) was first described in 1967 by Ashbaugh and colleagues [16], and came to prominence during the Vietnam conflict as trauma victims survived initial resuscitation only to succumb to progressive respiratory failure. ARDS remains prominent as a critical illness despite advances in understanding of pathology and many clinical trials of approaches to treatment. Two approaches to care have been confounded by large-scale cognitive errors.

In 1994, the NIH established a clinical network to carry out multi-center trials. Almost immediately, the ARDSNet community focused on the high ventilatory volumes and pressures popular at the time that seemed to exacerbate the ARDS injury. The investigators reasoned that protecting the lung from pressure-related injury during mechanical ventilation could improve outcomes. It was known that mammals, from mice to elephants and including man, have an ordinary tidal volume of 6.2–7.9 ml/kg during rest and ordinary activity [17, 18]. The ARDSNet investigators realized that some ARDS patients were being ventilated with tidal volumes of 12 ml/kg and higher, and decided to compare 6 and 12 ml/kg as ventilation strategies in ARDS. The results were astonishing. The lower tidal volume strategy was associated with a 22 % relative risk of death reduction [19]. Overnight, 6 ml/kg became the expected standard for ventilation for all patients, not just those with ARDS.

There was a problem: physicians in general practice outside the study rarely achieved the standard. Work by Kalhan et al. [20] and Mikkelsen et al. [21] suggested diagnostic uncertainty, avoiding patient discomfort and self-deception as prominent causes for the failure of the community to adopt the new standard.

An alternative explanation was offered by a group of NIH-based critical care physicians. They felt that the trial design itself was flawed. They suggested that the two tidal volumes of 6 and 12 ml/kg assigned to the two test arms were arbitrary and in fact neither arm represented a reasonable optimum. Rather, they suggested that a survey of general practice would have revealed a "wild-type behavior" somewhere between those extremes, and further that the wild-type behavior could well outperform the two extremes. The disagreement between the ARDSNet group and the NIH Critical Care Group has played out in the scientific literature with some drama [22, 23].

Whatever the specific reason, the standard of 6 ml/kg as a ventilation strategy that protects the lung has proven very difficult to achieve. While the ARDSNet investigators chose a low tidal volume entirely consistent with normal physiology, they made an implicit and unsubstantiated argument that it was the optimal tidal volume in the context of the very abnormal physiology of ARDS [24]. Identifying the better of two choices makes sense only when one of the choices is current best practice. Promulgating the "better choice" as optimal care has led to substantial confusion in the critical care community even while it has created a quality target that could be spurious and even harmful to some patients.

Steroids resurface with some regularity as a "magic bullet" for the prevention and/or treatment of ARDS. A pivotal appearance occurred in 1998 when Meduri and colleagues published a report in the Journal of the American Medical Association seeming to demonstrate a life-saving effect [25]. Only 24 patients were reported in the trial, of who only 16 received methylprednisolone. Nevertheless, the results seemed so compelling (5 of 8 placebo patients died, whereas only 2 of 16 treated patients died in hospital) that the trial was stopped prematurely because of the Lazarus-like effect of the drug.

Given the prominence of the journal and the amazing effect, therapy with the potent corticosteroid became standard care worldwide virtually overnight. Unfortunately, a subsequent larger trial using a similar strategy failed to show the salutary effect and suggests that in some circumstances the steroid treatment might be harmful [26]. Nor did earlier and more aggressive administration seem to help [27, 28].

Once again, a limited early trial with favorable results published in a high impact journal changed standard care more-or-less overnight. Subsequent larger trials showed the use of this magic bullet to be harmful, and data suggest that in the interim more patients may have been harmed than helped.

Renal/GU System

Renal dysfunction and renal failure are prominent in critical illness and predict poor outcomes. In 1964, a report appeared that infusion of the newly identified neurotransmitter dopamine could promote diuresis, at the same time promoting sodium excretion, glomerular filtration rate and renal blood flow in normal patients as well as those with congestive heart failure [29]. While dopamine was developed as a sympathomimetic amine for the treatment if shock, critical care physicians were excited about the potential role of dopamine administered in low doses to protect kidneys and even reverse renal injury.

Six years later, the first report appeared showing that dopamine could "reverse" renal failure [30]. This report was cited as a potential future use of the drug in a review article published by a distinguished pharmacologist in the *New England Journal of Medicine* [31]. Studies were quickly performed that appeared to show that the "magic bullet" had indeed been discovered [32–38]. With these apparent successes, patients with renal failure, at risk for renal failure, and having other organ failure were started on dopamine infusions as a standard practice in critical care.

Nearly two decades elapsed before detailed metaanalyses appeared showing that dopamine did not improve outcome from acute renal failure [39]. Hope persists: numerous trials are studying dopamine in combination with low dose loop diuretics to attenuate kidney injury despite the fact that neither class of drug alone has ever been shown effective.

Once again, a hint of a solution to a vexing and lethal problem prompted widespread adoption of practice in the absence of a clear and compelling clinical trial. Currently, the only FDA approved treatment for acute kidney injury is renal replacement therapy (dialysis).

GI/Nutrition System

Shock and critical illness cause a seemingly obligatory catabolic response. In 1932, Cuthbertson described and quantified the metabolic responses to serious injury, calling attention to the "ebb" and "flow" phases [40]. During the month-long ebb phase, patients would lose lean muscle mass and become weak. A great deal of descriptive science followed calling attention both to the loss of appetite and to the role of various systemic hormones in mediating the response. Force-feeding was unsuccessful in reversing the enervation and inanition.

By 1968, technology and applied science had evolved to allow for total intravenous feeding [41]. This technology proved lifesaving for both children and adults whose intestines were dysfunctional but were otherwise healthy. Cuthbertson's work was rediscovered and revived using modern measurement tools verifying the extent of nutritional deficiency in trauma and shock [42]. The idea of aggressively feeding shock/trauma patients with total intravenous feeding was quickly born. Remarkable claims to the effect that the body could use multiples of normal caloric intake were made [43]. Since feeding had to be good, aggressive feeding (read: overfeeding) was surely better. Parenteral alimentation quickly became parenteral hyperalimentation ("hyperal" was the argot of the era) and patients would receive four, five or even six thousand calories each day [44].

More than two dozen randomized trials of parenteral alimentation and hyperalimentation were ultimately performed. Overfeeding was discovered to cause significant and life-threatening complications [45]. Subsequent meta-analysis showed that parenteral nutritional support was generally ineffective, hyperalimentation was associated with complications and concluded that the gut should be used to provide ordinary caloric needs whenever possible [46]. Overfeeding was generally to be avoided regardless of route chosen.

The cognitive error here was a little different from those described in the prior vignettes. It simply "stood to reason" that the wasting syndrome following severe injury and other critical illness could be reversed if only adequate calories could be supplied. No consideration was ever given to the possibility that catabolism after injury might be adaptive.

Endocrine System

If nutritional goals needed to be kept in check, then certainly the endocrine milieu also needed to be kept in check. For decades, trauma surgeons and critical care physicians noted that stressed patients became hyperglycemic. Glucose concentrations twice normal were routinely observed and accepted as part and parcel of the "stress response" to severe injury. Complications were temporally associated with the hyperglycemia—especially infectious complications—but it was widely accepted that the complications caused the hyperglycemia and not vice versa.

In 2001, van den Berghe and colleagues published an extraordinary article in the *New England Journal of Medicine* [47]. The data showed that intensive insulin therapy—tightly controlling glucose levels to 80–110 mg/dl (which is a fasting level for most people) halved mortality among ICU patients who required mechanical ventilation. Virtually overnight, tight glucose control to the van den Berghe limits became standard care worldwide.

Closer read of the van den Berghe study would reveal that the patients were not general ICU patients but rather postoperative cardiac surgical patients receiving aggressive nutritional support including the aforementioned parenteral nutrition. Regardless, the advantage of tight glucose control was presumed to be generalizable. Five years later, van den Berghe attempted to reproduce her results in a medical ICU population [48]. The data failed to show improvement in mortality unless the patients were in a subset of patients requiring prolonged mechanical ventilation.

By this time, reports were appearing to suggest that the aggressive use of insulin was resulting in episodes of low blood sugar. This hypoglycemia was thought to have an adverse effect on patients. Thus the Normoglycemia in Intensive Care Evaluation–Survival Using Glucose Algorithm Regulation (NICE-SUGAR) trial was designed as a multi-center trial to test the hypothesis that intensive glucose control reduces mortality at 90 days. Forty-two hospitals enrolled over 6,000 patients. Mortality was higher in the intensive insulin therapy group [49]. A subsequent analysis found a tight association between hypoglycemia and excess mortality, but causality could of course never be proven owing to the study design [50].

Current best practice has been revised to include only modest control of glucose, typically to below 180 mg/dl. Once again, a "too good to be true" result published in a prestigious journal triggered a worldwide practice change that required another decade to be proven harmful.

Hematologic System

Anemia is common in critical illness. Surgery, trauma and medical hemorrhage (such as GI bleeding) cause acute blood loss anemia. Chronic illness can directly or indirectly (via treatments) cause production of red cells to fall and even fail entirely. Repeated phlebotomy for laboratory determinations causes a slower but equally important reduction in red cell mass. Transfusions are costly and harmful. It is therefore understandable that critical care physicians and their patients would value a strategy to increase red cell production.

As early as 1994, Krafte-Jacobs and colleagues noted that the levels of the hormone that stimulates red cell production, erythropoietin, are reduced in critical illness [51]. Given that Eschbach and colleagues had recently demonstrated erythropoietin to be effective at reversing the anemia of chronic renal failure it was a short step to speculate that administration of pharmacologic doses of erythropoietin would mitigate and even eliminate the anemia of critical illness [52].

Small reports quickly showed that critically ill patients could respond to erythropoietin [53]. Corwin and colleagues published two much larger formal trials in prestigious journals showing that, indeed, critically ill patients could have reversal of their anemia and require fewer transfusions [54, 55]. These promising results led to enthusiastic and rapid adoption of erythropoietin as a drug to treat and prevent anemias of critical illness. A post-hoc cohort analysis of the second study suggested that the benefit of erythropoetin might be specific for the trauma population, and reciprocally there might not be benefit for other critically ill patients.

A third study was therefore undertaken in which the patient class (medical, surgical, trauma etc.) was explicitly assigned. This study [56] showed three things. First, erythropoietin did not reduce transfusion utilization. Second, if there was a mortality benefit, it was restricted to the trauma population. Third, erythropoietin caused a significant increase in a harmful event, namely vascular thrombosis. The authors concluded "The use of (erythropoietin) is not supported for patients admitted to the ICU with a nontraumatic surgical or medical diagnosis, unless they have an(other) approved indication for erythropoietin."

Anemia remains a common problem in critical care. Intensivists have learned to tolerate significantly reduced hemoglobin levels as "normal" for critical illness with the exception of certain neurological conditions including traumatic brain injury, subarachnoid hemorrhage and ischemic stroke, where a slightly higher (but still anemic) hemoglobin level may produce a better outcome. In other words, anemia may be an adaptive response to critical illness.

Immune System

Among the most feared events in critical care is the appearance of an infection that overwhelms ordinary compensatory mechanisms. This condition – "sepsis"-- is frequent and often lethal. Among the most vulnerable are the very young, the very old, the injured and the immunosuppressed. Traditional treatments include fluids and antibiotics as well as drugs and devices to support failing hearts, lungs, kidneys and other vital organs.

The tools of molecular and cellular biology were applied to sepsis and revealed that the response to infection includes the elaboration of specific mediators and the proliferation of selected cell types. Septic patients were envisioned as the unfortunate vessels of unbridled inflammation. If only the inflammatory response could be tamed, lives might be saved.

Following a report that polyvalent immune sera raised against the endotoxin of a particular strain of E. coli significantly reduced mortality in patients with gram-negative sepsis [57], the race was on to identify what specific molecule was the culprit. Many molecular targets were identified. Many of those performed well in animal models. All failed in human trials [58]. All, that is, except one.

Activated protein C (drotecogin alfa, Xigris™) is a naturally occurring fibrinolytic protein that diminishes cellular adhesion. In 2001, the PROWESS trial showed a 20 % relative reduction in mortality when administered to patients with severe sepsis or septic shock [59]. Despite immediate concerns with the structure and conduct of the study, the FDA and other international regulatory agencies gave approval. The drug was quickly embraced as the only effective biological modifier to improve outcome from sepsis. There were adverse effects—the drug also acts as an irreversible anticoagulant so bleeding events were observed—but the critical care community now had an approved drug indicated for the treatment of severe sepsis and septic shock. The drug was used worldwide.

As adverse events accumulated, further trials were demanded. These were:

The ADDRESS trial, which evaluated activated protein C in less critically ill patients who nevertheless had severe sepsis [60] – it was terminated early for lack of efficacy

The RESOLVE trial, which looked at the responses of septic children—it too was terminated early for lack of efficacy [61].

The ENHANCE trial (an open-label study) focused on safety yet showed a higher bleeding rate than the PROWESS trial that led to approval [62]; and

The PROWESS-SHOCK trial (Prospective Recombinant Human Activated Protein C Worldwide Evaluation in Severe Sepsis and Septic Shock) which randomized 1,664 patients with septic shock and high risk of death to either the drug or placebo [63] and which showed no benefit to activated protein C.

Activated protein C was removed from the market in 2011, 10 years after its introduction. As of this writing, no biological response modifier has been proven effective in the treatment of severe sepsis and septic shock. The critical care community continues to rely on the traditional treatments of fluids, antibiotics and organ-specific support.

Conclusion

It is apparent that large-scale cognitive error in critical care is widespread. In every case described above, a common and serious clinical problem was reported to yield to a simple solution that could be rapidly (albeit in the case of drugs, expensively) implemented in critical care units world wide. Change was quickly implemented. Patients were likely harmed. The "new standard" turned out to be problematic and was either discarded or extensively modified.

In each case, the new standard involved a readily achievable change in practice. Such one-step solutions defy the fact that humans are not only complicated (meaning that they have multiple interacting parts) but also complex (meaning that the physiology of the whole cannot be predicted by summing the physiology of the component parts). To a great extent, critical care "works" because critical care physicians, nurses and allied health personnel create a safe context in which the patient can heal. This is very different than imagining caregivers identify and "fix" an abnormal component. Well-intended interventions may or may not have the desired effect. However with very high frequency, those interventions have unintended adverse effects. Owing to their rarity (if the adverse effects were common and prohibitive, they would have been recognized earlier on) substantial surveillance seems to be required following adoption of a new practice.

This should not be interpreted as nihilism. There are a few interventions that have proven successful in improving survival and functional outcome in critical illness. This chapter is an invitation to a more nuanced response to the apparent success of one or two "pivotal trials". Rather than a rush to embrace (much less "approve") any new "best practice," some sort of conditional acceptance that would encourage and support wider "real-world" testing and data collection seems appropriate.

We have come to understand that there are few one-size-fits-all "magic bullets." What is all-too-often lost in the denouement is that the drug, device or treatment actually was successful on a smaller scale in a precisely defined and selected group of patients. While there might not be a one-intervention-fits-all solution, there might well be a palette of interventions that work under certain circumstances. Personalizing critical care probably requires that we make the best match between the needs of a specific patient and a limited set of more tightly chosen options. It is at this precise point that the two general types of cognitive error can be abolished: recognizing that there is no single best treatment, and insuring that all available data have been considered to make the best choice for each particular patient.

> Men, it has been well said, think in herds; it will be seen that they go mad in herds, while they only recover their senses slowly, and one by one. – Charles Mackay
>
> (Extraordinary Popular Delusions and the Madness of Crowds is a history of popular folly by Scottish journalist Charles Mackay, first published in 1841.)

References

1. Einstein A, Calaprice A. The ultimate quotable Einstein. Princeton: Princeton University Press; 2011.
2. Endsley MR. Toward a theory of situation awareness in dynamic systems. Hum Factors. 1995;37(1):32–6.
3. Hurlbert RJ, Hadley MN, Walters BC, Aarabi B, Dhall SS, Gelb DE, et al. Pharmacological therapy for acute spinal cord injury. Neurosurgery. 2013;72(2):93–105.
4. Bracken MB, Collins WF, Freeman DF, Shepard MJ, Wagner FW, Silten RM, et al. Efficacy of methylprednisolone in acute spinal cord injury. JAMA. 1984;251(1):45–52.
5. Bracken MB, Shepard MJ, Collins WF, Holford TR, Young W, Baskin DS, et al. A randomized, controlled trial of methylprednisolone or maloxone in the treatment of acute spinal-cord injury- results of the second national acute spinal cord injury study. N Engl J Med. 1990;322(20): 1405–11.
6. Edwards P, Arango M, Balica L, Cottingham R, El-Sayed H, Farrell B, et al. Final results of MRC CRASH, a randomised placebo-controlled trial of intravenous corticosteroid in adults with head injury-outcomes at 6 months. Lancet. 2005;365(9475):1957–9.
7. Preliminary report: effect of encainide and flecainide on mortality in a randomized trial of arrhythmia suppression after myocardial infarction. N Engl J Med. 1989;321(6):406–12.
8. Engel G, Cho S, Ghayoumi A, Yamazaki T, Chun S, Fearon WF, et al. Prognostic significance of PVCs and resting heart rate. Ann Noninvasive Electrocardiol. 2007;12(2):121–9.
9. Shoemaker WC, Appel PL, Kram HB. Role of oxygen debt in the development of organ failure sepsis, and death in high-risk surgical patients. Chest. 1992;102(1):208–15.
10. Shoemaker WC, Appel PL, Kram HB, Waxman K, Lee TS. Prospective trial of supranormal values of survivors as therapeutic goals in high-risk surgical patients. Chest. 1988;94(6): 1176–86.
11. Shoemaker WC, Appel PL, Kram HB, Bishop MH, Abraham E. Temporal hemodynamic and oxygen transport patterns in medical patients- septic shock. Chest. 1993;104(5):1529–36.
12. Russell JA, Phang PT. The oxygen delivery/consumption controversy- approaches to management of the critically ill. Am J Respir Crit Care Med. 1994;149(2):533–7.
13. Velmahos GC, Demetriades D, Shoemaker WC, Chan LS, Tatevossian R, Wo CC, et al. Endpoints of resuscitation of critically injured patients: normal or supranormal? A prospective randomized trial. Ann Surg. 2000;232(3):409–18.
14. McKinley BA, Kozar RA, Cocanour CS, Valdivia A, Sailors RM, Ware DN, et al. Normal versus supranormal oxygen delivery goals in shock resuscitation: the response is the same. J Trauma. 2002;53(5):825–32.
15. Balogh Z, McKinley BA, Cocanour CS, Kozar RA, Valdivia A, Sailors RM, et al. Supranormal trauma resuscitation causes more cases of abdominal compartment syndrome. Arch Surg. 2003;138(6):637–42.
16. Ashbaugh DG, Bigelow DB, Petty TL, Levine BE. Acuterespiratory distress in adults. The Lancet, Saturday 12 August 1967.
17. Tenney SM, Remmers JE. Comparative quantitative morphology of the mammalian lung: diffusing area. Nature. 1963;197:54–7.
18. Stahl WR. Scaling of respiratory variables in mammals. J Appl Physiol. 1967;22:453–60.
19. Acute Respiratory Distress Syndrome Network. Ventilation with lower tidal volumes as compared with traditional tidal volumes for acute lung injury and the acute respiratory distress syndrome. N Engl J Med. 2000;342(18):1301–8.
20. Kalhan R, Mikkelsen M, Dedhiya P, Christie J, Gaughan C, Lanken PN, et al. Underuse of lung protective ventilation: analysis of potential factors to explain physician behavior. Crit Care Med. 2006;34(2):300–6.
21. Mikkelsen ME, Dedhiya PM, Kalhan R, Gallop RJ, Lanken PN, Fuchs BD. Potential reasons why physicians underuse lung-protective ventilation: a retrospective cohort study using physician documentation. Respir Care. 2008;53(4):455–61.

22. Deans KJ, Minneci PC, Cui X, Banks SM, Natanson C, Eichacker PQ. Mechanical ventilation in ARDS: one size does not fit all. Crit Care Med. 2005;33(5):1141–3.
23. Brower R, Thompson BT. Tidal volumes in acute respiratory distress syndrome-one size does not fit all. Crit Care Med. 2006;34(1):263–4.
24. Gattinoni L. Counterpoint: is Low tidal volume mechanical ventilation preferred for all patients on ventilation? Chest. 2011;140(1):11–3.
25. Meduri GU, Headley AS, Golden E, Carson SJ, Umberger RA, Kelso T, et al. Effect of prolonged methylprednisolone therapy in unresolving acute respiratory distress syndrome: a randomized controlled trial. JAMA. 1998;280(2):159–65.
26. Steinberg KP, Hudson LD, Goodman RB, Hough CL, Lanken PN, Hyzy R, et al. Efficacy and safety of corticosteroids for persistent acute respiratory distress syndrome. N Engl J Med. 2006;354:1671–84.
27. Bone RC, Fisher Jr CJ, Clemmer TP, Slotman GJ, Metz CA. Early methylprednisolone treatment for septic syndrome and the adult respiratory distress syndrome. Chest. 1987;92: 1032–6.
28. Luce JM, Montgomery AB, Marks JD, Turner J, Metz CA, Murray JF. Ineffectiveness of high-dose methylprednisolone in preventing parenchymal lung injury and improving mortality in patients with septic shock. Am Rev Respir Dis. 1988;138:62–8.
29. McDonald Jr RH, Goldberg LI, McNay JL, Tuttle Jr EP. Effect of dopamine in man: augmentation of sodium excretion, glomerular filtration rate, and renal plasma flow. J Clin Invest. 1964; 43(6):1116–24.
30. Talley RC, Forland M, Belier B. Reversal of acute renal failure with a combination of intravenous dopamine and diuretics. Clin Res. 1970;18:518.
31. Goldberg LI. Dopamine- clinical uses of an endogenous catecholamine. N Engl J Med. 1974; 291:707–10.
32. Henderson IS, Beattie TJ, Kennedy AC. Dopamine hydrochloride in oliguric states. Lancet. 1980;2:827–8.
33. Parker S, Carlon GC, Isaacs M, Howland WS, Kahn RC. Dopamine administration in oliguria and oliguric renal failure. Crit Care Med. 1981;9:630–2.
34. Davis RF, Lappas DG, Kirklin JK, Buckley MJ, Lowenstein E. Acute oliguria after cardiopulmonary bypass: renal functional improvement with low-dose dopamine infusion. Crit Care Med. 1982;10:852–6.
35. Lindner A. Synergism of dopamine and furosemide in diuretic-resistant, oliguric acute renal failure. Nephron. 1983;33:121–6.
36. Graziani G, Cantaluppi A, Casati S, Citterio A, Scalamogna A, Aroldi A, et al. Dopamine and furosemide in oliguric acute renal failure. Nephron. 1984;37:39–42.
37. Palmieri G, Morabito A, Lauria R. Low-dose dopamine induces early recovery of recombinant interleukin-2 impaired renal function. Eur J Cancer. 1993;29A:1119–22.
38. Flancbaum L, Choban PS, Dasta JF. Quantitative effects of low-dose dopamine on urine output in oliguric surgical intensive care unit patients. Crit Care Med. 1994;22:61–6.
39. Kellum JA, Decker JM. Use of dopamine in acute renal failure: a meta-analysis. Crit Care Med. 2001;29(8):1526–31.
40. Cuthbertson DP. Observation on the disturbance of metabolism produced by injury to the limbs. Q J Med. 1932;25:233–46.
41. Dudrick SJ, Wilmore DW, Vars HM, Rhoads JE. Long-term total parenteral nutrition with growth, development and positive nitrogen balance. Surgery. 1968;64:134–42.
42. Monk DN, Plank LD, Franch-Arcas G, Finn PJ, Streat SJ, Hill G. Sequential changes in the metabolic response in critically injured patients during the first 25 days after blunt trauma. Ann Surg. 1996;223:395–405.
43. Solomon JR. Nutrition in the severely burned child. Prog Pediatr Surg. 1981;14:63–79.
44. Owings JM, Bomar Jr WE, Ramage RC. Parenteral hyperalimentation and its practical applications. Ann Surg. 1972;175(5):712–9.
45. Klein CJ, Stanek GS, Wiles III CE. Overfeeding macronutrients to critically ill adults: metabolic complications. J Am Diet Assoc. 1998;98(7):795–806.

46. Heyland DK, Montalvo M, MacDonald S, Keefe L, Su XY, Drover JW. Total parenteral nutrition in the surgical patient: a meta-analysis. Can J Surg. 2001;44(2):102–11.
47. Van den Berghe G, Wouters P, Weekers F, Verwaest C, Bruyninckx F, Schetz M, et al. Intensive insulin therapy in critically ill patients. N Engl J Med. 2001;345:1359–67.
48. Van den Berghe G, Wilmer A, Hermans G, Meersseman W, Wouters PJ, Milants I, et al. Intensive insulin therapy in the medical ICU. N Engl J Med. 2006;354(5):449–61.
49. Finfer S, Chittock DR, Su SY, Blair D, Foster D, Dhingra V, et al. Intensive versus conventional glucose control in critically ill patients. N Engl J Med. 2009;360(13):1283–97.
50. The NICE-SUGAR Study Investigators. Hypoglycemia and risk of death in critically Ill patients. N Engl J Med. 2012;367:1108–18.
51. Krafte-Jacobs B, Levetown ML, Bray GL, Ruttimann UE, Pollack MM. Erythropoietin response to critical illness. Crit Care Med. 1994;22(5):821–6.
52. Eschbach JW, Egrie JC, Downing MR, Browne JK, Adamson JW. Correction of the anemia of end-stage renal disease with recombinant human erythropoietin. Results of a combined phase I and II clinical trial. N Engl J Med. 1987;316(2):73–8.
53. van Iperen CE, Gaillard CA, Kraaijenhagen RJ, Braam BG, Marx JJ, van de Wiel A. Response of erythropoiesis and iron metabolism to recombinant human erythropoietin in intensive care unit patients. Crit Care Med. 2000;28(8):2773–8.
54. Corwin HL, Gettinger A, Pearl RG, Fink MP, Levy MM, Shapiro MJ, et al. Efficacy of recombinant human erythropoietin in critically ill patients: a randomized controlled trial. JAMA. 2002;288:2827–35.
55. Corwin HL, Gettinger A, Rodriguez RM, Pearl RG, Gubler KD, Enny C, et al. Efficacy of recombinant human erythropoietin in the critically ill patient: a randomized, double-blind, placebo-controlled trial. Crit Care Med. 1999;27:2346–50.
56. Corwin HL, Gettinger A, Fabian TC, May A, Pearl RG, Heard S, et al. Efficacy and safety of epoetin alfa in critically ill patients. N Engl J Med. 2007;357(10):965–76.
57. Ziegler EJ, McCutchan JA, Fierer J, Glauser MP, Sadoff JC, Douglas H, et al. Treatment of gram-negative bacteremia and shock with human antiserum to a mutant Escherichia coli. N Engl J Med. 1982;307(20):1225–30.
58. Webster NR, Galley HF. Immunomodulation in the critically ill. Br J Anaesth. 2009;103(1): 70–81.
59. Bernard GR, Vincent JL, Laterre PF, LaRosa SP, Dhainaut J-F, Lopez-Rodriguez A, et al. Efficacy and safety of recombinant human activated protein C for sepsis. N Engl J Med. 2001; 344:699–709.
60. Abraham E, Laterre P-F, Garg R, Levy H, Talwar D, Trzaskoma BL, et al. Drotrecogin alfa (activated) for adults with severe sepsis and a low risk of death. N Engl J Med. 2005;353: 1332–41.
61. Nadel S, Goldstein B, Williams MD, Dalton H, Peters M, Macias WL, et al. Drotrecogin alfa (activated) in children with severe sepsis: a multicentre phase III randomised controlled trial. Lancet. 2007;369:836–43.
62. Bernard GR, Margolis BD, Shanies HM, Ely EW, Wheeler AP, Levy H, et al. Extended evaluation of recombinant human activated protein C United States Investigators extended evaluation of recombinant human activated protein C United States Trial (ENHANCE US): a single-arm, phase 3B, multicenter study of drotrecogin alfa (activated) in severe sepsis. Chest. 2004;125:2206–16.
63. Ranieri VM, Thompson BT, Barie PS, Dhainaut J-F, Douglas IS, Finfer S, et al. Drotrecogin alfa (activated) in adults with septic shock. N Engl J Med. 2012;366:2055–64.

Chapter 22
Newly-Acquired Complex Performance Competence and Medical Errors

Alan Lesgold

Introduction

Increasingly, the acquisition of competence is defined using learning progressions [1]. For conceptual bodies of knowledge, such progressions are reasonably straightforward. They state stages of understanding and capability that people pass through on the path to expertise. Generally, once each stage is fully mastered, performance at that stage is relatively less demanding of cognitive processing resources, leaving some capacity free to notice cues for routine required actions. In mission critical areas, including many areas of medicine, competence includes not only knowing how to deal with situations but also being reliable, while exercising that expertise, in carrying out critical routines (e.g., hand washing) even when overloaded when complex problems that must be solved. This chapter considers the circumstances during the course of progressing to expertise under which there is a danger of routine but critical actions being omitted and then discusses possible ways to minimize the likelihood of critical omissions.

Newly-Acquired Complex Performance Competence and Medical Errors

In everyday life, we tend to assume that with practice people become more competent. This even is the case for certain critical kinds of competence, such as driving a car. We assume that it is the novice who will miss stop signs and not respond quickly enough to a potential accident situation. In this chapter, I raise the possibility that certain kinds of critical performances may vary non-monotonically

A. Lesgold, PhD
School of Education, University of Pittsburgh, Pittsburgh, PA 15260, USA
e-mail: al@pitt.edu

V.L. Patel et al. (eds.), *Cognitive Informatics in Health and Biomedicine*,
Health Informatics, DOI 10.1007/978-1-4471-5490-7_22, © Springer-Verlag London 2014

during the course of learning, sometimes becoming less reliable for a period after previously having been pretty well established. To establish this argument, it is necessary to accept that learning of complex performance capability proceeds in stages, i.e., that it involves learning progressions.

The study of science learning was the source for the notion of learning progressions [1, 2]. A learning progression is an account of the stages that a learner goes through in gaining expertise. Perhaps the best known learning progression is Piaget's stages of cognitive development, which specifies the stages a child goes through in becoming more able to gain understanding from new situations, progressively gaining the ability to observe, then to manipulate, then to plan abstractly a set of manipulations that might help in understanding a new set of situations. Many learning progressions, though, involve smaller and somewhat more concrete domains of competence, such as understanding electrical circuits or understanding how to diagnose cardiovascular disease or knowing how to evaluate and treat traumatic blows to the head.

Non-monotone Aspects of Competence Development

So, for example, specific areas of medical diagnosis and treatment knowledge may pass through several stages as that knowledge develops. Students learn enough anatomy and physiology to be able to understand how a disease develops and progresses, after which they learn how to reason through a specific case to diagnose that disease. The left side of Fig. 22.1 illustrates this progression. It also can happen that a student might learn a rule that is conceptually less completely grounded but still embodies the high probability that a particular cluster of symptoms indicates the likelihood of a particular disease. This is shown on the right side of Fig. 22.1.

Going even further, when all goes well, these two capabilities – to quickly recognize a disease from its symptoms and to diagnose it through reasoning about what could produce the presenting information – become coordinated, so that correct diagnoses come quickly to mind but also are reflected upon to be sure that they make sense in the case at hand. Note that these stages may be reached independently for different disease clusters and symptom clusters. One might, for example, become adept at dealing with one specialty like cardiology without becoming as well prepared in another like orthopedics. Indeed, the very presence of so many medical specialists is an indication that these stages are not stages of overall medical competence but rather for coherent subsets of medical practice.

Ordinarily, one would see progression from the novice stage through the intermediate levels to the expert stage as representing improvement in medical knowledge. Each stage, when fully attained, after all, means added diagnostic capability. Interestingly, though, sometimes short-term setbacks occur along the path to greater capability. In some of my own work on radiological expertise, this was the case [3, 4]. Indeed, I can recall situations over the course of a year or two where the same person diagnosed a particular X-ray image correctly early in residency and

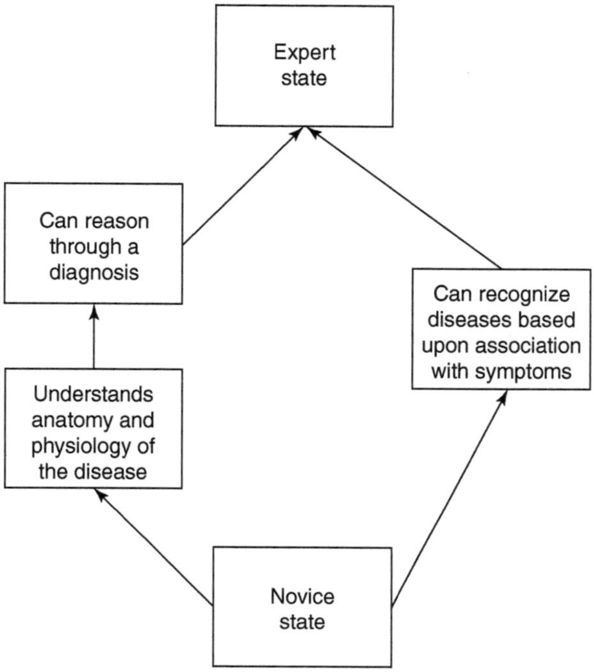

Fig. 22.1 Sample learning progression

incorrectly after months of additional experience. While setbacks are temporary and overall competence keeps growing, such setbacks do occur. Perhaps the most well-known brief setback occurs as children learn tenses of verbs. It is not unusual for a child who has just learned that past tense verbs often end in –ed to revert from saying "went" to saying "goed". A range of developmental progressions are well documented to include brief setbacks [5]. These reversals of apparent competence are interesting because they may, as suggested below, be openings for increased medical error. I first discuss current views about non-monotone competence development and then consider its implications.

Three general explanations have been advanced for non-monotone developmental occurrences [6], and these also should be considered for non-monotone competence acquisition. First, and particularly relevant to medical learning, acquiring a more systematic approach to problem solving might lead to a small number of cases where the new approach fails while a more superficial approach might succeed. For example, I might correctly diagnose a particular instance of Disease X because the case matches the experience of my Aunt Maude. When I learn more about Disease X, I might learn that its standard symptoms more often mean that the patient has Disease Y but not yet know enough to recognize and understand why the symptoms of the patient like Aunt Maude indicate Disease X. That could make me incorrect in diagnosing a case like hers until I learn even more and become able to correctly differentiate the situations in which the less common situation arises.

A second possibility according to Siegler is that the newly learned capability may overload cognitive capacity until parts of it become automated. What used to

Table 22.1 Principles of knowledge and competence development

1. People are endowed with an innate information-processing system
2. People form higher units from lower units. In other words the learning system is hierarchical.
3. Higher units serve as components for still-higher units.
4. There is a bias to process using highest-formed units
5. If, for some reason, higher units are not available, lower-level units are utilized.

be shoot-from-the-hip recognition may suffer when deeper diagnostic capability has just been acquired, simply because the new inferential capability isn't automated enough to fit within limited human processing capacity. In such a situation, a resident who "follows his instincts" might be correct in a diagnosis while he might fail if put in a situation in which his diagnosis must be defended. This second possibility is the one to which I return below.

Siegler suggests a third possibility as well. This is that different aspects of competence may grow at different rates, allowing one aspect to overshadow another with the other being dominant later. In infant development, for example, leg length and leg muscle strength develop on slightly different tracks, so when the leg grows faster than its muscles, apparent balance capability may briefly be lost. In medical learning, knowledge of different mechanisms may similarly show uncoordinated development, leading to diagnoses favoring whichever area of practice has been dealt with most recently, especially for medical students and interns/residents on rotating assignments.

The prevailing research view [6] is that the underlying accumulation of knowledge is monotone, i.e., that further learning or development does not destroy knowledge, even if certain capabilities may temporarily decrease. Nonetheless, for the purpose of patient safety, understanding setbacks is important. Before getting to that, it is worth considering what the basic principles of the development of knowledge are in the first place, since we may be better able to anticipate how cognitive overload will express itself if we consider those principles.

While many different sets of learning principles can be found, when considering the long-term development of medical expertise, it is worth attending to principles originating in the developmental psychology world. For example, Table 22.1 lists a set of principles [7] we might consider (in quoting these principles, I have replaced the word "infant" with the word "people" because of the focus of this chapter). The first three principles explain a little of how the learning at different stages is combined to create higher-order processing units. Most notably for medicine, direct statistical association of symptoms to diagnoses and deep understanding of the mechanisms behind diseases get integrated into higher-order units that encompass both knowledge sources, enabling experts both to quickly recognize diseases and to check their recognition against a set of expectations generated from their deeper understanding [8–10].

The fourth and fifth principles in Table 22.1 are especially important in understanding performance failures. Once a resident has acquired a reasonable level of

Table 22.2 Stages in formation of medical expertise [9]

1.	Development of elaborate declarative networks explaining the causes and consequences of disease in terms of general underlying pathophysiological processes
2.	Encapsulation of these declarative networks into a limited number of diagnostic labels, syndromes or high-level, simplified causal models, explaining signs and symptoms
3.	Transition into illness scripts through the acquisition of experience-based, contextual or enabling conditions knowledge
4.	Storage of interpreted instances of these scripts as exemplars of the particular illness

ability to reason about the meaning of symptom clusters in a given situation, we can expect him to use that ability. Sometimes, though, when that ability is just developed, the cognitive load imposed by deeper reasoning can interfere with successful recognition-based performance. More broadly, it can interfere with a range of clinical behaviors that otherwise might occur close to automatically. It is this paradox, that deeper understanding of why one's recognition-based decisions are right can interfere with making and acting upon those recognitions until the deeper understanding is automated, that I suggest merits a bit more attention. After all, at least in hospital settings, much of medical care is delivered by new physicians who have just acquired much of the knowledge they use every day.

This is the fundamental point I wish to remind about in this chapter. It is common in discussing errors, both in aviation and in medicine, to cite "human error" as the cause, implying that an actor at the scene should have tried harder. As the effort to reduce error has matured in each area where human performance is critical, we have learned that some human error, while predictable, cannot be contained by just pushing people to work harder. Shooting soldiers on guard duty who fell asleep did not make camps more secure in the eighteenth and nineteenth centuries. Blaming pilots who, generally, died as a consequence of the error being identified, did not make flying safer. We cannot expect that simply manipulating incentives for the erring actor will make medical errors less likely. Rather, changes in training and especially engineering of patient care environments – the topic of some chapters in this volume – are essential.

In considering the status of medical expertise in hospital settings, it is useful to keep in mind how that expertise develops. Table 22.2 quotes four stages of developing expertise put forward by Schmidt and Rikers [9]. These stages pretty much ignore the acquisition of specific recognition for symptom clusters that occurs alongside knowledge-driven recognition of diseases, but they nicely unpack some of the ways in which knowledge-driven diagnostic skill develops and the later stages in which it is integrated with memory of specific cases that become exemplars.

For purposes of this discussion, what is important is that a lot of learning takes place after medical students and new physicians have acquired both substantial understanding of disease and its manifestations – and consequently after much of their time as hospital house staff. Moreover, each stretch of existing knowledge produces a period of increased cognitive activity, including more extensive inference from primary medical knowledge [11], which can exhaust the cognitive capabilities of the new physician.

Cognitive Overload and Medical Errors

Given the concepts sketched above, it may be worth exploring some of the implications of cognitive overload that occurs as medical knowledge is expanding. Perhaps the most important implication is that initial demonstration of mastery within a restricted situation may be an overestimate of the reliability of knowledge. Sometimes this is mundane. For example, one might observe, in a restricted set of situations, that a resident always washes his hands upon entering a patient room. Even so, we might expect that on occasion, when the resident is extremely overloaded mentally, he may forget to wash before touching the patient. Given that this can occur even when the disposition to do the right thing is present, extensive learning has occurred, and mastery has been demonstrated, it makes sense to provide an efficient and effective means of reminding the resident to wash.

Many such approaches to reminding have been tried. Some are likely to fail because the reminders themselves become so commonplace as to not intrude into consciousness when one is overloaded. Others are more effective because they intrude more into consciousness. For example, at least for compromised patients who require masks and gowns, the placement of a rack near the room door with all of the apparel that is needed likely also will prompt hand washing, simply because it intrudes so completely. Interestingly, this might be a situation where well-meant efforts to move the rack of gloves, masks, and gowns out of the way to facilitate movement of equipment and patients in and out of a room could decrease the effectiveness of the rack as an intrusive warning to engage in actions that, in easy cases, might be automatic and assumed.

There are, of course, other situations in which errors occur that are more complex. Here again, the first approach to consider is probably to assure that the patient environment intrusively reminds health care workers to do the right thing. Intrusion is critical if cognitive overload is the problem, since attentional field is decreased under conditions of overload, so routine warnings not only are habituated to but also lose effectiveness since they may not be noticed when the cognitive capabilities of a health care worker are overloaded. Another useful form of intrusion is paraprofessional help. A culture in which it is acceptable for a nurse to remind a doctor about basic practices will likely do better in maintaining those practices, since while the doctor may be concentrating on a hard diagnosis, the nurse may not simultaneously be as overloaded.

While incentives to reduce errors may not be effective when arranged for the key actor in a medical situation, since that actor already may be overloaded cognitively, such incentives may work when provided to other health care workers who may not be as overloaded and hence more able to remind the key actor to carry out a required action such as hand washing. More broadly, though, it should be noted that what incentives do, in essence, is elevate one action to be more likely than others. Under conditions of cognitive overload, simply making a required routine act take over consciousness and interrupt more complex thinking will assure that the routine act is carried out but interfere with the action that depends upon the cognition that

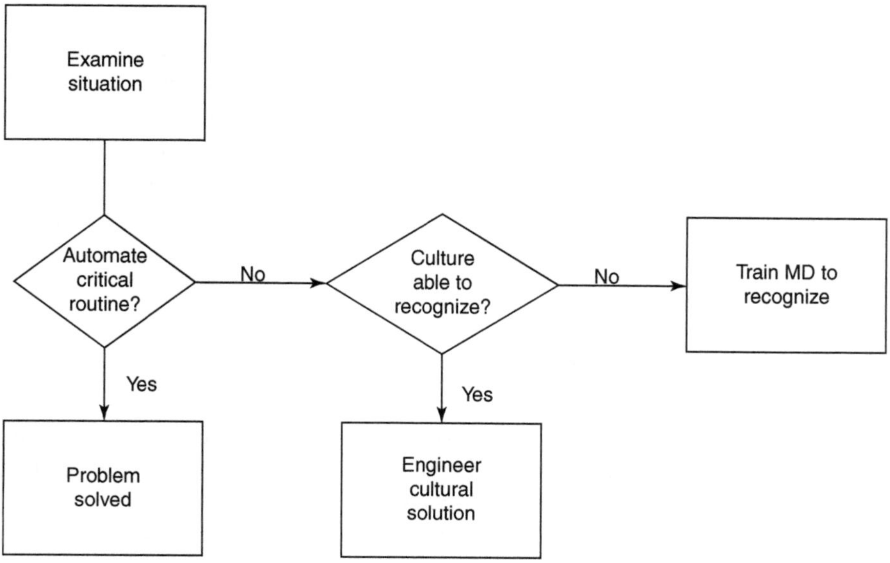

Fig. 22.2 Decision tree for preventing overload errors

produced the overload. This suggests that reminders alone may not always do the job. They will work best when they prompt a needed response, that response is highly automated (and thus not demanding of substantial cognitive resources), and the environment is engineered to best support an automated response.

When considering how best to assure that critical actions are performed, then, three basic possibilities should be considered, as suggested by Fig. 22.2. The best option, as just discussed, often is to automate the assurance of a critical function or make its achievement minimally demanding of cognitive resources. An example of this is the checklist. When a work protocol uses a checklist, there is a high level of certainty that each step in the checklist will be executed, at least when the step is understood by the work team. Moreover, a checklist serves as a temporary memory for work in progress, so the execution of a critical step will not erase the group's memory for steps that need to follow. For this reason, checklists are extremely useful. However, not all checklists are effective, and it is essential to design checklist and associated training well if they are to work [12]. For example, in order for a checklist to solve a problem, there has to be a trigger for its use. For example, the takeoff checklist used by pilots only works for takeoffs. If there is an emergent event in the air, it may or may not trigger a checklist type of protocol. Similarly, hospitals have code protocols (which really are somewhat more elaborated versions of checklists), which help assure that important actions are not overlooked in defined code situations. Such protocols work when there is a triggering event that causes them to be entered.

However, there are circumstances in which there is no triggering event, and there are also lapses in noticing the critical event and thereby triggering use of a protocol.

The simple hand washing case is an example of this. The cognitive overload that sometimes occurs in hospital settings tends to result in a person not noticing the appropriate trigger for hand washing. This can be overcome perhaps as suggested above, by making the cues for hand washing more intrusive. In essence, that is a variation of automating or engineering a solution to the problem. Sometimes, though, that is not completely possible. In that case, perhaps the next possibility to consider is enculturation of social processes that assure the triggering of appropriate routines.

Enculturation of Reliability

The aviation industry has gone through several generations of crew team training, and that training increasingly includes schemes of team protocols that assure that important routines are not ignored when complex situations occur [13]. Clearly, similar approaches are possible in medicine, and this book's chapters provide glimpses of this possibility.

One important element of such training is the development of shared understanding by the medical team of the effects of cognitive overload and the circumstances under which it is likely to arise. Another key element is likely to be identification of who in the team is most likely to not be overloaded and hence capable of assuring that critical routines are not missed. Finally, a team needs to practice engaging complex situations and moving into "crisis mode." In that crisis mode, part of the overt team activity is to split the needed tasks in ways that assure that critical tasks are not given to someone overloaded by even harder tasks, at least to the extent possible.

The aviation industry does this kind of training routinely, even though there are no fixed teams in aviation – individual pilots and cabin attendants are assigned individually, with only a modest force toward team continuity produced by union work rules and the accidents of particular personnel with seniority wanting to work together. Nonetheless, the team training works and, while the number of emergency cases has been extremely low both before and after training, such training seems to have reduced air disasters [14]. So, it seems worthwhile to consider medical team training across job levels (i.e., physicians, nurses, technicians) as an important part of an effort to remove medical errors.

It is important to realize, though, that situations of cognitive overload in the medical world are not restricted to emergency situations such as code calls. Aircraft crew deal with one flight at a time, and a flight lasts, on average, a couple hours. Medical practice is organized to involve almost continual parallel processing. Nurses have multiple patients to care for. While doctors in some specialty areas can make sequential rounds, seeing a patient at a time, even then it is not unusual for a doctor to see a patient, request data that takes time to collect, such as a lab test, and then be interrupted when the data become available. And, of course, there are practice areas, such as emergency department work, where parallel processing is pretty much the order of the day, at least at times. Even during office hours, it is not unusual for a physician to have overlap in the overall processing of patients, and the office team certainly has such overlap – a nurse or aide is positioning one patient to be seen after the patient the physician is seeing at the moment while also handling the orders of the patient already seen and being on call to assist the physician with the patient currently being seen.

One approach, consistent with some of the work reported elsewhere in this volume, is to do the needed team training and related training of individual health care roles on the assumption that medical settings are continually in an overload mode. In the airplane cockpit, most of the time activity is being handled by the plane itself, with one pilot monitoring the situation to detect potential issues. In contrast, medical care systems, with their emphasis on staffing efficiency, generally have most or all staff assigned enough critical work to pretty much fill their cognitive capacity, at least much of the time. Therefore, it is less critical for such staff to learn when to go into team collaboration mode and more critical for teams to have permanent arrangements in place to assure that cognitive overload does not lead to omission of critical actions.

How this can happen will vary as a function of how urgent certain actions are. Let us first consider situations in which it is problematic if certain actions are omitted for extended periods but where moment-to-moment changes do not generally require action. For example, after I had my hip replaced, it was important for someone to check periodically, but not continually, for signs of blood clots. If such checks did not occur in the past hour, the risk would be extremely low, but if there was no check for a day or two, this could be more problematic. Presumably, this kind of problem of things not being noticed in a timeline of a few hours could be handled by a checklist. So, for example, an electronic patient record system might prompt the duty nurse every few hours to verify that a set of checks had been made – such prompting already occurs for various routine actions. While this is partly an engineering solution rather than a training solution, it also is common to train nursing staff as well as resident physicians to ask a set of check questions whenever visiting a given patient – or every few hours when visits are continual or frequent.

It would be consistent with the results reported or referenced in this volume to develop further research on the efficacy of monitoring checklists of this kind. While much of checklist work has been done to assure that relevant actions are taken at a point of treatment, extending the concept to checklists that can be applied to monitor whether the longer term course of patient care is free of critical omissions makes a lot of sense. Personal experience suggests that for "quality of life" issues like food service in hospitals, this is pretty routine, but perhaps it is less well developed or systematic for medical actions that should occur regularly but are not critical at any given moment. So, for example, surgical residents routinely check themselves for certain complications on daily visits, as part of implicit or explicit protocols, but they may be less likely to check for the pattern of overall health care team attention to certain issues over the past day.

The Role of Reminders

It also can safely be predicted that scheduled actions will occur reliably but that unscheduled actions and checks may have higher chance of omission. While some of these unscheduled checks can be scheduled, by prompting a nurse to enter explicitly the results of a check just as there is prompting to deliver medication, there may be team activities that could supplement this, since there will never be a truly complete list of all the things that a nurse or physician should notice in a patient. In particular, team meetings might include discussion of what needs to be checked for in a particular class of patients, whether those checks are occurring reliably, and what evidence supports that belief. While much of this may be routine and part of training for different health care professionals, it also is likely that problems might emerge in such discussions and that discussion of those problems might lead to changes in systemic prompts for certain checks.

As noted above, there is a danger in automating reminders about routine checks. A check that tends to be made automatically requires minimal cognitive resources. While it is possible that without an automated reminder and under cognitive overload, the trigger that should prompt a check may fail to be attended, it also is possible, as discussed in this volume, that an extended array of automated reminders may produce cognitive overload and lack of attention to all of the warnings that might be posted. This volume reports work on dashboards for patient information display, and all of the problems associated with such dashboards also are present in any collection of automated warning systems meant to assure that routine checks are made and routine actions taken.

More broadly, the management of all of the routine as well as alarming data that is generated by or observable in a patient is itself a major source of cognitive overload. Systems that simply remind health care staff about checks needed or situations meriting a response are likely to contribute to cognitive overload and hence exacerbate the problem of omission of needed care activity. This volume includes discussion of efforts to improve dashboard displays so that the most relevant information is most salient and information is organized in manageable ways. While intelligent display management and prioritization of relevant information has great potential for improving the reliability and success of patient care, though, more may be required.

Specifically, some of the intelligence in data management will likely need to be provided by the health care worker, to supplement what can be done by machines. No matter how good automated prioritizing of warnings gets, it will not be perfect, and it will be critical to train personnel to find ways to work together to assure good outcomes.

Conclusion

To summarize, past research and the findings in this volume suggest that management of cognitive overload is a key requirement to assure that critical but routine actions are taken when needed. Engineering work environments and team work patterns is an important way to better prompt such actions and to assure that they are taken, when possible, by the health care worker whose overall activity will be least affected by the added cognitive load. Training teams to distribute work to minimize overload and to react positively to reminders from colleagues likely will contribute to improved reliability of critical actions. In some cases, though, it also will be necessary to train health care teams to review their own performance of the routine and mundane but critical and to consider ways to improve it. The work reported in this volume makes considerable progress on the research needed to elaborate and confirm the efficacy of these key steps.

Discussion Questions

1. Managing cognitive load is an important consideration in efficient and effective management of critical care activities. What impact do you think the health care technology will have in managing cognitive load?
2. What new skills do you think will be needed for competent performance in complex domain, as heath care technology becomes a part of our everyday clinical practice?
3. What aspects of training in team collaboration will be most useful in assuring reliability of health care in situations where some team members will experience high cognitive load?

References

1. Smith CL, Wiser M, Anderson CW, Krajcik J. Implications of research on children's learning for standards and assessment: a proposed learning progression for matter and the atomic molecular theory. Meas Interdiscipl Res Perspect. 2006;4:1–98.
2. Stevens SY, Shin N, Krajcik JS. Towards a model for the development of an empirically tested learning progression. In: Learning progressions in science conference, Iowa City, 2009.
3. Lesgold A, Rubinson H, Feltovich P, Glaser R, Klopfer D, Wang Y. Expertise in a complex skill: diagnosing X-ray pictures. In: Chi M, Glaser R, Farr M, editors. The nature of expertise. Hillsdale: Erlbaum; 1988. p. 311–42.
4. Lesgold AM. Acquiring expertise. In: Anderson JR, Kosslyn SM, editors. Tutorials in learning and memory: essays in honor of Gordon Bower. San Francisco: Freeman; 1984. p. 31–60.
5. Cashon CH, Cohen LB. Beyond U-shaped development in infants' processing of faces: an information-processing account. J Cogn Dev. 2004;5:59–80.
6. Siegler RS. U-shaped interest in U-shaped development – and what it means. J Cogn Dev. 2004;5:1–10.
7. Cohen LB, Chaput HH, Cashon CH. A constructivist model of infant cognition. Cogn Dev. 2002;17:1323–43.
8. Boshuizen HP, Schmidt HG. On the role of biomedical knowledge in clinical reasoning by experts, intermediates and novices. Cogn Sci. 1992;16:153–84.
9. Schmidt HG, Rikers RM. How expertise develops in medicine: knowledge encapsulation and illness script formation. Med Educ. 2007;41:1133–9.
10. Patel VL, Glaser R, Arocha JF. Cognition and expertise: acquisition of medical competence. Clin Invest Med. 2000;23:256–60.

11. Patel VL, Groen GJ, Arocha JF. Medical expertise as a function of task difficulty. Mem Cogn. 1990;18:394–406.
12. Hales B, Terblanche M, Fowler R, Sibbald W. Development of medical checklists for improved quality of patient care. Int J Qual Health Care. 2008;20:22–30.
13. Helmreich RL, Merritt AC, Wilhelm JA. The evolution of crew resource management training in commercial aviation. Int J Aviat Psychol. 1999;9:19–32.
14. Flin R, O'Connor P, Mearns K. Crew resource management: improving team work in high reliability industries. Team Perform Manag. 2002;8(3/4):68–78.

Chapter 23
Reflections on the Role of Cognitive Science in Biomedical Informatics

Edward H. Shortliffe

Introduction

Decision making is an inherent part of everything that health professionals do, and accordingly it is not surprising that cognitive science has relevance throughout all of patient care, health promotion, and disease prevention. Even the procedural specialties that depend on manual dexterity or similar skills, such as surgery, intrinsically depend on making good decisions about which procedures to perform, when to undertake them, and how best to prepare patients for what will be required. Many tough decisions carry over to prevention and public health: how best to advise patients, how best to encourage healthy behaviors, and how best to react when surveillance suggests that new attacks on the health and safety of the population may exist.

All such decisions depend on the knowledge of the decision makers, often augmented by their ability to weigh evidence and to access key information, either about the patient or about the phenomenon that is demanding attention. We often hear that biomedicine and health care, perhaps more than any other areas of human endeavor, are remarkably dependent on facile access to complete and accurate information that forms the basis for wise decisions about diagnosis, testing, treatment, or other management issues. The notion of "evidence-based medicine" has become a major focus of medical education and practice [1], a trend that is attempting to counter the high level of variation in clinical practices that has been shown to exist both regionally and among physicians within a single community [2].

The science of information and knowledge management in biomedical research, clinical practice, and public health is known as *biomedical informatics* [3]. It has recently been formally defined by the principal informatics professional society [4]

E.H. Shortliffe, MD, PhD, MACP
College of Health Solutions, Arizona State University, Phoenix, AZ 85004, USA

Department of Biomedical Informatics, Columbia University, New York, NY 10032, USA

Department of Public Health, Weill Cornell Medical College, New York, NY 10065, USA
e-mail: ted@shortliffe.net

V.L. Patel et al. (eds.), *Cognitive Informatics in Health and Biomedicine*, Health Informatics, DOI 10.1007/978-1-4471-5490-7_23,

as "the interdisciplinary field that studies and pursues the effective uses of biomedical data, information, and knowledge for scientific inquiry, problem solving, and decision making, motivated by efforts to improve health" [5]. There are a growing number of academic departments in biomedical informatics (BMI), most commonly in medical schools, offering graduate degrees, courses for medical or nursing students, and certificate programs for individuals who may be seeking intensive mid-career exposure to the field. Many graduates are also trained in one of the traditional health professions, but others view biomedical informatics alone as their health-professional training. The American Board of Medical Specialties approved a formal medical subspecialty of clinical informatics in 2011 and offered a board examination in the field for the first time in 2013 [6].

BMI research focuses on creating new methods, optimal processes, or theories that inform the field's evolution. Such work often draws on computer science or communications, but other component sciences include the decision sciences, cognitive science, statistics, information science, and management science. It has broad applicability across all of biomedicine, with applied work and practice that deal with molecules and cells (*bioinformatics*), tissues and organ systems (*imaging* or *structural informatics*), patients (*clinical informatics*), or populations and society (*public health informatics*). Because the field recognizes that people are the ultimate users of biomedical information, it also draws heavily on the social and behavioral sciences. Biomedical and clinical decisions are made in context of complex economic, ethical, social, educational, and cognitive factors; they are also embedded in complex organizational systems, such as research universities, hospitals, health systems, clinics, outpatient practices, or public health departments.

As this volume demonstrates, the field of cognitive science has much to offer to our understanding of how clinicians make decisions in complex healthcare environments. Without such insights, it is folly to design interventions, whether technological or procedural, that attempt to reduce decision-making errors, to improve the ways in which errors are handled once made, or to enhance the safety of patients. In the BMI community, where researchers and practitioners are often designing solutions intended to improve or support clinical decision making, the relevance of cognitive science has accordingly become clear [7]. Cognitive scientists are increasingly involved as collaborators on informatics research or development projects, and they play a particularly visible role in the field of human-computer interaction and usability testing [8]. We have accordingly seen the emergence of an important subfield of BMI known as *cognitive informatics*. In the remainder of this chapter, I will summarize some of my own experiences, as a clinician, biomedical informatics researcher, and educator, in coming to a belief that cognitive informatics is not only a desirable but a mandatory component of essentially all BMI research and development projects, as well as system implementations and evaluations.

Cognitive Science and Clinical Decision Making: The Early Years

As a medical student in the 1970s, I became aware of a growing body of work that highlighted the importance of decision science and cognition to the practice of medicine. I was already interested in computer-based decision-support tools for clinicians, focusing on this area for my doctoral work in informatics, and was introduced to formal decision science, probabilistic inference, and decision analysis notions. Dr. Barbara McNeil from Harvard Medical School published a series of influential papers on the subject in the *New England Journal of Medicine* [9–11], and these opened my eyes to formal decision science and its relevance to clinical practice (and to the development of decision-support software). Other authors saw the relevance of decision science to clinical practice [12] and they published papers showing how normative theory could be embodied in computer programs [13].

But I was working on a problem that seemed immune to a formal decision analytic approach: the selection of antibiotic therapy for patients with bacterial meningitis or bacteremia [14]. We developed methods for interviewing infectious disease experts to understand how they made such decisions, hoping that we could model our computer program after the kind of knowledge and reasoning that they exhibited (which explains why such programs became known as *expert systems* [15]). We did not realize it at the time, but our interviewing approach was very similar to the kind of "think-aloud" problem solving studies that were underway in the cognitive science community. The process of interviewing experts to understand how they solved problems and then to encode their knowledge for use by computer programs in time became known as *knowledge engineering* [16]. In the cognitive science community, this same notion has been dubbed *knowledge elicitation.*

At about the same time, however, Pauker and coworkers were taking a cognitive-science approach to studying clinical decision making, hoping that they too could develop programs that simulated expert decision making rather than pursuing a formal decision analytic approach. Their groundbreaking work in this area first appeared in 1976 [17].

The close-knit group of researchers working at this intersection of cognitive science, expert problem solving, and decision-support programs became known as the "artificial intelligence in medicine" community. Their work led in time to the creation of a journal (*Artificial Intelligence in Medicine*, Elsevier) [18], a European Society for AI in Medicine [19], an ongoing international research community, and retrospective analyses of the field and its impact [20–22].

I was working at Stanford University's medical school during this period, and it was a cognitive psychologist from our main campus who had perhaps the most far-reaching influence on our understanding of human problem solving in the context of medical decision-making. Amos Tversky was a dominant figure in decision research and his collaborative work with Daniel Kahneman, while not initially focusing on medicine, was immediately recognized in medical circles for its relevance [23]. Subsequently Tversky became involved with the Society for Medical Decision Making [24] and with medical school research at Stanford, often using medical examples to illustrate both the use of heuristics (which characterizes much of the work in medical AI) and biases (which explain many of the classical reasoning errors that can occur in clinical practice settings).

The discussion above demonstrates that cognitive-science research and researchers have been relevant and involved in biomedical informatics research and practice since the early days of the field (which emerged as a separate discipline in about 1970). In most cases, articles about the cognitive work were studied by clinicians or informaticians and the lessons were then incorporated into informatics research or the design of programs. It was in the 1990s, however, that some cognitive scientists identified medicine and biomedical informatics as areas of primary interest and moved into the field full-time. Similarly, informatics trainees increasingly became interested in cognitive topics and sought formal coursework and research experiences in the area. Accordingly we have seen a gradual involvement of cognitive scientists as full-time collaborators on research projects, in design or evaluation activities, as informatics teachers, and increasingly as faculty members in academic informatics departments.

Informatics Research as a Subject of Cognitive-Science Study

It was during the 1990s that I personally began to appreciate the central role of cognitive-science expertise in much that we do in biomedical informatics. Building on our group's ongoing interest in decision support, and having forged a relationship with the American College of Physicians and its major commitment to the development and dissemination of clinical guidelines [25], we became interested in how such guidelines could be implemented in computer programs and made available as part of normal workflow in clinical settings. As the Arden Syntax had demonstrated for clinical alerts and reminders [26], a standard method for encoding the logic of clinical guidelines would be highly desirable. Yet we knew that no single institution could propose a standard that would be embraced broadly by the community or industry. We accordingly joined forces with several other institutions to create a collaboratory of informatics investigators with the goal of developing methods for guideline representation that would be viewed as more broadly developed, openly made available, and therefore more acceptable to the community [27].

Our multi-institutional effort became known as the InterMed Collaboratory, with participation of individuals from Stanford, Columbia, and Harvard Universities. But we soon discovered that collaboration was difficult at a distance, although we scheduled frequent conference calls among participants and made regular use of email and shared documents via the Internet. We accordingly approached Professor Vimla Patel at McGill University, who had become known in the AI in Medicine community after her keynote presentation at the AIME meeting in Maastricht in 1991. We invited her and her group to join the InterMed Collaboratory and to help us to understand how best to develop effective collaboration at a distance. Dr. Patel readily agreed and applied her cognitive-science expertise to a rigorous analysis, using as study data the records of all email messages among InterMed participants, audio recordings of all phone calls, copies of the documents that we wrote collaboratively, and observations of interactions when we occasionally managed to meet in person. The early results of this work had a profound influence on how the individual site leaders managed their teams and the schedule and types of interactions [25]. The results revealed, for example, "that occasional face-to-face meetings are crucial precursors to the effective use of distance communications technology; that conference calls play an important role in both task-related activities and executive (project management) activities, especially when clarifications are required; and that collaborative productivity is highly dependent upon the gradual development of a shared commitment to a well-defined task that leverages the varying expertise of both local and distant colleagues in the creation of tools of broad utility across the participating sites" [28]. The success of this study of collaboration was instrumental in allowing the various groups to produce a uniform representation model (the Guideline Interchange Format, known as GLIF [29]) and participants all viewed the cognitive work, in which we served as subjects of study as well as collaborators, as an extremely important research result of the InterMed effort. Furthermore, as the cognitive work became more familiar, we found other ways in which the collaboration could benefit from cognitive expertise, and the Patel group at McGill made especially important observations about how guidelines are developed and interpreted during the encoding process, and why different people with different backgrounds will make different decisions about what a guideline means and how it should be encoded [30, 31]. We realized that these insights were important not only to the encoding process and any authoring software that we would offer, but also to understanding how differently a specialist and generalist might perceive the same guideline, given their differing mental models of both the disease and the patient. Such observations naturally play an important role in determining how guideline-based advice should be presented to users, for example.

Cognitive Approaches to Informing System Design and Content

Another lesson of the importance of cognitive informatics arose a few years later when I had moved to Columbia University and Dr. Patel had joined the informatics faculty there as well. There was a strong interest in New York City regarding how to reduce the risk-taking behaviors of young people regarding HIV and possible exposure to AIDS. Educational web sites began to appear, providing information regarding the virus, how it is transmitted, and what steps can be taken to reduce the risk of exposure. In discussions within our department at that time, however, we began to question whether such web-based interventions would be effective in altering behavior. After all, it is difficult to design an educational resource to change behavior if we have imperfect information about why people act the way that they do in the first place. Viewing this question as central in any effort to affect behavior, Dr. Patel and her team undertook studies with young adults and adolescents, enlisting subjects who kept detailed diaries and agreed to meet for confidential interviews on multiple occasions over a period of months. The resulting insights were striking. The subjects generally had excellent knowledge about HIV/AIDS, how it is transmitted, and why it is dangerous. They had heard about it in school or from friends. When they made bad decisions that exposed them to risk, it was essentially never out of ignorance about the disease. There was a variety of other psychosocial explanations for doing what they knew to be risky, including the desire to demonstrate their trust to their sexual partners [32, 33]. Such work provides an important informatics lesson: one needs to understand the minds and mental models of intended users before defining either the form or content of a computer-based resource that is intended to inform its users or to alter their behaviors.

Cognitive Science, Patient Safety, and Informatics

The cognitive unit in our informatics department gradually became involved in almost every project that we undertook. A cultural shift was underway as faculty and students began to realize that cognitive informatics was an important element in all that we did – whether designing systems, determining their usability, evaluating their impact, or defining what content was most important to include. After the IOM error report was released [34], and informatics units became increasingly involved in identifying informatics methods to reduce sources of medical errors, the cognitive informatics unit played a fundamental role in helping us to understand the nature of errors that do occur [35, 36] as well as suitable venues for trying to intervene appropriately and effectively [37]. They also helped us to ascertain methods that would assist in system evaluations, especially regarding usability [38].

Cognitive Science in the Education of Biomedical Informaticians

Courses on cognitive informatics topics also became extremely popular among our graduate students, and many were attracted to become involved in the kinds of projects that the cognitive unit was undertaking. Some of the lecture topics would focus on technology (with emphasis on topics such as usability testing, designing for effective human-computer interaction, cognitive walkthroughs in the design of technology, evaluation methodology, and safety issues in the design and use of clinical systems). Others would focus more on cognitive issues that had less direct (but still real) relevance to the design and implementation of computer systems. Examples include cognitive challenges in handing off patients between teams [39], workflow analysis and visualization [40], how lay people cope with information about disasters [41], or (as is emphasized in this volume) biomedical complexity and error [42]. In addition, cognitive studies of learning, especially in medical education, provide many lessons for those of us who are creating curricula, and devising instructional methods, for biomedical informatics degree programs [43].

Conclusion

In summary, cognitive science has always had a role to play in biomedical informatics research and education, even though it took a few decades before these relationships were formalized in a growing number of research and training programs. In the early days, informatics researchers were drawn to cognitive notions intuitively, and indeed there has always been an important role for psychology and cognition in computer science, especially in areas such as artificial intelligence, natural language processing, and visualization. Subsequently, cognitive informatics has moved into the mainstream, as people with formal training and experience in cognitive science have joined informatics research groups, learned about informatics concepts, and nurtured the growing discipline at the intersection. The greatest challenge at present is the relative lack of individuals who have excellent training in both cognitive science and the other core topics of biomedical informatics [5]. Vimla Patel was clearly a trailblazer in this area, and because we have worked together and I know her work well, I have emphasized her cognitive work in this chapter. Others who are trained in cognitive science and informatics, including those whom Dr. Patel has trained, are now creating their own units and research programs. But we need more such people and should accordingly encourage more young people to seek cognitive science and biomedical informatics training. The resulting bridging expertise, combined with the knowhow of computer scientists, informaticians, and clinicians, will have a profound influence on health and health care in the future: safer clinical environments, higher quality care, a healthier population, and improved design and implementation of technological tools and solutions.

References

1. Straus SE, Glasziou P, Richardson WS, Haynes RB. Evidence-based medicine: how to practice and teach it. 4th ed. New York: Churchill Livingstone; 2010.
2. Wennberg JE. Practice variation: implications for our health care system. Manag Care. 2004; 13(9 Suppl):3–7.
3. Shortliffe EH, Cimino JJ. Biomedical informatics: computer applications in health care and biomedicine. 4th ed. New York: Springer; 2013.
4. American Medical Informatics Association. Bethesda, MD. Available from: http://www.amia.org. Cited 7 Jul 2013.
5. Kuikowski CA, Shortliffe EH, Currie LM, Elkin PL, Hunter LE, Johnson TR, et al. AMIA board white paper: definition of biomedical informatics and specification of core competencies for graduate education in the discipline. J Am Med Inform Assoc. 2012;19(6):931–8.
6. Shortliffe EH. President's column: subspecialty certification in clinical informatics. J Am Med Inform Assoc. 2011;18(6):890–1.
7. Patel VL, Arocha JF, Kaufman DR. A primer on aspects of cognition for medical informatics. J Am Med Inform Assoc. 2001;8(4):324–43.
8. Horsky J, Schiff GD, Johnston D, Mercincavage L, Bell D, Middleton B. Interface design principles for usable decision support: a targeted review of best practices for clinical prescribing interventions. J Biomed Inform. 2012;45(6):1202–16.
9. McNeil BJ, Adelstein SJ. Measures of clinical efficacy: the value of case finding in hypertensive renovascular disease. N Engl J Med. 1975;293(5):221–6.
10. McNeil BJ, Keller E, Adelstein SJ. Primer on certain elements of medical decision making. N Engl J Med. 1975;293(5):211–5.
11. McNeil BJ, Varady PD, Burrows BA, Adelstein SJ. Measures of clinical efficacy: cost-effectiveness calculations in the diagnosis and treatment of hypertensive renovascular disease. N Engl J Med. 1975;293(5):216–21.

12. Schwartz WB, Gorry GA, Kassirer JP, Essig A. Decision analysis and clinical judgment. Am J Med. 1973;55(3):459–72.
13. Gorry GA, Kassirer JP, Essig A, Schwartz WB. Decision analysis as the basis for computer-aided management of acute rental failure. Am J Med. 1973;55(3):473–84.
14. Shortliffe EH. Computer-based medical consultations: MYCIN. New York: American Elsevier; 1976.
15. Duda RO, Shortliffe EH. Expert systems research. Science. 1983;220(4594):261–8.
16. Scott AC, Clayton JE, Gibson EL. A practical guide to knowledge acquisition. Reading: Addison-Wesley; 1991.
17. Pauker SG, Gorry GA, Kassirer JP, Schwartz WB. Towards the simulation of clinical cognition: taking a present illness by computer. Am J Med. 1976;60(7):981–96.
18. Artificial Intelligence in Medicine. Canada: Elsevier B.V. Available from: http://www.journals.elsevier.com/artificial-intelligence-in-medicine. Cited 7 Jul 2013.
19. Artificial Intelligence in Medicine. 2010. Available from: http://aimedicine.info/aime/. Cited 7 Jul 2013.
20. Schwartz WB, Patil RS, Szolovits P. Artificial intelligence in medicine: where do we stand? N Engl J Med. 1987;316:685–8.
21. Shortliffe EH. The adolescence of AI in medicine: will the field come of age in the '90s? Artif Intell Med. 1993;5(2):93–106.
22. Patel VL, Shortliffe EH, Stefanelli M, Szolovits P, Berthold MR, Bellazzi R, et al. The coming of age of artificial intelligence in medicine. Artif Intell Med. 2009;46(1):5–17.
23. Tversky A, Kahneman D. Judgment under uncertainty: heuristics and biases. Science. 1974;185:1124–31.
24. Society for Medical Decision Making. Available from: http://www.smdm.org/. Cited 7 July 2013.
25. Shortliffe EH, Barnett GO, Cimino JJ, Greenes RA, Huff SM, Patel VL. Collaborative medical informatics research using the internet and the World Wide Web. Proc AMIA Symp. 1996:125–9.
26. Hripcsak G, Ludemann P, Pryor TA, Wigertz OB, Clayton PD. Rationale for the Arden syntax. Comput Biomed Res. 1994;27(4):291–324.
27. Open Clinical KMfMC. Guideline Modelling Methods Technologies. New York, 2006. Available from: http://www.openclinical.org/gmm_glif.html. Cited 8 Jul 2013.
28. Shortliffe EH, Patel VL, Cimino JJ, Barnett GO, Greenes RA. A study of collaboration among medical informatics research laboratories. Artif Intell Med. 1998;12(2):97–123.
29. Ohno-Machado L, Gennari JH, Murphy SN, Jain NL, Tu SW, Oliver DE, et al. The guideline interchange format: a model for representing guidelines. J Am Med Inform Assoc. 1988;5(4):357–72.
30. Patel VL, Allen VG, Arocha JF, Shortliffe EH. Representing a clinical guideline in GLIF: individual and collaborative expertise. J Am Med Inform Assoc. 1998;5:467–83.
31. Patel VL, Arocha JF, Diemeier M, Greenes RA, Shortliffe EH. Methods of cognitive analysis to support the design and evaluation of biomedical systems: the case of clinical practice guidelines. J Biomed Inform. 2001;34(1):52–66.
32. Patel VL, Gutnik LA, Yoskowitz NA, O'Sullivan LF, Kaufman DR. Patterns of reasoning and decision making about condom use by urban college students. AIDS Care. 2006;18(8):918–30.
33. Patel VL, Yoskowitz NA, Kaufman DR. Comprehension of sexual situations and its relationship to risky decisions by young adults. AIDS Care. 2007;19(7):916–22.
34. Kohn LT, Corrigan JM, Donaldson MS. To err is human: building a safer health system. Washington, DC: National Academy Press; 2000.
35. Zhang J, Patel VL, Johnsen TR, Shortliffe EH. A cognitive taxonomy of medical errors. J Biomed Inform. 2004;37(3):193–204.
36. Horsky J, Zhang J, Patel VL. To err is not entirely human: complex technology and user cognition. J Biomed Inform. 2005;38(4):264–6.

37. Keselman A, Patel VL, Johnson TR, Zhang J. Institutional decision-making to select patient care devices: identifying venues to promote patient safety. J Biomed Inform. 2003;36(1–2): 31–44.
38. Kushniruk AW, Patel VL. Cognitive and usability engineering methods for the evaluation of clinical information systems. J Biomed Inform. 2004;37(1):56–76.
39. Abraham J, Kannampallil T, Patel VL. Bridging gaps in handoffs: a continuity of care approach. J Biomed Inform. 2012;45(2):240–54.
40. Vankipuram M, Kahol K, Cohen T, Patel VL. Toward automated workflow analysis and visualization in clinical environments. J Biomed Inform. 2011;44(3):432–40.
41. Keselman A, Slaughter L, Patel VL. Toward a framework for understanding lay public's comprehension of disaster and bioterrorism information. J Biomed Inform. 2005;38:331–44.
42. Kahol K, Buchman T, Patel VL. Biomedical complexity and error. J Biomed Inform. 2011;44(3):387–9.
43. Patel VL, Yoskowitz NA, Arocha JF, Shortliffe EH. Cognitive and learning sciences in biomedical and health instructional design: a review with lessons for biomedical informatics education. J Biomed Inform. 2009;42(1):176–97.

Epilogue

Paradigm Shifts in Complexity Thinking

Thomas Kuhn, in the often-cited philosophical treatise on the history of science, *Structure of Scientific Revolutions*, describe the paradigm shifts that happen during the development of a scientific discipline. These paradigm shifts are episodic and are driven by the identification of the anomalies in existing knowledge leading to re-thinking of the existing research approaches. At the start of this research endeavor on exploring cognitive complexity in the critical care work environment in 2007, our understanding on complexity had reached such a transitional state – much had been written and discussed regarding the contributors and its potential causal determinants to complexity in clinical settings, limited research insights were available regarding methods or approaches to study complex environments. The current thinking during the time was driven by theoretical perspectives on complexity that were drawn from domains such as physics (and complexity perspectives), and applied aspects from such as aviation and the military.

Our thinking was also influenced by the external influences that have shaped the healthcare system in recent decades. For example, we have seen several paradigmatic changes in healthcare systems, research and practice: technological advancements for patient care (including both medical devices and management tools such as the EHR and clinical decision support systems), incentivization of the use of health information technology, and increased focus on efficiency. In addition, there has been a strong emphasis on a culture of safety in clinical settings which has served to change the discourse about practice.

The fundamental changes that we attempted in order to study complexity in clinical settings were twofold: first, to further develop our approach for studying complexity, and second, to gain a better understanding of complexity as it manifests in critical care practice to inform the development of interventions to ensure efficient, effective and safe care of patients.

As cognitive scientists, we are concerned with the processes that lead to particular outcomes in task performance, a perspective that unifies the work presented in this volume. Adverse events are a possible outcome of a violation of the boundaries of safe practice, and we can characterize the individual and collective cognitive

V.L. Patel et al. (eds.), *Cognitive Informatics in Health and Biomedicine*, Health Informatics, DOI 10.1007/978-1-4471-5490-7, mechanisms that direct the evolution of error. Inconsistencies in information flow that can ultimately lead to the misinterpretation of critical patient data are assessed, in order to develop interventions that enhance the robustness of the handoff process. Efforts to regulate decision-making in complex environments are well intentioned, but have been found to be unpredictable and at times, harmful. All of these insights emerged from a focus on the individual and collective cognitive processes that underlie clinical decision-making and communication, and the contexts in which these processes are situated.

This perspective differs from the outcomes-oriented view that frequently prevails in patient safety research. While discrete measures taken at specific time points (e.g., efficiency or performance metrics) can provide insights into the nature of work activities, they may not address the complexities of human interaction within clinical environments. This is because most human interactions are sustained episodes of events that unfold over time among evolving networks of human actors. Such interactions can be used to trace the progressive effect of task interdependencies, challenges faced by users during the task (e.g., errors, breakdowns and other critical incidents), nature of the task flow, and strategies adopted during the task. This is especially relevant in clinical environments where the clinician's activities are often characterized as extremely challenging due to cognitive overload, need for multi-tasking, and often further complicated by less than friendly health information systems. In other words, analyzing sustained episodes of interaction sequences can provide a set of metrics (in terms of activities, tasks, and activities) that are crucial in characterizing a complex clinical work environment. Our approach to studying complexity conforms to *trace-based interactionist* approach that helps in identifying the nuances, constraints and interactions within the clinical system. A serendipitous outcome of utilizing the trace-based approach is its inherent ability to account for the social aspects of work activities. For example, interactions with the actors, artifacts and peers situate the activities within the contextual aspects of the work environment. This aspect of the trace-based approach is key to socio-technical analysis and design.

As exemplified by the 2011 IOM report, a socio-technical approach is instrumental in designing, incorporating and studying clinical contexts. One of the critical aspects of our approach is to understand the progression and evolution of human interactions with technology, collaborators and other artifacts. This led us towards utilizing a trace-based temporal approach that helps in capturing long-term interactions and their effects in a systematic manner. While the need for the use of socio-technical approach has been traditionally acknowledged in cognitive and social sciences, methodologies and technological innovations have influenced the effective capture of utilization of the socio-technical approaches. For example, we attempted to overcome the inherent limitations of ethnographic observation by a small number of human researchers with the use of radio-frequency sensors, and mobile data capture tools using the iPad/iPhone that provide convergent quantitative measures. While the technology is still evolving and our results are preliminary, we have attempted to shift the focus onto adapting available technology to develop effective tools that can aid in capturing holistic perspectives on the complex critical care environment.

In summary, adapting our process-oriented perspective to confront the complexity of the critical care workspace required methodological innovation, such as the development of new experimental paradigms to capture the process of error recovery, and the use of digital data capture tools to augment observation by human researchers. In addition, established methods were used to study aspects of the critical care work process that had received limited attention, such as the exigencies of imposed standardized protocols. These methodological innovations and shifts in the focus of our intention were guided by the complexity paradigm, with a focus on the characterization of the mechanisms that underlie the resilience of sociotechnical systems in the face of potentially harmful deviations in communication and decision making, and the unanticipated adaptations of these systems to attempts to standardize patient care. Characterization of these mechanisms allowed for the development of interventions that aim to either leverage this adaptive capacity, or regulate it at points where the harmful effects of variable behavior were readily apparent.

There are grounds for optimism that the culture of safety that is taking hold in healthcare will begin to transform patient care. The methods and empirical knowledge will contribute to the growing body of knowledge that informs new practices and innovative theoretically-grounded interventions. To quote Paul Starr from his much acclaimed work on the Social Transformation of Medicine (1982, p.3): "Modern Medicine is one of those extraordinary works of reason: an elaborate system of specialized knowledge, technical procedures, and rules of behavior." Every few decades, medicine expands on this elaborate system and undergoes a social transformation with profound consequences for public health. The time is ripe for a transformation in which we can more effectively leverage the tools at our disposable to move us ever closer to the realization of the promise of a culture of safety. This is not merely a lofty goal as it has been achieved in countless other disciplines. The problem is complex, but not intractable.

Vimla L. Patel
David Kaufman
Trevor Cohen
Thomas Kannampallil

Glossary

Abdominal aorta A major artery located in the abdomen.

Accelerometer Device that measures physical acceleration experienced by an object.

Adult respiratory distress syndrome (ARDS) An inflammation of the lungs that causes fluid to leak from the blood stream into the air spaces even when the blood stream is operating at low pressure.

Advance Trauma Life Support American College of Surgeons' official guidelines for the systematic treatment of patients in trauma critical care.

Adverse event When recovery from a medical error does not occur, the result may be an adverse event such as an anaphylactic reaction to a drug given to an allergic patient.

Anaerobic organisms Organisms that do not require oxygen for growth, such as the bacteria that colonize the colon.

Anchoring heuristic A tendency of clinicians to stick to an initial impression of a case and ignore evidence to the contrary.

Antecedent-consequent matrix Matrix that provides the counts of number of transitions between antecedent and consequent events.

Artifact analysis The analysis of the structure and content of an artifact and triangulation of findings across artifacts that results in a highly encoded representation that describes complex domain work.

Ascites Accumulation of fluid in the peritoneal cavity.

Availability heuristic Judgment on the basis of the readiness with which previous examples come to mind.

Balance Theory Model A multidimensional human factors model which can be used to characterize work systems such as the ICU in a way that more closely approximates its full complexity.

Base stations Stationary devices that provide radio coverage and tracking of the tags (Related to Tags).

Cardiac tamponade Mechanical restriction of cardiac function on account of accumulation of fluid in the pericardium, often with fatal consequences.

V.L. Patel et al. (eds.), *Cognitive Informatics in Health and Biomedicine*, Health Informatics, DOI 10.1007/978-1-4471-5490-7,

Care-delivery related deviations Deviations dealing with the care provided to the patient that may not be specified in guidelines.

Checklists A list of items required, things to be done, or points to be considered, and usually used as a reminder.

Clinical Decision Support (CDS) The provision of intelligently filtered clinical knowledge and/or patient-specific information with the aim of enhancing quality of care.

Clinician-centered approach A research approach predicated on understanding communication activity, within the global context of clinician workflow.

Coagulopathy Failure to form blood clots (and hence stop bleeding).

Cognitive artifact An artificial device designed to maintain, display, or operate upon information in order to serve a representational function. In the clinical setting, this may include a piece of paper-based or computer-based documentation, such as a note or a to-do list.

Cognitive bias A systematic departure from a standard of rationality or normative rational theory.

Cognitive informatics Multidisciplinary study of cognitive information and computational sciences that investigates all facets of human computing, including design and computer-mediated intelligent action.

Cognitive overload A situation where the learner (or the information processor) has too much information to process or too many tasks to learn simultaneously, resulting in the learner being unable to process this information. In this situation, the processing demands of an activity go beyond the processing limits of the learner.

Common ground Common ground refers to the knowledge shared by two or more individuals engaged in communication.

Communication error An error in the exchange or transmission of thoughts, messages, or information between sender and receiver.

Communication space A hypothetical construct that refers to the combined space across all communication modalities.

Complex Adaptive System A special case of complex systems, a complex adaptive system is a collection of individual agents with freedom to act in ways that are not always predictable, and whose actions are interconnected so that one agent's actions change the context for other.

Complex Cognitive System Non-deterministic and dynamically structured cognitive system, usually including multiple human agents and artifacts.

Complex Systems Non-deterministic and dynamically structured system.

Computerized Physician Order Entry System that enables the electronic entry of a clinician's instructions for the treatment of patients under his or her care.

Computerized Weaning Protocol (CWP) A weaning protocol provided by a computer.

Content model A structure for standardizing communication content during handoffs.

Continuity of care Continuity of care is the process by which care providers are cooperatively involved to coordinate ongoing patient care management toward the goal of high quality, cost-effective medical care.

Conversational grounding Common ground is often achieved through conversational grounding—a process that involves an act of conveying a message and an indication that the message has been understood by the recipient.

Core common ground Common sense, cultural sense, and formal sense; derives from the interlocutors' (speaker/hearer) shared knowledge of prior experience.

Critical care medicine A multidisciplinary healthcare specialty that cares for patients with acute, life-threatening illness or injury. Critical care medicine is practiced within the Emergency Care Department and Intensive Care Units within the hospital setting.

Declarative knowledge Knowing "that" (e.g., the diagnostic criteria for Rheumatoid Arthritis), as opposed to *procedural knowledge*, which is knowing "how" (e.g., how to insert a chest drain).

Descriptive decision theory Descriptive decision theories describe how individuals actually make decisions (including deviations from the norm).

Deviation as errors Deviations from the standard that: (i) violate a prescribed order of activities with a negative impact on workflow, (ii) result in (directly or indirectly) compromising patient care, or (iii) result in an activity being repeated due to failure in execution or a loss of information.

Deviations Steps performed that are not on an accepted pre-defined standard.

Deviations as innovations Deviations that potentially benefit the individual, team or patient by bringing novelty to the situation at hand.

Diaphragm The muscle that separates the thoracic and abdominal cavities.

Distributed cognition Cognitive theory originated by Hutchins that proposes cognition, rather than being confined to the mind of an individual, can be viewed in terms of its distribution across the minds of multiple individuals and external media.

Effectiveness Refers to the accuracy and completeness with which users achieve certain goals.

Efficiency Refers to the relationship between (a) the accuracy and completeness with which users achieve certain goals using the tool and (b) the resources expended in achieving them.

Emergence How complex behavior and patterns arise out of a multiplicity of relatively simple interactions.

Emergent common ground Shared sense and current sense; primarily derives from the interlocutors' individual knowledge of prior and/or current experience that is pertinent to the current situation.

Enrichment It is the process of accentuating the importance of certain aspects of information.

Error recovery Detection and correction of a committed error, such that adverse consequences are mitigated.

Erythropoietin A hormone manufactured by the kidney in response to low oxygen delivery that stimulates production of red blood cells in the bone marrow.

Extubation Removal of the endotracheal tube through which ventilation is provided.

Failure Mode and Effect Analysis (FMEA) A well-established engineering approach toward determination of the underlying cause of a system malfunction.

Figure-ground metaphor A research strategy based on a visual metaphor where an investigator chooses to shine a bright light on the foreground, illuminating a phenomenon of interest, and a dimmer light on the background (i.e. the context). In this regard, one never loses sight of the context and one may choose to bring different facets of context to the foreground in sharp view, as their relevance becomes apparent.

Formal communication events Events that include rounds and handoffs. These are scheduled events with a set of goals and expectations. This is in contrast to informal events which happen routinely, but are opportunistic.

Framing effects Occur in decisions that are biased by the manner in which information is presented.

Functional decomposition A research strategy in which complex systems can be decomposed into smaller functional components and the relations between them.

Functional Resonance Accident Method (FRAM) A methodology that aims to determine the underlying causes of an adverse outcome by studying the dependencies between different system functions, and the variability of these functions.

Glomerular filtration rate A measure of kidney function that estimates the volume of fluid that is filtered out of the blood for further processing by the kidney into urine.

Guideline A statement or other indication of policy or procedure by which to determine a course of action (Related to Protocols).

Handoff The process of transferring primary authority and responsibility for providing clinical care to a patient from one departing caregiver to one oncoming caregiver.

Handoff phase Transfer of information from outgoing to incoming clinicians.

Hematoma A localized collection of blood.

Heuristic A heuristic is a mental shortcut that allows individuals to solve problems and make judgments quickly and efficiently using readily available strategies. This rule-of-thumb strategy is helpful in most situations, but it can also lead to biases.

Hidden Markov Modeling (HMM) Probabilistic modeling tool that is usually employed for temporal sequence analysis.

Holter monitor A portable recorder that accumulates up to 24 h of continuous electrocardiogram data.

Hyperglycemia High levels of glucose in the bloodstream.

In situ studies or in vivo studies Studies that investigate naturally occurring phenomena in context with minimal external manipulation.

Individual deviations Deviations initiated by a single clinician.

Inferior vena cava A large vein located in the abdomen.

Information breakdowns A gap or disruption in the information flow between sender and receiver in a given process.

Information flow Information flow is the transfer of information between sender and receiver in a given process.

Information gain The rate of information gathered (or retrieved) from a source (or multiple sources) over a set period of time.

Information seeking The process of finding information that is distributed across multiple sources to complete a task at hand.

Information unit The smallest functional unit of clinically-relevant information described by the clinician.

Interdisciplinary The concept of something occurring between disciplines, often used in reference to activities that occur between individuals from different clinical disciplines. Examples of clinical disciplines include (but are not limited to): nursing, medicine, pharmacy, physical therapy, social work, nutrition, and respiratory therapy.

Intermediate effects People at intermediate levels of expertise may perform more poorly than those at lower level of expertise on some tasks, due to the challenges of assimilating new knowledge or skills over the course of the learning process.

In vitro or laboratory-based studies Studies in laboratory-based conditions with experimental manipulation

Joint Commission The Joint Commission (TJC), formerly the Joint Commission on Accreditation of Healthcare Organizations (JCAHO), is a United States–based nonprofit tax-exempt organization that accredits more than 19,000 health care organizations and programs in the United States.

July effect An increase in medical errors upon arrival of new residents to begin their training in July.

Just-in-time grounding The act of sharing only specific task knowledge at the time a discussion occurs based on the assumptions that there are no other reasons to talk to an agent, the task or encounter is rare, or there is not limited task time for grounding (sharing knowledge) at the time of the conversation.

Kardex A traditional nursing card indexing system and a paper-based semi-structured nursing tool that provides a synopsis of a patient and was historically written in pencil so that it could be updated easily for the purpose of communication between nursing shifts.

Latent and active failures Active failures are the "face" of an error; they represent the immediate effects of an error. Latent failures are the enduring, systemic problems that make errors possible but are less visible.

Learning progressions Descriptions of sophisticated ways of thinking about or understanding how learning progresses through various stages. They represent a promising framework for cognitive science research on how people learn in a given domain.

Local optimization Optimization is a process of selecting an appropriate activity (in this case, information) from a set of available alternatives. Local optimization involves utilizing sources of information that provide immediate (and quick) information that helps in solving the information problem at hand.

Mathematical coupling The source of systematic error in certain analyses, arising from having one variable either directly or indirectly containing the whole or components of a second variable. An example familiar to car buyers are the oft-published data regarding speed and fuel efficiency (miles per gallon). They are coupled through the weight of the vehicle.

Medical error Adverse effect of care, whether or not it is evident or harmful to the patient.

Medical knowledge hierarchy A hierarchical framework that characterizes the nature of medical knowledge. It is typically used to characterize how medical knowledge is used to solve clinical problems.

Medical Subject Headings (MeSH) A comprehensive controlled vocabulary for the purpose of indexing journal articles and books in the life sciences.

Mental models Mental models are used to describe how individuals form internal representations of systems. Mental models are designed to answer questions such as "how does this work?" or "what will happen if I take the following action?" or "why is the patient not more responsive to the medications he is currently receiving?"

Mistakes Errors resulting from attempted execution of an incorrect process, on account of incorrect or incomplete knowledge or interpretation.

Multi-professional rounds Multi-professional round (MPR) is a mechanism by which teams of different clinical professionals perform joint evaluation. For example, such multi-professional teams are often convened to evaluate quality and decision-making initiatives.

Naturalistic Naturalistic studies are a form of research which is conducted by observing and studying people in their natural environment. It is also characteristic of such studies that the activities in this environment are observed or investigated without attempting to influence or manipulate them.

Naturalistic clinical reasoning Nature of reasoning process in real-world healthcare practice in view of making decisions about diagnosis and management plan for the patient.

Naturalistic decision making A research paradigm or approach that studies decisions, sensemaking, situational awareness, planning – all of which emerge in natural settings and take forms that are not easily replicated in the laboratory. Decision-making in critical care medicine settings that include stress, uncertainty, time pressure and changing conditions exemplify such situations.

Near miss A violation of the consensual bounds of safe practice that is detected and managed before resulting in an adverse event.

Non-linear behavior Responses are disproportional to applied stimuli.

Normative decision theories Normative decision theories propose the manner in which people should make decisions in order to optimize an outcome. These theories assume an ideal decision maker, who is fully informed and rational, is able to process information with perfect accuracy, resulting in an optimal decision.

Ontology Formal representation of knowledge as a set of concepts within a domain and associated relationships between pairs of concepts.

Opensimulator An open source implementation platform for virtual world development (see virtual world).

Overlap In this context refers to the extent to which two or more communication events share common semantic content.

Paracentesis A procedure through which fluid is removed from the abdominal cavity, often for the purpose of microbiological studies.

Parenteral alimentation (Total parenteral nutrition) The administration of water, carbohydrates (sugars and starches), amino acids, fats, vitamins and micronutrients into large veins as the primary and even sole source of nutrition and hydration.

Pathfinder A method of network scaling developed by Roger Schvaneveldt. Pathfinder was originally developed to reveal patterns underlying conceptual relatedness data elicited from humans, but has subsequently been applied for other purposes such as citation network analysis.

Pathognomonic finding A clinical finding that indicates a particular diagnosis with certainty.

Patient safety The reduction of risk of unnecessary harm associated with health care to an acceptable minimum; also the name of a movement and specific research area.

Pericardium The membranous sac surrounding the heart.

Phlegmon A mass of inflammatory tissue.

Ping, Tag-base Information captured when a tag comes in close proximity to a base station.

Ping, Tag-tag Information captured when two tags come in close proximity to each other.

Post-turnover phase Oncoming clinician assumes care for patients.

Pre-emptive grounding The act of sharing knowledge prior to a specific conversational task, assuming that the knowledge will be needed in the future and that the time for the conversational task is limited. The communicators elect to bear the grounding cost ahead of time and risk the effort being wasted if the knowledge shared is never used.

Premature ventricular contraction A heartbeat that originates in the lower chamber of the heart prior to the normal conduction from the upper chamber of the heart. Three or more such contractions in a row is called ventricular tachycardia. Sustained ventricular tachycardia can degenerate into ventricular fibrillation, where the lower chamber does no effective pumping but rather vibrates incoherently.

Pre-post study design Requires collection of data on study participants' level of performance before the intervention took place (pre-), and collection of the matching data after the intervention took place (post).

Pre-turnover phase Outgoing clinician getting ready to go off-shift.

Priming In the context of our error experiments, "priming" refers to alerting participants beforehand to the presence of an error.

Principle of least collaborative effort Suggests that participants try to minimize their collaborative effort—the work that both do from the initiation of each contribution to its mutual acceptance.

Proactive deviations Deviations that occur when (i) an activity is performed (without compromising patient care) in anticipation of a future requirement (or lack thereof) when treating a patient or (ii) an activity (which may be out of the bounds of an individual's role in the trauma team) is performed in order to correct or prevent error occurrence.

Procedure-related deviations Deviations that deal with adaptations in the physical implementation (or procedure) of a specific step in the guideline.

Process-related deviations Deviations that may be related to how the guideline is implemented.

Prospective A prospective study, loosely defined, is a study that starts in the present and continues forward in time. It is differentiated from a retrospective study, which looks back from a known outcome, determining the factors that influenced the outcome. In other words, prospective studies attempt to capture phenomena of interest as they occur, where prospective studies of medical error require the observer to be present from the point in time at which the error is initiated.

Protocols A precise and detailed plan for a regimen of diagnosis or therapy. Most often it is evidence-based.

Radio-frequency identification (RFID) Wireless non-contact use of radio frequency to transfer data for the purpose of identifying and tracking tags attached to objects.

Rationality Rationality assumes that individuals are rational decision makers; that people make choices to maximize utility or self-benefit.

Reactive deviations Deviations that occur when an activity is performed in reaction to an unanticipated event or change in patient condition, diagnostic process or treatment plans.

Real-time location sensing (RTLS) Automatic identification and tracking of tags attached to objects or people in real-time.

Received signal strength (RSSI) Measurement of power present in received radio signal.

Reductionism The assumption that a complex system can be reduced to its component individual parts.

Re-intubation Reinsertion of the endotracheal tube through which ventilation is provided.

Respiratory therapist (RT) A healthcare professional with a focus on the respiratory system, often charged with maintaining mechanical ventilation for the purpose of life support.

Retrospective Retrospective studies attempt to elucidate the underlying cause of phenomena of interest after they have occurred. For example, retrospective studies of medical error may involve chart review and after-the-fact interviews.

Richmond Agitation Sedation Scale (RASS) A standardized instrument to measure the alertness of a sedated patient.

Schema A mental structure.

Sedation holiday A period in which sedatives are withdrawn from a ventilated patient, in anticipation of a Spontaneous Breathing Trial (SBT).

Semantic coding A method of coding based on the meaning of the content being coded.

Semi-naturalistic This term is used to describe studies that occur in context, providing ecological validity (for example in the context of critical care practice), but with some experimental constraints.

Sepsis A combination of total body inflammation and infection that leads to progressive organ failure ("severe sepsis") including cardiovascular collapse ("septic shock").

Shared Mental Models (SMM) Shared understanding of a group of individuals that, in this context, includes the underlying causes of a patient's current state, the overall plan of care, and the allocation of responsibilities among clinicians on the team.

Situation model An assessment of a patient case that develops in situ while the team is engaged in a patient care task or communication.

Slips Errors resulting from flawed execution of a correctly chosen process.

SMM Index A quantitative measure of overlap.

Spiral method A software development process combining elements of both design and prototyping-in-stages. Also known as the spiral lifecycle model (or spiral development), it is a systems development method (SDM) used in information technology (IT).

Split flow A type of emergency room management in which triage patients are either given expedited treatment for the seriously ill or in less severe instances patients are examined and sent to a resulting pending area.

Spontaneous Breathing Trial (SBT) A procedure through which the ability of a patient on a ventilator to breathe independently is evaluated by assessing his or her breathing without support.

Standard clinical practice A practice standard that reflects the behavior and performance levels expected in clinical practice.

Steroid (corticosteroid, glucocorticoid) A class of drugs that strongly inhibit inflammation. Their side effects include impaired wound healing and high blood sugar (glucose). Class members include prednisone, hydrocortisone and methylprednisolone.

Systems-centered approach Investigates phenomena in a broader context with a particular focus on converging factors across spans of time in explanations of causality.

Tags Mobile devices that when attached to objects can be used to identify and track objects (Related to Base Stations).

Team deviations Deviations involving more than one clinician in a team.

Temporal frames Reflects certain windows of time associated with particular activities (e.g., morning rounds).

Tool resilience The ability or tendency of the tool to cope with information breakdowns. This coping may result in the individual "bouncing back" to a previous state of normal functioning, or simply not showing negative effects.

Transition probability matrix See Antecedent-consequent matrix.

Trauma A serious physical wound caused by an external source.

Unified Medical Language System (UMLS) A compendium of controlled vocabularies as well as the map or translation between the vocabularies.

Ventilator weaning A process through which the dependence of a patient upon artificial ventilation is gradually reduced, and ideally eliminated.

Virtual reality Computer-simulated environments that can simulate physical presence of objects in the real world.

Virtual world A 3-D immersive computer-generated environment explored by users in the guise of animated computational characters, or avatars.

Weaning Protocol (WP) A prescribed sequence of steps through which to accomplish ventilator weaning.

Work Domain Ontology An ontology that captures the concepts for a particular domain of work.

Workflow Depiction of a sequence of operations, declared as work of a person or group, an organization of staff, or one or more simple or complex mechanisms. It may be seen as any abstraction of real work.

Working knowledge Knowledge related to the performance of practical tasks at hand.

Index

A

Adaptive behaviors
- aviation and nuclear power, 148
- chart review process, 148
- checklists, 177–178
- classification schemas, deviations
  - cognitive decision making process, 176
  - concordance with original classification, 175–176
  - immersion process, 176
  - inter-rater agreement, 175
  - Kappa statistics, 174–176
  - replication and rating/coding, 174
  - training phases, 174
  - video recording, 176
- complex adaptive system (*see* Complex adaptive system)
- ED and ICU, 149
- educational tool, 178
- experts' knowledge, 177
- extended classification, deviations
  - A(×4) model, 166
  - care delivery-related, 164–166
  - chi-square p-values, pair-wise relationships, 167
  - and clinician role, 172–174
  - errors, 162–163, 165
  - and expertise of trauma leader, 167–169
  - field observations, 166
  - GCS and ISS, 166
  - individual, 165, 166
  - innovations, 163, 165
  - proactive, 163–165
  - procedure-related deviations, 164, 166
  - process-related deviations, 164, 166
  - reactive, 164, 165
  - team, 165, 166
  - time-stamped observation, 166
  - in trauma care, 162
  - trauma standard protocol, 169–172
- gaining experience, 177
- HIT, 148
- implications, informatics and cognition, 178–179
- insurance companies, 147–148
- intervention types, 148
- IOM, 148
- protocols and standards, 176–177
- quality of care, 148
- top-down reasoning strategy, 161–162
- trauma critical care (*see* Trauma critical care)
- zero-tolerance environment, 177

ADDRESS trial, 450

Adult respiratory distress syndrome (ARDS), 445

Advanced trauma life support (ATLS), 436
- description, 156
- each time-stamped observation, 166
- initial assessment and management, 158
- initial survey and management, 153, 154
- trauma critical care, 153
- trauma scenario, 155

ARDS. *See* Adult respiratory distress syndrome (ARDS)

ATLS. *See* Advanced trauma life support (ATLS)

B

Barcode medication administration systems (BCMA), 345

BCMA. *See* Barcode medication administration systems (BCMA)

V.L. Patel et al. (eds.), *Cognitive Informatics in Health and Biomedicine*, Health Informatics, DOI 10.1007/978-1-4471-5490-7, © Springer-Verlag London 2014

C

The Cardiac Arrhythmia Suppression Trial (CAST), 443–444
Cardiac intensive care unit
CTICU, range of patients, 321–322
handoff artifact analysis
content analysis, IHIC framework, 324
dimensions, 324
Nemeth's method, 324
research methods to analyze handoffs
observations, 322–323
patient responsibility, 322
Cardio-thoracic ICU, 39
Cardiothoracic Intensive Care Unit (CTICU), 295, 321
CAST. *See* The Cardiac Arrhythmia Suppression Trial (CAST)
CDSS. *See* Clinical decision support system (CDSS)
Clinical artifacts
artifacts, use by clinicians
artifacts from the CTICU, 325
CVVHD, 327–328
hand-written notes, 328
information flow of patient data, 328
nurse admission Kardex, 325–326
Nurse personal handoff sheet, 327
presence of codes by type of artifact, 331
resident computer-based handoff print-out, 329
resident/PA computer-based handoff artifact, 328
resident/PA handoff artifact, 325
Clinical Communication Space Theoretical Framework, 319
as communication tools
checklists, 332
medication information, 333
paper artifacts, 332
structuring of handoff data, 332
summarization, 332
complexity, variables, 318
content overlap, patient safety
coding artifacts, 333
commonality of information, 334
computer-based tools, 334
IHIC coding, 333–334
interdisciplinary nature, 333
between nurses and physicians, 335
coordination, multidisciplinary team, 318
e-artifacts
computer-based tools, 330
transcription and siloed information, 330
handoff
communication, 317
definition, 317
EHR handoff tool, 319
increased frequency, 318
information and comparison
element, definition, 329
handoff artifacts, 329
inter-coder reliability, 329
interdisciplinary codes, overlap, 330
unique code, 329
prior handoff and communication research, 319
computer-based documentation, 319
CSCW, 320
Distributed Cognition, 319
IHIC framework, 321
intra-disciplinary activities, 320
paper-based documentation, 320
'parallel play' process, 320
standardization, 319
standardization of nursing handoffs, 319
types, 319, 320
transitions of care, 317
Clinical decision-making
complex and challenging, 424
healthcare delivery system, 424
heuristics, 425–426
Clinical decision support system (CDSS)
adherence and compliance, 187
complex adaptive environments, 187
computerized alerts and electronic clinical guidelines, 186
and CWP, 186, 187
and HIT, 187
medical errors, 187
and WPs, 186–187
Clinical rounds structuring
content of the rounds
differences in duration, 417
group attrition, 417
data collection
clinical staff during round, 413
communication themes, 414
content of rounds: qualitative analysis, 413
group composition and contributions, 412
identifying information, 413
socializing, 412
time spent during rounds, 412
duration, comparison, 415–416
impact of interdisciplinary rounds, 417
participants

additional clinical team members, 411
verbal consent, 411
rounding procedure, 410
setting
composition of the team, 411
semi-structured format, 410
team communication, 409
team theater, 410, 411
time spent on rounds, 414–415
Cognitive error in critical care medicine
best practice, 441–442
description, 441
drug allergy, 441
endocrine system, 448–449
GI/nutrition system, 447–448
heart and vascular system, 443–445
hematologic system, 449
identification, 441
immune system, 450–451
neurological system, 442–443
one-intervention-fits-all solution, 451
pivotal trials, 451
pulmonary/respiratory system, 445–446
renal/GU system, 446–447
Cognitive heuristics and biases, critically ill care
'Address Problem' steps, 227
ascertained physicians' view, 204
ascertaining physicians' perspectives, 228
biomedical informatics, 229
Bounded Rationality, 205
Clinicians' view, 218–219, 226
computer-based modules, 204
critical care, 219–220, 223–225
critical patient care, 220–223
data analysis
clinicians' view, 212
naturalistic clinical reasoning, 212–216
data collection
clinicians' view, 211–212
description, 211
ER and ICU, 211
literature review, 211
naturalistic clinical reasoning, 212
diagnostic process and use, 207–211
differential diagnosis, 226
emergency departments/intensive care, 228
experts discontinue, 206
framework development and validation
critical care settings, 216–217
framework validation, 217–218
medicine, 216
real-world critical care environment, 216
generalizability, 227–228
health information technology, 228
humans, 205
individuals actually and observed, 205
literature review, 218
medicine, 203, 204
naturalistic clinical reasoning, 219
non-critical state, 226
patient's symptoms and clinical data, 226
patient's treatment and management plan, 226
pre-existing condition, 227
primary categories, 204–205
real-world clinical observations, 226
reasoning errors and patient outcomes, 225
theoretical foundation, 206–207
therapeutic phase, patient care, 227
Cognitive informatics (CI)
communication in critical care
failures during handoff, 8–9
HAND-IT (Handoff Intervention Tool), 9
handoff artifacts from CTICU, 9
Handoff Information Coding (IHIC), 10
mental models, 9
patient care in intensive care settings, 9
SOAP note, 9
error recovery
ability to correct errors, 7
clinicians in an Emergency Department (ED), 7–8
Computerized Weaning Protocol (CWP), 8
critical care settings, 8–9
'error in evolution', 6
innovations, 8
NDM approach, 8
OpenSimulator development, 7
quest for zero defect, 6
real-world clinical rounds, 7
standardized protocols, 7–8
utility and limitations of standardization, 8
weaning protocol, 8
interdependencies and open-endedness, 2–3
methodological imperatives
clinician-centered approach, 5
"day in the life" approach, 5
figure-ground (FG) research strategy, 3–4
flow of activity, 5
functional decomposition (FD), 3–4

Cognitive informatics (*cont.*)
human-intensive observation, 4–5
study of error recovery, 4
technological tools, 5
workflow, 4
performance in critical settings, 3
property of emergence, 3
systems-centered approach, 3
work and information flow
bedside rounding practice, 11
3D virtual reality environments, 11
dynamics of team interaction, 11
information seeking process, 11
radio identification tags, 11
team theater, 11
work for education and training, 12
Cognitive science in BMIs
academic departments, 468
and clinical decision making
"artificial intelligence in medicine" community, 469
computer-based decision-support tools, 468–469
expert systems, 469
formal decision analytic approach, 469
full-time collaborators, 470
knowledge engineering and elicitation, 469
research and researchers, 469
complex organizational systems, 468
computer science/communications, 468
decision making, 467, 468
education, 472
evidence-based medicine, 467
human-computer interaction and usability testing, 468
informatics research, 470–471
informing system design and content, 471–472
optimal process/theories, 468
patient safety and informatics, 472
principal informatics professional society, 467–468
research and training programs, 472–473
Common computerized weaning protocol (CWP), 436
Common performance conditions (CPCs), 189, 192
Communication and complexity
clinical communication space, 235, 236
common ground, 239–240
electronic health records, 235
handoff process (*see* Handoff process)
morbidity and mortality, 235
systems-centered approach, 236
Complex adaptive system
behavior assessment
aviation, 152
black box analysis, 152
checklists, 151
cockpit, 152
complex social system, 151
CRM, 151
emergency landing, US Airways flight, 151–152
error definition, 151
root cause, errors, 150–151
healthcare
analyzing process, 150
data collection, 150
description, 149
dynamic network, 150
emergence of stable strategies, 150
observers, 150
positive and negative feedback, 150
workflow document, 150
Complexity in critical care environment
communication, care transitions
care transitions (or handoffs), 351
handoff intervention tool, 351
SMM, 352
effects of complexity
components, specific combinations, 347–348
computability, 347
range, degree of interrelatedness, 347–348
errors recovery and correction
naturalistic clinical environment, 351
nature of errors, 351
functional decomposition, 350
methodological approaches
SMM in communications, 352–353
systems complexity perspective, 352
properties
cause and effects, 344
complex problems, 343
emergence, 344
functional decomposition perspective, 345
openness, 344
self-organization, 344
sources
complexity of natural systems, 345
engineered complexity, 345
factors, 345
study approach
emergence, 346
Focus+Context, 350
functional decomposition, 349

identify components, 349
interactions/interrelatedness, components, 346
linearity, 346
non-decomposability, 346
nonlinear behavior, 346
research objectives, 350
system behavior, 350
Computer-based physician order entry systems, 87
Computerized provider order entry (CPOE), 184, 345
Computerized weaning protocol (CWP)
components, 192
CPC-based checklist, 192
FRAM-based normative model, 190
implementation and safe use, 187
misinterpretation, 198
and MV, 186
patient's eligibility, 185
sedation assessment, 192–193
shadowing sessions, 195
standardized solutions, 197, 198
weaning sessions, 194
Computer-supported cooperative work (CSCW), 87, 320
Continuous Veno-Venous Hemodialysis (CVVHD), 327
Conversational analysis
case management categories, 101–102
decision flow diagram, 102, 103
frequency and percentage, clinician errors, 102
CPCs. *See* Common performance conditions (CPCs)
CPOE. *See* Computerized provider order entry (CPOE)
Crew resource management (CRM), 151
Critical care
academic setting, 26
case management, 29
characteristics, 251
clinician-centered approach, 251–253
complex cognitive systems, 24
data analysis, 253–255
data collection, 253
decision-making, 24
error management, 28
PED, 21
preliminary study, 21
Critical care, handoff process
handoff communication, 264
hospital settings, 249–250
Human Computer Interaction, 263
methodological approach, 263
MICU workflow terminology, 250–251
participants, 250
physician, 251
pre-turnover and post-turnover phases, 264–265
sequential approach, 264
theoretical rationale (*see* Critical care)
Critical care medicine
clinical decision-making, 424–426
description, 423
error management, 426–429
error-ridden and failure-prone system, 424
hand-offs, 429–432
healthcare system grows in size and complexity, 438
and ICU (*see* Intensive care unit (ICU))
immediate and accurate information availability, 424
information seeking behavior, 433–435
injury and harm risks, 424
life-threatening conditions, 423
protocol-based practice, 435–437
workflow, 432–433
CRM. *See* Crew resource management (CRM)
CSCW. *See* Computer-supported cooperative work (CSCW)
CTICU. *See* Cardiothoracic Intensive Care Unit (CTICU)
CVVHD. *See* Continuous Veno-Venous Hemodialysis (CVVHD)
CWP. *See* Computerized weaning protocol (CWP)

D

Data analysis
descriptive statistics, 98, 99
qualitative
case management categories, 98–100
clinician and utterance types, 98
error and error correction categories, 98–100
Data coding
audio recordings, 96
case management, data analysis, 97
categories, error codings, 97–98
description, 96
errors in communication, 97
utterance, 96
Decision flow
clinical round transcript segment, 104–106
coding process, 102
sequence of conversation over time, 102, 103
sequence of utterances, 103–104
temporal events in narrative text, 103

Descriptive statistics, 98, 99
Detection ratio (DR), 120
Diabetic ketoacidosis (DKA), 64–65
DKA. *See* Diabetic ketoacidosis (DKA)
DR. *See* Detection ratio (DR)

E

E-artifacts
computer-based tools, 330
transcription and siloed information, 330
EC. *See* Error correction (EC)
Egregious errors
anchoring heuristic, 36
attempted murder, 43–44
availability heuristic, 36
clinical practice, 55
clinical scenarios, 44–45
clinicians, 56
cognitive mechanisms, 36
contraindicated colonoscopy, 49
diagnosis by students, 37
dialysis nursing, 51–54
disease schemata, 37
error recovery (*see* Error recovery)
expert-like manner, 55
experts (*see* Experts)
framing effects, 36–37
hematoma, 50
heuristics lies, 36
high-profile medical malpractice cases, 36
holistic perspective, 35
human error, 35
inappropriate antibiotics, 48–49
individual error, 49
laboratory based experiments, 54–55
makeshift laboratory settings, 44
medicine reveal experts, 36
mismanaged diverticulitis, 42–43
natural language protocol analysis, 46
nurses and non-expert nurses, 54
participants, 45
pericardial sonogram, 50
prerequisites, 44, 45
recall and inference analysis, transcripts, 46
transcribed protocol, 46
undiagnosed ureteral injury, 50
x-ray and CT scan, 49
EHR. *See* Electronic health records (EHR)
Electronic health records (EHR), 345
Embedded errors
dialysis nursing, 51–52
expert and non-expert participants, 47
knowledge-based errors, 52–53
prerequisites, 43, 44
Emergency care
description, 128
EDs, 127
EHR systems, 142
healthcare, 127
HIT, 143
implementation effects
decreasing opportunities, 140
methods, 140
split flow layout, hospital, 139, 140
task transition patterns, 141–142
teaching institution, 141
trauma cases, 142
workflow and physical layout, 142
layered complexity, 127
task transition decisions (*see* Task transition decisions, emergency care)
WDO (*see* Work domain ontology (WDO))
EMT. *See* Error management training (EMT)
Endocrine system, 448–449
ENHANCE trial, 450
Environmental factors, task transition decisions
break in task, 137, 138
frequent types, 138
opportunistic decisions, 137–139
PACS station, 139
planned decisions, 136–137
Error correction (EC)
composition and communication team, 100
and decision flow, 102–106
and error categories, 98, 99
and generated
clinician types, 101
frequencies examination, 101
residents and attending physicians, 100–101
and propagation, 104–107
team interaction transcript, 99–100
Error detection in simulated clinical rounds. *See* Simulated clinical round error detections
Error etiology and recovery, 88
Error management
individuals
cognitive demands, 428
critical care physicians, 428
error recovery *in vivo*, 427
expertise in knowledge and skills, 428

experts and non-experts commit errors, 427
in vitro study of error detection and recovery, 427
OpenSim, 427
patient safety, 426
traditional approach, 426–427
teams
improved decision-making, 429
learning, 429
mean, 429
performance, 429
power and value, distributed cognition, 429
semi-naturalistic approach, 428–429
Error management training (EMT), 122–123
Error recovery
anesthesiology, 23
aviation, 20–22, 37
clinical round roles
audio recording analysis, 114
daily routine, 114
and error detection in medical settings, 114
ethnographic observations, 114
paper-based scenarios, 114–115
PED, 114
retrospective data, 114
study design, 115
cognitive model, 38–39
critical clinical information, 22–23
data analysis, 98–100
data coding, 96–98
data collection, 96
decision-making responses, 38
domains, 38
3D virtual world, 27
eradicate error, 32
error corrections (*see* Error correction (EC))
error perception, 28–29
errors in clinical problems, 108
ethnographic and interview data, 24
evaluation, 29
experimental paradigm, 30–31
handoffs at shift change, 25
healthcare environment, 109
healthcare practice, 31
human agents and technology, 24
human error, 31
Hutchins' work, distributed cognition, 23–24
indicators, 39–40
individual accountability, 18–19
individual cognition, 28
interpretation, 29
knowledge types, 25
learning, 26
medical error, 17
MICU (*see* Medical intensive care unit (MICU))
misperception, 30
naturalistic paradigm, 28, 92
Norman's model, 28
operational priorities, 30
paper-based case scenarios, 30–31
participants, 95–96
PEDs, 24
pilot study, 107–108
psychiatric emergency data, 24
Rasmussen's characterization, 22
retrospective studies, 27, 41–42
semi-naturalistic environment, 27–28, 91–92
study site, 95
teaching/patient rounds, 109
traditional approaches, 17–18
training, 122–123
web-based tutoring system, 123–124
zero defects, 19–20
Ethnographic methodologies, 87
Experts
and complex errors, 50–51
correction and justification, 51
diagnostic reasoning, 37
expertise and expectations, 46–47
and non-expert participants, 47
subjects and non-expert subjects, 47, 48

F

FRAM. *See* Functional resonance accident method (FRAM)
Functional resonance accident method (FRAM)
approximate adjustments, 188
and CDSS tools, 189
and CPCs, 189, 190
critical care
classification, weaning sessions, 194–195
evaluation study, 195–196
misinterpretation, sedation scale, 195
description, 188
emergence, 188
parameters, 189
potential variability, 189
reinforce, 188

Functional resonance accident method (*cont.*)
variability characterization, 189–190
and WPs
and CWP, 190–191
feedback and impact monitoring system, 194
monitoring interventions, 193
RASS score, 192–193
training and education, 193
variability checklist, 192

G

GI/nutrition system, 447–448

H

HAND-IT. *See* Handoff intervention tool (HAND-IT)
Handoff, artifacts
communication, 317
content analysis, IHIC framework, 324
definition, 317
dimensions, 324
EHR handoff tool, 319
increased frequency, 318
Nemeth's method, 324
nurse personal handoff sheet, 327
prior handoff and communication research, 319
computer-based documentation, 319
computer-supported cooperative work (CSCW), 320
Distributed Cognition, 319
IHIC framework, 321
intra-disciplinary activities, 320
paper-based documentation, 320
'parallel play' process, 320
standardization, 319
standardization of nursing handoffs, 319
types, 319, 320
research methods
observations, 322–323
patient responsibility, 322
resident computer-based handoff print-out, 329
resident/PA computer-based handoff artifact, 328
resident/PA handoff artifact, 325
structuring of handoff data, 332
Handoff communication
barriers, 246–248
communication errors, 244
content and structure, tools, 272
critical care (*see* Critical care, handoff process)
critical clinical and organizational process, 244
decision making breakdowns, 284
definition, 243–244
description, 271
design, tool (*see* Handoff intervention tool (HAND-IT))
effect, expertise, 284–285
electronic tools, 272
features, design, 285
formal inter-departmental, 246
handoff solutions, 248
implications, practice, 286
individual, 244
information breakdowns, 283–284
intra-professional, 244
medication management, 246
and MICU (*see* Medical intensive care unit (MICU))
nursing handover, 246
paper-based tools, 272
patient safety, 271–272
phases, 286
practices, consideration, 246
researchers and hospital quality, 244
research motivation, 248–249
resilience, 284
SOAP and SBAR, 273
survey-based and self-reported measures, 286–287
synchronous, 244
theoretical framings, 245, 273–274
Handoff intervention tool (HAND-IT)
content standardization and content summarization, 275
data analysis, 282–283
design, 275–277
development, 275
evaluation, 275
information categories, 275, 277
measurement, evaluation, 281–282
MPR, 279–280
organization, 285
participants, 278–279
patient care information, 275
procedure, 280–281
requirements, 274
study design, 279

Handoff process
  communication and complexity
    accentuate a system-oriented approach, 241
    analytic foci, 238
    artifacts and electronic health records, 238
    Balance Theory Model, 236
    complex adaptive systems, 237
    complex contexts, 240
    distributed approach, 238
    ICU, 236
    immense complexity, 237
    miscommunication, 241
    organizational conditions, 236
    patient trajectory, 238
    physical environment, 236
    practitioners, 237
    pre-post design, 238–239
    quality of h, 241
    semi-naturalistic and naturalistic environments, 237
    socio-natural system, 237
    study performance and plan interventions, 237
    system behavior, 237
    system-centered approach, 238
    tools and technologies, 236
Hand-offs, critical care medicine
  clinician-centered approach, 430
  description, 429–430
  document types, 430
  facilitation, 430
  feedback, 431–432
  HAND-IT, 431
  outcomes, 430
  phases classification, 430
  poor, 431
  SOAP note, 430–431
  standardization, 431
  tools/materials, 430
  transitions of care settings, 431
Health information technology (HIT), 86, 143, 187, 198, 199, 345
Heart and vascular system
  abnormalities *vs.* identifying and mitigating, 444
  CAST, 443–444
  circulatory shock, 444, 445
  electrocardiographic data, 443
  Holter monitors, 443
  mathematical coupling, 444
  pulmonary artery catheter, 445
  PVCs, 444
  supranormal resuscitation, 444–445
  validation, 444
Hematologic system, 449
Heuristics and biases, diagnostic process
  attraction effect, 209
  availability, 207
  clinical data, 207
  clinical scenario, 208
  cognitive processes, 210
  confirmation bias, 208, 209
  empirical studies, 208
  extrapolation, 208
  hypothesis generation, 207
  omission and outcome bias, 208
  omission bias, 210
  osteoarthritis, 209
  overconfidence bias, 208
  premature closure, 208
  representativeness, 207
  search satisficing, 208
  sunk cost bias, 210
  support theory, 208
Heuristics, clinical decision-making
  advantages, 425
  availability and planning fallacy, 425
  characterize physicians' use, cognitive heuristics, 425
  cognitive de-biasing strategies, 426
  confirmation and in-group bias, 425
  cookbook approach to medicine, 426
  high velocity environments, 425
  ICU environment, 426
  immediate need assessment and addressing problem, 425
  incorporation, 426
  patient management and deformation professional, 425
  proof-of-concept study, 425
  semi-structured questionnaire, 425
Hidden Markov Modeling (HMM)
  activity list and clinical descriptions, 365
  disadvantages, 363
  evaluation and results, 367
  quantitative data, 364
  received signal strength indication (RSSI) value, 364
  recognition accuracy, 367
  sparse matrix of tag-base encounters, 366
  temporal sequence of events, 363
  testing, 364, 366
  training, 364
HIT. *See* Health information technology (HIT)
HMM. *See* Hidden Markov Modeling (HMM)

The Hybrid Method to Classify Interruptions and Activities (HyMCIA), 134
HyMCIA. *See* The Hybrid Method to Classify Interruptions and Activities (HyMCIA)

I

ICU. *See* Intensive care unit (ICU)
Immune system, 450–451
Information seeking behavior, critical care medicine
  characterization, 435
  clinicians and hospital leadership, 434
  data collection, 434, 435
  data loss and misinterpretation, 435
  data retrieved types, 434–435
  distributive nature of clinical data, 435
  electronic medical records, 433–434
  information capture, 434
  monitor changes in process/structures, 434
  Morbidity and Mortality Conference/multi-disciplinary rounds, 434
  physicians in complex environment, 434
  plan resource, 434
  sensor-based technology, 434
Information use, sub-optimal patterns
  clinical decision making and reasoning
    data-driven approach, 405
    hypothesis-driven reasoning strategy, 405
    information filtering, 405
    iterative back-and-forth switching, 404
  effectiveness of information seeking, 389
  enriching the external representation, 404
    EHR, 404
    enrichment of source, 404
    reading the physician notes, 404
  focus, 391
  information seeking
    distributed nature of information, 398
    electronic records, 398
    increased patient diagnosis, 390
    information gain *versus* time spent, 401
    knowledge utilization, 401–402
    loss of information, 390
    optimal rate of information gain, 400–401
    rate of information gain, 399–400
    redundancy of available information, 390
    sources and utilization of resources, 399
    time spent on sources, 399
  medical knowledge
    categories and examples, 397
    coded transcripts, 396
    diagnosis, 396
    empirium, 396
    levels of, 396
    observations, 396
  method
    Charnoff's marginal value theorem, 395
    data analysis, 393–394
    data collection, 392
    information unit, 393–394
    iPad application, 393
    overall rate, 394
    participants, 391
    procedure, 391
    rate of information gain, calculation, 395
    scoring mechanism, 395
  patient-based approach, 406
  source and organization, 390, 392
  source-based approach, 406
Intensive care unit (ICU)
  breadth and depth, complex healthcare system, 424
  cardio-thoracic, 39
  care disrupt continuity, SMM, 298–299
  clinical decision-making, 424–425
  cookbook approach, 426
  CTICU, 295
  data collection method, SMM analysis, 296
  divergent frames and priorities, 296–297
  dynamic complexity, 429
  embedded errors, 427
  environment, 426, 428
  errors during practice, 40
  handoff, 430
  in-depth interviews, clinicians, 296
  multi-disciplinary ICU team model, 424
  patient care, 293
  patients' safety and outcomes, 435
  reducing waiting times, 432
  SMM, rounds, 297–298
Intensive medical care, 59

K

Kappa statistics, 174–176
Knowledge
  gaps
    cognitive psychologists, 196
    concept-mapping methodology, 196

conceptual gaps, 197
description, 196
knowledge elicitation methodology, 197
MICU clinicians, 197
pathfinder network, 196–197
RASS score, 197
target, 196, 197
limits
average score, 120–121
clinicians listening to clinical rounds, 122
DR, 120
error detection, 120, 121
mean DR with and without priming, 121–122
primed and unprimed state, 120

L

Learning progressions
cognitive overload and medical errors
checklists, 461
decision tree, 461
hand washing case, 462
incentives, 460–461
initial demonstration of mastery, 460
intrusion, 460
definition, 455
electrical circuits, 456
engineering and team work, 464–465
non-monotone aspects
competence acquisition, 457
developmental occurrences, 457
diagnostic capability, 458
infant development, 458
intermediate levels, 456
knowledge and competence development principles, 458–459
monotone, 458
sample learning progression, 456, 457
setbacks, 457
stages in formation, medical expertise, 459
symptoms and diagnose, 456
X-ray image, 456–457
Piaget's stages, cognitive development, 456
reliability enculturation
airplane cockpit, 463
code calls, 462
crisis mode, 462
efficacy, monitoring checklists, 463
electronic patient record system, 463
emergency department work, 462
identification, 462
lab test, 462
reminder roles, 463–464
team training, 462, 463

M

Mechanical ventilation (MV), 184, 186, 194, 195
Medical error
complexity of system, 18
conventional approaches, 17
July Effect, 19
temporal evolution, 22–23
Medical intensive care unit (MICU)
care based approach, 255
complexity, resolving patient case, 260–261
data collection, 96, 254
environment, 107
handoff breakdowns, 259–260
handoff communication model, 256–257
handoff process and interdependencies, 257–259
participants, 95–96
physician handoffs, 251
pre-turnover coordination activities, 261–263
semi-structured interviews, 253
standardization, 261
study site, 95
team member roles and responsibilities, 250
workflow terminology, 250–252
Methylprednisolone (MP)
administration, 443
clinical benefits, 443
post-hoc analysis, 442
steroids resurface, 446
MICU. *See* Medical intensive care unit (MICU)
Misconception, 26
MP. *See* Methylprednisolone (MP)
MPR. *See* Multi-professional round (MPR)
Multi-professional round (MPR), 279–280
MV. *See* Mechanical ventilation (MV)

N

NASCIS. *See* The National Acute Spinal Cord Injury Study (NASCIS)
The National Acute Spinal Cord Injury Study (NASCIS), 442

Naturalistic decision-making (NDM)
categorizing physicians' behaviors, 132
cognitive science and decision-making research, 93
contextual models, 132
decision errors, 93
description, 92
human error research, 92–93
military domain, 93
NDM. *See* Naturalistic decision-making (NDM)
Neurological system
higher risk of systemic infections, 443
magic bullet, 443
MP, 442, 443
NASCIS, 442
pharmacological therapy, 442
randomized controlled trials, 442
SCI, 442
The Normoglycemia in Intensive Care Evaluation-Survival Using Glucose Algorithm Regulation (NICE-SUGAR) trial, 448

O

OpenMetaverse library, 116
Opensimulator (OpenSim), 116

P

PED. *See* Psychiatric Emergency Department (PED); Psychiatric emergency department (PED)
Piaget's stages, cognitive development, 456
Premature ventricular contractions (PVCs), 443, 444
Protocol-based practice, critical care medicine
ATLS, 436
CWP, 436
description, 435–436
deviations, 436
FRAM, 436, 437
healthcare, 436–437
ineffective use, 437
non-beneficial deviations, 437
SMM characteristics, 436
socio-technical factors, 436
standardized polices, 436
tight glucose control, 437
weaning protocol, 437
PROWESS-SHOCK trial, 450
Psychiatric Emergency Department (PED), 21, 24, 40, 114
Pulmonary artery catheter, 445
Pulmonary/respiratory system
ARDS, 445
magic bullet, harmful, 446
NIH-based critical care physicians, 445–446
steroids resurface, 446
ventilation strategy, 446
PVCs. *See* Premature ventricular contractions (PVCs)

R

Radio-frequency identification (RFID)
clinical work activities: evaluation studies, 362–363
clinical workflow (*See* HMM, activity modeling)
complexity and critical care workflow
complex cognitive system, 359
human-intensive ethnographic methods, 359
paradigmatic complex system, 358
exploratory investigations of clinician activities, 358
framework for studying errors
errors, origin and propagation, 384, 385
monitoring using sensors, 384
IRB-regulated protocols, 385
real time location systems (RTLS)
active RFID system, 360
entity activity recognition, 360
IP-Lite radio connection protocol, 360
MASCAL. RFID sensors, 360
patient arrival at a trauma unit (example), 360, 362
signal strength index (RSSI), 360
tag-tag and tag-base configuration, 360–361
real-time monitoring in ED, 383
tracking clinicians (*See* Tracking clinicians, emergency care activities)
visualization of workflows
online 3-D virtual environments, 383
virtual reality (VR) visualizations, 382
virtual trauma unit for workflow visualization, 382
Radio identification technology (RID), 432
RASS. *See* Richmond agitation sedation scale (RASS)
Registered Nurses (RNs), 30
Renal/GU system, 446–447

RESOLVE trial, 450
Respiratory therapist (RT)
assessment, 194–195
and CWP, 185
dayshift and nightshift, 186
RASS score, 197
and SBT, 185
weaning protocol, 185
RFID. *See* Radio-frequency identification (RFID)
Richmond agitation sedation scale (RASS)
knowledge structure of RTs, 197
RTs misinterpreted, 195
sedation assessment, 186, 190, 192–193
RID. *See* Radio identification technology (RID)
RNs. *See* Registered Nurses (RNs)
RT. *See* Respiratory therapist (RT)

S
SBAR. *See* Situation, Background, Assessment and Recommendation (SBAR)
SBT. *See* Spontaneous breathing trial (SBT)
SCI. *See* Spinal cord injuries (SCI)
Semi-naturalistic data collection, 84
Shared Mental Model index (SMMi), 304
Shared mental models (SMM)
advantages, teamwork, 292
communication errors, 310–311
comparison with rounds, 305–306
convergence and divergence, 311
critical care, 291
description, 292–293
Handoffs and team communication, 293–295
ICU, 295–303
limitations, 312–313
medical errors, 291–292
patient conversations, 303
Pyramid Method, 303
quantification, 311–312
resident-to-resident and charge nurse-to-charge nurse, 304–305
shared mental models, 304–310
SMMi, 304
team members, communication and coordination, 291
Simulated clinical round error detections
description, 113–114
in error recovery (*see* Error recovery)
failed detection, 118
limits of knowledge, 120–122
participants and case construction
clinical plausibility, 119
errors, case scenarios, 119
MICU, 118–119
paper based questions, 119
virtual ICU
ethnographic data, 118
OpenMetaverse library, 116
Opensimulator (OpenSim), 116
screenshot, resulting rounds, 116, 117
scripting languages, 116
Second Life, 116
virtual rounds, steps, 116, 117
virtual world, 115
web-based tutoring system, 123–124
Situation, Background, Assessment and Recommendation (SBAR), 272, 273
SMM. *See* Shared mental models (SMM)
SOAP. *See* Subject, Objective, Assessment and Plan (SOAP)
Spinal cord injuries (SCI)
NACSIS-II trial, 442
treatment, 443
Spontaneous breathing trial (SBT)
eligibility and readiness, 185
and RASS, 186
screening assessment, 185, 190
and sedation holiday, 184
Subject demographics, 64
Subject, Objective, Assessment and Plan (SOAP), 273, 278, 279, 282, 284

T
Task transition decisions, emergency care
breaks in task, 135
canonical activities in EDs, 133
categorizing, 134
dashboard displays systems, 136
decision making, 132–133
distributed cognition, 132
environmental factors, 136–139
methodology, 133–134
NDM, 132
non-deterministic environments, 132
observation, 135
opportunistic decisions, 135
patient assessment, observation and communication, 133
physicians decisions, 134–135
Team decision-making
in domains outside of medicine, 93–94
in medicine (ICU and ER), 94–95

Teamwork and error management
analysis of errors, cases, 69–70
apprentice training process, 60
classification, newly generated errors, 71–72
clinical case development, 65–67
clinical environment, 60
cognitive research, 62
cultural shift, 85
detection and correction, schematic representations, 60, 73–80
detection factors
interaction, 82–83
nature, 82
person attributed, 81
semi-naturalistic *vs.* laboratory-based studies, 83
diagnosis, 63
generation and progress, 70, 71
ICU, 60
monitoring mechanism, 62–63
nature, critical care, 63–64
participants, 64
procedure, 67–68
progression and occurrence, medical error, 70, 71
qualitative nature, 72–73
recovery, embedded errors, 61–62
team-based care activities, 86
teamwork and error detection, 62
text analysis and coding, 68
well-organized knowledge structures, 63
Tracking clinicians, emergency care activities
data analysis
antecedent-consequent matrix, 373
interaction, 373
location-based transition probability matrix, 373
mechanism, aggregation and dispersion, 375
movement of clinicians and interactions, 371
pair-wise interactions, 374
time spent and proximity, 372
transitions between locations, 372–373
data collection, 370–371
ED environment, 368
participants, 369
results
collaboration: aggregation and dispersion, 379–380
collaborative activity., 380
co-location of nurses, 376
correlation between location, 376
pair-wise co-location probability, 379
Pearson moment-correlation, 375
team size dispersion, 380
time spent and proximity, 376–377
transition between locations, 377–379
validating sensor and shadowing data, 375
sensor-based technology, 368
sensor setup
good signals, 370
spatial orientation of the base stations in the ED, 369
threshold signal strength, 370
shadowing
time-stamp, 370
UObserve suite of data logging tool, 370
study setting
care team for trauma ED, 368
physical set-up, 368
Trauma Center of an Emergency Department (ED), 368
Trauma critical care
acuity/case type indicator, 155
ATLS guideline, 153, 154, 156–157
classification, severity, 155–156
deviations, classifications
clinician expertise and distribution, 160
distribution and severity, 158–160
field observations, 157–158
initial assessment and management, 158
mean deviations per trauma case, 158, 159
patient outcome, 161
proactive and reactive, 160–161
dynamic and unpredictable environment, 152
primary survey and resuscitation, 156
secondary survey, 156
team structures, 153
tertiary survey and definitive care, 156
trauma scenario walkthrough, 154–155
x-rays and CT scans, 153–154

U

UMLS. *See* Unified medical language system (UMLS)
Unified medical language system (UMLS)
adding in objects, 131
code constraints, 132

description, 130
emergency department WDO, 130
Upper gastro-intestinal bleeding, 64–65
Utterance categorization, 101–102

W
WDO. *See* Work domain ontology (WDO)
Weaning protocols (WPs)
barriers, CDSS, 186–187
and FRAM (*see* Functional resonance accident method (FRAM))
healthcare standardization, 183–184
HIT, 199
in MICU
and CWP, 185
decision support characteristics and MV, 184
and RASS, 187
and RT, 186
and SBT, 184
standardization tool evaluations, 187–188
Web-based tutoring system
description, 123
error detection
component, 123, 124
training, 123
performance report, 124
Work domain ontology (WDO)
action/operation, 128
analysis methods, 129
building out, 130
components, 129
constraints, 128–129
data collection methods, 129
framework, 128
goals, 128
identifying operations, 130, 131
implementation-independent description, 128
objects/required components, 128
partial work domain, 129–130
and UMLS, 130–132
Workflow, critical care medicine
description, 432
HMM, 432
information displays/handoff process, 433
interruptions, 432–433
multidimensional concept, 432
observational study, 432
RID, 432
sterile cockpit, 433
WPs. *See* Weaning protocols (WPs)

MIX
Papier aus verantwortungsvollen Quellen
Paper from responsible sources
FSC® C105338

If you have any concerns about our products,
you can contact us on
ProductSafety@springernature.com

In case Publisher is established outside the EU,
the EU authorized representative is:
Springer Nature Customer Service Center GmbH
Europaplatz 3, 69115 Heidelberg, Germany

Printed by Libri Plureos GmbH
in Hamburg, Germany